James E. Klein
6-18-76

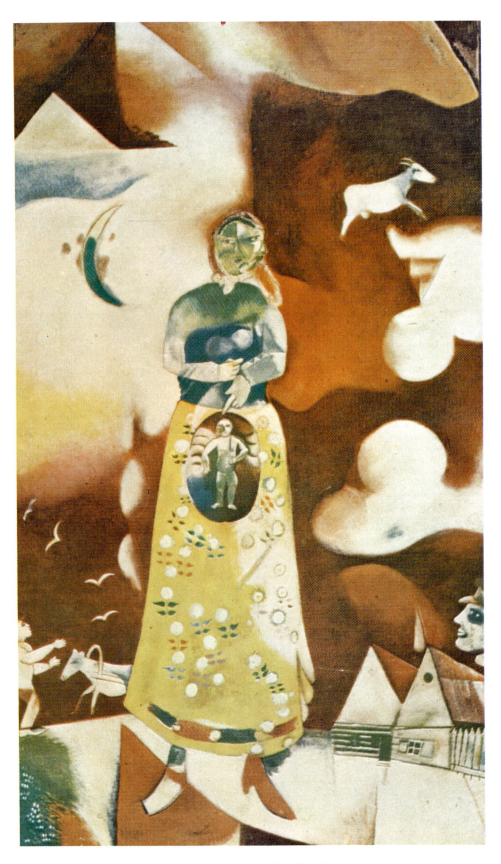

Maternité, 1913, by Marc Chagall (1889-   ).

ICONOGRAPHIA GYNIATRICA

ICONOGRAPHIA GYNIATRICA

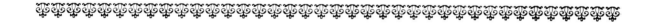

A Pictorial History of Gynecology and Obstetrics

HAROLD SPEERT, M.D.

F. A. DAVIS COMPANY, Philadelphia

© 1973 by F. A. DAVIS COMPANY

Copyright under the International Copyright Union. All rights reserved. This book is protected by copyright. No part of it may be reproduced, stored in a retrieval system, or transmitted in any form or by any means, electronic, mechanical, photocopying, recording, or otherwise, without written permission from the publisher. Manufactured in the United States of America.
Library of Congress Catalog Card Number 71-167953.
ISBN-0-8036-8070-8.

Dedication

To the women in my life: my wife, the memory of her mother and mine, my daughters, my sisters, and my patients.

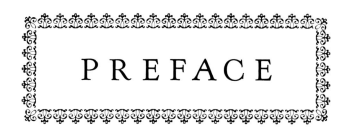

PREFACE

"HISTORY IS BUNK," said Henry Ford. Not that he meant to abjure all record of the past; he only denigrated written history. "By looking at things people used and that show the way they lived," the great industrialist insisted, "a better and truer impression can be gained than could be had in a month of reading." Nearly five centuries earlier Leonardo da Vinci, one of the first advocates of graphic illustration, similarly expressed his disaffection with verbal exposition. "Oh writer! — with what words would you describe a heart without filling a book?"

Man has recorded his observations and impressions in images for about 30,000 years. These figures were largely supplanted by the written word in historical documentation during the early centuries that followed Gutenberg's invention of printing from movable type, in the mid fifteenth century. In recent years pictures and objects have regained status as adjuncts, even alternatives, to words in providing insight into manners, customs, and attitudes of which no other evidence may be available. "Pictures made without any medical intent," wrote Henry Sigerist, "by reflecting the customs of the time, become revealing documents that tell us how physicians dressed or what the leper's costume was; they permit us to look into the sick room, into the room of the woman in childbirth, into the doctor's office, the apothecary's shop or the barber's bathhouse. We thus obtain information on subjects that are rarely discussed in the literature." Pictures, in addition, although ambiguous at times, can produce an emotional impact rarely achieved by the printed paragraph.

Manifold are the subjects of pictorial histories already in print: the Bible, the carrousel, the cinema, the circus, costume, crime, embroidery, flight, the American Indian, inventions, magic, morals, music, the American Presidents, various religions, ships, sports, the United Nations. Several authors have covered the broad field of medicine graphically, and Curt Proskauer has produced an elegant pictorial history of dentistry. The present volume, the first attempt to record the history of obstetrics and gynecology primarily through pictures, encompasses in broad perspective, extending back to prehistory, topics relating to woman and her role in reproduction, including female anatomy, early midwifery, embryology, scenes of pregnancy and birth, labor and its complications, obstetric instruments, cesarean section, the newborn infant, monsters, nursing, control of conception, and gynecologic surgery.

The history of obstetrics and gynecology has been written in painting, pottery, parchment, paper, and plaster, rock drawings, wood-carvings, coins, tapestries, mosaics, gravestones, and sculpture. Graphic records reach back into the Paleolithic age. The earliest known medical papyri, from about 3000 BC are devoid of illustrations, although scenes of obstetric delivery and of circumcision were depicted in sculptural relief on the Egyptian tombs at Saqqara, about the twenty-fifth century BC. Not until about 500 AD, when manuscripts became established as a medium of medical record and communication, were illustrations used in medical texts; but only a few appeared in the manuscripts of Western civilization during the first millennium AD. The ensuing years of the Middle Ages witnessed an unprecedented burst of ornament and color illustrations, often full-page but known nonetheless as miniatures because of the vermilion pigment, called minium, with which the figures were made.

From all these sources, from the clay vessels of early civilizations, the manuscripts and textbooks of the past thousand years, the paintings of the Renaissance and the modern world, the engravings of the nineteenth century, and the cartoons of the twentieth, have I drawn material. Dealing only with topics amenable to pictorial representation, this work does not purport to cover all aspects of obstetric and gynecologic history. Bypassed, for example, is anesthesia for childbirth, a dramatic chapter in the history of obstetrics but one that provides little record in pictures.

Gratefully do I record my thanks to the museums, libraries, publishers, photographers, authors, and collectors who have granted permission to reproduce figures to illustrate this volume; to the reference staff of Columbia University's Medical Library, for obtaining much of my source material; to Mrs. Alice Weaver, head of The New York Academy of Medicine's Rare Book Room, for help in identifying the sources of old illustrations; and to my wife, Kathryn H. Speert, for her editorial assistance and for typing the manuscript.

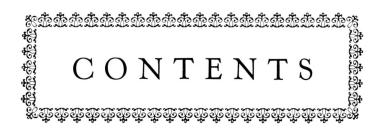

CONTENTS

1. THE FEMALE ANATOMY — 1
2. PREGNANCY: *Diagnosis, Scenes, and Garb* — 43
3. THE MIDWIVES — 67
4. BIRTH SCENES — 79
5. THE ANATOMY OF PREGNANCY — 153
6. MAN'S BEGINNINGS: *Embryology* — 187
7. THE OBSTETRIC PELVIS — 211
8. LABOR AND ITS COMPLICATIONS — 223
9. ACCOUTERMENTS OF THE BIRTH CHAMBER — 265
10. PUERPERAL FEVER — 289
11. CESAREAN SECTION — 297
12. THE NEWBORN: *Resuscitation, Swaddling, Circumcision, and Baptism* — 317
13. NURSING — 333
14. MONSTERS AND MYTHS — 361
15. MULTIPLE PREGNANCY AND BIRTH — 377
16. FERTILITY AND ITS CONTROL — 409
17. GYNECOLOGY — 455
18. HOSPITALS FOR WOMEN — 495
19. OBSTETRIC AND GYNECOLOGIC TEXTS — 511

PICTORIAL CREDITS AND SOURCES — 523

INDEX — 529

Ye Mothers, in your name, who set your throne

In boundless Space, eternally alone,

And yet companioned! All the forms of Being,

In movement, lifeless, ye are round you seeing.

Whate'er once was, there burns and brightens free

In splendor — for 't would fain eternal be;

And ye allot it, with all-potent might,

To Day's pavilions and the vaults of Night.

Life seizes some, along his gracious course;

Others arrests the bold Magician's force;

And he, bestowing as his faith inspires,

Displays the Marvellous, that each desires.

—From Goethe's *Faust,* translation by
Bayard Taylor (1870)

Chapter 1

THE FEMALE ANATOMY

The earliest representations of the human body, in the form of cave drawings and stone figures, date back to the Middle Aurignacian period (40,000–16,000 BC). Not until many millennia later do existing records show evidence of any serious attempt at the study of human anatomy. Rare are anatomic illustrations from ancient times. Even the illustrious Aristotle (384–322 BC) confessed that the interior of the human body remained unknown to him.

Only by dissection could anatomic structure be revealed. Until the sixteenth century, however, corpses were hard to obtain and the conditions for their dissection were rigidly prescribed by the civil authorities. As a result, very little advance was made between the time of Galen (second century AD) and the anatomic renaissance ushered in by the famous quintet of the 1600s—Sylvius, Vesalius, Fabricius, Eustachius, and Falloppius. Indeed,

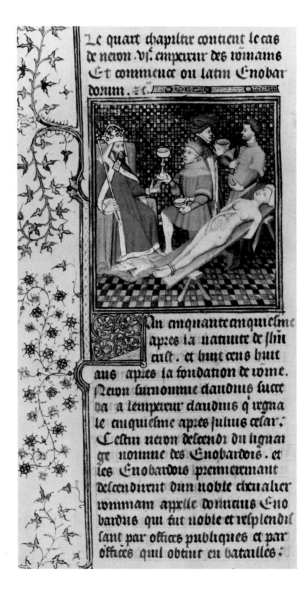

Fig. 1-1. A medieval concept of female anatomy. Emperor Nero, having murdered his mother, Agrippini, witnesses her autopsy. Miniature from a collection of stories by Giovanni Boccaccio: *Le cas des nobles hommes et femmes,* about 1410. Bibliothèque de l'Arsenal, Paris.

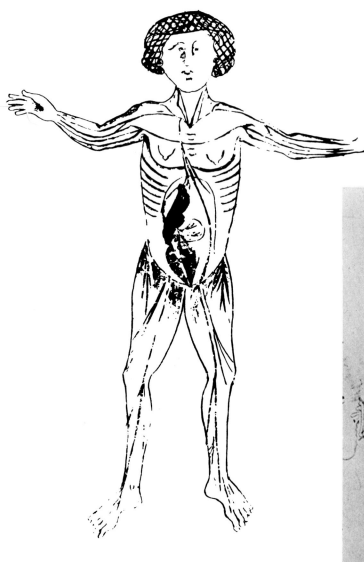

Fig. 1-2. Anatomy of the female internal genitalia. Illustration from a Provençal manuscript of the late thirteenth century.

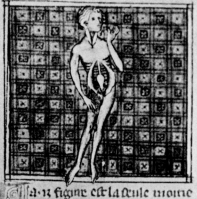

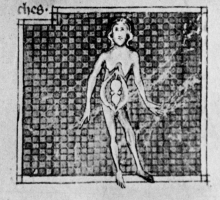

Fig. 1-3. Woman's reproductive organs. On either side of the uterus is shown a *female testicle,* as the ovary was called. Miniature from a Parisian manuscript, dated 1314, of Henri de Mondeville, 1260–1320.

the intervening 1500 years have been termed the dark ages of anatomy. In Bologna, home of Europe's oldest university, the students themselves had to procure the cadavers and stand the expense of the anatomic demonstrations until 1442, when the city assumed this responsibility. Even then, only the bodies of executed criminals who had been born at least 30 miles distant could be used. As a result, only one or two dissections were performed each year and female cadavers were rare. The authority of Galen prevailed, although he too had but scant knowledge of the internal anatomy of the human; and his teaching, based on his dissections of lower animals, was studded with error.

Before the sixteenth century, therefore, human anatomic illustrations were few and schematic. With the Renaissance and its emphasis on realism, the human form received new attention, but mainly from the master artists like da Vinci and Michelangelo, who were interested primarily in art itself rather than medicine. Earliest of the anatomic illustrators was Giacomo Berengario da Carpi (1470–1530) who produced the first human anatomic drawings made from direct observation in two works published in 1521 (*Commentaria supra anatomia Mundini*) and 1522 (*Isagogae breves*). Only two decades later, in 1543, from the dissections and authorship of Andreas Vesalius (1514–1564) and the illustrations of his artist, Jan Kalkar, *De humani corporis fabrica* appeared. Based on Vesalius' dissections of at least nine female corpses, this work, an unprecedented combination of scholarship and art, has been acclaimed as the foundation of modern human anatomy.

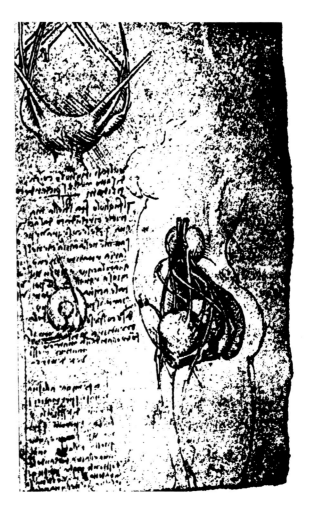

Fig. 1-4. The female organs of generation. By Leonardo da Vinci (1452–1519). Of him Sir William Osler wrote,

"Insatiate in experiment, intellectually as greedy as Aristotle, painter, poet, sculptor, engineer, architect, mathematician, chemist, botanist, aeronaut, musician and withal a dreamer and a mystic, full accomplishment in any of one department was not for him! A passionate desire for a mastery of nature's secrets made him a fierce thing, replete with too much rage! But, for us, a record remains . . ."

Most of da Vinci's writings were locked away for years; his anatomical drawings, some 779 in number, notable for their simplicity, clarity, and accuracy, lying forgotten in Windsor Castle from the time of Charles I (1625–1649) until their rediscovery in 1778.

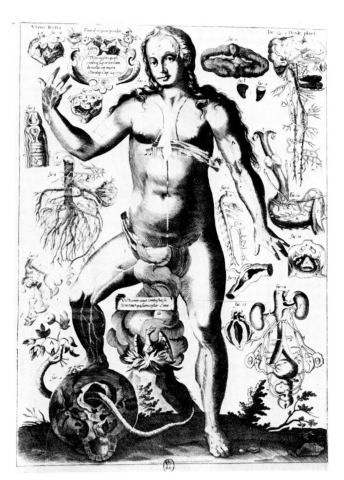

Fig. 1-5. The human female form. Anatomical plate with mobile shutters, providing access to the viscera, from Johann Remmelin's *Kleiner Welt-Spiegel*, a group of three plates intended to reveal the entire human anatomy. Shown is an allegorical representation of woman, with her foot resting on a skull with serpent and with a cloud of smoke rising before her from the burning nest of the holy phoenix. This work was first published in 1613 in Latin as *Catoptron microcosmicum*, in 1634 as *Pinax microcosmographicus* under the name of Stephan Michael Spacher, and in subsequent editions as *Kleiner Welt-Spiegel* under Remmelin's own name.

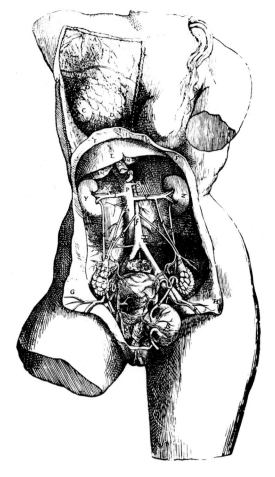

Fig. 1-6. The female pelvic viscera. From Vesalius' *De humani corporis fabrica*, 1543. It contained the first good illustrations of the female internal genitalia.

THE FEMALE ANATOMY 5

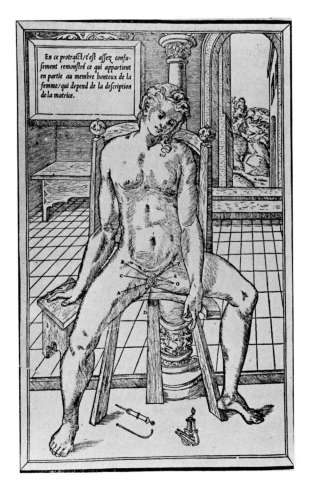

Fig. 1-7. An anatomic plate showing the external female genitalia. The subject points to a vaginal speculum, catheter, and syringe on the floor. From *De dissectione partium corporis humani*, published by Charles Estienne (Etienne) in Paris in 1545. The French language edition appeared the following year. Estienne (1503–1564), known also as Carolus Stephanus, was a contemporary of Vesalius but began his work independently; some of his illustrations were printed before the publication of Vesalius' *Fabrica*.

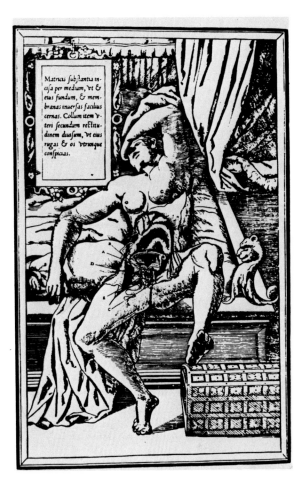

Fig. 1-8. Female internal genitalia. From the anatomy of Charles Estienne, *De dissectione*, 1545.

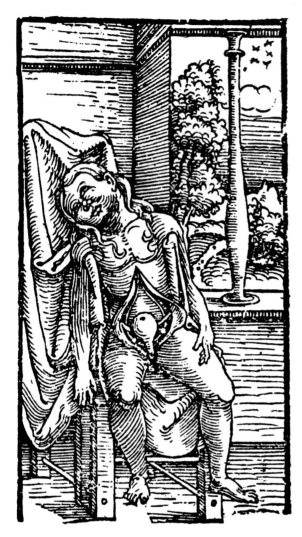

Fig. 1-9. The female body and internal genitalia. From the *Arzneispiegel* (1547) of Johann Dryander (real name Eichmann), an anatomist and mathematician of Marburg, Germany. This figure was adapted, with little more change than the addition of a background, from a woodcut of Berengario da Carpi, published a quarter century earlier. In 1682 Antonius Novarini reproduced the same figure in his *Anatomia curiosa*, making only trivial additional changes in the background scene. Thus, for more than a century and one-half essentially the same illustration of the female organs appeared in anatomic texts.

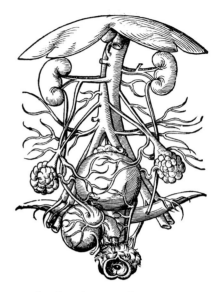

Fig. 1-10. The female reproductive tract. As illustrated in Jacob Rueff's *De conceptu et generatione hominis*, Frankfurt, 1580.

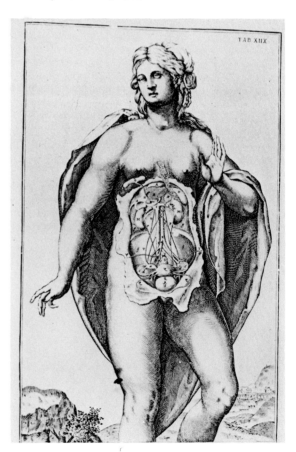

Fig. 1-11. The female abdominal and pelvic viscera. Plate from Julius Casserius, *Placentini tabulae anatomicae*, Venice, 1627. A student of Fabricius, Casserius portrayed the female form with beauty and accuracy.

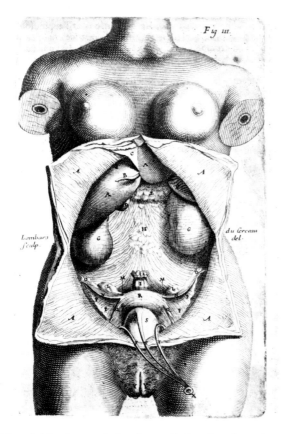

Fig. 1-12. Anatomical plate of the female pelvic organs. From the 1681 edition of François Mauriceau's *Traité des maladies des femmes grosses, et de celles qui sont accouchées.*

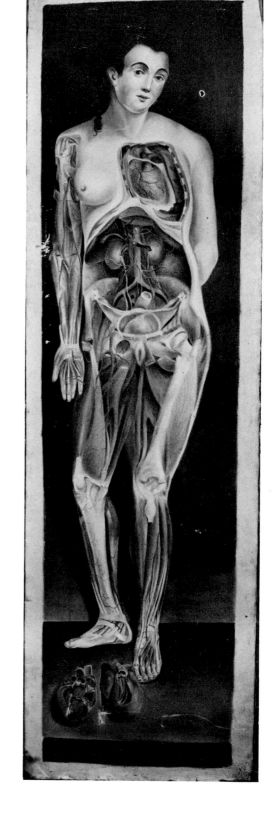

Fig. 1-13. The female anatomy. Painting by Jacques-Fabien Gautier-d'Agoty (1710–1781). Musée de Dijon, France.

THE GENITAL ORGANS

Early medical records, dating back to the Ebers Papyrus (1550 BC), regarded the uterus as an independent animal, capable of movement within the host. It was portrayed, elsewhere, in a variety of forms resembling a tortoise, a newt, or a crocodile. Aretaeus the Cappadocian, eminent Greek physician of the second century AD, wrote in his *Causes and Indications of Acute and Chronic Diseases,*

"In the middle of the flanks of women lies the womb, a female viscus, closely resembling an animal, for it is moved of itself hither and thither in the flanks, also upwards in a direct line to below the cartilage of the thorax, and also obliquely to the right or the left, either to the liver or the spleen; and it likewise is subjected to prolapse downwards, and in a word is altogether erratic. It delights also in fragrant smells and advances toward them, and it has an aversion to fetid smells and flees from them; and on the whole the womb is like an animal within an animal."

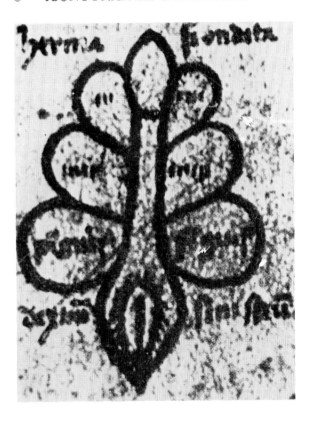

Fig. 1-14. Human uterus. As illustrated in an early medieval manuscript showing the seven cells or chambers. Biblioteca Ambrosiana, Milan.

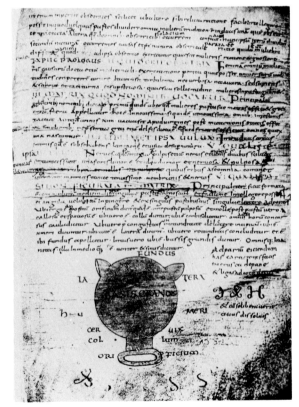

Fig. 1-15. The human uterus. As illustrated in the ninth century manuscript of Moschion. The corpus (*Basis grandis*) is sharply demarcated from the cervix.

According to Hippocrates, about six centuries earlier, the uterus often went wild when not fed with male semen.

Replacing this animalistic concept of the uterus in the early centuries of the Common Era was the *seven cells* doctrine, a morphologic myth which visualized the uterine corpus as divided into seven compartments, three on either side and one in the middle. Male embryos were believed to develop in the cells on the right, females on the left, while the middle cell was reserved for hermaphrodites. This doctrine remained popular in the medical teachings of the middle ages, until exposed by the light of anatomic dissection.

An ingenious analogy between the male and female parts was proposed by Guy de Chauliac, famous French surgeon of the early fourteenth century, who compared the uterus with the penis.

"The uterus is like a penis turned inside out ... it has in its upper part two arms with the testicles ... like the scrotum ... a common body in the middle ... a collum with a canal in it like the shaft ... and the vulva is like glans and preputium."

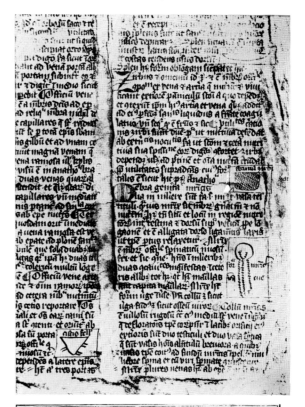

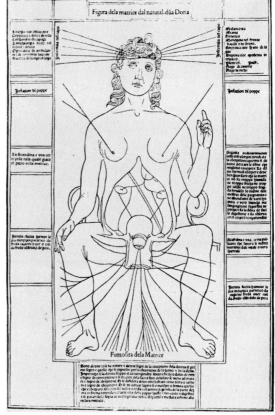

Fig. 1-16. Latin manuscript page of Henri de Mondeville, 1304, containing diagram of uterus, lower right. The Y-shaped zig-zag line represents the endometrial cavity and cervical canal; the lateral zig-zag lines, the vaginal rugae; the round smooth line, the serosal surface of the uterus. The other illustrations represent the gallbladder, spleen, and omentum.

Fig. 1-17. Woodcut of the female figure. From Ketham's *Fasciculus medicinae*, Venice, 1491. The uterus, apparently drawn from the object, is authentically represented here for the first time in a printed book. Ketham is a corruption or pen name of Johannes von Kirchheim (1460–1491), a Swabian physician. His text, a miscellaneous collection of popular Latin medical tracts, mostly of the fourteenth century, is regarded as the first illustrated medical work; its figures, the first didactic medical woodcuts.

Fig. 1-18. Diagram of the human uterus. From the *Anthropologium* of Magnus Hundt, Leipzig, 1501. (*Testiculus* = ovary, *Vasa seminalis* = oviduct, *Os matricis* = cervical os, *Os exterius* = vaginal introitus, *Via vesice* = urethra). Copied from the *Anothomia* (1316) of Mundinus (Mondino dei Luzzi, c. 1270–1326), this figure perpetuated the seven cell concept of the uterus. Of this organ Mundinus wrote,

"It is made chiefly for conception, and consequently to cleanse or purge the whole body from superfluous undigested blood. This is the case in human beings only. Other animals do not menstruate, and in them such superfluities are consumed by the production of hide, fur, claws, beaks, and feathers and the like, of which man is deprived."

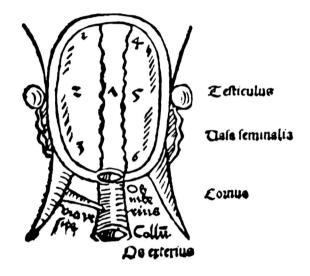

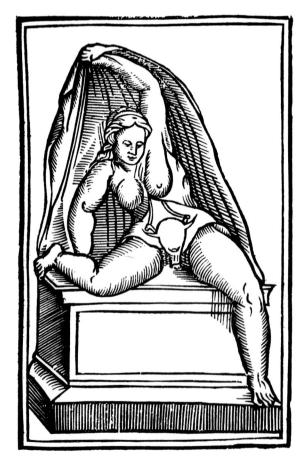

Fig. 1-19. Woodcut. From Berengario's *Carpi commentaria cum amplissimis additionibus super Anatomia Mundini*, Bologna, 1521. He stated,

"You have in this figure the uterus intact with horns. You see how the seminal vesicles go to the testicles and from the testicles to the uterus, but the testicles are not in their natural place, for this is below the horns. . . . You see also in this figure how the mouth of the uterus is above the neck . . ."

Fig. 1-20. Woodcut. From Berengario's *Commentaria*, Bologna, 1521. The woman in the figure points to the opened cavity of her extirpated uterus, to demonstrate its unilocular structure, while putting a foot on the contemporaneous anatomic texts to indicate contempt for their tradition-bound errors. The black dots on the endometrial surface Berengario interpreted as "the heads of the veins which are called cotyledons." Commenting on the text of Mundinus and the seven cell concept of the uterus he embraced, Berengario wrote, "*Tamen est purum mendatium dicere quod matrix habeat septem cellulas . . .* (It is a sheer lie to say that the uterus has seven compartments.)"

Fig. 1-21. The human uterus. From Berengario's *Isagogae breves*. The organ's anterior and posterior aspects are shown and the opened uterus with the endometrial surface exposed (center). *Testiculus* designates the ovary, *vas spermaticum* the ovarian artery (vein). The uterine *horns,* perhaps an inaccurate representation of the round ligaments, are shown attached to the uterus at the level of the cervix. In the writings of Berengario, Vesalius, and others of their era, *collum,* or neck, usually refers to the vagina; and *os externum,* or external os, to the vaginal introitus, in contrast to modern terminology. These figures of the uterus were copied by other anatomists for the next century and one-half. Berengario wrote, "The uterus, also called vulva, has two parts, that is, a receptacle, or sinus or cavity, and a cervix, or neck.... The substance of its receptacle is sinewy ... compased of one tunic surrounded by the peritoneum.... All of its cavity is moved to the center in the reception of the sperm, which it embraces and touches with its sides. The substance of its cervix, or neck, is of muscular flesh, like cartilage with some fat; it has wrinkle upon wrinkle which give delight by rubbing in coitus.... The form of the cervix is oblong, round, concave ... [the receptacle] has a single cavity or cell, which somewhat near its fundus is divided into two parts, as if there were two uteruses terminated at one neck. In its right part most often males are bound fast, in the left part, females." [J. Berengario da Carpi: *A Short Introduction to Anatomy (Isagogae breves)*, L. R. Lind, trans. University of Chicago Press, Chicago, 1959.]

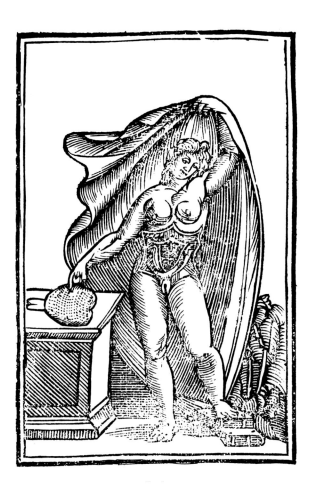

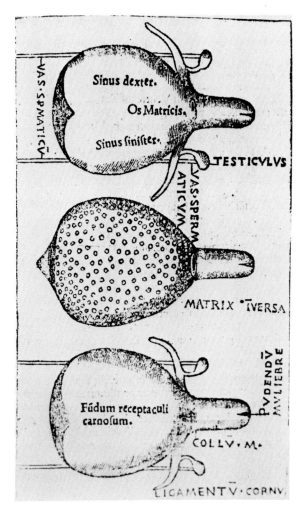

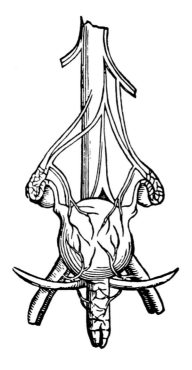

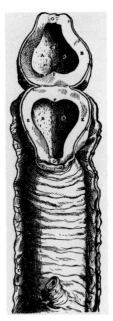

Fig. 1-22. The human uterus. From the *Tabulae anatomicae* of Andreas Vesalius, 1538. When this work was published Vesalius, newly appointed as professor at Padua, was but 23 years old. The prominence he gave to the *uterine horns* in this figure has been interpreted by some as an act of diplomatic deference to the prevailing teaching of Galen. Vesalius' later illustrations of the uterus fail to show these structures. Vesalius pictured and gave the first good description of the oviduct, although erring in his belief that the uterine tube was attached to the female gonad. In Liber V of his *Fabrica* he wrote,

"The vessel that conveys the semen from the testis to the uterus originates from the body of the testis...just as in the male. However, it surrounds the testis like a circle instead of being attached only to its posterior surface....Continuing its course it...develops several convolutions. Finally it proceeds toward the uterus in serpentine fashion and ends in the midst of the uterine cornu."

The uterine tubes were later described more accurately by Vesalius' student, Gabrielle Falloppio (1523?–1562), for whom these structures are now named, in the latter's *Observationes anatomicae*, Venice, 1561.

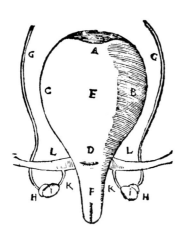

Fig. 1-23. The female internal genitalia. From the *Anatomia Mundini* of Johannes Dryander, Marburg, 1541. Dryander showed the uterus with "a certain carneous tuberosity [at A] by which the uterus is seen to be bifid," but he denied that it had other cells or compartments. Like Vesalius, Dryander endowed the uterus with horns. The gonads are shown with epididymes, with "vessels carrying semen to the uterus around the cornua."

Fig. 1-24. The uterus and vagina. As depicted by Vesalius in his *Fabrica*, 1543. The organs, from a parous woman, have been opened longitudinally; the urethra, at bottom, is shown incorrectly, opening into the vagina; A and B are designated *sinuses of fundus uteri*. Either the subject possessed an arcuate uterus or Vesalius was not yet ready to reject completely the doctrine of uterine compartmentation. Gone, however, are the uterine horns and the fanciful seven cells of antiquity.

THE FEMALE ANATOMY 13

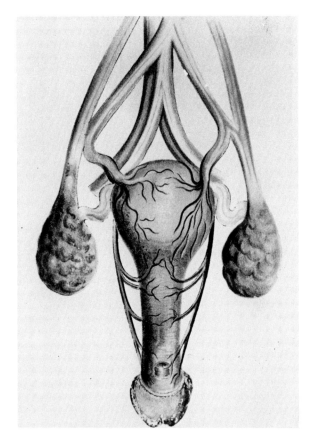

Fig. 1-25. The female reproductive organs. From the *Kunstbuch*, 1575, of Georg Bartisch (1535–1607?), Königsbrück ophthalmologist and surgeon. Striking is the phallus-like representation of the female genitalia. The uterine blood supply is shown inaccurately, and as in the Vesalian figure, the urethra is incorrectly pictured opening into the vagina.

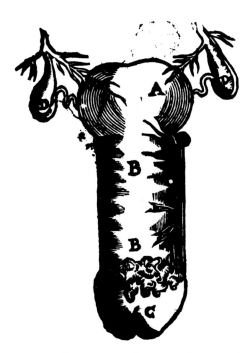

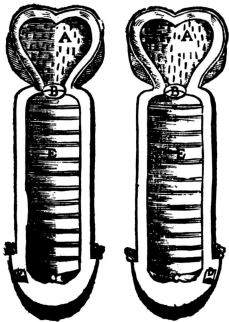

Fig. 1-26. Illustrations of uterus, adnexa, and vagina. From Scipione Mercurio's *La Commare O'Raccoglitrice*, first published in 1595. The uterine cavity was still shown in bipartite form. Unmistakable is the phallic simulation of the female genitalia.

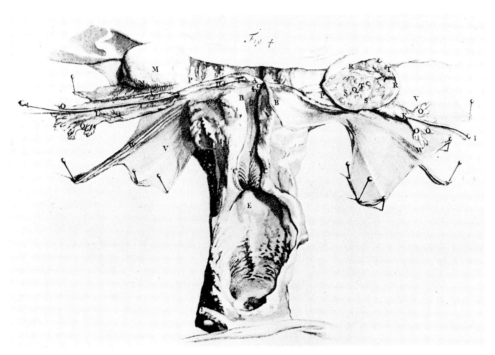

Fig. 1-27. Dissection of the female genitalia. By Govert Bidloo (1649–1713) from his *Anatomia humani corporis,* Amsterdam, 1685. Accurately represented are the pinned-out broad ligaments, the round ligaments designated by W, the probed fallopian tubes, the opened endometrial cavity, the capacious vagina with its rugae, the narrower cervix with its *plicae palmitae,* and the ovaries, one bisected, showing graafian follicles.

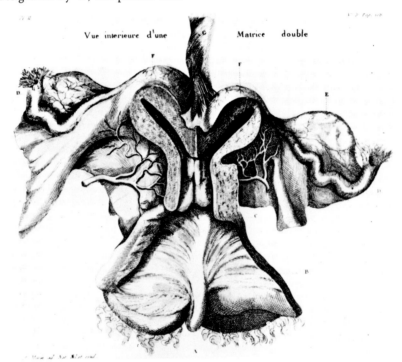

Fig. 1-28. Double uterus (uterus didelphys unicollis). One of the earliest representations of this anomaly, from J. L. Moreau, *Histoire naturelle de la femme,* Paris, 1803.

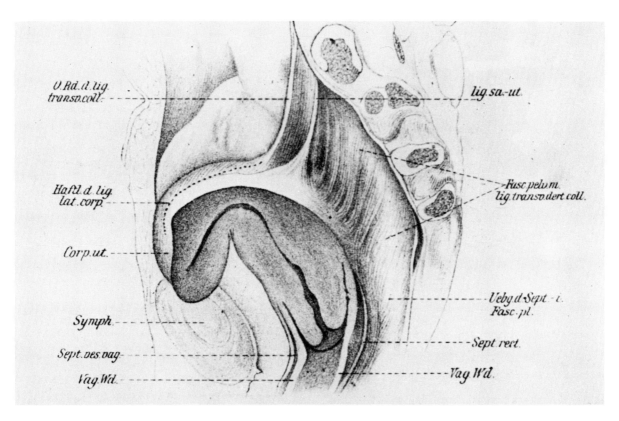

Fig. 1-29. The transverse cervical, or cardinal, ligament, principal support of the uterus. As illustrated by Alwin Mackenrodt (1859–1925) from his dissection of a fetus of eight months. Mackenrodt wrote,

"... firm, bandlike, fibrous processes can be isolated, which attach directly to the uterine cervix, vagina, rectum, and bladder. These bands, arranged systematically, carry complex muscular elements as well as numerous bundles of elastic fibers.... This whole ligamentous apparatus appears so excellent and extensive that it is quite surprising that it has not been recognized previously.... These masses of fibers extending from the pelvic fascia to the side of the cervix assume an important and independent position, so that we must sharply separate them generically from the broad ligament of the corpus.... Because of the anatomic and physiologic differences we no longer speak of the whole lateral ligamentous structure simply as the broad ligament, but only the peritoneal duplication attached to the corpus; while we designate the lateral ligamentous structure of the cervix as the transverse or lateral cervical ligament ... the principal means of support of the uterus, and in its upper edge it conducts the principal blood vessel of the uterus, the uterine artery.... The closure of the inferior pelvic aperture of the female is ... pictured as a complex but extremely effectively arranged apparatus of ligaments and membranes, which extend from the pelvic fascia and come together at the uterus.... The transverse cervical ligaments carry the brunt of the load, aided by the uterosacral and pubo-vesico-uterine ligaments.... Descensus of the genitalia is attributable to atrophy of the ligaments of the internal pelvic musculature."

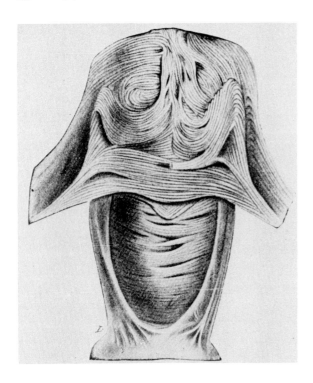

Fig. 1-30. The uterine musculature, external layer, anterior aspect, with serosa and bladder removed. From L. T. Hélie, *Recherches sur la disposition des fibres musculaires de l'utérus développé par la grossesse,* Paris, 1864. After 12 years' investigation Hélie concluded that the myometrium consists of three main layers, each further divided. The external layer, he maintained, contains two longitudinal parts with a transversely arranged sheet of muscle fibers between them; the internal, two triangular, one on the anterior and one on the posterior wall of the uterus, connected by an arch at the fundus. The middle or principal layer, he stated, consists of an interlacing network of fibers curved as figures-of-eight, perforated by blood vessels. Myometrial contraction thus resulted in constriction of the blood vessels, as by a ligature.

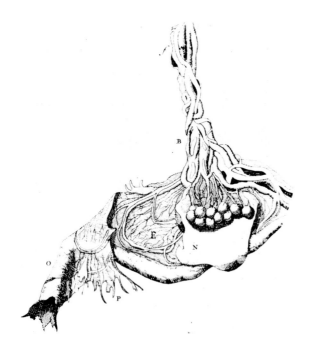

Fig. 1-31. The human ovary, its berry-like ovula fed by branches of the spermatic artery. From Jan Swammerdam's *Miraculum naturae sive uteri muliebris fabrica,* Leyden, 1672. The presence of vesicles in the female testes had been mentioned in the sixteenth century writings of Vesalius and his disciple Falloppio, but these Paduan anatomists had no notion of the function of the fluid-filled follicles. Falloppio's successor, Fabricius ab Aquapendente, described the hen's ovary and, recognizing it as the organ of egg formation, named it *ovarium.* The long prevalent teaching of Aristotle persisted nonetheless, that the human egg was formed in the uterus.

THE FEMALE ANATOMY 17

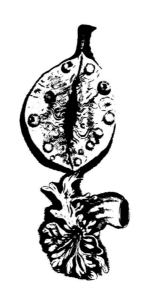

Fig. 1-32. Bisected human ovary, with follicles and fimbriated end of oviduct. From Reinier de Graaf's *De mulierum organis,* Leyden, 1672. The latter part of the seventeenth century witnessed a resurgence of the idea, already voiced by Fabricius and even earlier by Gian Matteo de Gradi of Milan, known also as Ferrari d'Agrate (d. 1480), that the mammalian female testes, like the ovaries of birds, are the site of egg formation. Jan Swammerdam and Jan van Horne, working together in Leyden, and the Danish anatomist Niels Stensen independently developed this theory in relation to the human in 1667, but their proposed book was never published because of personal bickering and the death of van Horne in 1670. Two years later de Graaf's classic volume appeared, describing the female testes and, with due credit to the unfinished manuscript of van Horne, presenting the evidence that the female gonad is indeed an ovary, the producer of eggs. The ovarian follicle, pictured by de Graaf, has been designated ever since by his name.

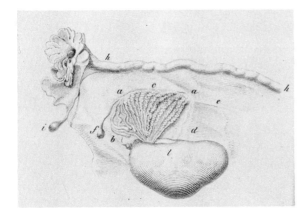

Fig. 1-33. The parovarium. As illustrated by George Ludwig Kobelt (1804–1857) in *Der Neben-Eierstock des Weibes*, Heidelberg, 1847. Tafel 1, Fig. 3, opp. p. 52. The mesonephric remnant, or Wolffian body, was first described in the human in 1802 by Johann Christian Rosenmüller (1771–1820) in a pamphlet of 12 pages on the development of the fetal ovary. Rosenmüller wrote,

"Seen between the ovary and tube are innumerable vessels, which branch from a stem behind the round ligament of the uterus and course toward the ovary between the peritoneal folds, having a relation to the tube similar to that of the mesenteric vessels to the intestine. For, connected to one another, they form an arc . . . the observed structure appeared conical in the cadavers of all the born fetuses I have seen. In an infant of 12 weeks I found that it consisted of many little canals, extensively convoluted at the base of the conical structure, these canals merging toward the upper extremity of the ovary where, after narrowing and coming closer together, they united and disappeared. I counted about 20 of these little canals."

This remnant of the Wolffian body in the female has been designated as the epoophoron, the parovarium, and the *organ of Rosenmüller;* its component ducts, as the *tubules of Kobelt*.

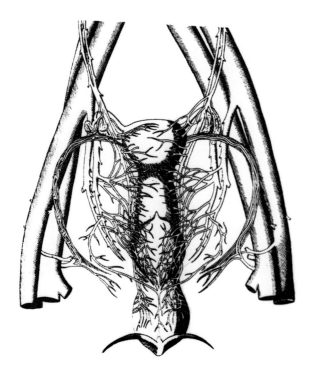

Fig. 1-34. The uterine blood supply. A sixteenth century concept from the *Tabulae anatomicae* (1552) of Bartolommeo Eustachio (1520?–1574). Branches of the hypogastric and ovarian arteries are shown leading to the uterus, bladder, and clitoris, prominently depicted with its two crura. Eustachio, who injected the blood vessels with colored fluids, was able to demonstrate numerous anastomoses in the pelvic vasculature. Figure from *Explicatio tabularum anatomicarum Bartholom. Eustachii,* Leyden, 1742, by Bernhard Siegfried Albinus (1697–1770), foremost anatomic illustrator of his time.

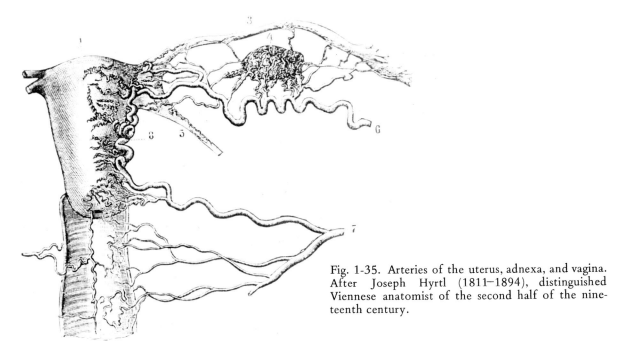

Fig. 1-35. Arteries of the uterus, adnexa, and vagina. After Joseph Hyrtl (1811–1894), distinguished Viennese anatomist of the second half of the nineteenth century.

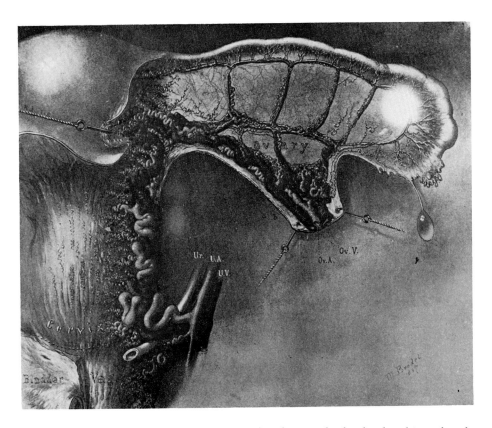

Fig. 1-36. The uterine and ovarian vessels, 1897. By Max Brödel (1870–1941). He founded the Department of Art as Applied to Medicine in the Johns Hopkins Medical School and introduced a new standard of excellence to medical illustration.

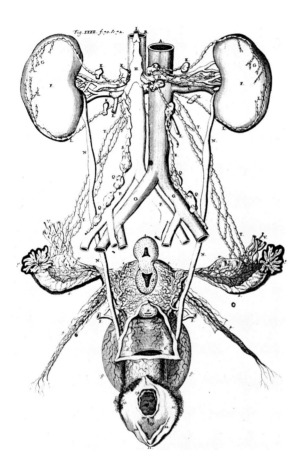

Fig. 1-37. The lymphatics of the female urogenital system. From *Adenographia curiosa et uteri foeminei anatome nova,* Leyden, 1691, of Anton Nuck (1650–1692). Distinguished Dutch anatomist and surgeon, Nuck demonstrated the lymphatic vessels, nodes, and their connections by injections with air, mercury, wax, and a variety of colored solutions. Chapter 8 of his *Adenographia* contains the first description of the lymphatic network of the ovary. At first Nuck believed that the lymphatic vessels originated from the arterial capillaries and that the nodes consisted of conglomerates of tiny blood vessels, but his autopsy studies ultimately led to a correction of this error.

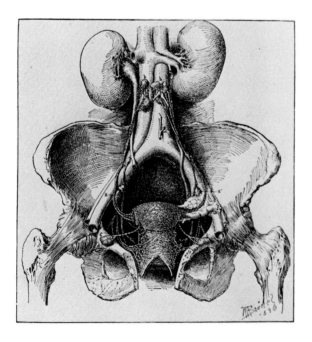

Fig. 1-38. The lymphatics of the female pelvic organs. By Max Brödel, 1896.

Fig. 1-39. Innervation of the female pelvic organs. From R. Lee's *On the Ganglia and the Other Nervous Structures of the Uterus,* London, 1842, showing posterolateral aspect of the uterus in the fourth month of pregnancy with the great uterocervical ganglion and its neural connections to the uterus, vagina, rectum, and bladder. From the sixteenth century, anatomists had claimed that they were able to trace the pelvic nerves into the uterus, but their descriptions were inadequate and their illustrations schematic. Frustrated by his inability to demonstrate a nerve supply to the uterus, Friedrich Osiander stated in 1829, in his textbook of obstetrics, that he had been deceived by the authority of the earlier anatomists but now felt quite certain that the nerves of the human uterus had never been seen, by him or anyone else. Yet every obstetrician of experience had felt against his arm the great contractile force of which the uterus is capable in response to the stimulation of internal version. Of the existence of nerves in so irritable an organ there could be no doubt. Robert Lee (1793–1877), a British obstetrician, presented the first good description of the nervous structures of the uterus on June 17, 1841, before the Royal Society of London; publication was made the following year. The innervation of the uterus, its plexuses, and its ganglia, were described in greater detail a quarter of a century later, in a monograph by Ferdinand Frankenhäuser (1832–1894) in *Die Nerven der Gebaermutter und ihre Endigung in den Glatten Muskelfasern,* Jena, 1867. The uterocervical ganglion and plexus have since been identified eponymicly with the names of both Lee and Frankenhäuser.

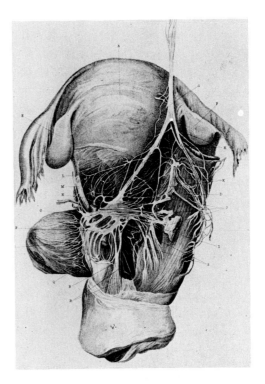

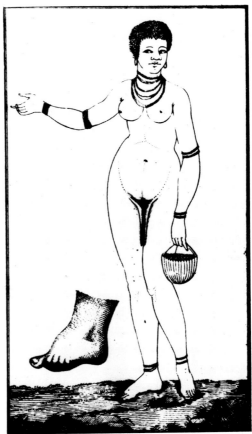

Fig. 1-40. The Hottentot Apron of the labia minora. Francesco Plazzoni (d. 1622) wrote, "*Nymphae vocantur vel quod sint castitatis praesides, vel quod sponsum primo intermittant, vel quod aquis prosilientibus praesint.*" Restated by Sir Charles Bell (1774–1842), "The most modest of the uses ascribed to them is that of directing the stream of urine." Among the Hottentots, of South Africa, labial size figured largely in a woman's sexual attractiveness. Artificial elongation by friction, stretching, and even hanging heavy weights from them, became a part of the daily routine of many Hottentot girls, some from early infancy, leading to the hypertrophy that came to be known as the *Hottentot apron.* Engraving from J. L. Moreau (de la Sarthe) in his *Histoire de la femme,* Paris, 1803.

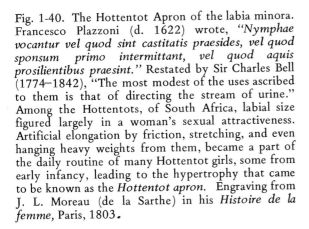

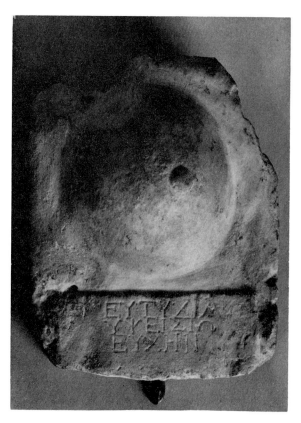

Fig. 1-41. Ex-voto in the form of a breast. Recovered from the northern slope of the Acropolis in Athens. Staatliche Museen, Antikenabteilungen, East Berlin.

THE BREAST

"The shape of the breasts is like a gourd. They are round for holding blood to be changed into milk...they have teats, that the new born child may suck therefrom.

Second, as to substance. They are of glandular flesh, since superfluous blood prepared in them must be transformed into milk. This change is wrought by cooling...

Third, as to size. They are larger in a woman than in a man for two reasons. One is that they may produce milk, but not so in man. Second, that they may reflect back to the heart by repulsion the heat which they receive from it. This is more needed in women, for they have less heat round the heart than men.

Fourth, observe their number. They are two in human beings as in every animal that beareth one or two young. In animals that bear many the breasts are more in number.

Fifth, observe their place and connection.... In man they are situated on the chest but not so in other animals.... For the breasts are made to generate milk, and milk is formed from the superfluity of well-digested blood. But the great quantity of such superfluous blood in other animals doth form horns, fur, claws, teeth, and so forth.... The veins which go to the womb should go, as Galen hath said... by a winding course, so that the blood might be ever refined and well digested.... They [the breasts] are connected with the heart and the liver by an ascending vein.... They are connected too with the womb by veins..." [From a translation of the Latin text of the Anatomy of Mundinus, 1316 AD]

Symbol of sex, determinant of fashion, inspiration for poetry and art, as well as source of sustenance for her young, woman's cherished asset, the breast, has also proved one of her major liabilities, prey to cults of mutilation and a fertile field for tumor growth.

THE FEMALE ANATOMY 23

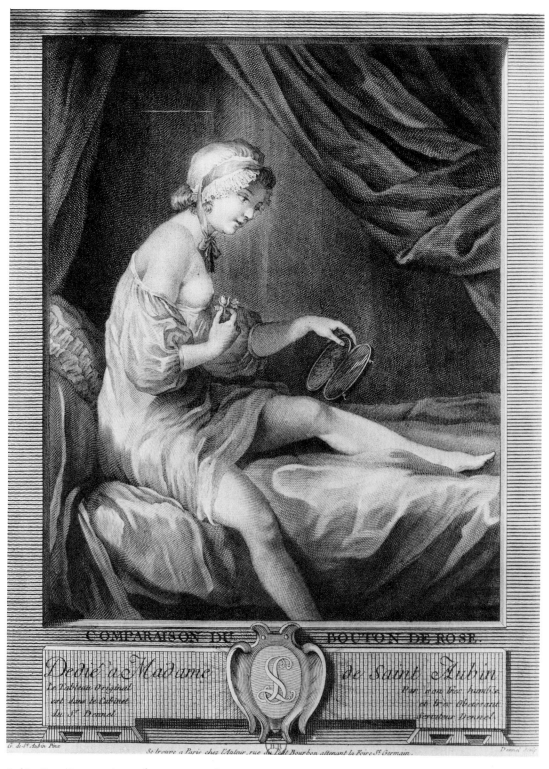

Fig. 1-42. *La Comparaison du Bouton de Rose* (Comparison with a Rosebud). By the Parisian artist Gabriel Jacques Saint-Aubin (1724–1780), dedicated to his wife. This theme was popular in the art and literature of the eighteenth century.

24 ICONOGRAPHIA GYNIATRICA

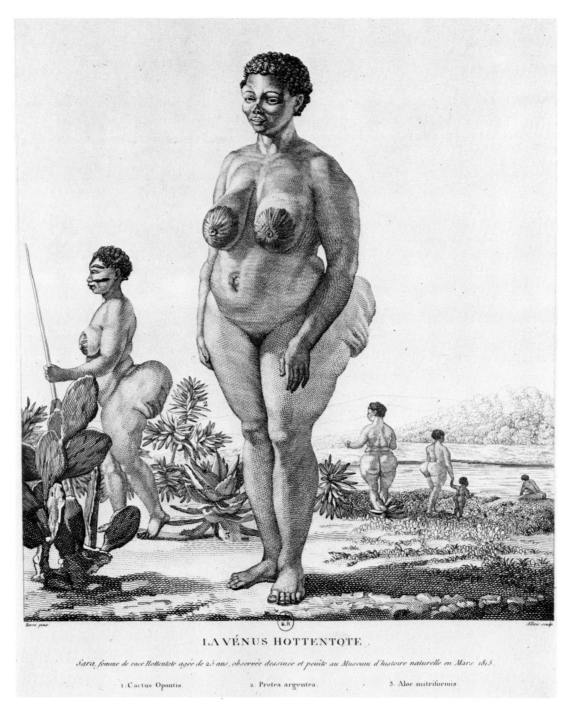

LA VÉNUS HOTTENTOTE.

Sara, femme de race Hottentote agée de 25 ans, observée dessinée et peinte au Museum d'histoire naturelle en Mars 1815.

1. Cactus Opontia.   2. Protea argentea.   3. Aloe mitriformis.

Fig. 1-43. The "Hottentot Venus" Sarah Baartman at age 25. Engraving from a painting, made from life in 1815, at the *Museum d'Histoire Naturelle* in Paris. Describing this embodiment of the Hottentot ideal of feminine beauty, Georges Cuvier (1769–1832) wrote in his *Mémoire*,

"Her breasts, which she was in the habit of raising and pressing against her clothing, when left naturally showed their great pendulous mass, each capped obliquely with a darkish areola more than four inches in diameter, creased with radiating furrows, and near the center of which was a nipple, so flattened as to be almost invisible."

Bibliothèque Nationale, Paris.

THE FEMALE ANATOMY 25

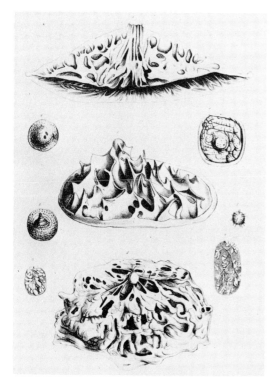

Fig. 1-44. Illustrations (Plate IV), from *The Anatomy and Diseases of the Breast,* 1845, by Sir Astley Paston Cooper (1768–1841), distinguished British anatomist and the foremost surgeon of his time. (1) Anatomical preparation showing how the suspensory ligaments extend from the breast to the inner side of the skin, (2) the breast dissected to show the ducts and lobules, (3) the mammary gland sectioned through the nipple. Cooper wrote of the mammary fascia, the ligaments of which were subsequently named for him,

"This is divided into two layers; the superficial, and the deeper layer of the breast, between which the gland of the breast is included.... The anterior or superficial layer passes upon the anterior or cutaneous surface of the breast: here it forms a fibrous covering, but not a true capsule ... passing between the gland and the skin; but it also enters the interior of the secretory structure. Here it sends out two sets of processes of a fibrous nature from its two surfaces.... By these processes, the breast is slung upon the forepart of the chest, for they form a moveable but very firm connexion with the skin, so that the breast has sufficient motion to elude violence; yet by this fibrous tissue it is, excepting under age, lactation, or relaxation, prevented from much change of place."

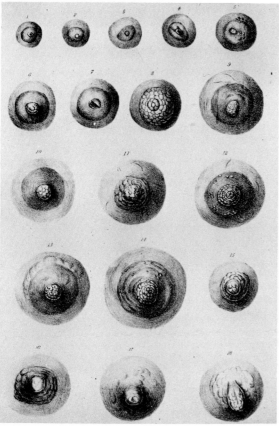

Fig. 1-45. The human nipple. Illustrations (Plate I) from Sir Astley Cooper's *The Anatomy and Diseases of the Breast,* 1845. (1-10) the nipple at various developmental stages, from age 2 to 20 years, (11) the nipple of a parous woman of 24 years, (12) the nipple of a pregnant woman, age 26, (13) the nipple of a woman of 28 years after 9 months' lactation, (18) the nipple of a multipara in old age.

26 ICONOGRAPHIA GYNIATRICA

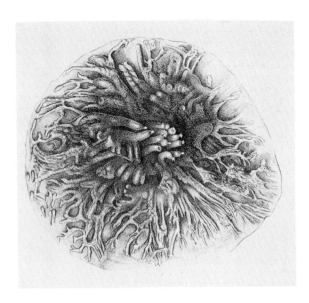

Fig. 1-46. Lactiferous ducts. Anatomic preparation, injected with wax, from a woman who died while lactating. Plate V, Figure 1 from Sir Astley Cooper's *The Anatomy and Diseases of the Breast*, 1845.

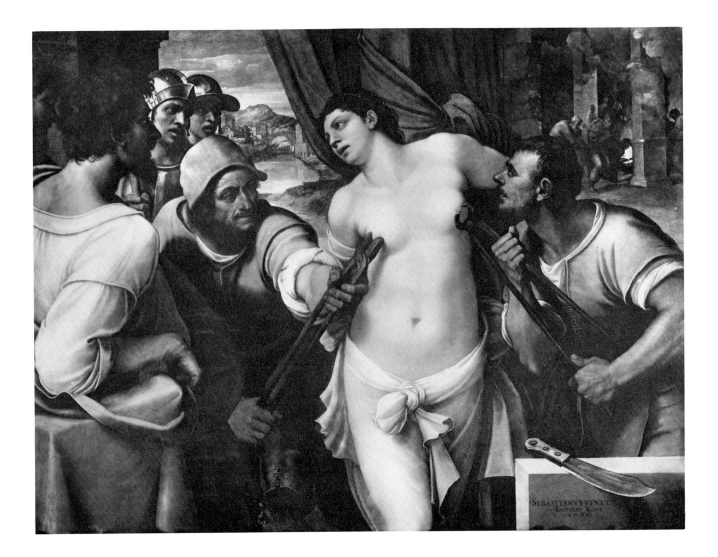

THE FEMALE ANATOMY   27

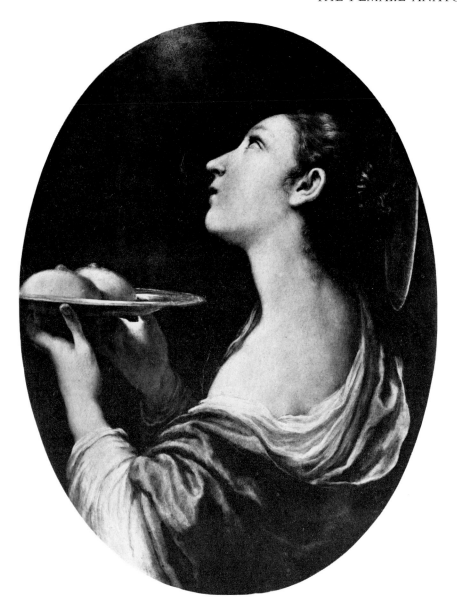

Fig. 1-48. St. Agatha offering her ablated breasts to God, symbolizing her martyrdom. Painting by Lorenzo Lippi (1606–1665). Galleria degli Uffizi, Florence.

Fig. 1-47. The martyrdom of St. Agatha, protectress against diseases of the breast. Painting by Sebastiano del Piombo (1485–1547). According to legend, this beautiful virgin of Catania, Sicily, was tortured, her breasts crushed and amputated, because she resisted the advances of Quintianus, Roman governor of Sicily. Sentenced to burning at the stake, she was released by the people when an earthquake occurred as the fire was lit. Agatha was then confined to prison, where she was visited by St. Peter, who performed a miracle and made her whole again. She died on February 5, AD 251, subsequently celebrated as her festival date. The later rescue of Catania from fire during an eruption of Mt. Etna was ascribed to St. Agatha's veil. Her intercession was also credited with the sparing of Malta from Turkish conquest in 1551.

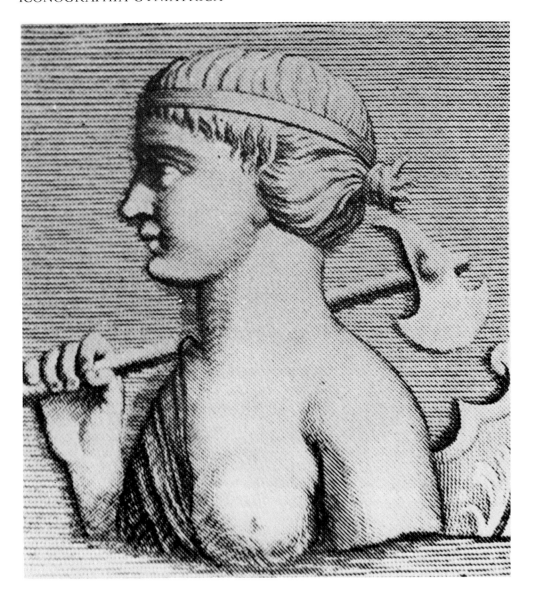

Fig. 1-49. An Amazon, her right breast absent, according to her tribe's custom of its early ablation. Engraving by an unknown artist. Hippocrates told of these legendary women in his *Airs, Waters and Places,* "In Europe there is a Scythian race called Sauromatae ... different from all other races. Their women mount on horseback, use the bow, and throw the javelin from their horses, and fight with their enemies as long as they are virgins; and they do not lay aside their virginity until they kill three of their enemies.... Whoever takes to herself a husband, gives up riding horseback unless the necessity of a general expedition obliges her. They have no right breast; for while still of a tender age their mothers heat strongly a copper instrument constructed for this very purpose, and apply it to the right breast, which is burnt up, and its development being arrested, all the strength and fullness are determined to the right shoulder and arm."

Ptolemy wrote in his *Judgments Derived from the Heaven,*

"The men are timid and submissive ... on the contrary, most of the women are vigorous, imperious, and militant, because of the ascension of the Moon and their majestic mien. Such are the Amazons, who avoid having contact with men, who apply themselves to weapons, and who make their daughters hardy from childhood, cutting off their right breast in order that they may be better fitted to military exercises, and who uncover this portion of their bosom in exploits of war and in combats, so as to reveal their natural vigor and male courage."

THE FEMALE ANATOMY 29

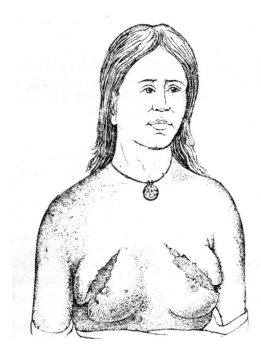

Fig. 1-50. Multilation of the breasts. As practiced in centuries past by the Skoptsy, a sect of the Russian Raskolniki, who also mutilated the labia and clitoris to sanctify their female children. "Blessed are the barren, and the wombs that never bare, and the paps which never gave suck." (St. Luke 23:29)

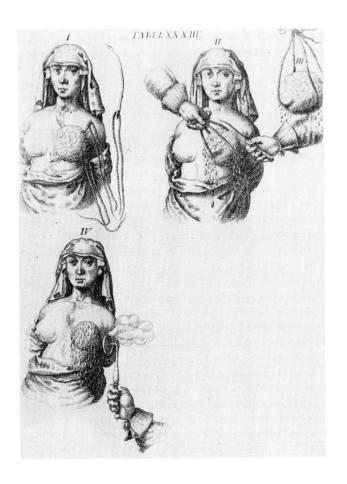

Fig. 1-51. Amputation of the breast. Differing greatly in purpose but only slightly in manner from ritualistic mutilation was therapeutic mutilation of the breast, reintroduced in the thirteenth century by Lanfranc of Milan (d. 1315), who brought to France the attainments of Italian surgery. Centuries earlier the Greeks had treated mammary cancer by excision, but with little success. Lanfranc advocated total amputation. Illustrated, from the seventeenth century surgery of Scultetus (1595–1645) (Table 38 [number misprinted in original plate] in his *Armamentarium chirurgicum,* 1655) are four steps in the operation. Legends from the English translation, 1674,

"Fig. I. represents a breast affected with an ulcerated Canker, the basis whereof is thrust through with two needles... drawing after them a twisted flaxen thread; Fig. II shews how the Chyrurgian takes hold, with his left hand, of the ends of the threads... and with his right hand... he cutteth the Canker out by the roots; Fig. III shews a Canker cut from the breast, weighing six Physical pounds; Fig. IV. shews how the Chyrurgian, after the cutting off of a breast ulcerated, doth lightly cauterize the place with a red hot iron..."

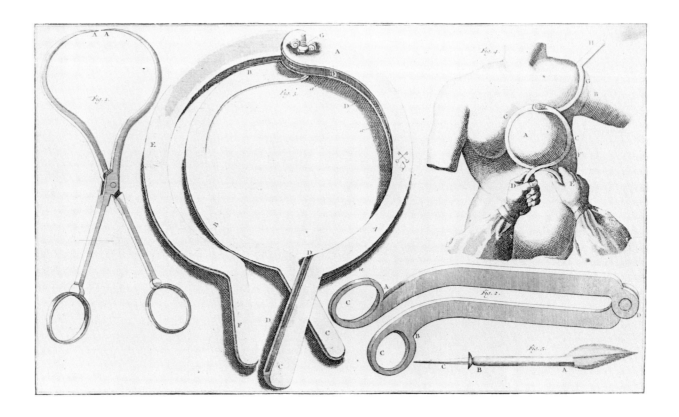

Fig. 1-52. A so-called improved method of amputating the cancerous breast. Contrived by the Dutch surgeon Helvetius and shown in Table 23 of Lorenz Heister's *Institutiones chirurgicae,* 1739, regarded as the best illustrated surgical text of the eighteenth century. Legends from the English translation *A General System of Surgery*, 1757, vol. 2, pp. 64–65, "Fig. 1. is the Pliers or Tenaculum of Helvetius, serving to... hold up the cancerous Breast.... Fig. 2. Exhibits another steel Tenaculum... to compress the Breast; Fig. 3. Represents a new Instrument for amputating cancer'd Breasts. AA, a semi-circular and double brass Plate, joined so as to leave a Space DDD between, to receive and direct the falciform Knife E F.... B B is another semi-circular and single brass-plate to act against the former, compress, and elevate the Breast.... Fig. 4. Represents the left Breast of a Woman, cancerous, and going to be amputated...."

The surgery of benign mammary tumors in Heister's day is well exemplified in one of his case reports. The patient, aged 30, had known of a lump in her breast, the size of a hen's egg, for three years. Heister recommended its removal before it changed into cancer. Heister wrote,

"I ordered a barber, who came with her to me, to prepare a good quantity of lint, a linen compress, and a long roller with two heads, one ounce of alcohol vini, a cordial julep, and some Hungary-water for smelling to. The next morning, at the appointed time, the barber came with two of his journeymen. I seated her in the chair, and ordered one of them to hold her round the shoulders and breast, and to raise her upwards; then making an incision with a knife through the skin, I dissected the tumor gradually, and at length cut it out, the wound bleeding but very little; then filling up the wound with lint, moistened with the alcohol vini, I laid a compress over it, and applied the two-headed roller, fixing the compress by circular turns round the breast, and ordered her to be put to bed giving her some of the cordial julep, and Hungary-water to smell to."

THE FEMALE ANATOMY 31

INTERSEX

"... the sexes were originally three in number ... there was man, woman, and the union of the two, having a name corresponding to this double nature; they once had a real existence, but it is now lost, and the name only is preserved as a term of reproach." [Plato: *Symposium*. Translation by Benjamin Jowett, 1871.]

"There is no such biological entity as sex. What exists in nature is a dimorphism within species into male and female individuals, which differ with respect to contrasting characters, for each of which in any given species we recognize a male form and a female form, whether these characters be classed as of the biological, or psychological, or social orders. Sex is not a force that produces these contrasts; it is merely a name for our total impression of the differences." [Frank Lillie: General biological introduction, in E. Allen (ed.): *Sex and Internal Secretions*. Williams & Wilkins Co., Baltimore, 1932.]

Hermaphroditos, a minor Greek divinity, half man and half woman, was first mentioned in literature by Theophrastus (died c. 287 BC) in his *Characters*. Of this ambisexual deity a later author of unknown name wrote,

To men I am Hermes; to women I appear as
  Cypris.
I bear the emblem of both my parents.
So it was quite proper for them to put me,
  Hermaphroditos, in mixed baths since I am
  an ambiguous child.

In art Hermaphroditos has been depicted in a variety of media—marble statues, paintings, vase decorations, gems—most of these works dating back to the Hellenistic-Roman period. Murals in private homes and public baths, from the fourth century BC, showed Hermaphroditos as a beautiful youth with full fe-

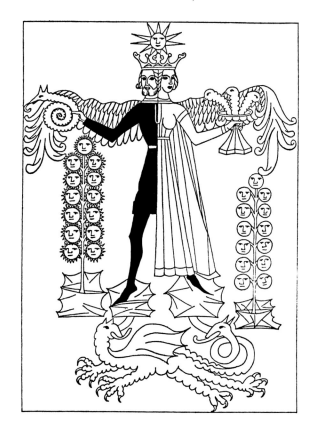

Fig. 1-53. Winged King-Queen hermaphrodite or androgyne. Drawing from the manuscript of Michael Cochen (c. 1530). Standing on the double-headed flying dragon of Nature, between the tree of the sun and the tree of the moon, the King holds a coiled serpent, Life; the Queen, a cup containing the heads of three young snakes or dragons representing Life's components: Spirit, Soul, and Body. The "Hermetic Androgyne" is a representation of the alchemical philosophy of Thoth or Hermes Trismegistos, the Egyptian god to whom is attributed the sacred books of wisdom, the *Corpus Hermeticum*, which pictured life as generated by equal and opposite forces. Stadtbibliothek Vadiana, St. Gallen, Switzerland.

male breasts, well rounded hips, and male genitalia. In real life, however, far from objects of veneration, the unfortunate possessors of mixed sexual characters were met with scorn and violence. The latter-day Greeks, it is said, cast them into the sea; the Romans abandoned them at birth, on a desert island. Regarded by some as a manifestation of sorcery, hermaphrodism led to the burning at the stake of Michael Servetus (1511–1553), Spanish theologian and discoverer of the pulmonary circulation.

The scientific study of hermaphrodism began with Albrecht von Haller (1708–1777), who critically reviewed all reported cases and the previously held theoretical explanations of their origins. The pathological anatomy of genital malformations became intelligible through the embryologic studies of the late eighteenth and the nineteenth centuries. Genetic, hormonal, psychiatric, and surgical aspects of hermaphrodism present a continuing challenge to the biologists and physicians of the late twentieth century.

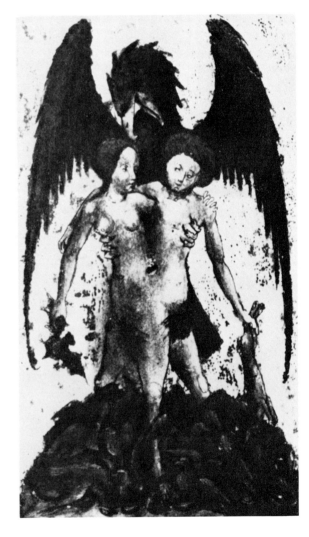

Fig. 1-54. Union of the primordial male and female forces. Illustration from an ancient alchemical manuscript. The eagle represents the male-female quicksilver, harmoniously perfect; the bat and hare, the subtle and the corporeal. Zentralbibliothek, Zürich.

THE FEMALE ANATOMY 33

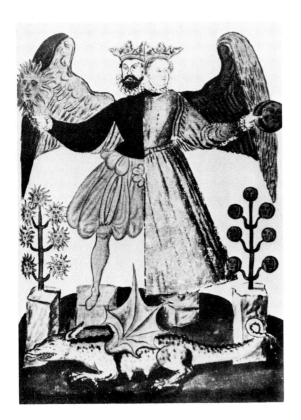

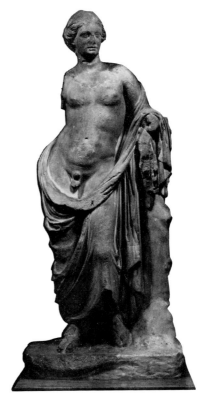

Fig. 1-55. "The Hermetic Androgyne." Miniature from a late seventeenth century German manuscript, *Dritter Pitagorischer Sinodas von der verborgenen Weisheit.*

Fig. 1-56. Hermaphrodite. Antique statue from Pergamon. Istanbul Archaeological Museums.

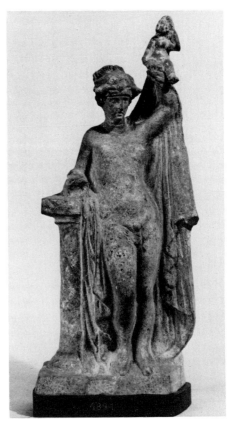

Fig. 1-57. Hermaphrodite. Terra cotta statue. National Archaeological Museum, Athens.

34 ICONOGRAPHIA GYNIATRICA

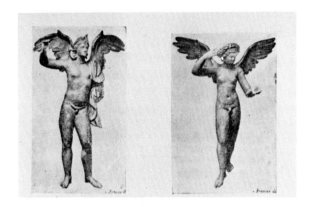

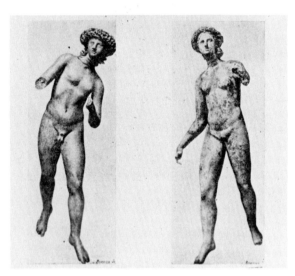

Fig. 1-58. Hermaphrodites. Terra cotta figures excavated from the subterranean tombs of the necropolis of Myrina, ancient town of Aeolis, in northwest Asia Minor. All four statuettes are fashioned in the form of a young woman merged with that of a yound man: well-formed breasts, female fat distribution, delicate head and neck, combined with small male external genitalia.

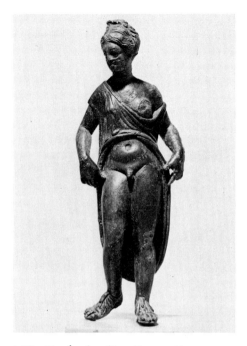

Fig. 1-59. Hermaphrodite. Bronze Roman statuette. Musée du Louvre, Paris.

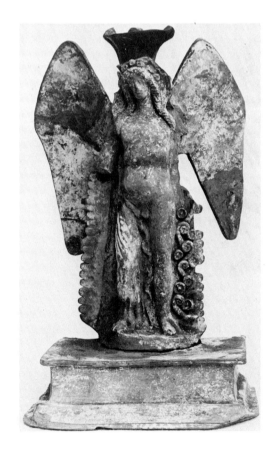

Fig. 1-60. Eros, Greek god of love. Depicted as an hermaphrodite. Greek terra cotta perfume vase which was shattered within the Musée Bonnat, Bayonne, France, by a violent hailstorm.

THE FEMALE ANATOMY 35

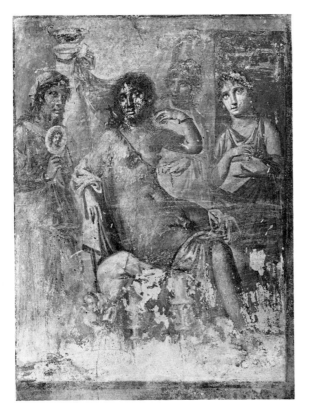

Fig. 1-61. Hermaphrodite. Fresco from Pompeii.

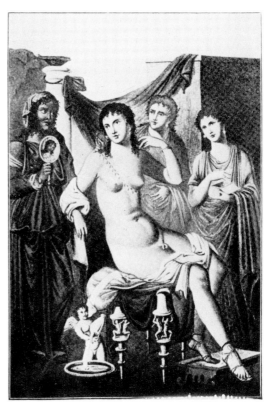

Fig. 1-62. Hermaphroditos and attendants. A Pompeian mural. In left background is depicted a bearded woman; in lower foreground, an hermaphroditic winged angel.

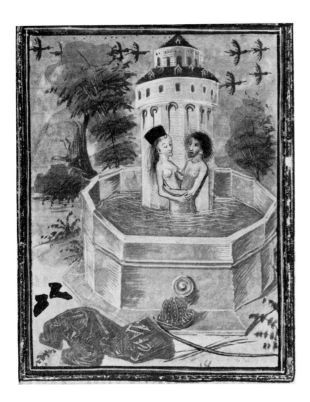

Fig. 1-63. Hermaphrodism. Figure from a fourteenth century French manuscript, *Les métamorphoses d'Ovide,* illustrating the legend of Salmacis. "O my father, and my mother," prayed Hermaphroditos to the god Mercury and the goddess Venus after he was seduced and inseparably entwined by the nymph Salmacis while bathing in a wooded pool, "Grant this prayer to your son, who owes his name to you both: if any man enter this pool, may he depart hence no more than half a man, may he suddenly grow weak and effeminate at the touch of these waters!" According to Ovid's legend, both parents were so moved by compassion for Hermaphroditos, who was now but half male and half female, that they infected the fountain of Salmacis with this horrible magic power.

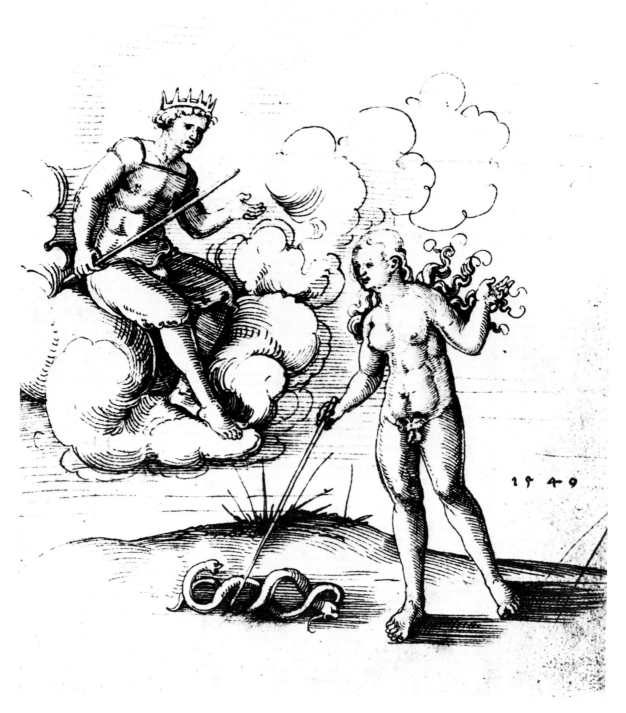

Fig. 1-64. "Hermaphroditus." Drawing by Erhard Schön, 1549. Erlangen Universitätsbibliothek, Germany.

THE FEMALE ANATOMY 37

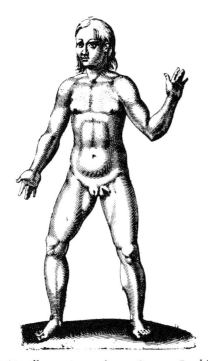

Fig. 1-65. Illustration, from Caspar Bauhin's *De hermaphroditorum,* Frankfurt, 1600 (1614), an early work dealing with the theological, legal, medical, and philosophical aspects of hermaphrodism; showing hermaphrodite with the external genitalia of both sexes.

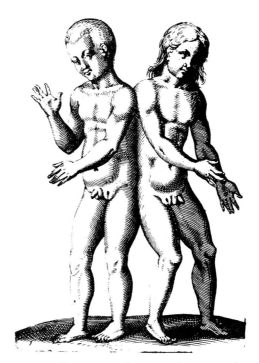

Fig. 1-66. Illustration, from Bauhin's *De hermaphroditorum* showing hermaphroditic conjoined twins, born near Heidelberg, Germany, in 1486.

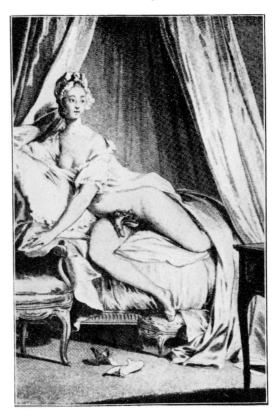

Fig. 1-67. Marie Ange, a pseudohermaphrodite of uncertain sex. Copper engraving, early nineteenth century.

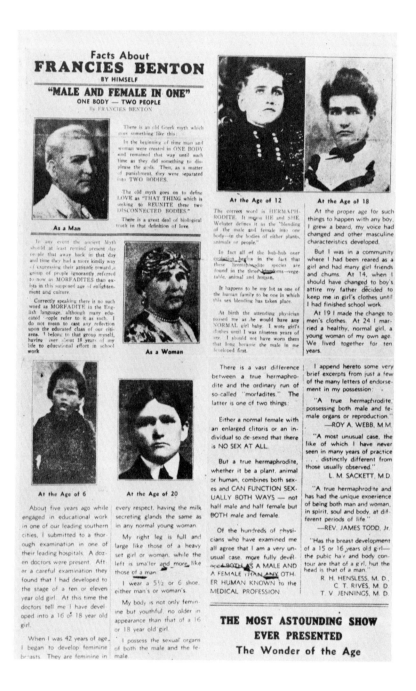

Fig. 1-68. Broadside, distributed by Francies Benton, a so-called practicing hermaphrodite, who was examined in 1936, at age 50, by Dr. Hugh H. Young, Director of The Johns Hopkins Hospital's Brady Urological Institute. Possessing full breasts, a heavy beard, and both a penis and a vagina, Benton made a living through circus exhibitions, and was able to copulate as either man or woman.

THE FEMALE ANATOMY 39

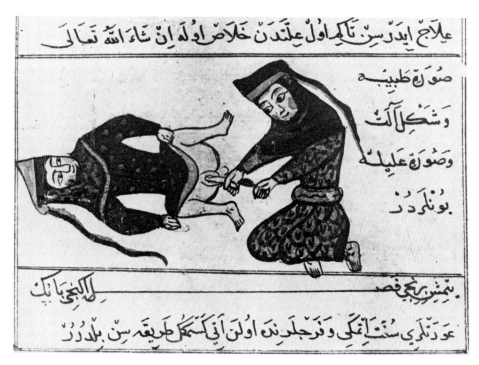

Fig. 1-69. Operation on an hermaphrodite by a midwife. Drawing from a twelfth century Persian treatise, *Imperial Surgery*, Baghdad, translated into Turkish in the fifteenth century by Sapoundji Oghlou. Bibliothèque Nationale, Paris.

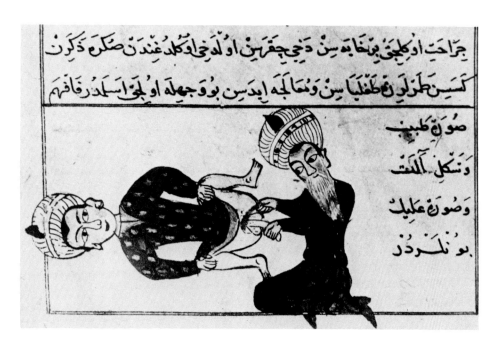

Fig. 1-70. Amputation of the penis by a surgeon. Drawing from the Turkish translation of the twelfth century Persian manuscript, *Imperial Surgery*. Widely publicized in the fall of 1966 was the establishment of a special clinic in The Johns Hopkins Hospital for the surgical alteration of sex. Thus was revived on a large scale a practice at least eight centuries old. Bibliothèque Nationale, Paris.

HIRSUTISM

"You should be women, and yet your beards forbid me to interpret that you are so." [*Macbeth*]

Prominent among the manifestations of masculinization is excessive growth of body hair. The cause of hirsutism can be traced in some cases to abnormal production of androgenic hormones by the gonads or adrenals, resulting from hyperplasia or tumor. In others, in which no explanation can be found, the condition is called *constitutional hirsutism,* a label of medical ignorance.

Masculinized women were described by Hippocrates in the sixth book of his *Epidemics*: Phaetusa, housekeeper for Pytheus of Abdera, a city of ancient Thrace; and Nanno, wife of Gorgippus of Thasos, a Greek island in the North Aegean Sea. Each grew a beard and acquired a deep voice after the menopause. Morbid interest in such unfortunates has never waned; circus side shows of the twentieth century continue to feature so-called bearded women. Despite their male features, many have married and have borne children.

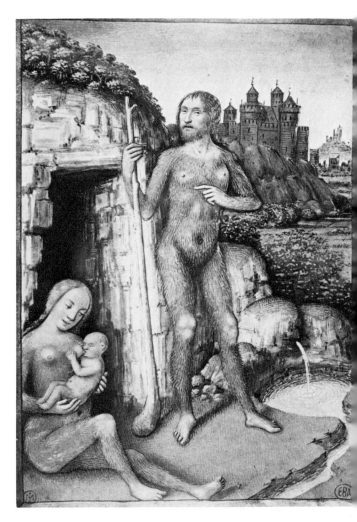

Fig. 1-71. *L'État Sauvage.* Painting, about 1510, by Jehan Bourdichon (c. 1457–1521), emphasizing the hypertrichosis of primitive man. Ashley Montagu (J.A.M.A. 187, 1964) has suggested that the subsequent reduction in man's body hair has been associated with his adoption of the active life of the hunter, with its dependence on massive sweating for maintenance of constancy of the body temperature.

THE FEMALE ANATOMY 41

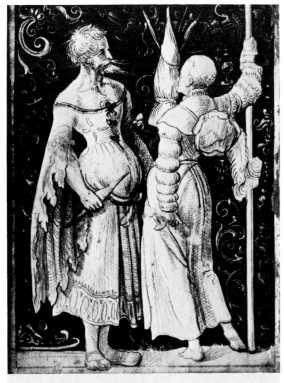

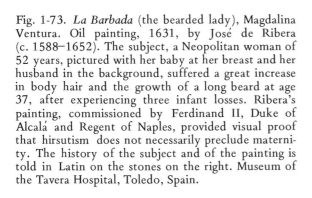

Fig. 1-72. *Femme Enceinte et Barbue* (bearded pregnant woman). By Niklaus Manuel Deutsch (1484–1530), one of a group of six drawings entitled *Le Monde Renversé*.

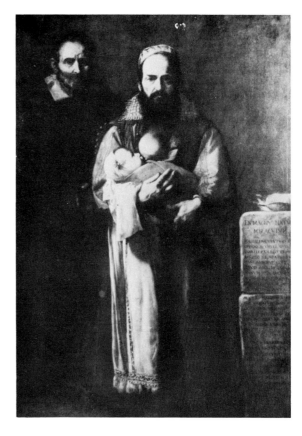

Fig. 1-73. *La Barbada* (the bearded lady), Magdalina Ventura. Oil painting, 1631, by José de Ribera (c. 1588–1652). The subject, a Neopolitan woman of 52 years, pictured with her baby at her breast and her husband in the background, suffered a great increase in body hair and the growth of a long beard at age 37, after experiencing three infant losses. Ribera's painting, commissioned by Ferdinand II, Duke of Alcalá and Regent of Naples, provided visual proof that hirsutism does not necessarily preclude maternity. The history of the subject and of the painting is told in Latin on the stones on the right. Museum of the Tavera Hospital, Toledo, Spain.

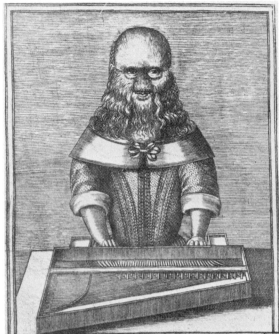

Fig. 1-74. Barbara Urslerin. Born in Augsburg in 1633, with long blond beard at age 20.

Fig. 1-75. Madame Fortune Clofullia, the Bearded Lady from Switzerland. Born Josephine Boisdechene in Versoix in 1831, she had a beard of fully 2 inches by age 8, 5 inches at age 14. In 1853 P. T. Barnum discovered her in London, brought her to America, placed her on exhibit in his New York Museum. Immediately she was haled into court under charges of fraud, brought by a William Charr, disgruntled over the 25 cents he had paid to see her. Three doctors examined the Bearded Lady, vouched for her female sex. Also her husband, a French artist, father of her two children, came to testify. The entire affair, it is believed, was arranged by Barnum as a publicity stunt. The great showman's scheme succeeded: the Bearded Lady appeared prominently in the press, and the paying public flocked to see her. Her surviving son, unusually hairy even for a boy, was appropriately named Esau. (Gleason's Pictorial Drawing-Room Companion, Harvard College Library, Theatre Collection.)

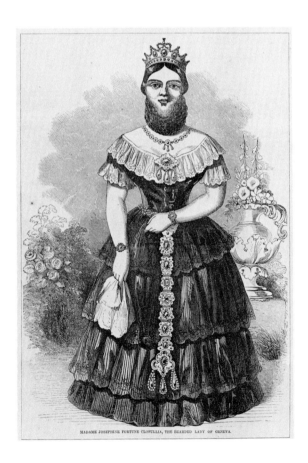

Chapter 2

PREGNANCY
Diagnosis, Scenes, and Garb

PREGNANCY DIAGNOSIS

"If the veins within her arm beat against thy hand, thou shalt say: she is pregnant." [Brugsch (Berlin) Papyrus, 1350 BC]

Impatient with Nature's slow answer to his perennial question, man has ever sought a reliable test for pregnancy's early diagnosis. Hippocrates (c. 460–370 BC) instructed the woman who had missed her period to drink a solution of honey in water before retiring. If pregnant, she would soon suffer painful abdominal distention; if not pregnant, she would sleep undisturbed. Many distinguished physicians who came after *the father of medicine,* including Avicenna (c. 979–1037) and Savonarola (c. 1384–1462), as well as countless charlatans, claimed to be able to diagnose pregnancy from the woman's urine. The ancient Egyptians, as early as the fourteenth century BC, had, in addition, resorted to this fluid for diagnosing fetal sex. Grains of wheat and barley, in separate bags, were moistened daily with the woman's urine. Germination of either indicated pregnancy: the wheat, a male child; the barley, a female.

Uroscopy, for the diagnosis of pregnancy as of almost all human ailments, enjoyed great favor during the Middle Ages. A cult of practi-

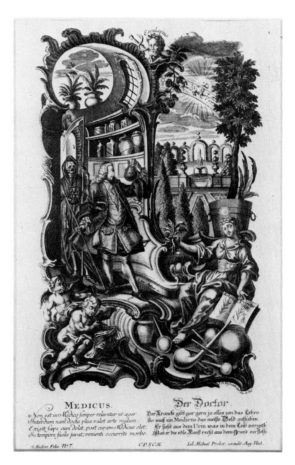

Fig. 2-1. Uroscopy. A seventeenth century engraving, Augsburg, Germany. Thomas Brian wrote, in 1637, "*Urina est meretrix, vel mendax:* The urine is an Harlot, or a Lier. It were farre better for the Physician to see his Patient once than to view his Urine twenty times." (*The Pisse-Prophet, or Certaine Pisse-Pot Lectures,* London, 1637.)

tioners arose, known as *piss-prophets,* who limited their craft to urinary diagnosis. Albertus Magnus (c. 1193–1280) taught that pregnancy urine would float milk; and Jakob Rueff (c. 1500–1558) said that it would coat an iron needle with black spots. Urinary diagnosis, which fell into disrepute toward the middle of the seventeenth century, was revived briefly in France in 1831 with a flurry of excitement over the *Kyesteine pellicle,* a whitish, opaque, granular layer that was said to form on the surface of pregnancy urine allowed to stand for two to six days. Although hailed by *The Lancet* as "a new and highly valuable mode of detecting pregnancy," neither the constancy nor the specificity of this pellicle could be confirmed in the urine of pregnant women, and the enthusiastic claims for it were soon forgotten.

In contrast to the poorly controlled or frankly fraudulent tests that preceded, a sensitive and specific method of pregnancy diagnosis was announced in 1928 by Selmar Aschheim (1878–1965) and Bernhard Zondek (1891–1966), based on the presence of gonadotrophic hormone in the urine. This epochal discovery won immediate and universal acclaim; and although the original procedure of Aschheim and Zondek has since undergone many modifications, gonadotrophin tests for pregnancy, irrespective of technique and including the most recent immunologic methods, are still commonly designated generically as *A-Z tests.*

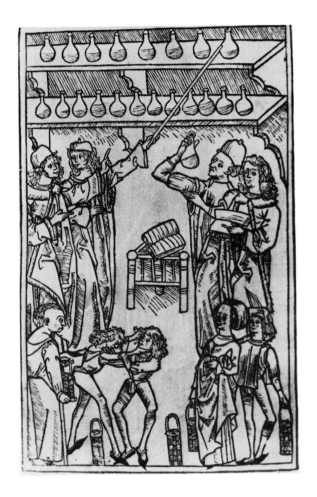

Fig. 2-2. Uroscopy in the diagnosis of pregnancy. Woodcut, Strasbourg, late fifteenth century.

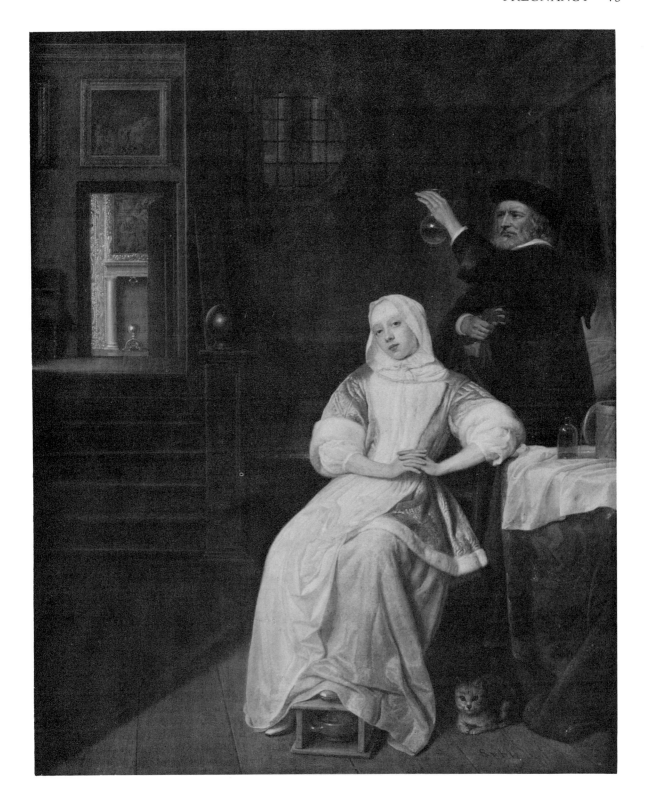

Fig. 2-3. The Sick Lady. Painting by Samuel van Hoogstraten (1627–1678). Rijksmuseum, Amsterdam.

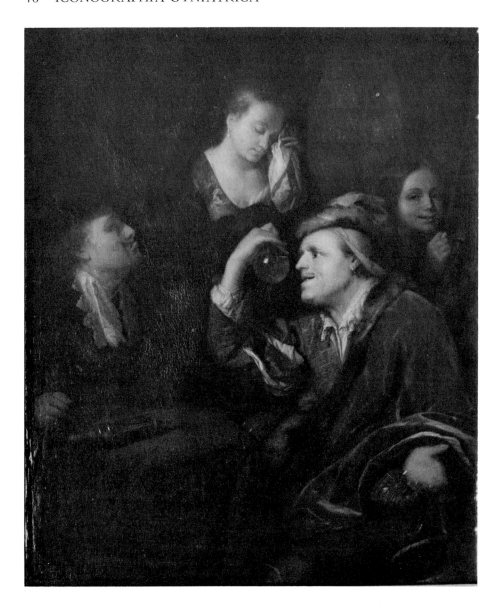

Fig. 2-4. *La Consultation Indiscrète*. Painting by Godfried Schalcken (1643–1706). Faintly outlined in the flask of urine that the doctor examines is a small figure, the embryo. On the left sits the irate father, scowling at his weeping, erstwhile virginal, daughter. Mauritshuis, the Hague.

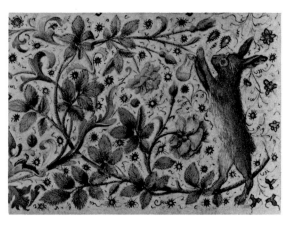

Fig. 2-5. A rabbit physician performing uroscopy. From a Franco-Flemish manuscript of *Hours of the Virgin*, early fifteenth century. The doe herself was later to serve as a test object in pregnancy diagnosis (Friedman test). Pierpont Morgan Library, New York.

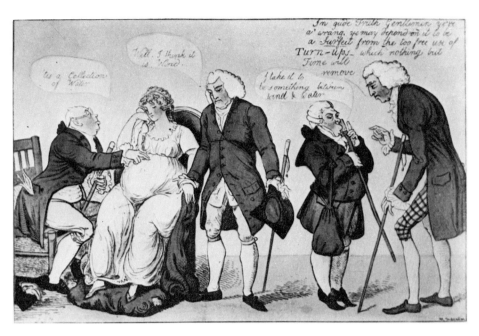

Fig. 2-6. "Time the Best Doctor." English print, 1804. The young patient, obviously pregnant, is surrounded by four doctors in consultation, each holding a different opinion of the cause of her abdominal enlargement: "a collection of water," "wind," "something between wind and water," and "a surfeit from the too free use of turn-ups—which nothing but time will remove." Clearly intended by the last consultant was a play on words, for turnips were then considered an emetic.

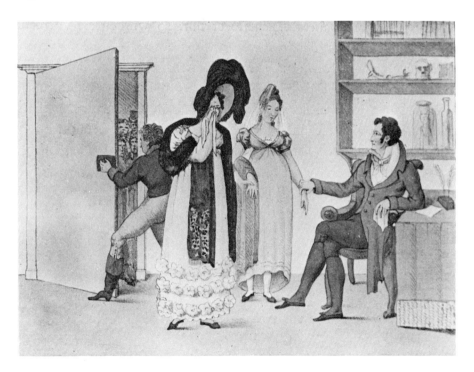

Fig. 2-7. *La Consultation des Piqûres.* French satire, nineteenth century. In the guise of a diplomat, the doctor contemplates his young patient with protuberant abdomen and her weeping mother, reassuring them, "It's not so bad; all will be well again in due time."

48 ICONOGRAPHIA GYNIATRICA

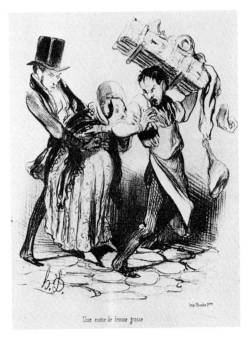

Fig. 2-8. *Une envie de femme grosse* (Craving of a pregnant woman). By Honoré Daumier (1808–1869), no. 15 in his series *Moeurs conjugales* (married life). The capricious appetites of the pregnant woman have long been treated humorously. Extreme perversions of taste and morbid cravings for unusual foods or indigestible substances are known as pica, after the omnivorous magpie (genus *Pica*). Daumier has pictured his pregnant subject preferring the arm of the butcher over the choice cuts of meat he carries.

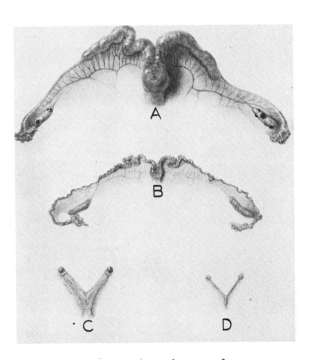

Fig. 2-9. Urinary gonadotrophic tests for pregnancy, twentieth century. (A) Positive Friedman test, rabbit (1929). (B) Negative Friedman test. (C) Positive Aschheim-Zondek test, mouse (1928). (D) Negative Aschheim-Zondek test. From E. C. Hamblen: *Endocrine Gynecology*, 1939. Courtesy of Charles C Thomas, Publisher, Springfield, Ill.

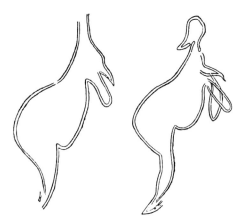

Fig. 2-10. Pregnant women. Drawn in clay by finger. These crude figures, about 60 cm high, recovered from the caves of Pech-Merle in southwestern France, are among the earliest known works of art, dating back to the Aurignacian age, about 16,000 BC.

PREGNANCY SCENES

"Provident nature is wonderfully kind to pregnant women; and when she is properly consulted, attended to, and obeyed from the beginning; nor weakened by excess of any kind; nor thwarted and put out of her course by preposterous mismanagement in her progress, will, nine hundred and ninety-nine times out of a thousand, carry her votary safely through all the wonderful changes of this eventful period." [Samuel Bard: *A Compendium of the Theory and Practice of Midwifery*. New York, 1812.]

PREGNANCY 49

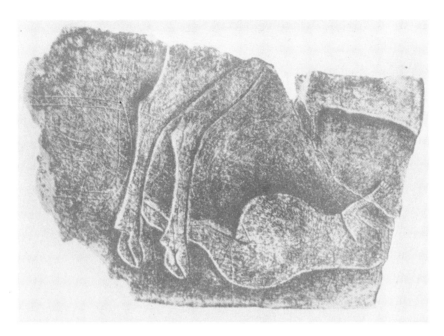

Fig. 2-11. Pregnant woman lying under a reindeer. A relic of the Paleolithic era, fragments of a carving on the sacrum of a reindeer, recovered from Laugerie-Basse, Dordogne, France. This figure may represent a magic rite. The animal, some scholars suggest, was believed to impart strength to the woman by walking over her.

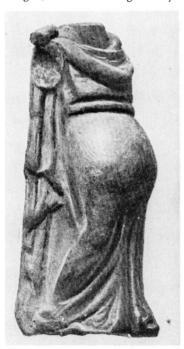

Fig. 2-12. Statue of a pregnant woman. Antedating the second century BC, discovered near Izmir on the Gulf of Smyrna, an inlet of the Agean Sea. The gravida's characteristic posture, or *pride of pregnancy* is well shown.

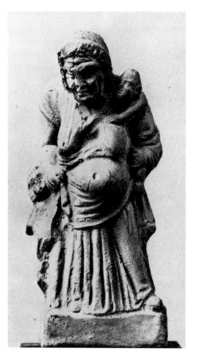

Fig. 2-13. Pregnancy. Ancient terra cotta figure. Staatliche Museen, East Berlin.

50   ICONOGRAPHIA GYNIATRICA

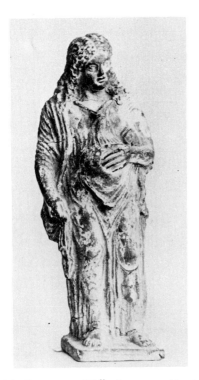

Fig. 2-14. Pregnancy. Hellenic terra cotta statue.

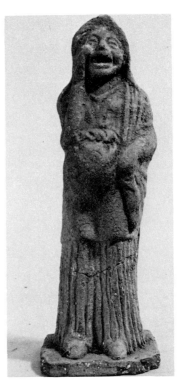

Fig. 2-15. Sobbing pregnant woman. Attic terra cotta figure, third century BC. National Archaeological Museum, Athens.

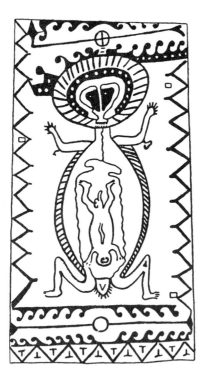

Fig. 2-16. Pregnant woman with male fetus. Painted woodcarving on a door, north coast of Dutch New Guinea, late nineteenth century.

Fig. 2-18. The Annunciation with Donors and St. Joseph. In the Mérode altarpiece of the Master of Flémalle (Robert Campin?, 1406–1444), probably painted between 1425 and 1428. The figures shown in the fully furnished interior of this domestic scene help tell the tale of the Virgin's conception and pregnancy: the lilies in the center symbolizing Mary's purity; their white petals enfolding a heart, the infant in her womb; the seven rays of light entering the room, the seven gifts of the Holy Spirit; the brightly polished kettle above the angel's head, Mary as "the vessel most clean." The Divine Light, a burning candle, has been snuffed at the moment of the Annunciation, when God assumed the flesh of man. Metropolitan Museum of Art, New York.

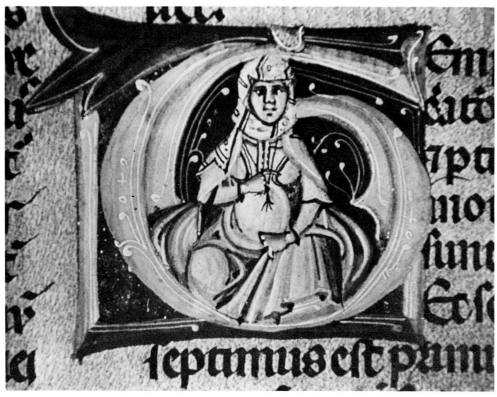

Fig. 2-17. A pregnant woman baring her abdomen for examination. Miniature from a fourteenth century manuscript of Gerard of Cremona's Latin translation of Avicenna's *Canon of Medicine*. Vatican Library, Urbino.

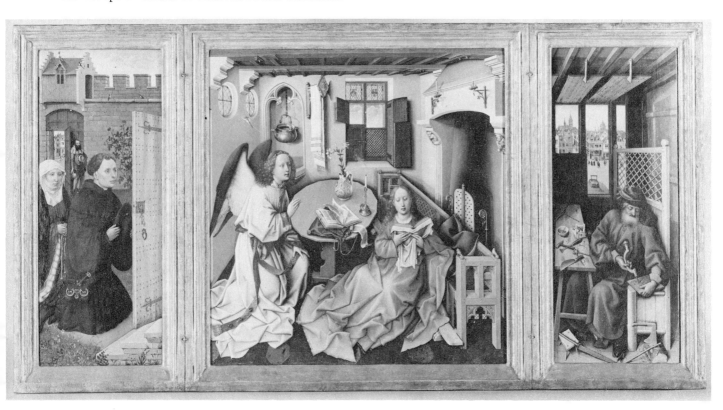

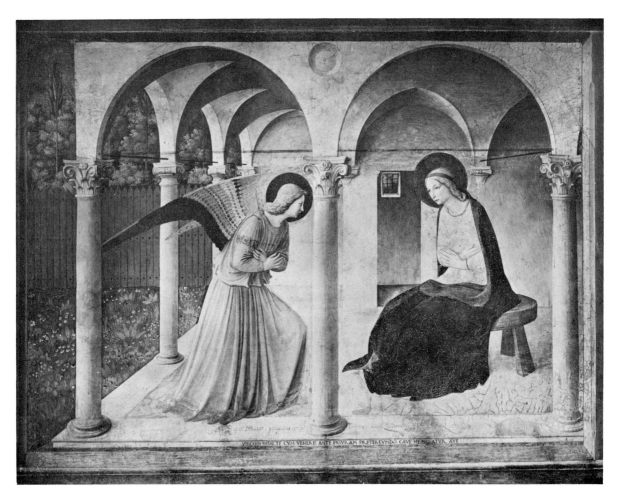

Fig. 2-19. The Annunciation. By Fra Angelico (1387–1455). Mary and Gabriel meet in an arcaded loggia, bordered by a flowering lawn and garden fence. Museo San Marco, Florence.

THE ANNUNCIATION

"In the sixth month the Angel Gabriel was sent from God to a city of Galilee named Nazareth to a virgin betrothed to a man whose name was Joseph, of the house of David; and the virgin's name was Mary. And he came to her and said, 'Hail, O favored one, the Lord is with you!' But she was greatly troubled at the saying, and considered in her mind what sort of greeting this might be. And the angel said to her, 'Do not be afraid, Mary, for you will conceive in your womb and bear a son, and you shall call him Jesus.'" [St. Luke 1:26-31]

Fig. 2-20. The Annunciation. By Jan van Eyck (1390?– 1440) and helpers. The scene is outside a church, on the doorstep of which are inlaid the opening words of an Easter hymn, "Queen of Heaven, rejoice." In a vase at the church entrance are the lilies symbolizing the Virgin's purity. Metropolitan Museum of Art, New York.

PREGNANCY 53

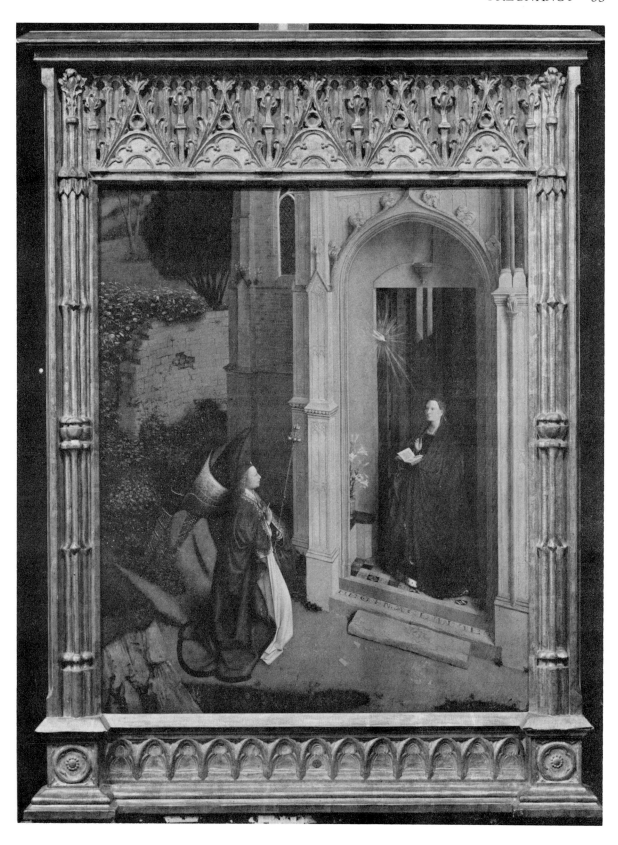

54 ICONOGRAPHIA GYNIATRICA

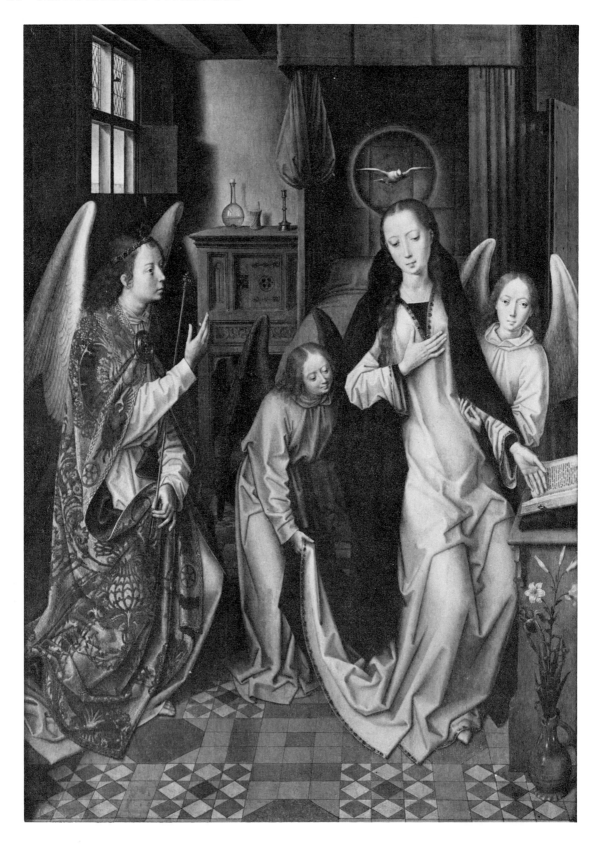

PREGNANCY 55

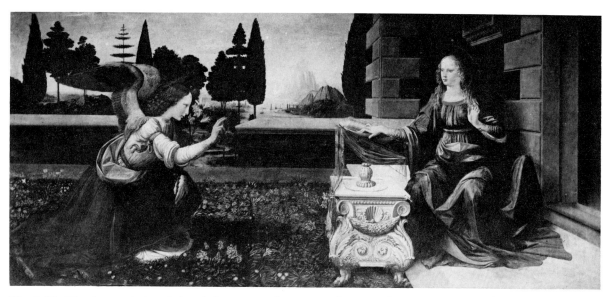

Fig. 2-22. The Annunciation. Painted about 1472 for the Convent of Monte Oliveto near Florence, Italy. Its artist is unknown, but it is generally considered to be an early work of Leonardo da Vinci. Galleria degli Uffizi, Florence.

Fig. 2-23. Saint Joseph and the Virgin. Ivory carving, fourteenth century. Musée de Cluny, France.

Fig. 2-24. The Holy Virgin, vessel of the Divine Infant. A German painting, 1524. In religious art of this era the pregnant uterus was usually shown in simple oval outline, containing a stylized version of the infant.

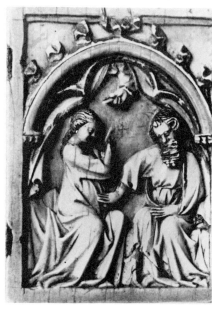

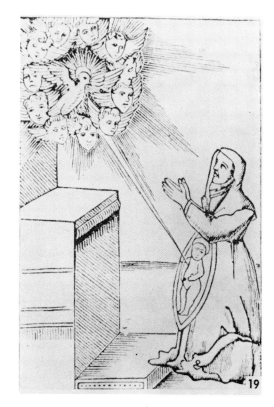

Fig. 2-21. The Annunciation. By Hans Memling (d. 1494). The setting is a well-furnished Flemish chamber, the bed draped in red, the floor ornately tiled. At the left the winged Gabriel alights. The lilies of purity stand in a vase at the Virgin's feet; the dove, symbolizing the Holy Spirit, hovers over her head. The Lehman Collection, New York.

56 ICONOGRAPHIA GYNIATRICA

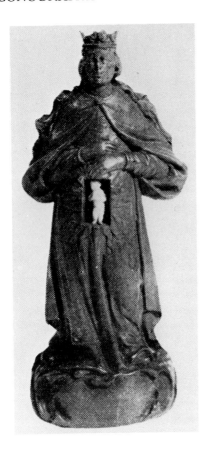

Fig. 2-25. The Virgin, her uterus opened to show the Infant Jesus. Spanish statuette, seventeenth century. Bibliothèque Municipale, Amiens, France.

THE VISITATION

"In those days Mary arose and went with haste into the hill country, to a city of Judah, and she entered the house of Zachariah and greeted Elizabeth. And when Elizabeth heard the greeting of Mary, the babe leaped in her womb; and Elizabeth was filled with the Holy Spirit and she exclaimed with a loud cry, 'Blessed are you among women, and blessed is the fruit of your womb! And why is this granted me, that the mother of my Lord should come to me? For behold, when the voice of your greeting came to my ears, the babe in my womb leaped for joy.'" [St. Luke 1:39-44]

To her cousin's exultant greeting the Virgin responded with what has come to be known as "The Song of Mary." (St. Luke 1:46-55)

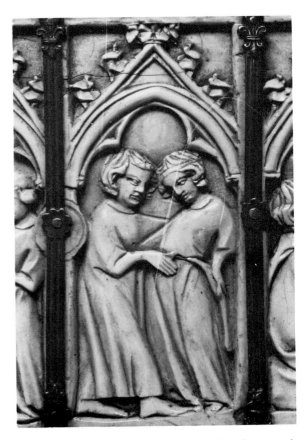

Fig. 2-26. The Visitation. Ivory carving, fourteenth century. Musée du Louvre, Paris.

PREGNANCY 57

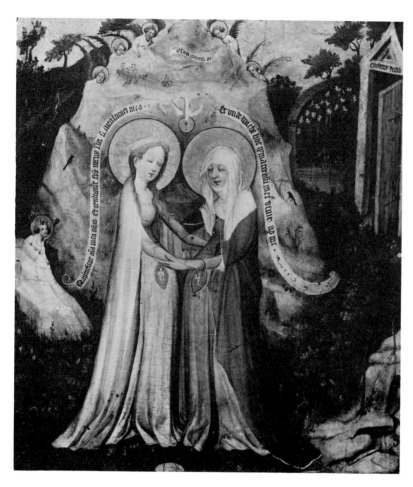

Fig. 2-27. Mary and Elizabeth: The Visitation. Oil painting by a master of the Cologne School, about 1410. Oval windows in the robes of the pregnant cousins permit a view of fetal John in the womb of Elizabeth, and of the Christ-child within Mary. Aartsbisschoppelijk Museum, Utrecht, Netherlands.

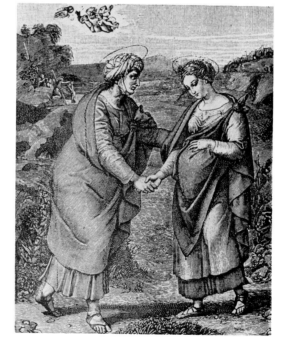

Fig. 2-28. The Visitation. Painting by Giulio Romano (real name Giulio Pippi) (1492–1546). This and other representations of Mary's visit to her cousin Elizabeth have been criticized by Biblical scholars for showing the Virgin with protruding abdomen; for, according to the text of St. Luke, Mary was then pregnant only a short time. Museum of Madrid.

58　ICONOGRAPHIA GYNIATRICA

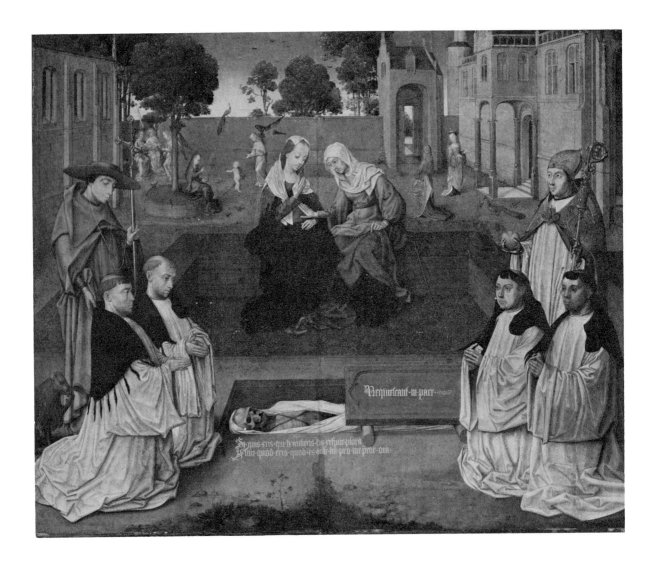

Fig. 2-29. *Spes Nostra*. Allegory on the vanity of human life. In the center, Elizabeth palpates the abdomen of the pregnant Virgin; in the foreground, priests kneel in prayer at man's grave; while in the background, Mary and Jesus play, angels sing, and on the wall is shown a peacock, symbol of resurrection. Rijksmuseum, Amsterdam.

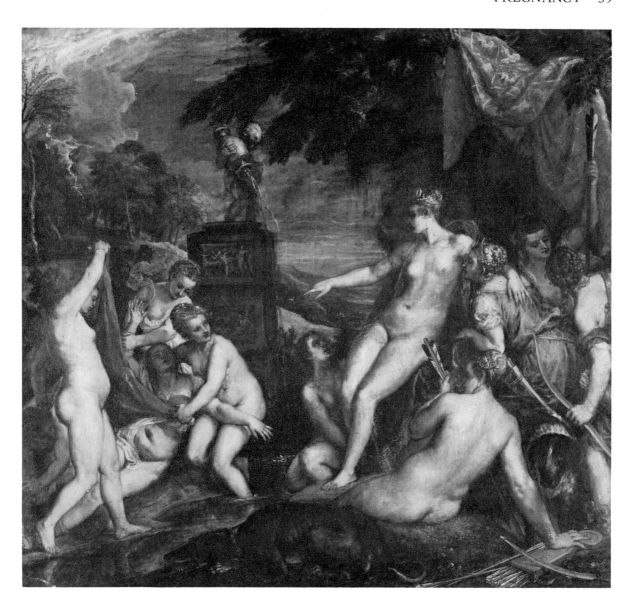

Fig. 2-30. Diana and Callisto. Painting by Tiziano Vecellio (1489?–1576), showing the discovery by Diana of Callisto's pregnancy. The pregnant nymph, left, reclines by the holy spring as her veil is torn from her.

According to ancient Greek legend, recounted later by Ovid, Callisto, the daughter of Lycaon, a king of Arcadia, became a follower of Diana, whom she accompanied in the hunt. Zeus fell in love with the maiden; but when Hera, his wife, learned of their tryst and of the ensuing birth of Arcas, the jealous goddess turned Callisto into a bear. When Arcas was full grown and out hunting, Hera brought before him Callisto in her ursine guise, intending that the lad, ignorant of his mother's identity, would shoot her. But the all-powerful Zeus snatched the bear away and established her among the stars, where she became known as Ursa Major, the Great Bear. Arcas, later placed beside her, was called Arcturus, the Lesser Bear. Still angered at her rival, Hera prevailed upon Poseidon, god of the sea, to forbid the Bears to enter the ocean, as did the other stars. Henceforth, the Greeks and Romans observed, the Bears alone, of all the constellations, never set below the horizon. (Only in the southern hemisphere is their setting to be seen.)

As a motif for the portrayal of pregnancy, the myth of Callisto found favor among classical artists, second only to the Visitation theme. National Gallery of Scotland.

60 ICONOGRAPHIA GYNIATRICA

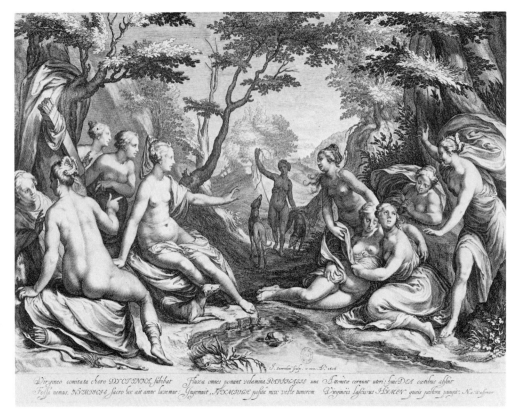

Fig. 2-31. Diana and Callisto. Engraving by Jan Pietersz Saenredam (1565–1607). The nymphs reveal Callisto's pregnancy to Diana. Bibliothèque Nationale, Paris.

MATERNITY GARB

The enlarging contours of woman's abdomen during pregnancy demand corresponding adaptations of her clothing. In all cultures the outer garments have typically been loose-fitting and draped. Underneath, from the time of the early Greeks and Romans, women have worn special girdles, binders, brassieres, and belts. In some societies these undergarments and devices were designed solely for their mechanical effect; in others, they were endowed with certain cultural values and even supernatural powers, as for protecting against the hazards of pregnancy and the injuries of labor.

The women of early Rome wore an abdominal binder in late pregnancy, beginning

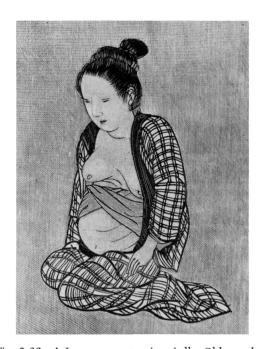

Fig. 2-32. A Japanese maternity girdle. Old woodcut.

usually in the eighth month, to expedite delivery. This Roman fashion had a persistent effect on European medicine into the Middle Ages; Ambroise Paré, for example, advocated the binder as late as the sixteenth century. Soranus of Ephesus (first and second centuries AD), on the other hand, restricted the binder to the earlier months of pregnancy, for uterine support, which he considered particularly important for active women. During the last two months Soranus permitted no binders, for he thought the weight of the unrestricted fetus would be more effective in hastening the birth process.

Similar counsel was proffered in the Orient. Chinese physicians prescribed binders to strengthen the loins of the pregnant woman and to help hold her body together. "And when it is undone," one wrote, "as it must be before confinement, then the abdomen expands and the fetus thus gets room to turn around." In nineteenth century Japan the midwife usually bound the expectant mother's abdomen tightly with a cloth, from about the fifth month of pregnancy until the onset of labor, to prevent excessive growth of the fetus. The women of Burma likewise wore a tight abdominal binder, from the seventh month, to minimize the ascent of the uterus. Thus, they reasoned, would the travel distance of the fetus be diminished, and the pain of labor correspondingly reduced.

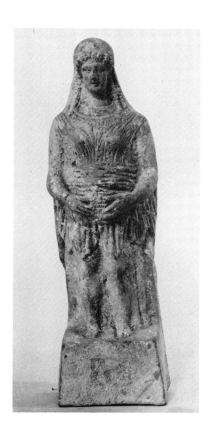

Fig. 2-33. Pregnant woman with abdominal binder. Hellenic terra cotta figure. National Archaeological Museum, Athens.

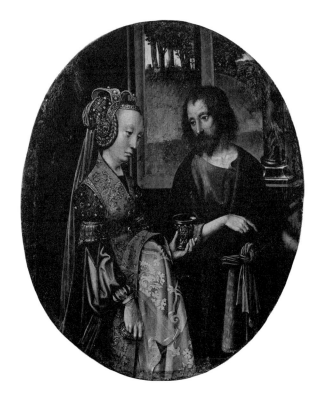

Fig. 2-34. Mary Magdalen, in maternity garb, with John the Baptist. By Cornelius Engelbrechtsen (1468–1533). Suermondt-Museum, Aachen, Germany.

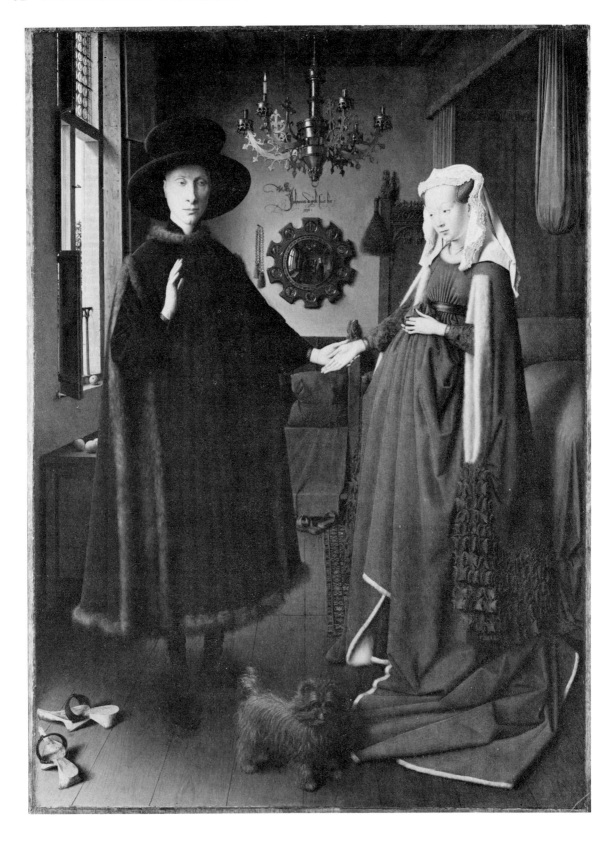

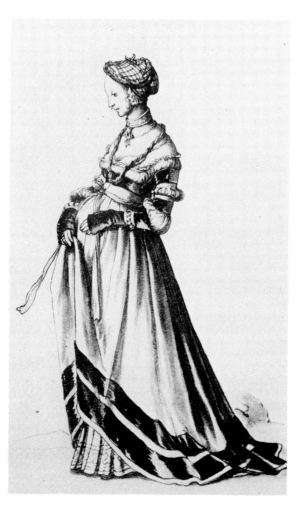

Fig. 2-36. A lady of Basel, Switzerland, in maternity dress. By Hans Holbein, the Younger (1497?–1543).

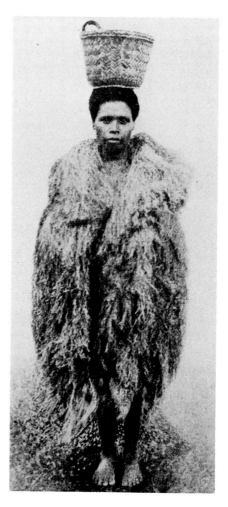

Fig. 2-37. Grass garment worn after childbirth by the women of Kiriwina, former name of the Trobriand Islands, in the Solomon Sea. The placenta was carried in a basket on the mother's head.

Fig. 2-35. Marriage portrait, 1434, Giovanni Arnolfini and his pregnant bride, Giovanna Cenami. By Jan van Eyck (1390?–1441). The Arnolfini marriage had already been consummated, in complete solitude, as was permitted at that time by canon law. Van Eyck was commissioned later to record the event. His painting served as the marriage documentary, he himself as the witness. On the wall, above the mirror, appears his signature, *Johannes de eyck fuit hic* ("Jan van Eyck was here"). Symbolizing faithfulness is the dog; purity, the mirror; the fruit in the left background, the fruit of the Garden of Eden; the carved figure on the chair, St. Margaret, patron saint of childbirth; the single burning candle, a wedding procession, an oath, and the all-seeing eye of God. The discarded pattens, in left foreground, recall the Biblical injunction, "Put off thy shoes from off thy feet, for the place whereon thou standest is holy ground." The National Gallery, London.

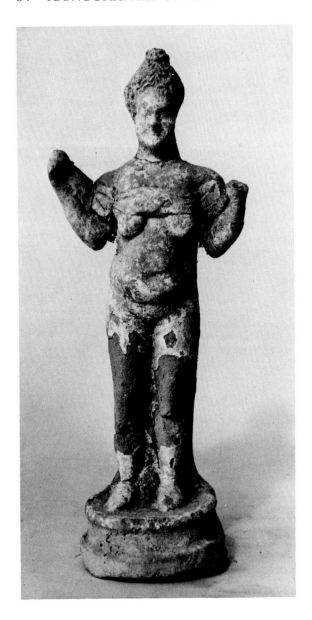

Fig. 2-38. Application of a breast binder. Terra cotta statuette from Tanagra, ancient city of central Greece. National Archaeological Museum, Athens.

Fig. 2-39. Nursing brassiere or breast binder, sixteenth century. From Scipione Mercurio's *La Comare*, Venice, 1596.

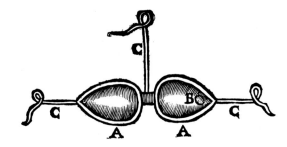

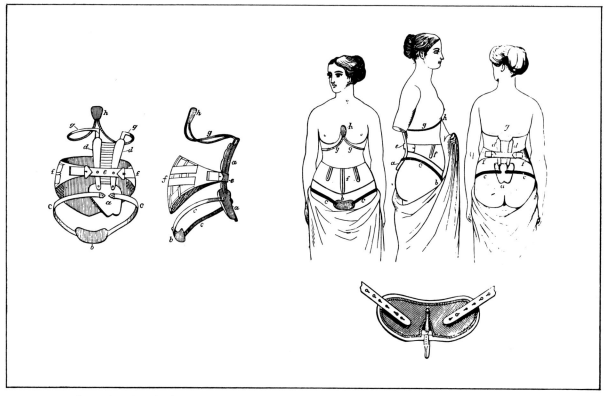

Fig. 2-40. The *pelvic band* of Dr. Protheroe Smith (1809–1889), designed as an aid to parturition. Smith explained, "A fixed point is secured for the exercise of mechanical force by means of, as it were, an artificial skeleton, the immobility of which is secured by two pads, one sacral, the other pubic, retained in their respective places by lateral springs, which embrace the pelvis below the cristae iliorum. . . . Then, a fixed point having been gained, attached to the sacral pad are two vertical levers, and one horizontal, the former . . . end each in a costal spring, embracing the thorax, and united by a sternal pad, so arranged as not to incommode the chest in respiration; the latter or horizontal is a powerful spring, buckled to a belt closely adjusted to the abdominal walls, and connected above to the costal springs and below to the pelvic band by elastic rings. It is thus constructed, so as to act in the manner of the abdominal muscles. During the parturient pains, this belt is readily tightened at will to assist, or supply the place of the voluntary muscular contractions, and is as readily relaxed in the interval of pains. When required, it may be made to maintain a steady uniform pressure, as is often needed *post partum*. This force, reacting upon the sacral pad, affords to the patient that support in the lumbar region which is so much called-for during labor . . ." [An aid to parturition and to the treatment of displacements of the uterus by a new mechanical appliance. *Brit. Med. J.* 2:580, 1896.]

66 ICONOGRAPHIA GYNIATRICA

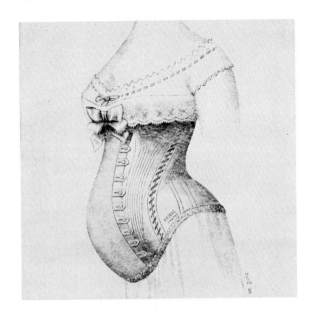

Fig. 2-41. Maternity girdle. French, late nineteenth century.

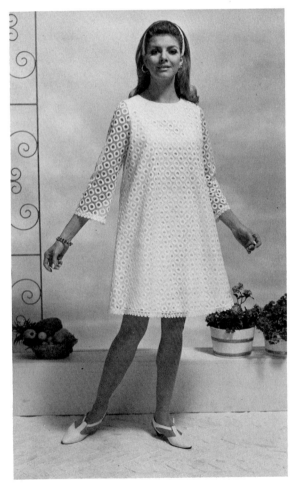
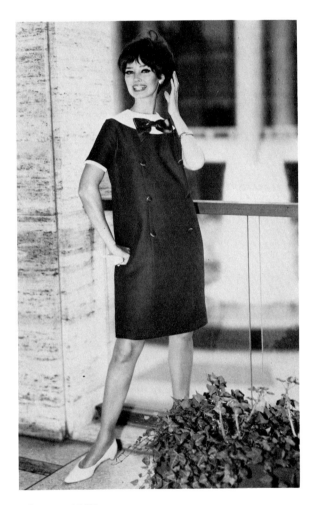

Fig. 2-42. Maternity dresses, 1967.

Chapter 3

THE MIDWIVES

As old as civilization is the history of midwifery. In every age and culture special attendants have proffered aid to the woman in labor, assuaging her pain, assisting her delivery, and tending her newborn. Reserved by tradition to females, the role of birth helper was known in English as *midwife* (with-woman), in French as *sage-femme* (wise woman), in German as *Hebamme* (lifting, relieving, or receiving nurse), in Spanish and Portugese as *comadre,* and in Latin as *cummater.* The view of Roderigo a Castro, expressed in 1594, was prevalent until the eighteenth century: *Haec ars viros dedecet* (This art is not suitable for men.) Physicians considered care of the parturient beneath their dignity.

The Bible records the part of the midwife in the second labor of Jacob's wife Rachel (Genesis 25:17) and in Tamar's delivery of twins (Genesis 38:28). When the Hebrews were enslaved in Egypt and their high birth rate threatened the security of the Pharaoh, he ordered the midwives to destroy all the male Hebrew infants at birth.

" 'When ye do the office of a midwife to the Hebrew women, and see them upon the stools; if it be a son, then ye shall kill him: but if it be a daughter, then she shall live.' But the midwives feared God, and did not as the king of Egypt commanded them, but saved the men children alive.... Therefore God

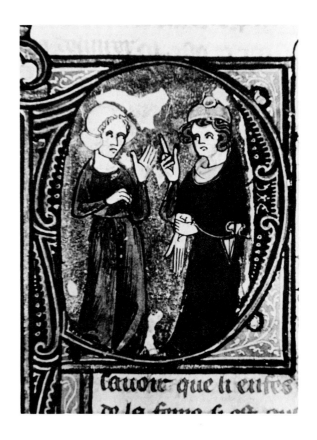

Fig. 3-1. Midwife, on left, receiving instructions from physician, on right. Miniature from a fourteenth century manuscript, *Régime du corps,* by Aldobrandin of Siena. Although physicians of this era often taught and supervised midwives, attendance in the birth chamber was restricted to the latter.

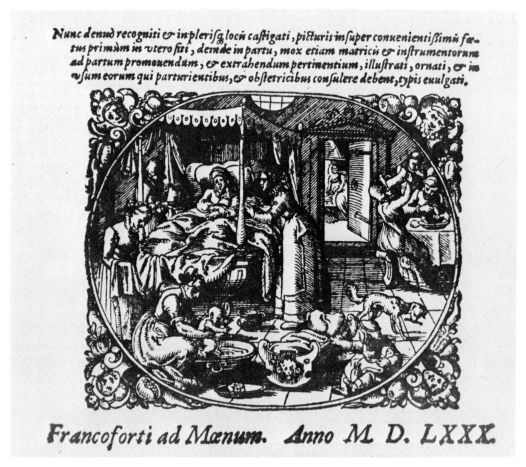

Fig. 3-2. A birth chamber, sixteenth century. From title page of Jacob Rueff's *De conceptu et generatione hominis,* Frankfurt, 1580. The midwife, at right, regales herself with a draught from her tankard.

dealt well with the midwives.... And it came to pass, because the midwives feared God, that he made them houses."

The recalcitrant Egyptian midwives Shiphrah and Puah explained, after balking at their ruler's decree that "the Hebrew women . . . are lively, and are delivered ere the midwives come unto them." (Exodus 1:15-21)

Most of these early self-styled specialists received no training; many were careless, dirty, and meddlesome. Their ethical standards were varied. At the fall of the Roman Empire, Eusebia, wife of the Emperor Constantius, being jealous of her fecund sister-in-law Helen, wife of Julian the Apostate, induced the midwife to murder Helen's child by allowing it to bleed from the umbilical cord.

Earliest of the male practitioners of obstetrics in Europe were the barber-surgeons, some of whom were trained by the midwives themselves. Subsequently known as man-midwives these men were widely ridiculed; their intrusion into an erstwhile forbidden domain was resented by many of their female counterparts. John Blunt (probably the pseudonym of S. W. Fores, a London bookseller) wrote,

"Such a man ought to be treated with as much indignity, as if he undertook to clear

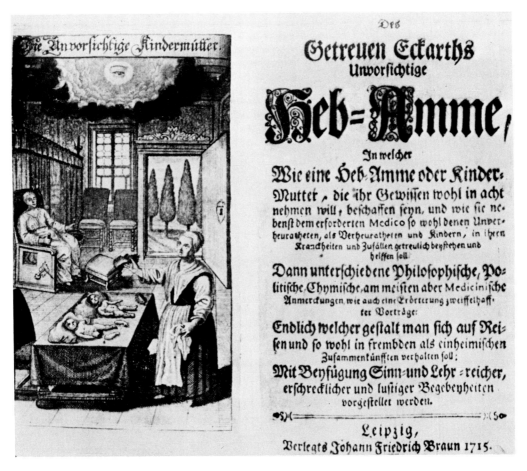

Fig. 3-3. Frontispiece from a German textbook for midwives, titled *Die Unvorsichtige Heb-Amme* (The Careless Midwife), by an unknown author writing under the pseudonym of Eckarth, published in Leipzig in 1715. The midwife stands before a table on which lie the mutilated bodies of two infants, an arm and leg shorn from one, the head from the other.

Explaining the scene, a poem begins,

See carelessness must lead here to the worst,
The midwife becomes a murderess of children,
This woman is crueler than Striges or Harpies,
And sacrifices many to Hecate.

She tears a piece from the uterus of the pregnant woman,
And even head, foot, and arms from her children.
The image of Lilith tortures the parturient
On her martyr's stool, and sends her to the grave.

But, continues the poem, the midwife will not go unpunished, for,

The eye of God has seen the evil deed,
Although the bodies are covered with earth,
A severe judgment will surely befall her,
Before which her brazen spirit quivers with fear and lamentation.

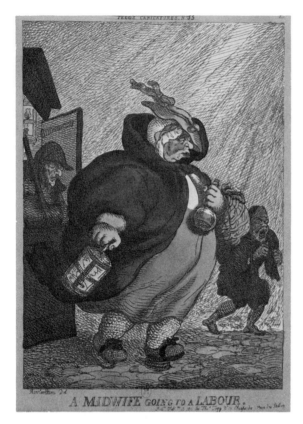

Fig. 3-4. "A Midwife Going to a Labour." A caricature, 1811, by Thomas Rowlandson (1756–1827). Wearing pattens to keep her shoes free of the mud through which she must wade, the midwife starts out with her traditional accouterments, lamp and flask. Thus were the midwives of the eighteenth and nineteenth centuries characterized:

Taking snuff, drinking gin and tea,
And the midwife's half-crown fee.

Charles Dickens, in his *Martin Chuzzlewit,* described the midwife, Mrs. Gamp, as,

"a fat old woman ... with a husky voice and a moist eye, which she had a remarkable power of turning up, and only showing the white of it.... She wore a very rusty black gown, rather the worse for snuff, and a shawl and bonnet to correspond.... The face of Mrs. Gamp—the nose in particular—was somewhat red and swollen, and it was difficult to enjoy her society without becoming conscious of a smell of spirits."

starch, hem a ruffle, or make a bed; yea, and with much greater; because in all these he is not called to handle the sacred parts of other men's wives ... man-midwifery is a personal, a domestic, and a national evil." [*Man-Midwifery Dissected,* London, 1793, pp. 62, 173.]

The French barber-surgeons who took up the practice of obstetrics were called *sage-femmes en culottes* (midwives in breeches). Most famous among them were Ambroise Paré (1510–1590), Jacques Guillemeau (1550–1609?), and François Mauriceau (1637–1709). Not until the middle of the eighteenth century were man-midwives accepted in England. Best known among them were James Douglas (1675–1742), his pupil William Hunter (1718–1783), and William Smellie (1697–1763).

Formal regulation of midwives was begun in England in the sixteenth century; but during this and the ensuing hundred years the main and often the sole qualification certified by the license was the good character of the recipient. Any reference to professional competence was usually limited to the length of the midwife's experience. "John Blunt" wrote in 1793 that "the principal business of a midwife in natural labors ... is only to press the palm of the left hand against the perinaeum during the birth ... " Only in complicated or neglected cases was a barber-surgeon summoned for help. Mutilation of both mother and child often followed.

Training for midwives was instituted by Hippocrates, in the fifth century BC, but for several centuries thereafter efforts to elevate their standards were sporadic and ineffectual. Self-taught or instructed by older midwives, most remained ignorant of the simple principles of obstetrics. The celebrated text of Soranus (AD 98–138), the leading Greek authority on obstetrics and gynecology during the reign of the emperors Trajan and Hadrian, was noteworthy as a guide for midwives. No significant contribution was made toward the education of midwives until 400 years later, when Eucharius Rösslin's *Rosengarten* appeared, a German language text, based in part on the early work of Soranus.

Regulation of midwives, by municipal or state examinations and formal licensure became increasingly widespread in Western Europe during the seventeenth century. The following *examen obstetricum,* given in Amsterdam in 1700, is representative:

1. Name the different parts of the uterus.
2. List the signs for diagnosis of pregnancy.
3. What signs permit the differentiation among a fetus, a mole, and an abortion?
4. How can one know that labor has begun?
5. What preparations must be made before labor?
6. How should the parturient be positioned during labor?
7. Describe the course of normal labor.
8. What measures are necessary if the fetus is in an abnormal position?
9. At what stage of labor should the woman be urged to bear down?
10. What should be done if the membranes do not rupture but a large amount of blood is expelled, resulting in loss of strength?
11. What should be done if the membranes rupture but delivery does not ensue?

Academic courses of instruction for student midwives were initiated in conjunction with European medical schools or hospitals during the first half of the eighteenth century—in Leiden in 1725, in Edinburgh in 1739, in Vienna in 1748. In France, a course for midwives was established in 1745 under the auspices of the Faculty of Medicine of Paris with Jean Astruc (1684–1766) as lec-

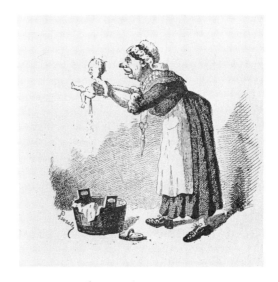

Fig. 3-5. *Sage-femme de Campagne* (Country Midwife). By the Parisian caricaturist and lithographer Lavrate (d. 1888). The umbilical cord shears hang from the midwife's neck.

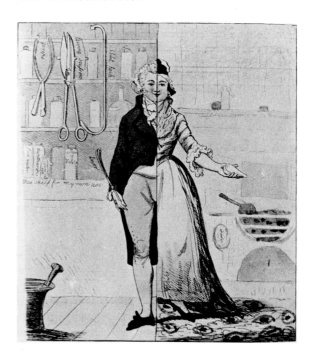

Fig. 3-6. "A Man-Mid-Wife, or a newly discovered animal, not known in Buffon's time." Frontispiece from *Man-Midwifery Dissected* by John Blunt, London, 1793. Shown in this caricature are the male midwife's instruments—the forceps, the *boring scissors,* and the blunt hook. Beneath them are vials of aphrodisiacs labeled "love water, cantharides, and cream of violets," with the subscript, "This shelf for my own use."

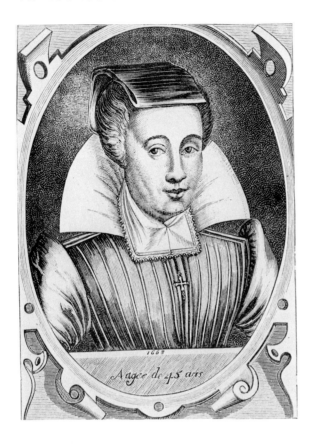

Fig. 3-7. Loyse Bourgeois Boursier (1563–1636). At age 45, from frontispiece to her textbook *Observations diverses sur la sterilité,* Paris, 1626 (ed. 1, 1609). Married to a barber-surgeon, Martin Boursier, Loyse Bourgeois became interested in the study of midwifery after the birth of her first child. After receiving instruction from her husband and his master, Ambroise Paré, she began practice among the poor of her neighborhood in Faubourg St. Germain; and after five years' experience, became a licensed midwife in Paris. She served as midwife to the French Court and royal family for 27 years, and delivered all the children of Marie de' Medici; but her glory came to an abrupt end in 1627 with the death from puerperal sepsis of the princess Marie de Bourbon-Montpensier.

turer. This inaugurated a new movement in French medicine which gathered momentum rapidly; and at the turn of the century a midwifery school was founded at the Maternité Hospital, which soon attracted young women from all parts of France to study there. In Germany, as in France, the training of midwives, as well as their licensure, was centrally controlled by the government.

Among the first midwives to migrate to Colonial America were Tryn Jansen and her daughter Anneke, who arrived in New Amsterdam in 1630, and Anne Hutchinson, who settled in Boston four years later. Supervision was haphazard, and although some midwives obtained licenses to practice, the unlicensed, unhampered by the authorities, were also permitted to ply their craft in most of the Colonies. Physicians in increasing number soon began to undertake the care of parturients, but the midwife remained in the ascendancy through the nineteenth century. As recently as 1909, New York's 3,000 midwives attended 40 per cent of the births in that city.

William Shippen (1736–1808) offered lectures to midwives, as well as medical students, in Philadelphia in 1765; and 52 years later, in 1817, Thomas Ewell, of Washington, D.C., appealed for voluntary contributions toward a lying-in hospital for the instruction of midwives. Without governmental support, however, all attempts to establish schools for midwives in America were frustrated by financial lack. Nearly all women who practiced midwifery did so out of economic necessity. Samuel Bard, in his *Compendium of the Theory and Practice of Midwifery* (1807), took note of their inability to afford even the standard textbooks.

At the end of World War I, the New York

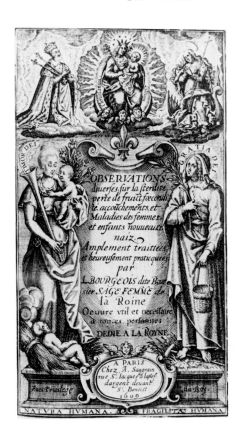

Fig. 3-8. Title page of Loyse Bourgeois' obstetric text. First published in Paris in 1609, subsequently translated into German and Dutch and widely quoted by English authors. Although obstetrics had been practiced exclusively by women, this was the first significant contribution to the obstetric literature by a female midwife. Loyse Bourgeois advocated the induction of premature labor for contracted pelvis and gave original descriptions of prolapsed umbilical cord and face presentation and their management.

Academy of Medicine's Public Health Relations Committee commented on the disturbing disparity between the city's maternal death rate, which had long remained stationary, and the progressively declining mortality from all other preventable causes. A subsequent study of the factors in 2,041 maternal deaths led to widespread reforms in obstetric practice throughout the nation. Sixty per cent of the preventable deaths were attributed to incapacity in the attendant: lack of judgment, lack of skill, or carelessness. The midwives, held up to the light of public scrutiny for the first time, were sharply criticized. Their numbers rapidly declined, from 1,197 in 1934, the year following the Committee's report, to 270 in 1939, to 2 in 1957. The last of New York's licensed midwives, having performed her final delivery in 1961, retired in 1963. In that year midwives attended but 0.3 per cent of the white births in the United States but still conducted a large part of the Negro deliveries in the South—41.1 per cent in Mississippi, 35.4 per cent in Alabama, and more than 20 per cent in Arkansas, South Carolina, and Georgia. Superseding this unlamented guild of quasi-professional accoucheuses, a new species of medically trained nurse-midwives is appearing on the American scene in increasing number, conducting hospital deliveries in cooperation with obstetric authorities.

Nurse-midwifery in the United States originated in New York in 1932 with the opening of the School of the Association for the Promotion and Standardization of Midwifery, which became part of the Maternity Center Association of New York three years later. High standards were established at the outset. A group of superior young women, most of

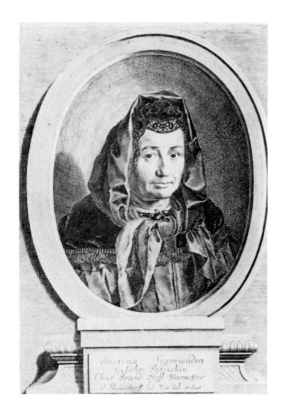

Fig. 3-9. Justine Dittrichin Siegemundin (1650–1705). Most famous of the German midwives, comparable in stature to the French Loyse Bourgeois, was Siegemundin, née Dittrichin, often referred to as *pious Justine* because of her frequent references to the Deity. Inscribed under her portait, on the frontispiece of her book, stand the lines:

An Gottes hilff und Segen
Geschickten Hand bewegen
Ist all mein Tuhn gelegen.

(My skillful hand and all my achievements are attributable to God's help and blessing.)

Recognizing her obstetric skill, which Siegemundin demonstrated as midwife to the city of Liegnitz, Friedrich III appointed her court midwife of Brandenburg, and in 1701 court midwife of Prussia. From the careful notes she kept of her cases, Siegemundin published in 1690 her *Die Chur-Brandenburgische Hoff-Wehe-Mutter*, an authoritative obstetric text in the form of a dialogue between two midwives, Justine (herself) and Christina (a pupil).

whom had already graduated from college, and many of whom held master's degrees were attracted to this school. Trained during the school's first two decades were 231 nurse-midwives. By March 1969 the American College of Nurse-Midwifery listed 711 members actively engaged in practice, education, or maternal and child health services, including instruction in family planning. These dedicated women continue to carry their teaching to all parts of the world, forming nuclei for the dissemination of higher obstetric standards wherever they go.

A questionnaire study of 174 countries, published in 1966 as a report of the International Confederation of Midwives, noted 600,000 midwives in 153 countries, covering 75 per cent of the world's population. Conspicuously lacking were data from mainland China, representing 23 per cent of the earth's people. A world total of 700,000 to 800,000 practicing midwives, professional and other, was estimated in 1966.

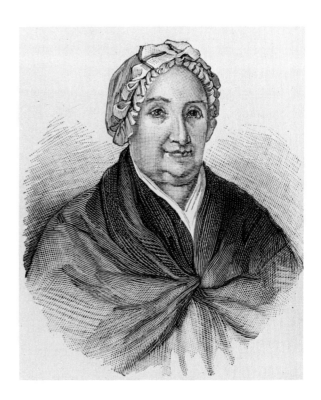

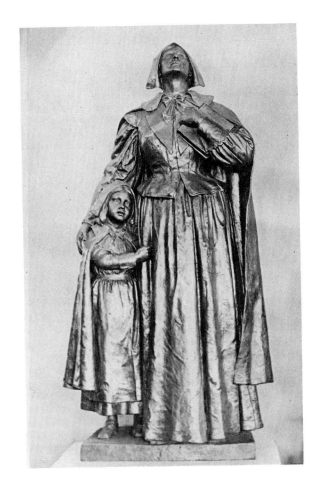

Fig. 3-11. Anne Hutchinson (1590?–1643). Statue by Cyrus E. Dallin before the General Court of Massachusetts, Boston. The most colorful and best remembered of Colonial American midwives Anne Hutchinson, a cousin of the English poet and dramatist John Dryden, emigrated from England to Boston with her husband in 1634. As a midwife she was said to be a "woman very helpful in the times of childbirth, and other occasions of bodily infirmities, and well furnished with means for those purposes." She also held religious meetings in her house where heretical views were often expressed. When one of her patients was delivered of an anencephalic monster, the neighbors' suspicions of the midwife were heightened; fear of witchcraft filled the air. Mrs. Hutchinson was summoned before the General Court of Massachusetts, excommunicated, and banished. In Rhode Island, her next home, she is said to have given birth to a hydatidiform mole. Soon she came into conflict with the Governor to whom she had been described as "of haughty and fierce carriage, of a nimble wit and active spirit and a very voluble tongue, more bold than a man, though in understanding and judgment inferior to many women." After the death of her husband, Mrs. Hutchinson moved to Long Island, then to Pelham or New Rochelle, New York, where she and all but one of her children were murdered in an Indian raid in 1643. Named for her is the Hutchinson River and its Parkway in New York's Westchester County.

Fig. 3-10. Elizabeth Nihell (1723–?). Most famous of the English midwives. Born in London, she was trained in midwifery at the Hôtel-Dieu in Paris. Mrs. Nihell is best known for her vituperative attacks upon the man-midwives, especially William Smellie, whose large hands she described as "the delicate fist of a great horse god-mother of a he-midwife." Smellie's disciples she referred to as,

"broken barbers, tailors, or even pork butchers... who, after passing half his life in stuffing sausages, is turned an intrepid physician and man-midwife... and what are those arms by which they maintain themselves, but those instruments, those weapons of death!"

In response to her letters attacking man-midwives came the angry retort from "Old Chiron":

"Midwives cram their patients with cordials, keeping them intoxicated during the time they are in labour, driving poor women up and down stairs, notwithstanding their shrieks, and shaking them so violently as often to bring on convulsion fits on pretence of hastening their labours, laughing at their cries, and breaking wretched jests upon the contortions of the women, whose torments would make a feeling man shudder at the sight."

The obstetric forceps Mrs. Nihell recognized as the principal threat to the midwives, for instruments were restricted to surgeons, exclusively male. Indeed, few women possessed the strength to use the forceps effectively in obstructed labor. She died at about age 50. Her book, *A Treatise on the Art of Midwifery,* London, 1760, is believed to have been written by her husband.

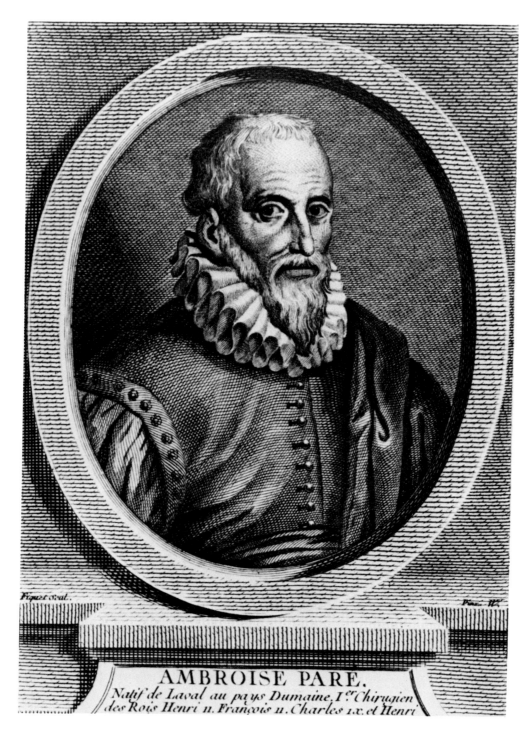

Fig. 3-12. Ambroise Paré (1510–1590). French barber-surgeon and most famous of the early man-midwives. Engraving by Etienne Ficquet (1719–1794) after a portrait by "W." He reintroduced the operation of podalic version which had been practiced centuries earlier but long since neglected or forgotten, recommended cesarean section on the living in addition to the dead or dying parturient, and helped achieve for obstetrics a new dignity. National Library of Medicine, Bethesda, Maryland.

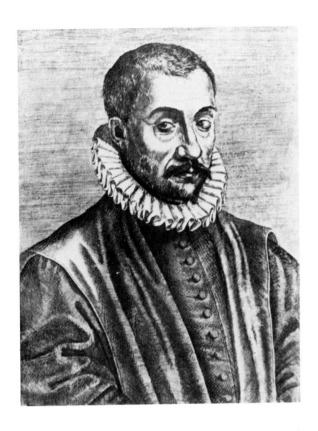

Fig. 3-13. Jacques Guillemeau (1550–1609?). Distinguished French accoucheur. Engraving by Antoine Vallée, 1585. From Paré, Guillemeau learned the technique of podalic version which he introduced as a method of treatment for placenta previa. His textbook *De la grossesse et accouchement des femmes* "corrected and enlarged by Charles Guillemeau," his son, and published in 1621, described a technique for delivery of the aftercoming head in breech presentation.

"... Turn the body of the infant upside down gently, placing it face downward.... Working the head loose by moving it up and down in this situation, and holding the infant with one hand, and with the index finger of the other hand placed in the infant's mouth, it will be easy to extract [the head] with the body."

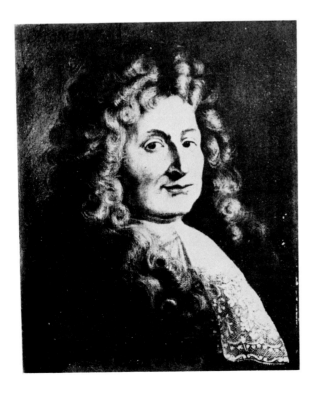

Fig. 3-14. François Mauriceau (1637–1709). French barber-surgeon, who became the dominant figure in obstetrics of the seventeenth century. His textbook *Traité des maladies des femmes grosses, et de celles qui sont accouchées,* 1668, which was translated into English, German, Dutch, Italian, Latin, and Flemish, helped establish obstetrics as a speciality. Mauriceau advocated antisyphilitic treatment during pregnancy, amniotomy for placenta previa, primary suture of perineal lacerations, and popularized a method of delivering the aftercoming head earlier described by Jacques Guillemeau, subsequently referred to as the *Mauriceau maneuver.*

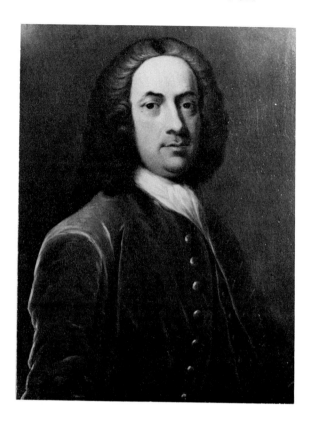

Fig. 3-15. William Smellie (1697–1763). Often called *the master of British midwifery,* and named by Fasbender, the distinguished obstetric historian, as "one of the most important obstetricians of all times and countries." Smellie gave a lucid description of the mechanism of labor, measured the diagonal conjugate of the pelvis, invented a number of obstetric instruments, produced a beautiful and accurate atlas of obstetric figures (*A Sett of Anatomical Tables,* London, 1754), and an excellent three volume obstetric text (*A Treatise on the Theory and Practice of Midwifery,* London, 1752–1764). Royal College of Surgeons of Edinburgh.

Chapter 4

BIRTH SCENES

From the crude cave drawings of the ice age to the elaborate sculpture and delicate detail of the Renaissance, man has used every medium of art to represent birth. Revealed in birth scenes, in addition to the obstetric techniques of the era, the roles of the attendants, delivery postures, and the accouterments of the birth chamber, are contemporary cultural concepts of the diety, of royalty, and of life and death.

In almost all early birth scenes the attendants are depicted as women. Males were usually barred from the birth chamber. Not until the eighteenth century did men begin to achieve recognition as accoucheurs. In most birth scenes the midwife stands, sits, or kneels

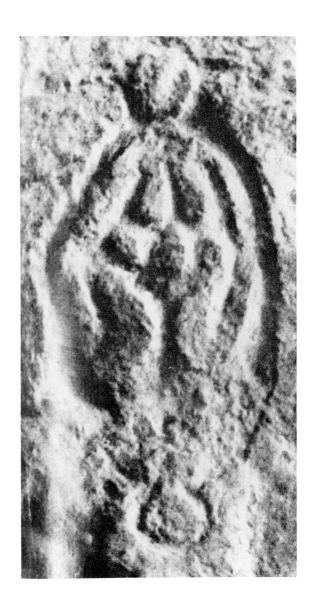

Fig. 4-1. Ice Age illustration of a birth. Bas-relief, 21 cm high, recovered in 1911 among the relics from the latter part of the Ice Age, on a cliff at Laussel, Dordogne, France. Excavations in this region, sometimes called *the cradle of prehistory,* have produced evidence of a succession of industrious peoples who thrived there despite the rigors of a subarctic environment, living in caves and subsisting mainly on caribou, over a span of 17,000 years, from about 32,000 to 15,000 BC. The woman is holding her flexed legs, against which she presses her abdomen, to aid her efforts to expel the child, whose head and shoulders have already been born. This figure is believed to be the earliest known representation of a birth scene.

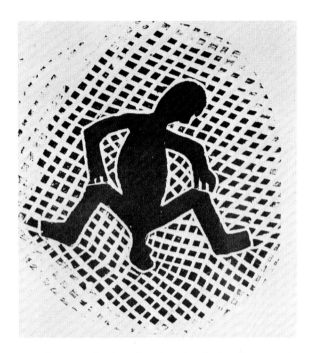

Fig. 4-2. Crude clay drawing simulating the preceding scene. From the Gold Coast of Africa, 1899 AD, showing a woman giving birth in the squatting position, her hands grasping or pressing against her thighs or knees, the infant's head protruding from her vulva. Staaliches Museum für Völkerkunde, Munich.

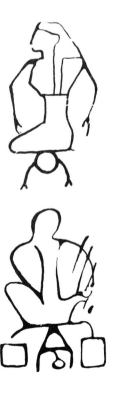

before the parturient, while one or more additional attendants lend support from behind. In primitive societies the parturient usually assumed one of several positions to enhance her expulsive efforts, which were often augmented by abdominal pressure applied manually by the attendants. After delivery, while the newborn was being bathed and swaddled, food and drink were brought to the mother; but flowers never were to be seen in the parturient's room.

Although the head of the newborn measures about one fourth of its body length, in most of the early birth scenes the infant is shown as a miniature adult, without regard for the true proportions of head to body. By the latter half of the fifteenth century the great artists had begun to paint the infant Jesus in the correct proportions of a human newborn, but not until the end of the seventeenth century did medical illustrations reflect a cognizance of the changing relations of head to trunk with growth of the infant.

The scenes that follow have been grouped to show (1) births in various ages and cultures, (2) births of Biblical and religious characters, (3) royal births, (4) births in legend, (5) birth as a source of joy and grief, and (6) the puerperium.

Fig. 4-3. Egyptian hieroglyphs meaning "to give birth." In the upper, the infant is being born by the vertex; in the lower, by the breech. In both, delivery is accomplished with the mother in the squatting position.

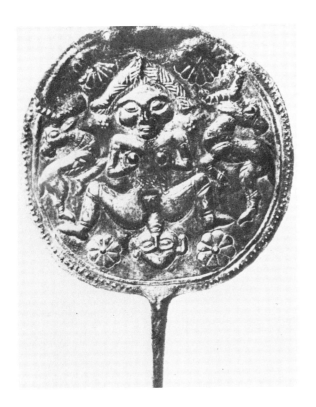

Fig. 4-4. Birth scene showing squatting mother, flanked by animals, and head of infant already born. Head of silver pin from Luristan, mountainous province of western Iran, first millennium BC. Thames & Hudson Archive, London.

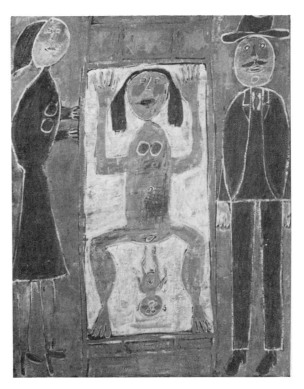

Fig. 4-5. *L'Accouchement*. Childbirth, 1944, by Jean Dubuffet (1901–   ), oil on canvas. Interpreted by Peter Selz, "This painting captures the naïveté of votive pictures; it is like those thank offerings found in pilgrimage churches and presents a comparable aspect of ritual, of 'emotion recollected in tranquility.'" Pierre Matisse Gallery, New York.

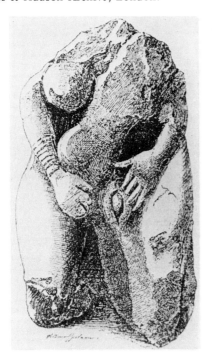

Fig. 4-6. Early birth scene. Remains of stone figure recovered in Ripač, Bosnia. The parturient is shown kneeling, her vulva distended by the infant's presenting part; behind and to the right the midwife also kneels, assisting in the delivery.

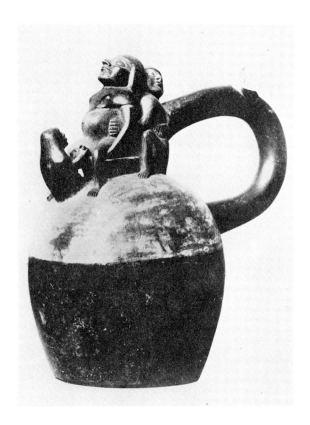

Fig. 4-7. Yuncan birth scene. Pre-Columbian stirrup-spout vase or funeral urn from the northern coast of Peru. In the top of the handle is an aperture. Two midwives assist delivery: one, sitting behind the parturient, presses her abdomen; the second, kneeling between the mother's legs, holds the infant's emerging head. Museum für Völkerkunde, West Berlin.

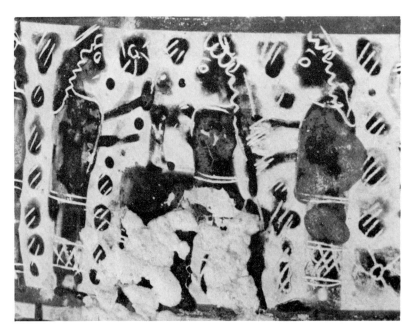

Fig. 4-8. Birth scene. Corinthian vase. The parturient, seated on the obstetric stool, receives the newborn infant into her arms from the midwife. Bibliothèque Nationale, Paris.

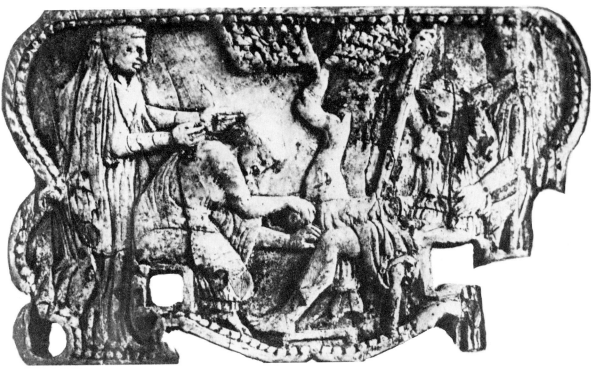

Fig. 4-9. Birth scene. Ancient ivory carving from Pompeii. The parturient, leaning against an attendant who stands behind her, supports herself with a staff in her right hand, grasps the attendant's shoulder with her left. Seated before the mother, the midwife, sponge in hand, assists the delivery of the emerging infant. Behind the midwife stands a priest or matron, with outstretched arms, either giving a benediction or waiting to receive the newborn. Museo Nazionale, Naples.

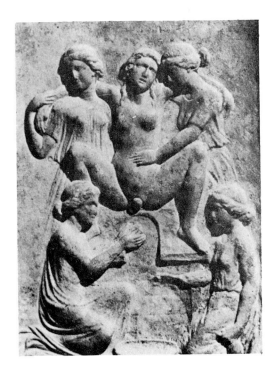

Fig. 4-10. Birth scene. Early Greek relief. The nude parturient is supported on either side by attendants, one of whom presses against her uterus; while the midwife and another assistant, kneeling before the birthstool, await the infant, whose head is presenting through the vulva.

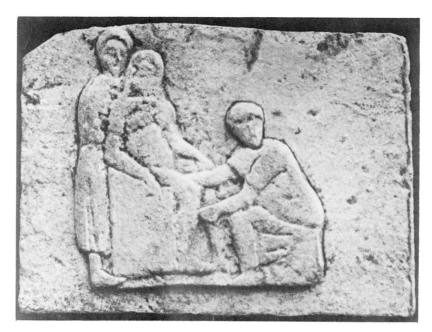

Fig. 4-11. Birth scene. Bas-relief, recovered near Rome in 1932. Seated on a birthstool is the nude parturient, supported from behind by an attendant, who presses over the uterus with her right hand. The midwife, on a small stool before the parturient, controls the infant's egress.

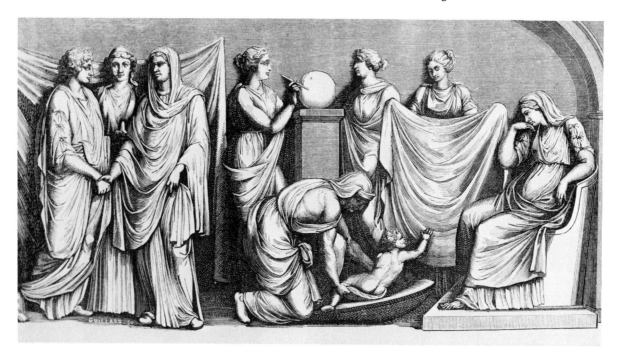

Fig. 4-12. Roman marble bas-relief depicting marriage and birth. On the left stands Juno, between bride and groom, presiding at their marriage. On the right, seated on the birthstool, the young mother regards her newborn babe being placed in, or taken from, a basin by the midwife; while an aide waits with open towel or wrapping to receive the infant. Two other women stand by a column supporting a globe on which one is inscribing the date and hour of birth which the Romans recorded with great precision.

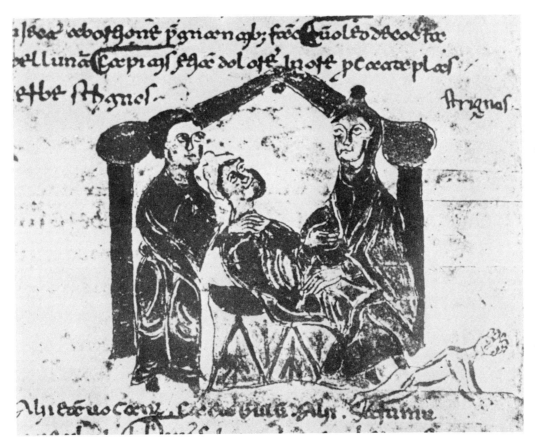

Fig. 4-13. Birth scene. Miniature from a twelfth century Cassinese manuscript. The woman has just given birth on a small table, attended by a man standing behind her and supporting her shoulders, and the midwife standing at her side. The newborn infant on the floor appears to be doing a push-up. Biblioteca Nazionale, Turin, Italy.

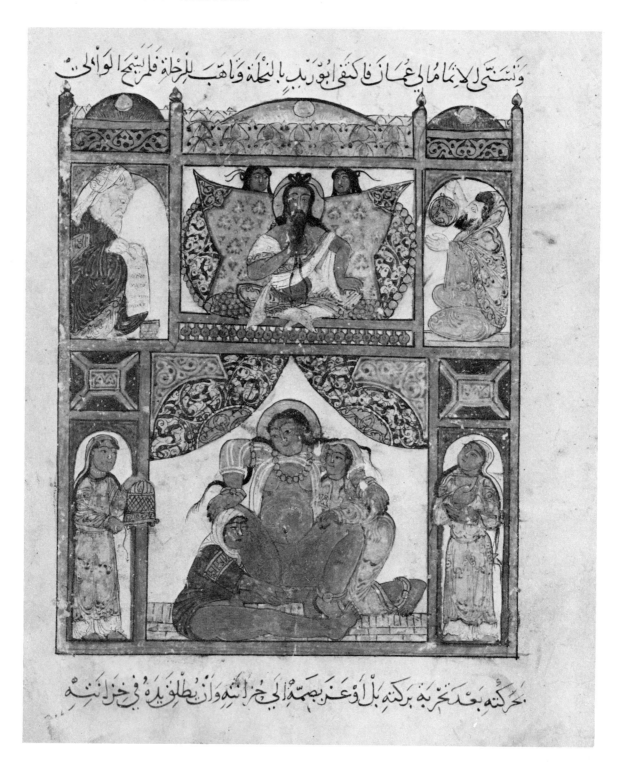

Fig. 4-14. Arabic birth scene. Early thirteenth century Baghdad miniature by Al-Wasiti from the 1237 manuscript *Maqamat* of Abu Mohammed al-Kisim al-Hariri (or Harizi). At upper left a scribe records the time of birth; at upper right an astrologer reads the horoscope of the newborn infant. Bibliothèque Nationale, Paris.

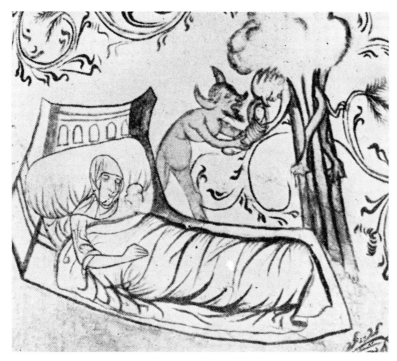

Fig. 4-15. Medieval Danish birth scene. Chalk drawing from Undløse (or Ondløse), on the island of Zealand. The devil, in the background, is about to exchange the newborn infant for another. Danish National Museum, Copenhagen.

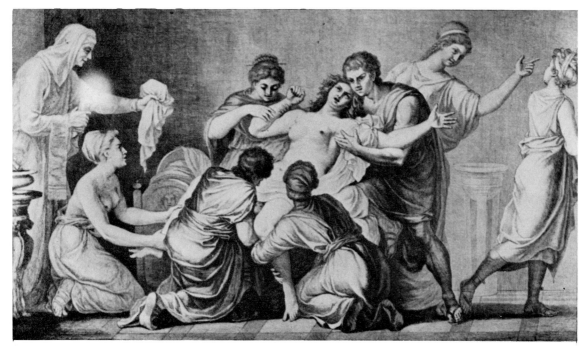

Fig. 4-16. Birth scene. Ancient Greece, painting and engraving by Esprit-Antoine Gibelin (1739–1813). The semi-recumbent parturient is supported from behind by a man, and her legs are held apart by two female attendants, as the midwife performs the delivery.

88 ICONOGRAPHIA GYNIATRICA

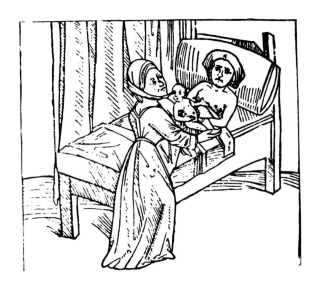

Fig. 4-17. Birth scene. Fifteenth century Germany, woodcut from Johannes Lichtenberger's *Prognasticatio in Latino,* Strassburg, 1488. The parturient lies on a wooden bed, her head and shoulders supported by a bolster. The midwife, in characteristic garb, stands at the foot of the bed holding the newborn.

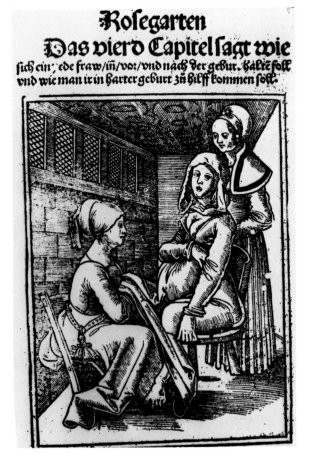

Fig. 4-18. Birth scene. From Eucharius Rösslin's *Rosengarten,* 1513. The parturient on the birthstool is supported by a female attendant while the midwife, seated in front, conducts the delivery under the folds of her subject's dress.

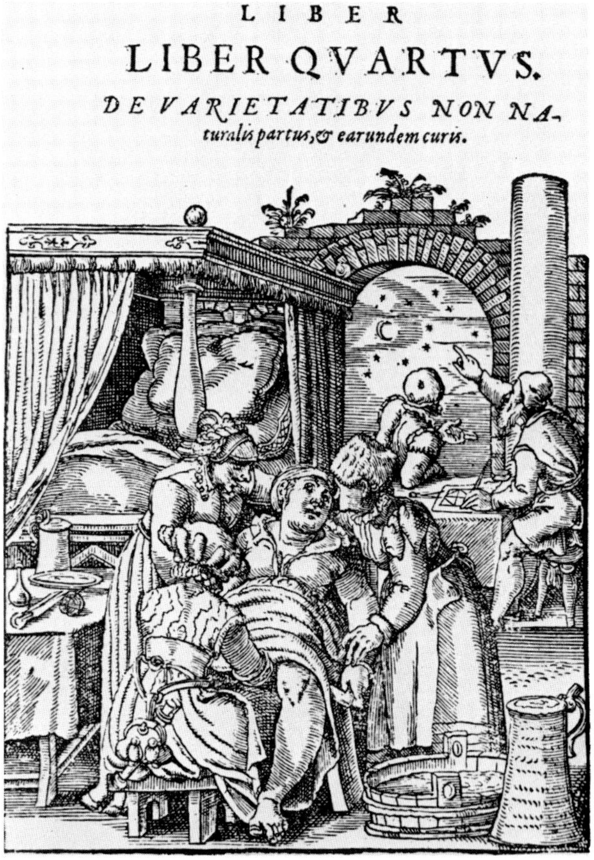

Fig. 4-19. Birth scene. From Jacob Rueff's *De conceptu et generatione hominis,* Frankfort am Main, 1580. The parturient on the birthstool is flanked by female attendants as the midwife performs the delivery. On the left before the patient's canopy bed, the table is set for the postpartum repast, in the right foreground the pitcher and the tub for the newborn's bath, in the background an astrologer studies the stars to foretell the infant's future.

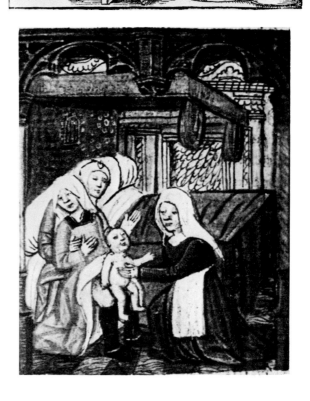

Fig. 4-20. French birth scene. Early sixteenth century, from Guillaume Alexis' *Passe-temps de tout homme,* Paris, 1505. The parturient, supported by an attendant, is seated on the birthstool beside her canopy bed; the kneeling midwife holds the newborn infant.

90 ICONOGRAPHIA GYNIATRICA

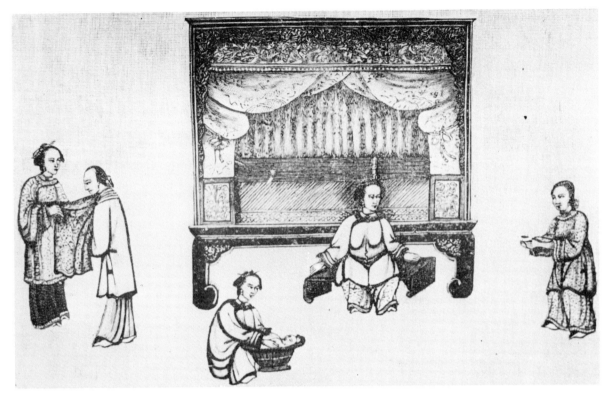

Fig. 4-21. Chinese birth scene. The parturient, recently delivered and still seated on the birthstool, is about to be served refreshment by the attendant at right. The newborn infant, being bathed in the foreground, is about to be wrapped in the cloth held by the two women at left.

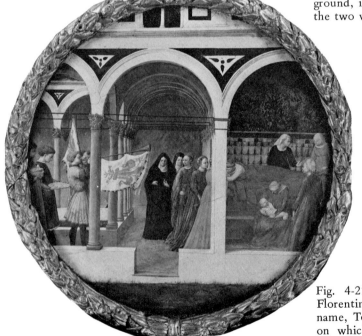

Fig. 4-22. Birth chamber of a fifteenth century Florentine lady. *Desco da parto* by Masaccio (real name, Tommaso Guidi, 1401–1428), a painted disc on which presents and food were brought to the parturient. Staatliche Museen Gemäldegalarie, Berlin-Dahlem.

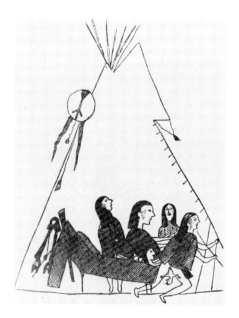

Fig. 4-23. Birth in a tepee. Kiowa Indians of Texas, native drawing, mid nineteenth century.

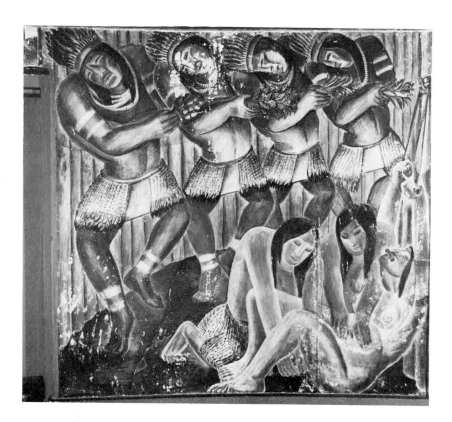

Fig. 4-24. California Indian birth scene. Mural by Bernard Borouch Zakheim (1898–   ), one of a series, 1937, symbolizing the early history of medicine in California. Assisting at a difficult birth are two squaws, one pressing on the mother's abdomen, the other delivering the infant, while the parturient pulls on ropes overhead to augment her expulsive efforts. In the background four men holding herbs perform a ceremonial dance. University of California Medical Center, San Francisco.

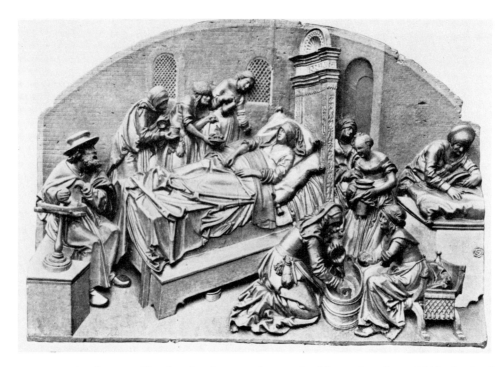

Fig. 4-25. A German birth scene. Woodcarving by an unknown Swabian artist, about 1510. At the foot of the parturient's bed sits an astrologer.

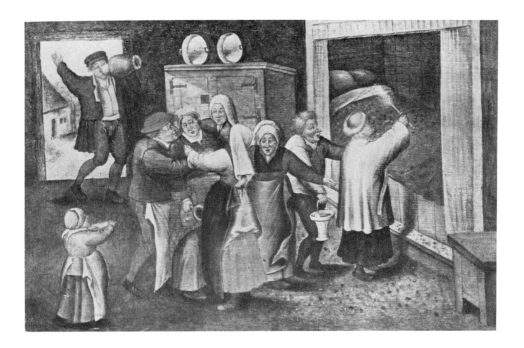

Fig. 4-26. A priest blesses the birth. Humorous painting by the Belgian artist Pieter Brueghel, the Elder (c. 1530–1569). The clergyman besprinkles the bed with holy water in anticipation of the blessed event, while the parturient's husband and several women, all drunk, struggle to help the laboring woman, jug in hand, to her bed.

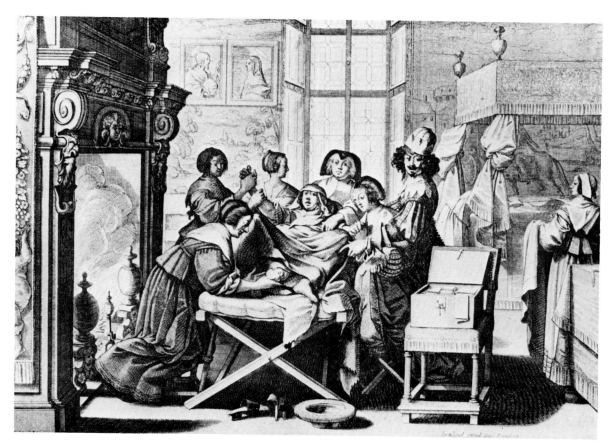

Fig. 4-27. Birth scene. Home of a French patrician, seventeenth century, during the reign of Louis XIII. Etching by Abraham Bosse (1602–1676), made in Paris, 1633. The birth table, surrounded by family and attendants, has been placed before the blazing hearth. *Dramatis personae:* the mother, the midwife, the husband, and the friend of the family (devout woman). Each recites a quatrain, engraved in French below the picture.

The mother: "Alas, I can do no more; the pain possesses me, enfeebling all my senses; my body is dying, and there is no remedy for the pangs I feel."

The midwife: "Madame, have patience, do not cry out so; soon it will all be over; by my faith, you will be delivered of a fine son."

The husband: "That news comforts me; all my grief has vanished; carry on, dear heart, have courage, your pain will soon be gone."

The devout woman: "From this painful effort, so unlike any other torment, deliver her, oh Lord, and be of help in her childbirth."

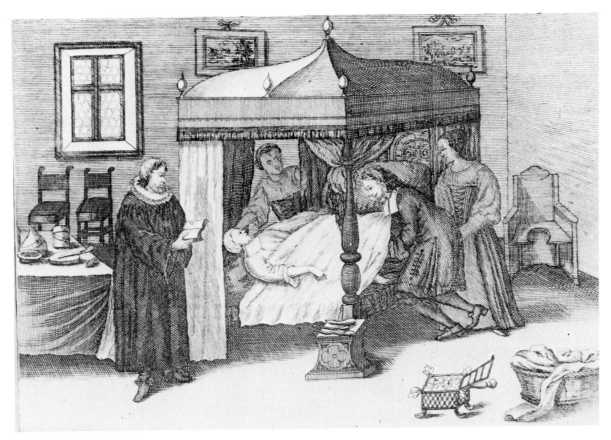

Fig. 4-28. Delivery of a dead infant. Early eighteenth century illustration from C. Völter's textbook for midwives, *Neueröffnete Hebammenschule,* Stuttgart, 1722, Chapter 10, entitled "How a dead fetus should be delivered, with skill, to preserve the life of the mother." For this difficult delivery, a physician or man-midwife has been engaged, the parturient placed on her bed in lieu of the birth-chair which is seen in the right background, and a priest summoned.

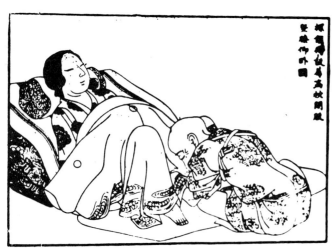

Fig. 4-29. Japanese birth scene. Nineteenth century, the obstetrician operating under the sheet, from Yoshihiro Mizuhara's atlas *Sanka zushiki,* 1837.

BIRTH SCENES 95

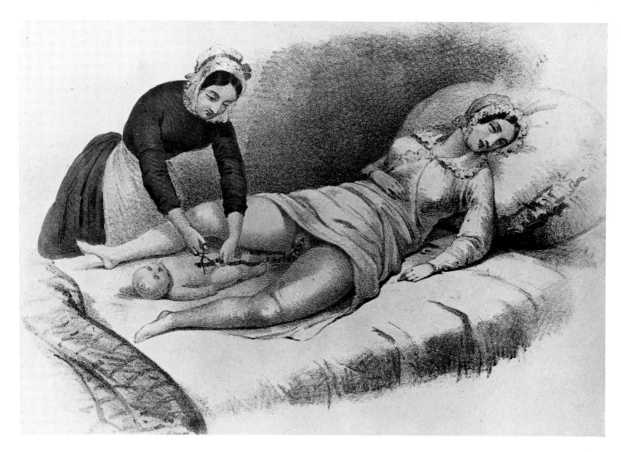

Fig. 4-30. American birth scene. Mid eighteenth century, from W. Beach, *Improved System of Midwifery*, 1848.

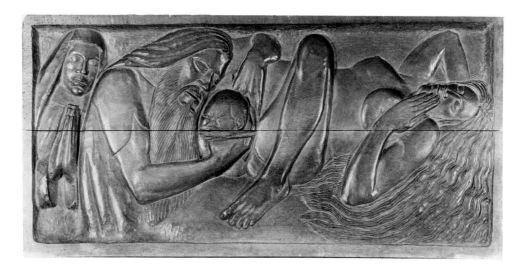

Fig. 4-31. *La Naissance de l'Homme* (The Birth of Man). Woodcarving on bed panel by Georges Lacombe (d. 1916).

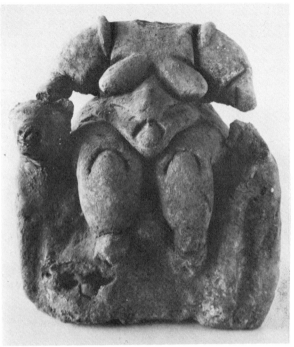
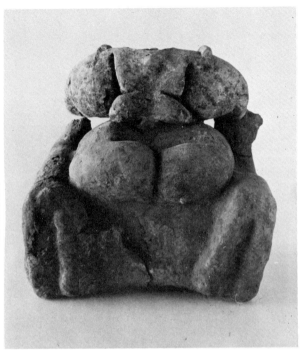

Fig. 4-32. Goddess giving birth. Clay statue, about 8 inches tall, excavated by James Mellaart in 1961 from the ruins of Çatal Hüyük, a neolithic city of about 7000-5000 BC, on the Anatolian plateau of Turkey.

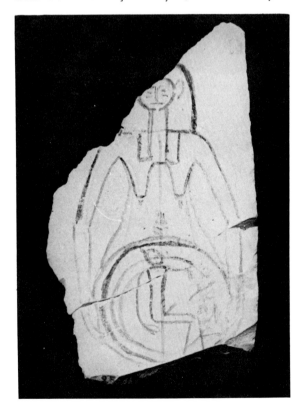

Fig. 4-33. Goddess giving birth to the sun. Ancient Egyptian drawing. Egyptian Museum, Cairo.

Fig. 4-35. Queen Ahmes giving birth to the sun, with the help of two divinities with bovine heads. Votive bas-relief of the Ptolmaic era (323–30 BC) recovered from Dendera, an ancient city of Upper Egypt. Egyptian Museum, Cairo.

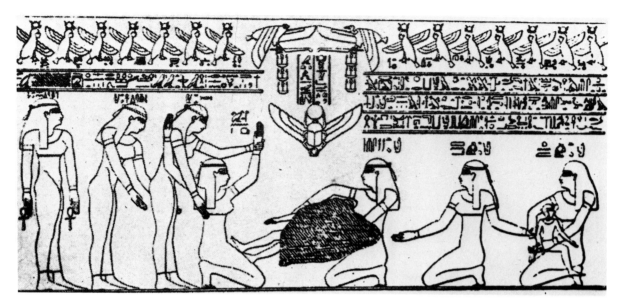

Fig. 4-34. The birth of Re. Drawing of an ancient Egyptian relief which no longer exists. The parturient goddess Ritho, kneeling at left of center, is supported from behind by a midwife, while another of three midwives, kneeling before the goddess, receives the infant Re, Egyptian god of the sun. Amhotep IV, who reigned in the fourteenth century BC, regarded Re as the only god who ruled over the whole world. Worship of Re during this era is considered by some as the beginning of monotheism in the Near East.

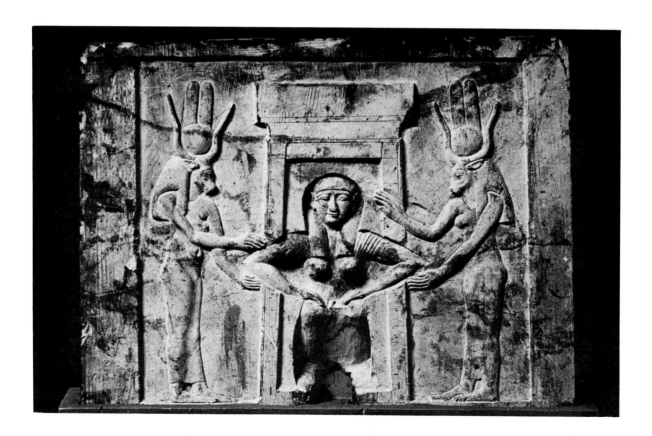

98　ICONOGRAPHIA GYNIATRICA

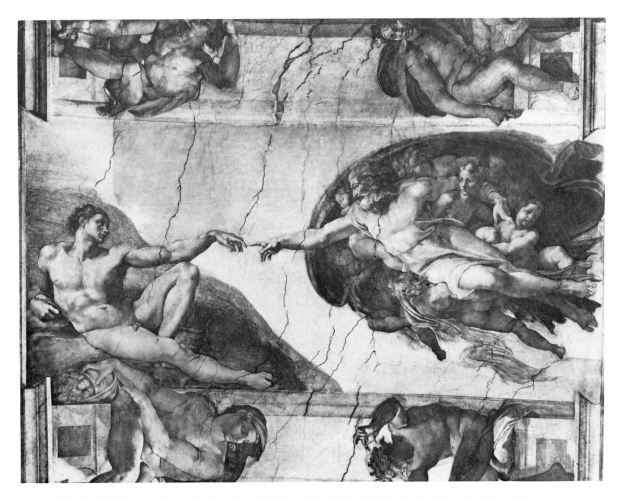

Fig. 4-36. The creation of Adam. By Michelangelo (1475–1564). Sistine Chapel ceiling, Vatican.

THE CREATION OF MAN

"And God said, Let us make man in our image, after our likeness: and let them have dominion over the fish of the sea, and over the fowl of the air, and over the cattle, and over all the earth, and over every creeping thing that creepeth upon the earth. So God created man in his own image, in the image of God created he him; male and female created he them." [Genesis 1:26-27]

"And the Lord God said, It is not good that the man should be alone; I will make him an help meet for him.... And the Lord God caused a deep sleep to fall upon Adam, and he slept: and he took one of his ribs, and closed up the flesh instead thereof. And the rib, which the Lord God had taken from man, made he a woman, and brought her unto the man. And Adam said, This is now bone of my bones, and flesh of my flesh: she shall be called Woman, because she was taken out of Man." [Genesis 2:18, 21-23]

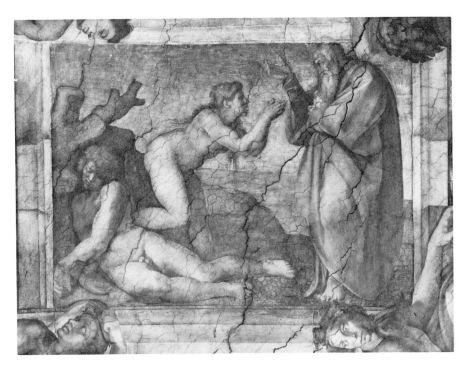

Fig. 4-37. The creation of Eve. By Michelangelo (1475–1564). Sistine Chapel ceiling, Vatican.

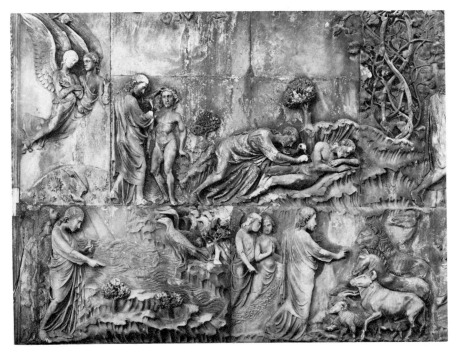

Fig. 4-38. The creation of man and of the world. Relief, probably by Lorenzo Maitani (c. 1275–1330), under whose direction the cathedral at Orvieto was built. God, on left, holds a hand over Adam's head and gazes intently at him, perhaps for hypnosis. At right, God cuts a rib from sleeping Adam. This fantasy was ascribed at one time, probably erroneously, to Giovanni Pisano (1245–1320?). Cathedral at Orvieto, Italy.

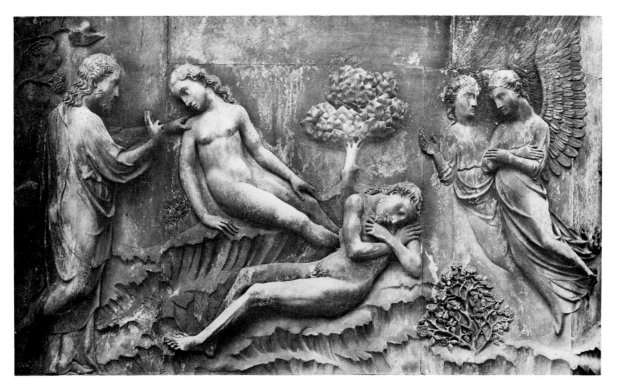

Fig. 4-39. The creation of Eve. Relief by Lorenzo Maitani (c. 1275–1330). Holding Eve by the right shoulder, God extracts her from Adam's side. Cathedral at Orvieto, Italy.

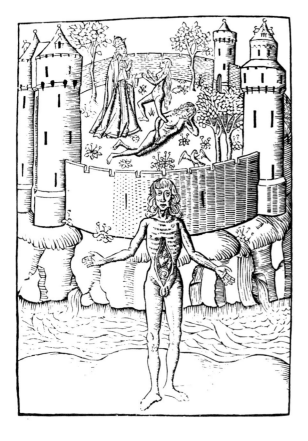

Fig. 4-40. The creation of Eve and the structure of man. From B. Glanvil's *Incipit prohemium de proprietatibus rerum fratris Bartholomei Anglici,* Haarlem, 1485. God, above in royal garb, receives Eve as she emerges from the side of sleeping Adam.

BIRTH SCENES 101

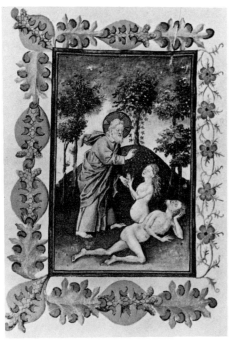

Fig. 4-41. The creation of Eve. Miniature by an unidentified Dutch master of the fifteenth century, in the *Book of Hours* produced for Catherine of Cleves on the occasion of her marriage to the Duke of Guelders.

Fig. 4-42. The creation of Eve. Painting by an unknown French artist of the early sixteenth century. In the background in the Garden of Eden, the snake looks from the apple tree as Eve hands Adam the forbidden fruit. Musée Royaux des Beaux-Arts de Belgique, Brussels.

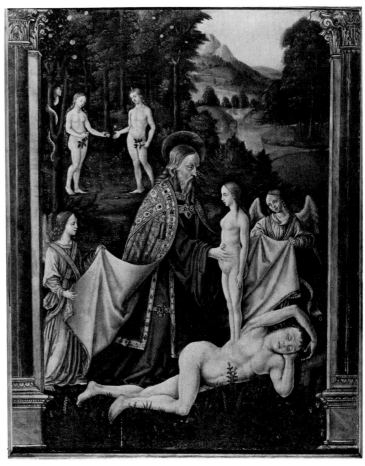

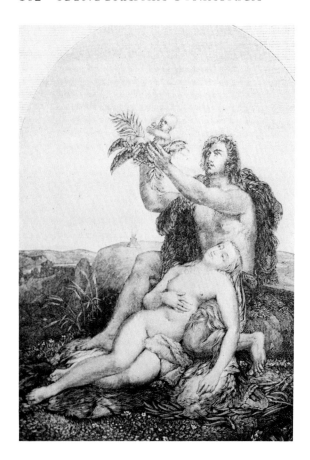

Fig. 4-43. "And Adam knew Eve his wife; and she conceived, and bare Cain, and said, I have gotten a man from the Lord." (Genesis 4:1) The first birth. By Theophile Auguste Vauchelet (1802–1873). Adam holds aloft newborn Cain. Critics have called attention to Eve's umbilicus.

THE BIRTH OF MARY

"And, behold, an angel of the Lord came to her and said: 'Anna, Anna, the Lord has heard your prayer. You shall conceive and bear, and your offspring shall be spoken of in the whole world.' And Anna said: 'As the Lord my God lives, if I bear a child, whether male or female, I will bring it as a gift to the Lord my God, and it shall serve him all the days of its life.'

... And her six months [her months] were fulfilled, as (the angel) had said: in the seventh [ninth] month Anna brought forth. And she said to the midwife: 'What have I brought forth?' And she said: 'A female.' And Anna said: 'My soul is magnified this day.' And she lay down. And when the days were fulfilled, Anna purified herself from her childbed and gave suck to the child, and called her Mary." [The postevangelium of James, in *New Testament Apocrypha,* W. Schneemelcher, ed., English trans. ed. by R. McL. Wilson. Westminster Press, Philadelphia, 1953.]

In the year 431 the Council of Ephesus, repudiating the doctrine of the Nestorian Christians, which denied the divinity of the man Jesus, declared Mary as the Mother of God. A popular subject for artists since has been the Virgin's birth.

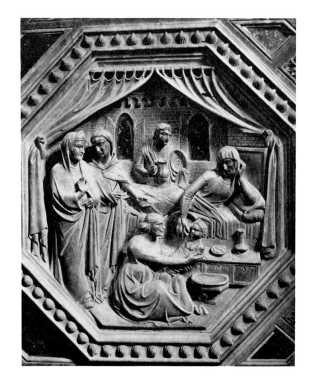

Fig. 4-44. The birth of the Virgin. Bas-relief by Andrea Orcagna (real name di Cione), 1308–1368. Tabernacle in Or San Michele, Florence.

Fig. 4-45. The birth of the Virgin. Fresco by Giovanni da Milano, about 1360. The parturient Anna washes her hands before partaking of the food being brought her by the attendants on the left. Renuccini Chapel, Church of Santa Croce, Florence.

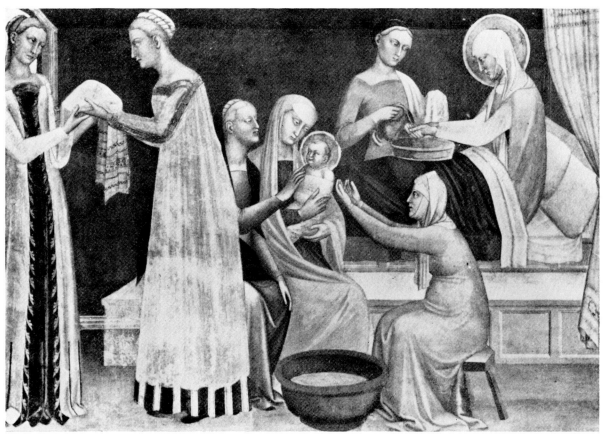

104 ICONOGRAPHIA GYNIATRICA

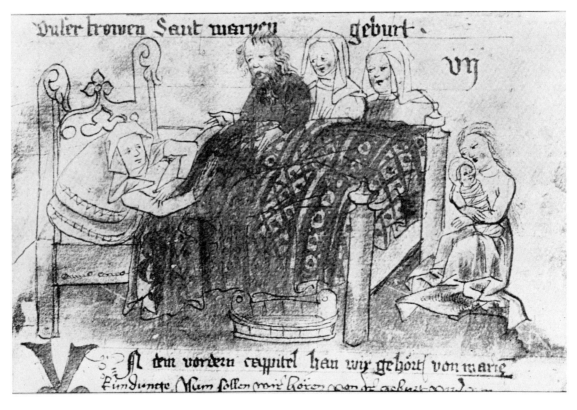

Fig. 4-46. The birth of Mary. From a fifteenth century German manuscript. The event is depicted in contemporary setting, the Virgin shown in a simple four-poster bed.

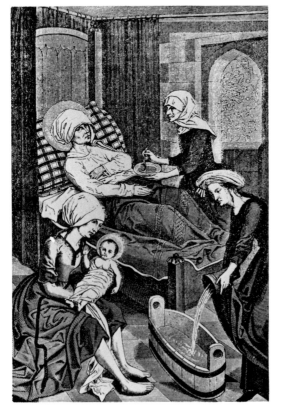

Fig. 4-47. The birth of the Virgin. By Bartholomäus Zeitblom (c. 1450–1517). The features of a fifteenth century German birth chamber are represented in a theme of great simplicity. Mother Anne, propped up in bed, is being served postpartum refreshment. Holding the newborn Mary, the nurse is about to test the temperature of the bath with her bare feet.

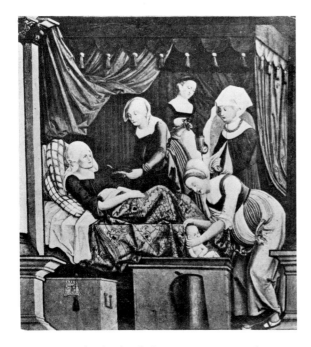

Fig. 4-48. The birth of the Virgin. Painting by Hans von Kulmbach (real name Süss), 1476–1522. In contrast to the preceding scene by his contemporary Zeitblom, von Kulmbach has depicted the birth of Mary in the house of a patrician, attested by the canopy bed with its elaborate drapes, the richly brocaded bed cover, and the bedside chests fitted with locks. Identical, however, are the essentials of the two scenes: the propped parturient receiving her postpartum collation, and the newborn infant its bath.

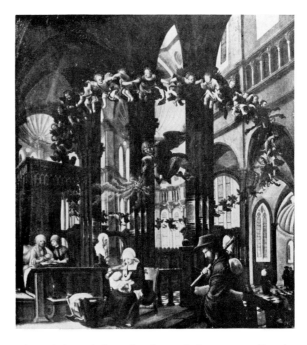

Fig. 4-49. Birth of the Virgin. By Albrecht Altdorfer (1480–1538), a figurative painting in which the grandeur of the church and the fantasy of the archangels dominate the simplicity of the birth scene.

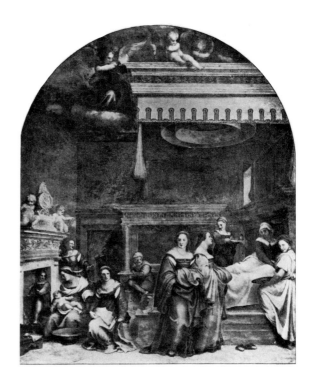

Fig. 4-50. Birth of the Virgin. Fresco by Andrea del Sarto (real name d'Agnolo), 1486–1531. Depicted is the birth chamber of an affluent Florentine lady of the fifteenth century, characterized by the high ceiling, elaborate canopy over the parturient's bed, and the marble fireplace, with mantel bearing the family crest, flanked by two angels. Church of St. Annunziata, Florence.

106 ICONOGRAPHIA GYNIATRICA

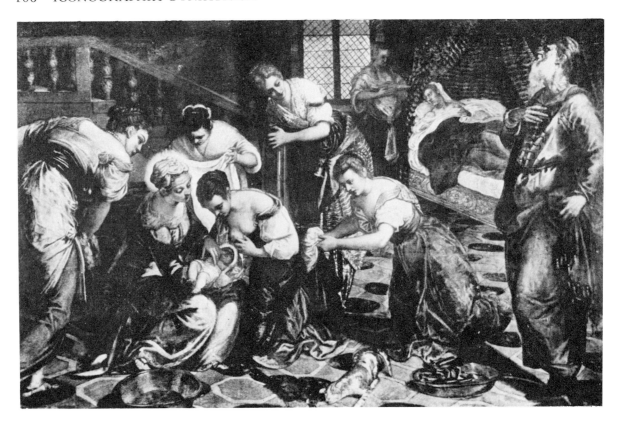

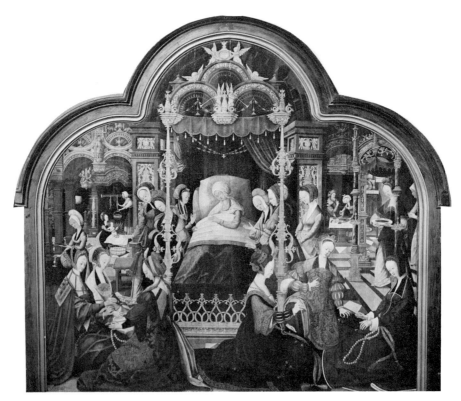

BIRTH SCENES 107

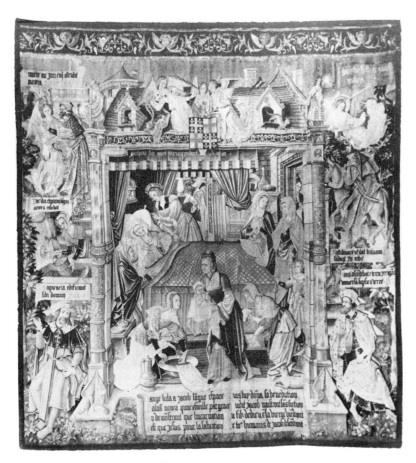

Fig. 4-53. The birth of Mary. Early sixteenth century tapestry depicting various scenes in the Virgin's life. Atelier de Reims, France.

Fig. 4-54. Birth of the Virgin. Altar woodcarving by an unidentified Dutch master. The hearth with kettle, on right, imparts an air of domesticity to the scene. Cathedral of Lübeck, Germany.

◀ Fig. 4-51. The confinement of Mother Anne. Painting by Il Tintoretto (real name Jacopo Robusti), 1518–1594. Elizabeth holds the newborn Mary while the wet nurse expresses milk from her breast for the infant. Jacob affects a theatrical pose, at the extreme right. The Hermitage, Leningrad.

Fig. 4-52. The birth of the Virgin. Attributed to an unknown Antwerp master, c. 1525. Groeninge Museum, Brussels.

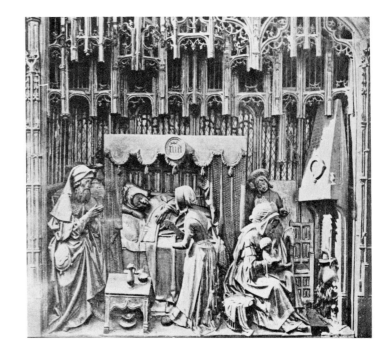

108 ICONOGRAPHIA GYNIATRICA

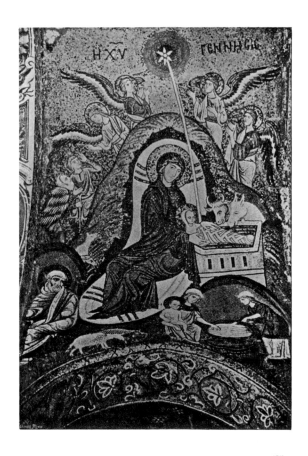

Fig. 4-55. The birth of Christ. Twelfth century mosaic. Recounted in this composite scene is the full Nativity sequence. Mary reclines alongside the crib, holding her newborn infant, wrapped diagonally in the characteristic fashion of the tenth to thirteenth centuries. Peering over the crib are the ever-present ox and ass. Joseph, who had gone for the midwives, observes remarkable phenomena on his return: a cloud arising from the ground, and a brilliant light filling the room. Praying angels hover over the scene. The Infant appears again in the foreground, about to be placed in the bath, the temperature of which an attendant is testing with her hand. Church of the Martyrs, Palermo, Italy.

THE NATIVITY

"And when the blessed Mary entered, the cave lit up with a resplendant glow as of the sixth hour of the day. This divine light did not diminish in splendor all day and night during Mary's sojourn there, and there she brought into the world a male child, who was surrounded from birth by adoring angels who said: 'Glory to God on high and peace on earth to men of good will.'" [Gospel of Pseudo-Matthew, chap. 13]

From the earliest simple representations of the Nativity, subsequently reinterpreted by the Byzantine craftsmen, the masters of the Renaissance, the artists of the Enlightenment, and most recently by the creators of the crude crèches of the twentieth century, the birth of Jesus has inspired probably more artistic efforts than have all other birth scenes combined. The details of the Nativity have been pieced together from liturgical passages, not all in agreement. According to the Gospels, the Virgin birth occurred in a stable. A story in the Apocrypha tells of Mary's confinement in a cave, attended by the midwives Zelemi and Salome who were brought there by Joseph. The latter version is represented in Byzantine art; the stable setting was adopted by western society. By the time of the Renais-

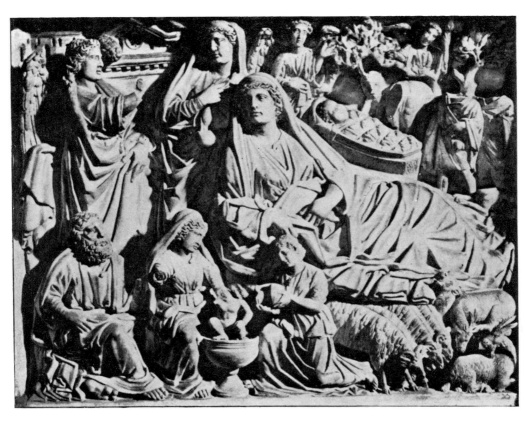

Fig. 4-56. The birth of Christ. Marble relief by Nicola (Niccolo) Pisano (c. 1208-1280). The subjects are depicted as classic Greek figures. The parturient Mary reclines in regal fashion on her chaise, the swaddled Christ child in the crib behind her. Broken off are the heads of the ox and ass. Shown again in the foreground is the Child, being bathed in a baptismal basin. Baptismal Pulpit, Pisa, Italy.

sance in Europe, the Byzantine cave concept had been almost entirely abandoned in favor of an open barn or stable which permitted a view of the manifold details of the outside world. In virtually all scenes of the Nativity the ox and ass are shown, as symbols of simple domesticity. Mary herself came to Bethlehem on an ass. Of the Virgin's appearance, Nicephorous Callixtus in the fourth century wrote, "The Madonna was of middle height, her face oval, her eyes brilliant and of olive tint, her eyebrows arched and black, her hair was pale brown, her complexion as fair as wheat."

Figuring prominently in most of the Nativity scenes are the three magi or wise men wearing identical capes and Phrygian caps. Many Renaissance artists painted them in royal garb, their relative ages being indicated by their respective beard lengths. In sharp contrast, humble shepherds were often shown.

While attempting to retain the solemnity of the Nativity, a number of Renaissance artists paid tribute to their sponsors by incorporating them in the scene, which thus became secularized to varying degrees. The whole Medici family, for example, appears in a Nativity painting of Boticelli; and in the works of some of the Dutch and Flemish masters, the Nativity is portrayed with the realism of a contemporary event.

110   ICONOGRAPHIA GYNIATRICA

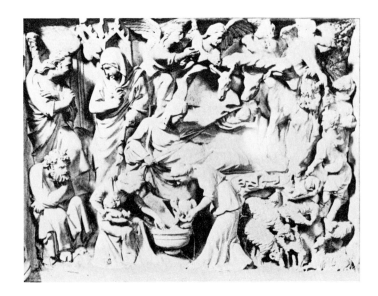

Fig. 4-57. The birth of Christ. Marble sculpture by Giovanni Pisano (1245–1320?), son of Nicola Pisano. Remarkably similar to his father's composition but more natural in execution, the younger Pisano's interpretation of the Nativity scene shows the reclining parturient as a tender mother rather than a proud princess, gently lifting the cover from the sleeping infant's crib. Pulpit, Church of San Andrea, Pistoia, Italy.

Fig. 4-58. The birth of Christ. Fresco by Taddeo Gaddi (1300?–1366). Sitting on a sack of straw in the stable, Mary holds the newborn Infant who is shown again in the foreground, having just been bathed and swaddled. Joseph is seen in the lower left corner. Several sheep, as well as the ox and ass, contemplate the holy event. Church of St. Francis, Assisi, Italy.

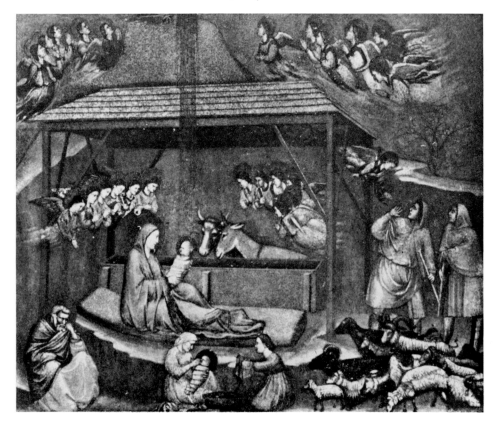

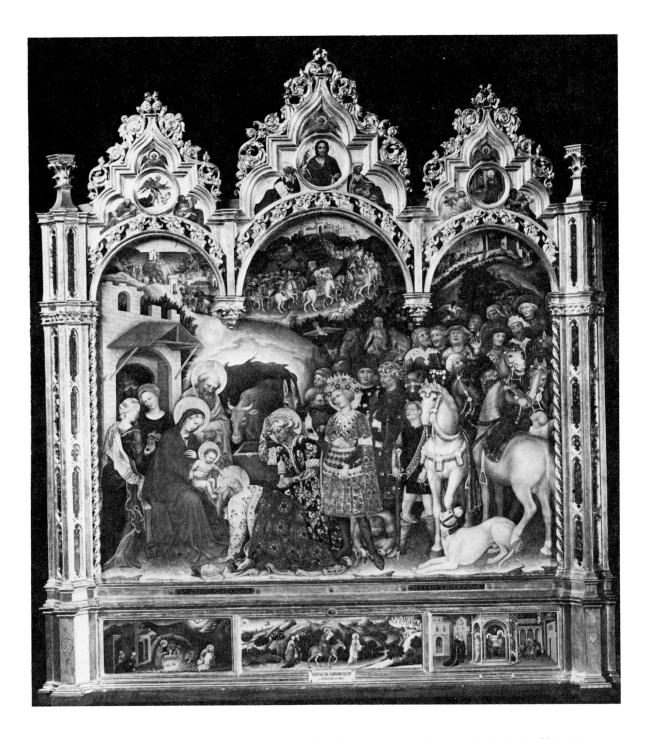

Fig. 4-59. The Nativity. Altarpiece panel by Gentile da Fabriano (1370?–1427?). Galleria degli Uffizi, Florence.

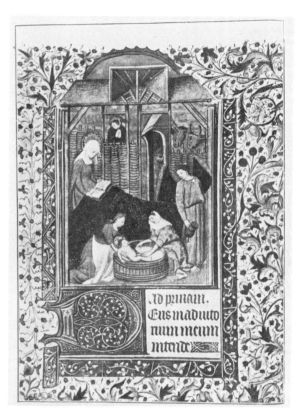

Fig. 4-60. The Nativity. From a miniature in a fifteenth century manuscript of the *Book of Hours*. Mary, wearing a golden robe and sitting up in bed reading a book, is apparently unconcerned with the activities about her. In the left background Joseph is seen in an attitude of prayer, in the right, the ox and ass. In the foreground the midwives bathe the Infant in a wooden tub. On the right, an angel carrying a pitcher represents the divine source of the water for the Infant's first bath. This is one of the few representations of the Nativity in which Mary is shown in bed. Bibliothèque de la Ville de Lyon, France.

Fig. 4-61. The Nativity. By Piero della Francesca (c. 1420–1492). Five angels make music as the Virgin, a strand of pearls about her neck, kneels and adores the Infant. The National Gallery, London.

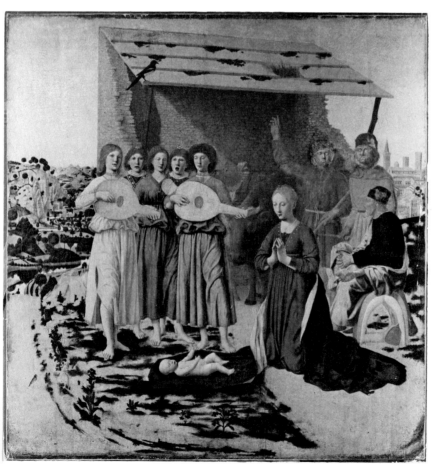

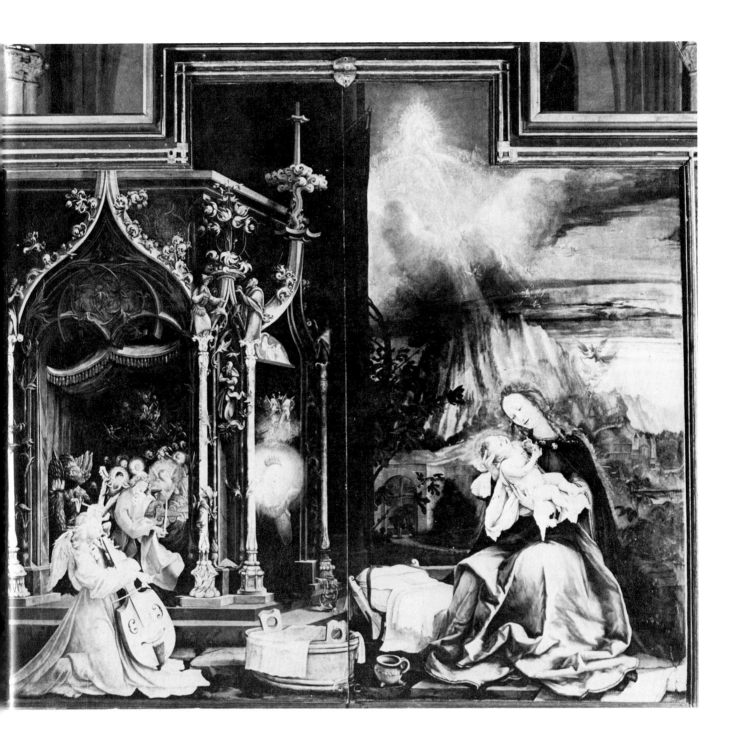

Fig. 4-62. The Nativity. By Mathias Grünewald, early sixteenth century German painter. Central panel from the altar of Issenheim, a small village in Alsace. The Virgin, in a rich setting, sits at the foot of her bed holding the newborn Babe, about to be bathed. Missing from the scene are the ox and the ass. Musée d'Unterlinden, Colmar, France.

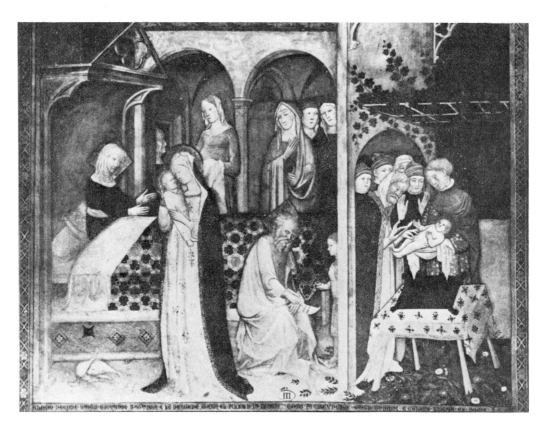

Fig. 4-63. The birth of John. Fresco by Lorenzo and Giacomo Salimbeni da San Severino, 1416. The parturient Elizabeth, sitting upright in a Gothic style bed with head canopy, holds forth her arms to receive her swaddled son from an attendant, while Zacharias, sitting on a chest at the bedside, records the child's name. Depicted in the scene on the right is the circumcision ritual. Chapel of San Giovanni Battista, Urbino, Italy.

THE BIRTH OF JOHN

"And there appeared unto him [Zacharias] an angel of the Lord standing on the right side of the altar of incenses, and when Zacharias saw him, he was troubled, and fear fell upon him. But the angel said unto him, Fear not, Zacharias: for thy prayer is heard; and thy wife Elizabeth shall bear thee a son, and thou shalt call his name John.... Now Elizabeth's full time came that she should be delivered; and she brought forth a son.... And it came to pass, that on the eighth day they came to circumcise the child; and they called him Zacharias, after the name of his father.... And his mother answered and said, Not so, but he shall be called John." [St. Luke 1:11-13, 57, 59, 60]

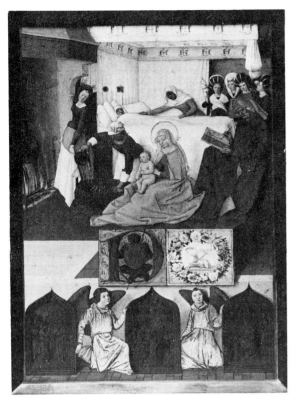

Fig. 4-64. The birth of Saint Jean-Baptiste. Miniature by Jean Fouguet (1415?–1480?) depicting a fifteenth century birth chamber. The drapes are embroidered with the initials E. C. for Étienne Chevalier, who commissioned the painting. The parturient Elizabeth lies under the bed covers, only her face showing. The Holy Virgin holds the infant John, while a nurse tests the temperature of his bath. Zacharias sits at the foot of the bed, recording his son's name. Musée Condé, Chantilly, France.

Fig. 4-65. The birth of Saint Jean-Baptiste. By an unknown artist of the Upper Rhine school, late fifteenth century. Elizabeth hands the naked newborn to Mary, while the midwife at the foot of the bed prepares the infant's bath. On a small table is set the postpartum collation of berries and wine. In the lower left corner Zacharias records the infant's name. Musée d'Unterlinden, Colmar, France.

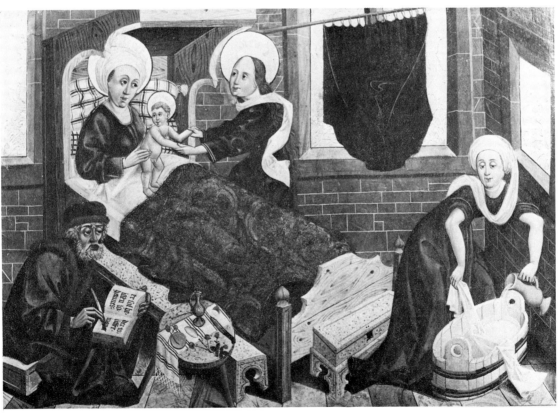

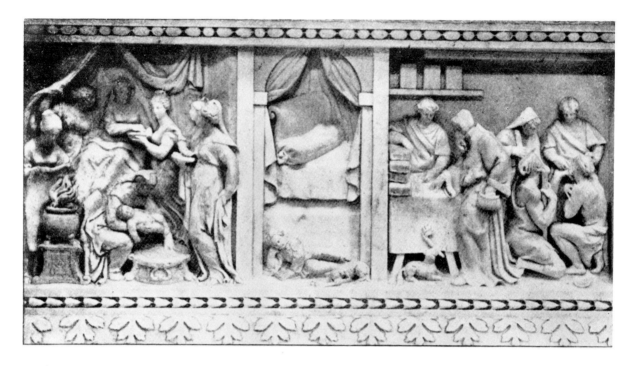

Fig. 4-66. The birth of Saint Dominic (1170–1221). Marble relief on his tombstone, by Lorenzo Lombardi, 1532. The parturient Joanna of Aza (Guzman) on the left, washes her hands in anticipation of the postpartum repast while the newborn Dominic is bathed. Monastery of St. Dominic, Bologna, Italy.

THE BIRTH OF BUDDHA

In the sixth century BC, according to Buddhist belief, there lived in northern India, near the Himalayas, the rich, powerful, and wise Prince Suddhodano and his virginal wife Maya, flawless in beauty and spirit. Miraculous as was her conception, when in a dream a great white elephant pierced her side with his tusk, so was her confinement, placed by Ceylon scholars in the year 544 BC. Under an embracing tree, attended by heavenly hosts, she gave birth to Siddhartha, the future Buddha. According to one version of the event, the infant emerged from his mother's right flank. (See chapter on cesarean section.)

It was prophesied at his birth that the young prince would renounce the world and all its earthly comforts, on seeing an old man, a sick man, and a corpse. This he did at age 19, when riding beyond the royal park. Dismissing his servants and doffing his princely raiment, Siddhartha entered upon a life of asceticism, practicing fasting and contemplation. Six years later he sat down under a bo tree (*Ficus religiosa*), vowed not to move until he had solved the riddle of life. After 49 days he attained enlightenment; hence the name Buddha, "the enlightened." Emancipated from his suffering, he devoted himself thereafter to helping others: "I teach sorrow, and the uprooting of sorrow."

BIRTH SCENES 117

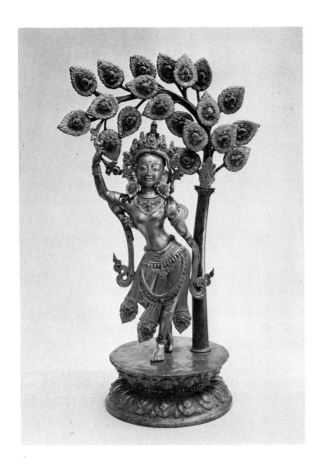

Fig. 4-67. The birth of Buddha. Gilded bronze from Nepal. Queen Maya stands under a flowering tree about to give birth to Siddhartha. Musée Guimet, Versailles.

Fig. 4-68. The birth of Bodhisattva, title for a future Buddha or savior of the world. Tibetan painting. Musée Guimet, Versailles.

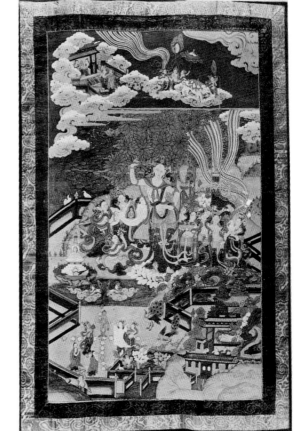

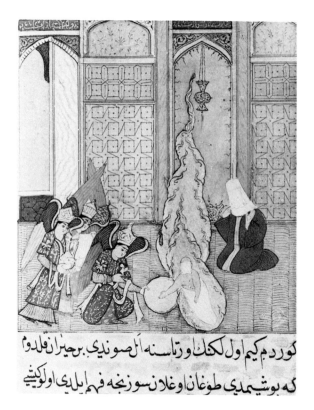

Fig. 4-69. The Birth of Mohammed. Miniature from *Siyer-un-Nebi* (Progress of a Prophet) a manuscript of 1368 copied in 1594 by Mustafa b. Yusuf b. Omer Erenzi Dariri. The infant Mohammed appears in a golden flame, the Turkish counterpart of the halo in Western religious art. Veiled are the faces of young Mohammed and his mother Amine, as are the faces of many holy figures in Turkish miniatures.

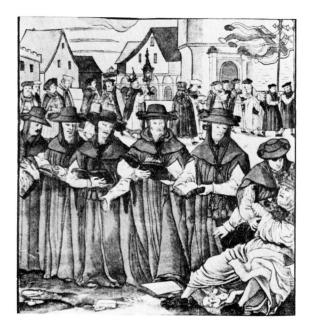

Fig. 4-70. The parturition of Pope Joan. Broadside by "Fraw Gilberta" showing the delivery during the papal procession. Berliner Königliche Kartensammlung, Berlin.

THE PARTURITION OF POPE JOAN

The myth of Pope Joan was contrived in the middle of the thirteenth century by Steven of Bourbon, a French Dominican, in his *Seven Gifts of the Holy Spirit.* Joan was born, the legend stated, in Ingelheim or Mainz, Germany of English parents. Falling in love with a Benedictine monk, she disguised herself as a man and fled with him to Athens where they studied together and Joan attained distinction as a scholar. After the death of her lover, Joan, still in male guise, proceeded to Rome, where she soon was named cardinal and ultimately elected pope, as John VIII, in the year 855, between the papacies of Leo IV and Benedict III. She died in childbirth during a papal procession. Subsequent popes, according to Giovanni Boccaccio's fourteenth century account, turned away at the halfway point in their processions with the clergy, in order to bypass the shameful site where Joan gave birth. The legend of Pope Joan provoked heated debate for many years. Refutation of the hoax was completed in 1863 with the publication of Johann Dollinger's *Papstfabeln des Mittelalters.*

Fig. 4-71. The parturition of Pope Joan. Woodcut from a German edition of Boccaccio's *Illustrious Women,* Ulm, 1473.

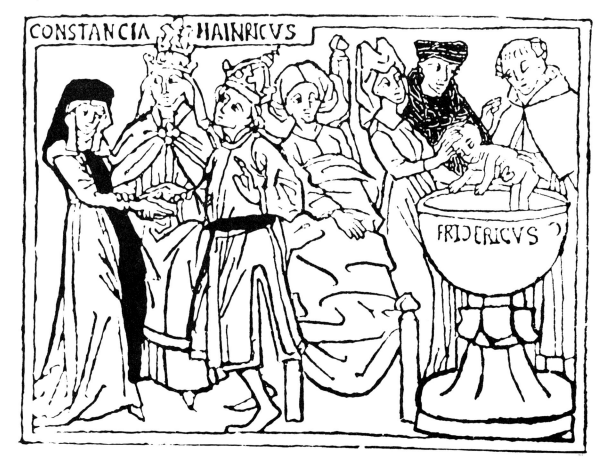

120 ICONOGRAPHIA GYNIATRICA

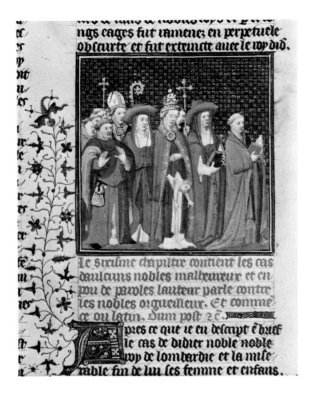

Fig. 4-72. The parturition of Pope Joan. Fifteenth century miniature. Bibliothèque Nationale, Paris.

Fig. 4-73. The parturition of Pope Joan. Woodcut from Joannes Wolf's *Lectionum memorabilium et reconditarum Centenarii XVI*, 1600.

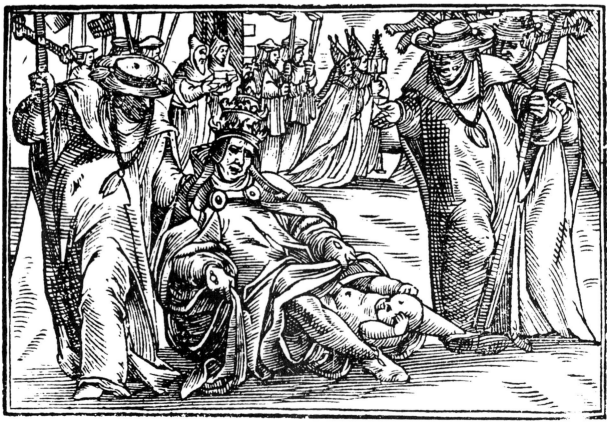

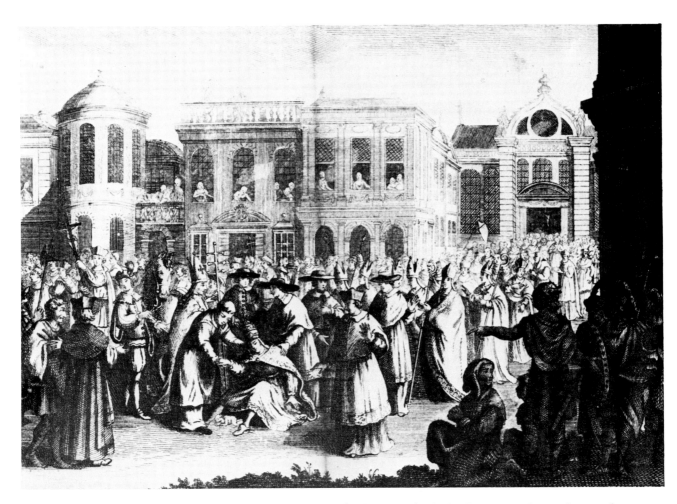

Fig. 4-74. The parturition of Pope Joan. Folding plate from F. Spanheim, *Histoire de la Papesse Jeanne fidelment tirée de la dissertation latine de Mr. de Spanheim*, 1736.

122 ICONOGRAPHIA GYNIATRICA

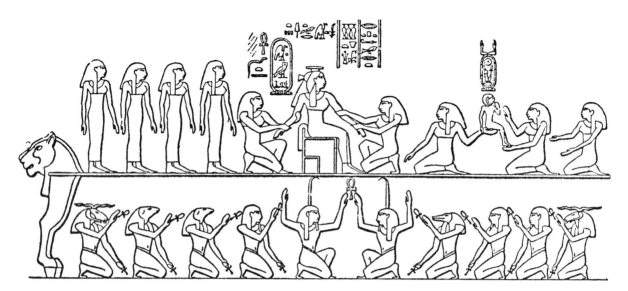

Fig. 4-75. The parturition of an Egyptian queen. Relief from the temple of Luxor, in Upper Egypt, on the east bank of the Nile, fourteenth century BC. The parturient sits on the birthstool attended fore and aft by female divinities acting as midwives, two of whom hold the queen's arms. The newborn prince is being passed along to the last attendant who waits with outstretched arms.

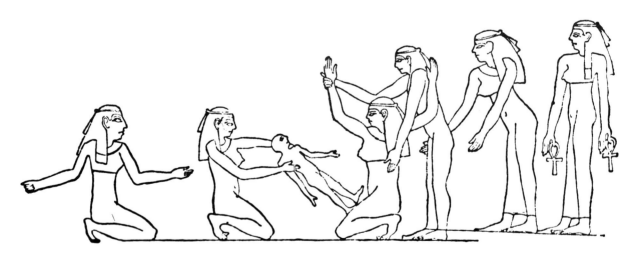

Fig. 4-76. The accouchement of Cleopatra. Relief from the temple of Esna, a town on the Nile, in Upper Egypt. The queen is giving birth in the kneeling position, supported by an attendant standing behind her. This figure bears a striking similarity to the mural depicting the birth of Re, the Egyptian sun god (Fig. 4-34).

BIRTH SCENES 123

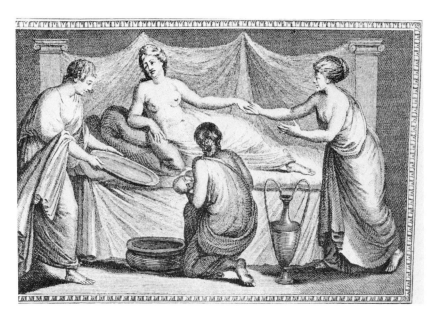

Fig. 4-77. The birth of Titus (Flavius Sabinus Vespasianus). Born in AD 40, Emperor of Rome, AD 79–81, Titus commanded a legion in the Judaean campaign taking Jerusalem in the year 70 after a bitter siege. The Colosseum was completed under his direction and the Roman public baths were named in his honor.

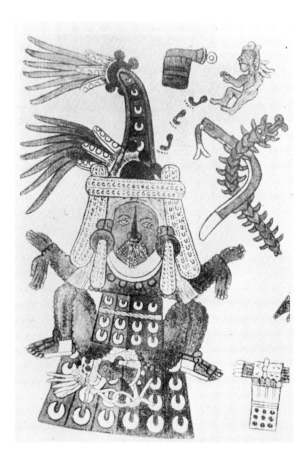

Fig. 4-78. Tlacolteotl in conception and parturition. Mexican queen regent of the thirteenth tonalamatl, a period of 260 days in the Mayan calendar. The descent of the child from heaven, in response to the queen's sacrifice, is indicated by the footprints over the chalchihuitl, the crown of precious stones worn by the queen.

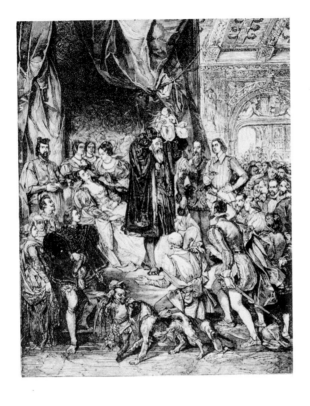

Fig. 4-79. The Birth of Henry IV. By Eugène François Marie Joseph Devéria (1805–1865). Born in 1553, Henry of Navarre became the first Bourbon king. A Protestant leader in the war of the Three Henrys, he realized that he could restore peace only if he himself embraced Catholicism. Accordingly, after abandoning the Protestant faith in 1593, he joined the Roman Catholic Church and made his triumphal march to Paris. He issued the Edict of Nantes in 1598, granting religious concessions to the Huguenots and was assassinated in 1610 while preparing for war against Spain. In Devéria's painting, placed on exhibition in 1827, the parturient Jeanne d'Albret, duchess of Bourbon and of Vendôme, is shown reclining while her father Henri d'Albret holds his newborn grandson aloft in proud display to his subjects.

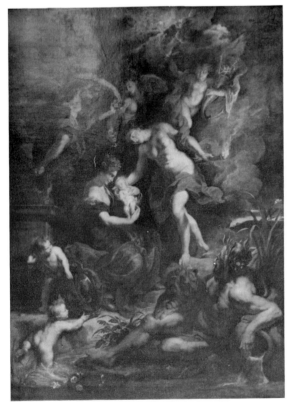

Fig. 4-80. The birth of Marie de' Medici. By Peter Paul Rubens (1577–1640). Lucina, goddess of childbirth, places the newborn princess in her mother's arms. An angel holds the horn of plenty containing crown and scepter, symbols of royalty, which foretell the infant's great destiny. In the foreground flows the River Arno, in Florence, locale of the birth scene. To date the event Sagittarius the centaur rides aloft with bow and arrow, but Rubens is believed to have erred in this representation for Sagittarius, the ninth sign of the Zodiac, symbolizes late November and early December, whereas Marie was born April 25, 1573, under the sign of Taurus. The second wife of French King Henry IV, after his assassination in 1610, Marie de' Medici became regent for their son, Louis XIII and promptly set about to reverse Henry's policies. She was also the mother of Henrietta Maria, queen of Charles I of England. Musée du Louvre, Paris.

BIRTH SCENES 125

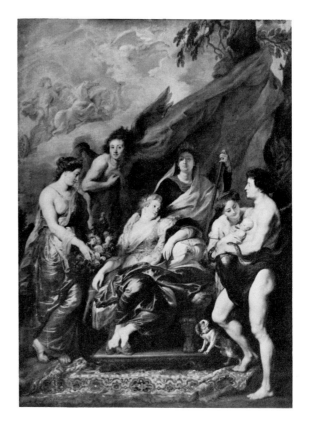

Fig. 4-81. The birth of Louis XIII. By Peter Paul Rubens (1577–1640). On the right holding the newborn, is the winged angel of wisdom with his symbolic snake; by his side fondling the infant, the goddess of justice. Behind the parturient queen stands her protectress, on the queen's right the goddess of fertility, her horn of plenty filled with flowers whose blossoms are depicted as the heads of the five children the queen is yet to bear. Above, in the guise of a horseman rides Castor of the constellation Gemini.

Born at Fontainebleau, September 27, 1601, Louis XIII succeeded his father Henry IV as King of France in 1610 under the regency of his mother Marie de' Medici. Prolonged discord prevailed between mother and son. In 1617 he drove her out; reconciled with her five years later, he entrusted the government to her favorite, Richelieu, but in 1630 sent her again into exile. During the reign of Louis XIII the French Academy was established. Musée du Louvre, Paris.

Fig. 4-82. The Birth of the Dauphin, Louis XIV of France, at Saint-Germain, September 5, 1638. The son of Louis XIII, whom he succeeded to the French throne in 1643 at age 5, Louis XIV enjoyed a reign of 72 years, the longest in modern European history, and became known as the Grand Monarch, or Louis the Great. His mother Anne of Austria acted as regent until 1661 when Louis assumed the role of absolute monarch, boasting, *"L'état c'est moi"* (I am the State). While engaging in four major wars, he also fostered his country's literature and art. In French history the seventeenth century has been called the Century of Louis XIV. Bibliothèque Nationale, Paris.

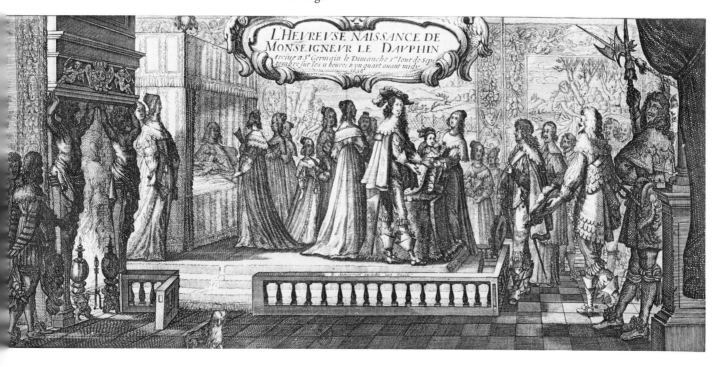

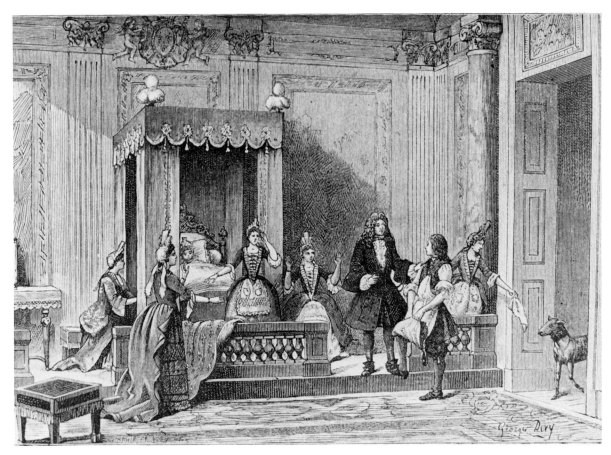

Fig. 4-83. Confinement of the Dauphiness, Anne-Marie-Victoire of Bavaria, at the birth of the Duke of Bourgogne, grandson of Louis XIV, August 6, 1682. Lithograph by G. Devy. To aid symphyseal spread during her prolonged labor, the accoucheur Jules Clément (1649–1729) is about to apply the skin of a lamb to the abdomen of the dauphiness. At the entrance to the birth chamber stands the bleeding animal, whose skin the butcher is delivering to the accoucheur. The pelts of freshly-skinned animals were also applied postpartum in some cases of dystocia during the seventeenth century. Madame Bourgeois advocated in her popular textbook for midwives, "As soon as a woman is delivered, after a long labor, she should be put into the skin of a black sheep that has been flayed alive; and, as warm as possible, it should be placed against the small of her back; this will strengthen it greatly. And to the abdomen should be applied the skin of a hare that has also been flayed alive, its throat then cut, and the blood rubbed into the skin, which is then applied very warm to the woman's abdomen. This corrects the dilatations made by pregnancy, and the melancholic blood [of the hare] drives out the bad and melancholic blood from the woman." [L. Bourgeois: *Observations diverses sur la sterilité,* Paris, 1626.]

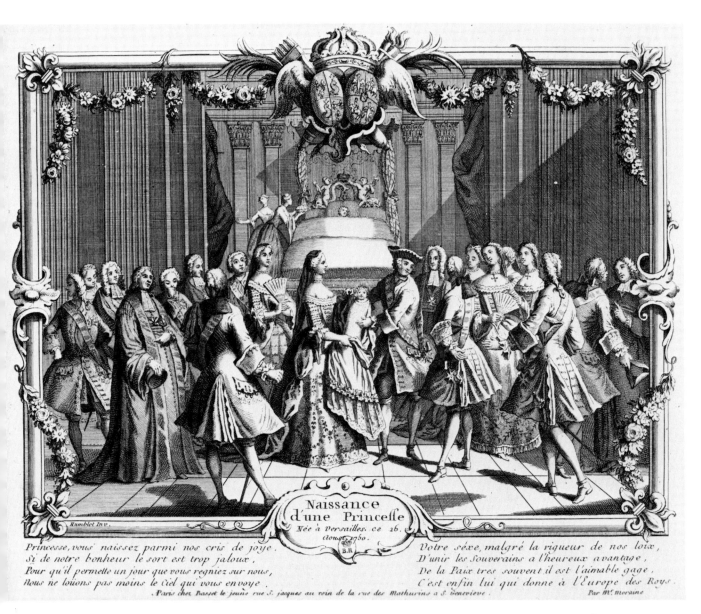

Fig. 4-84. Birth of a Princess, August 26, 1750, at Versailles, France. Princess Zephyrina (1750–1755), the fourth of 12 daughters of Marie Thérèse (daughter of Philip V of Spain) and Prince Louis (son of Louis XV of France). Bibliothèque Nationale, Paris.

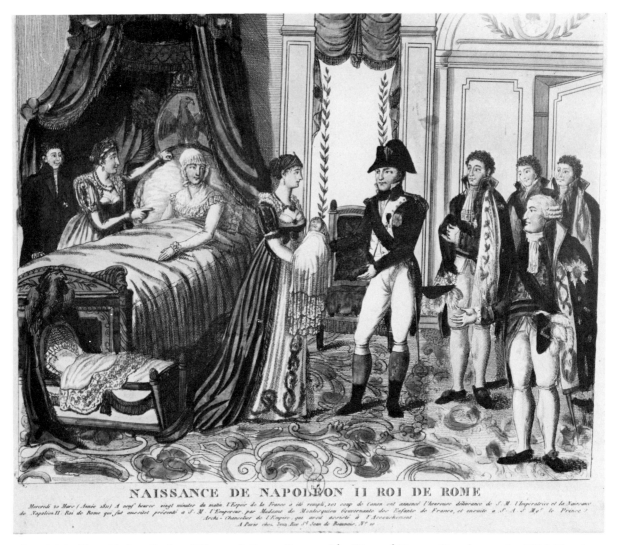

Fig. 4-85. The Birth of the "King of Rome." Napoleon I presents the King of Rome to grand dignitaries. After obtaining an annulment of the childless marriage to his Creole wife Josephine de Beauharnais, Napoleon married the Archduchess Marie Louise, daughter of Emperor Francis I of Austria, in 1810. A son Francis Joseph Charles was born the following year, March 20, 1811, to whom Napoleon gave the title King of Rome. Overthrown in 1814 Napoleon abdicated in favor of his young son, and after the Waterloo debacle the next year, proclaimed his heir Napoleon II. The French, however, ignored the youth and in 1818 his mother's family bestowed upon him the title of Duke of Reichstadt. Bibliothèque Nationale, Paris.

Fig. 4-86. Leda and the Swan. Free copy of a lost painting by Leonardo da Vinci, about 1506. According to Greek legend, Leda the wife of the Spartan King Tyndareus, bore him two mortal children, Castor and Clytemnestra. Zeus, king of the gods, in the guise of a swan symbolizing perhaps a phallus, visited Leda, and in due time she produced again: of this union, the immortal Pollux and Helen, the latter to become the heroine of Troy. Castor and Pollux, thus half brothers, were sometimes called sons of Zeus or the *Dioscouri,* sometimes sons of Tyndareus or *Tyndaridae.* Shown emerging from their eggshells are Leda's offspring. Spiridon Collection, Rome.

BIRTH SCENES 129

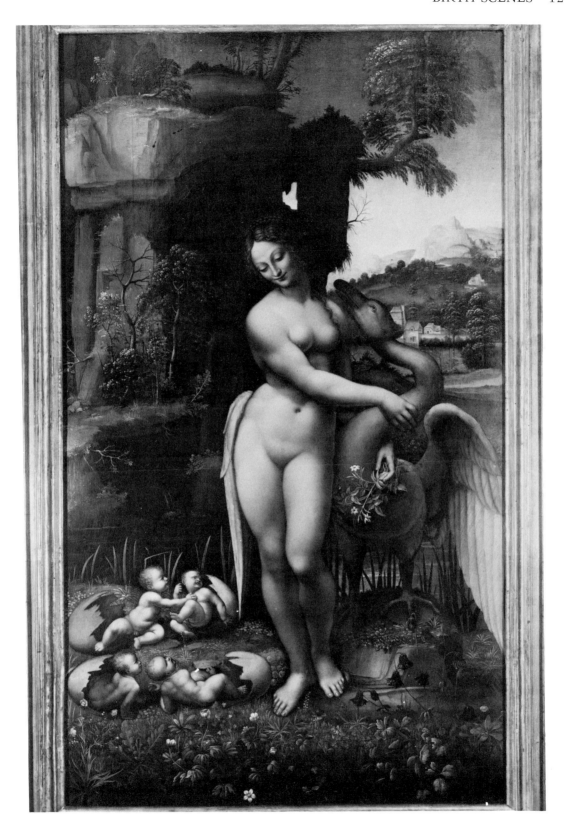

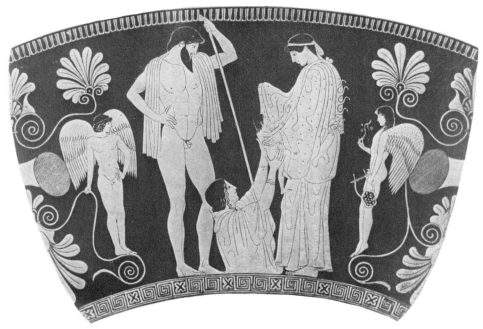

Fig. 4-87. The birth of Erichthonios. From a red-figured stamnos or widemouthed vase, about 500 BC. The newborn Erichthonios is being entrusted to Athene by Ge, or Gaea, the earth goddess emerging from the ground, while the bearded Hephaistos, father of the infant, looks on. On either side stand the winged Erotes who presided over the union of the gods and goddesses. Known also as Erechtheus, Erichthonios was a god of agriculture. Jointly with Athene he had a temple, the Erechtheum, on the Acropolis.

THE BIRTH OF VENUS

The goddess of love and beauty, Venus or Aphrodite came to life in the *Iliad* as the daughter of Zeus and Dione. According to later legend, Venus arose from the foam of the sea, near Cythera, from whence she was wafted to Cyprus. Of the "beautiful, golden goddess" one of the Homeric hymns tells,

The breath of the west wind bore her
Over the sounding sea,
Up from the delicate foam,
To wave-ringed Cyprus, her isle.
And the Hours golden-wreathed
Welcomed her joyously.
They clad her in raiment immortal
And brought her to the gods.
Wonder seized them all as they saw
Violet-crowned Cytherea.

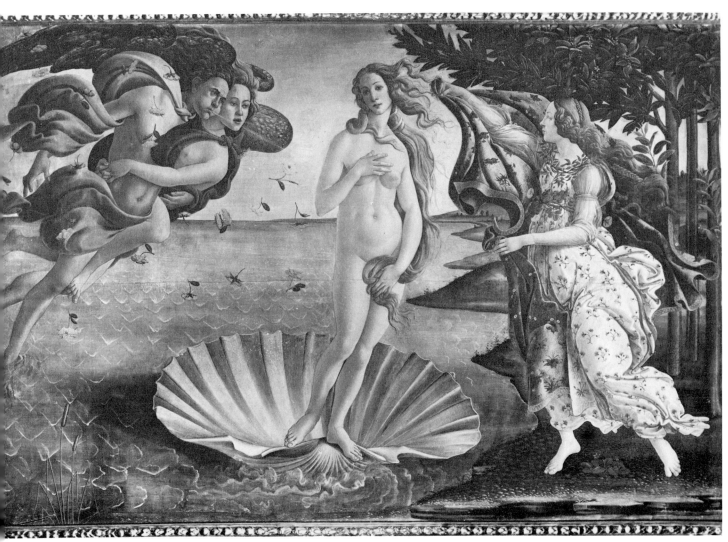

Fig. 4-88. The Birth of Venus. By Sandro Botticelli (Allesandro di Mariano dei Filipepi), 1444–1510. In contrast to his usual medium of wooden panels, Botticelli painted this scene, about 1480, on canvas. Venus is about to step out from the sea shell on which she has been blown ashore from the Aegean Sea by the zephyrs as one of the Hours moves to drape her in a star-studded robe. The scene has been endowed by some with quasi-religious meaning: the celestial Venus born of the sea symbolizing the Virgin Mary, source of divine love; the zephyrs, or wind gods, resembling angels; the Hour personifying spring and welcoming Venus ashore, recalling the relation of St. John to Jesus at the latter's baptism, or *rebirth in God*. Botticelli's "Birth of Venus" thus evokes man's hope for rebirth, the spirit of the Renaissance. Galleria degli Uffizi, Florence.

132 ICONOGRAPHIA GYNIATRICA

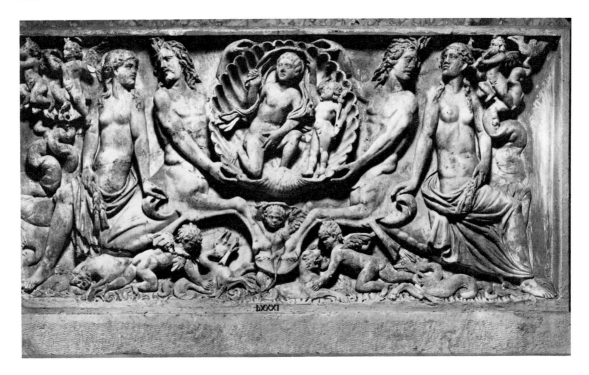

Fig. 4-89. The birth of Venus. Antique bas-relief. Galleria Borghese, Rome.

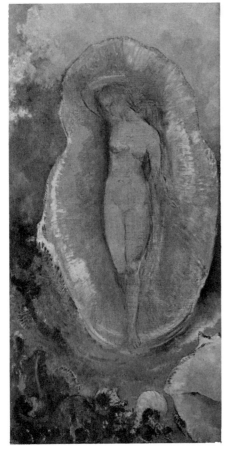

Fig. 4-90. Birth of Venus. Oil painting by Odilon Redon, about 1912. Stephen Higgons Collection, Paris.

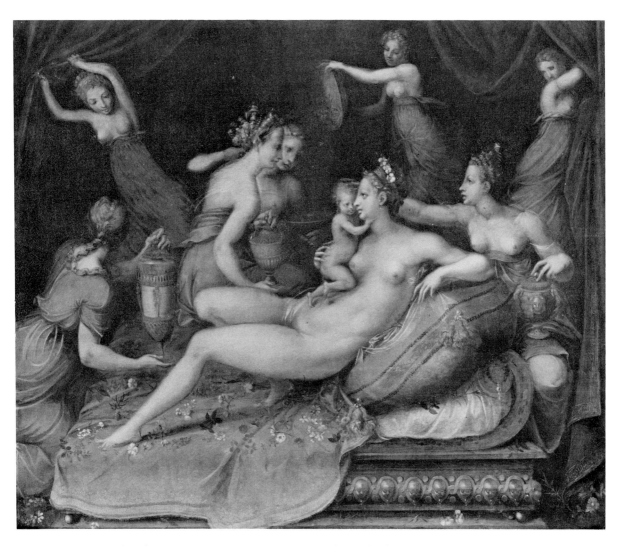

Fig. 4-91. The birth of Cupid. Painted by an unknown artist, school of Fontainebleau, between 1540 and 1560. Holding her newborn infant Cupid the god of love, Venus reclines on a couch strewn with flowers attended by the three Graces and the four Hours. Metropolitan Museum of Art, New York.

THE BIRTH OF ADONIS

Under the influence of Aphrodite, Myrrha became impregnated by her own father, Cinyras; then, dishonored, she was put to death by him. The gods, having compassion on her, transformed Myrrha into a tree, *Balsamodendron myrrha.* Nine months later, it opened up and gave forth a youth of great beauty, Adonis. Loved by both Aphrodite, the goddess of love and beauty, and Persephone, the queen of the dead, Adonis spent six months of the year with each. From the netherworld he returned each spring, symbolizing the rebirth of nature. Fond of hunting, Adonis was one day wounded by a wild boar, and as his life slipped away Aphrodite lamented,

Fig. 4-92. The birth of Adonis. Engraving by an unknown artist, in *Ovidius Herscheppinghe,* by Joost van den Vondel (1587–1679), (*Dichterlijke Werken van Joost van den Vondel,* Amsterdam, 1820–24).

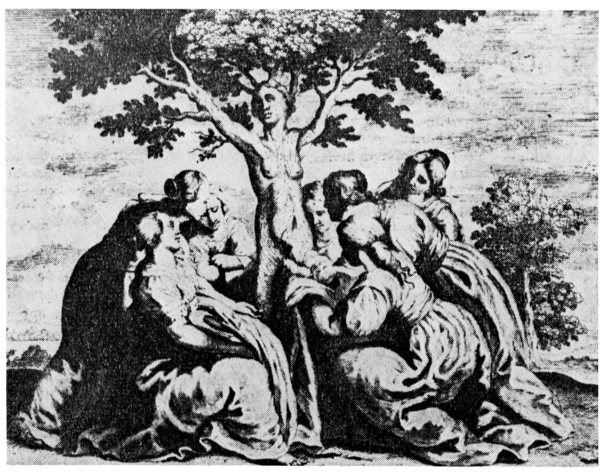

You die, O thrice desired
And my desire has flown like a dream.
Gone with you is the girdle of my beauty,
But I myself must live who am a goddess
And may not follow you.
Kiss me yet once again, the last, long kiss,
Until I draw your soul within my lips
And drink down all your love.
The mountains all were calling and the oak trees answering,

Oh, woe, woe for Adonis. He is dead,
And echo cried in answer, Oh, woe, woe for Adonis.
And all the Loves wept for him and all the Muses too.

Each drop of Adonis' blood that stained the earth Aphrodite changed into a crimson anemone. For another version of the birth of Adonis, see Figure 11-3, in Chapter 11.

Fig. 4-93. The birth of Adonis. Painting, artist not designated.

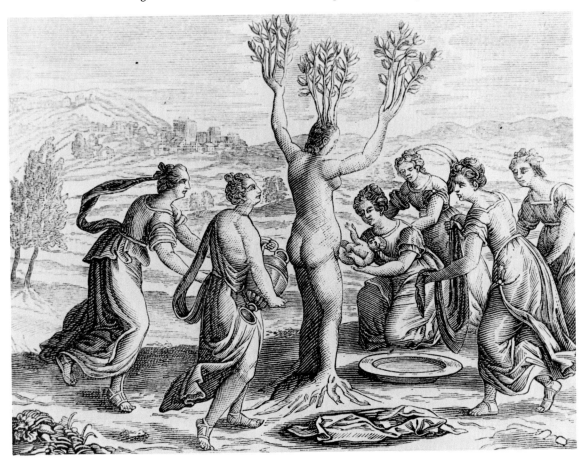

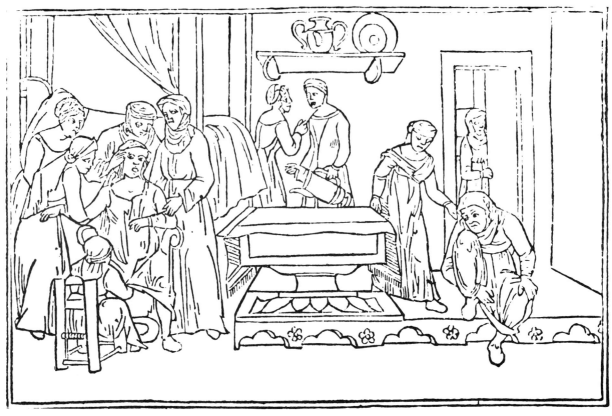

Fig. 4-94. The birth of Hercules. From a 1497 edition of Ovid's *Metamorphoseos vulgare*, Venice. According to the legend, Zeus visited Alcmene disguised as her husband Amphytryon during the latter's absence. The result: Hercules. This illustration probably inspired the woodcut introducing the fourth chapter of Rösslin's *Rosengarten*, published in 1513 (see chap. 19), in which the same postures and relations of the parturient, midwife, and attendants are shown.

THE CUNICULAR CONFINEMENT OF MARY TOFT

One day in April, 1726 Mary Toft, the illiterate wife of a poor journeyman clothier of Godalming in Surrey, England about 30 miles southwest of London, believing herself six weeks pregnant, was startled by a rabbit while weeding her garden. She soon developed a craving for rabbits. About five months later she miscarried, but for some weeks thereafter she continued to bleed and expel fragments of tissue; her thoughts meanwhile remaining with rabbits. In early November the entire community was startled by word that Mary Toft had given birth to a rabbit; and when 12 more rabbits appeared within the next week, John Howard, the local man-midwife, communicated the sensational news to a friend in London where it spread like wildfire. King George I promptly ordered an investigation, to be conducted by Nathaniel St. André, a Swiss anatomist attached to the royal court. Unbeknown to St. André, Mary kept inserting into her vagina pieces of rabbit that she had hidden in her pockets. Duped, St André reported that he "delivered her of the entire Trunk, strip'd of its skin, of a Rabbet of about four months' growth." On November 26 several of Mary's rabbit offspring were brought to St. James Palace for demonstration to the King, who thereupon ordered further enquiry. To the task were appointed the distinguished man-midwives Sir Richard Manningham and James Douglas who, suspecting a ruse from the start, extracted a confession from Mrs. Toft under the threat of a painful experiment. Of her confession Sir Richard wrote,

"... on Wednesday December 7, in the Morning, in the Presence of ... Dr. Douglas and myself, she began her Confession of the Fraud; and in her Confession she own'd, That upon her miscarrying she was seized with violent Floodings, and the womb was then ... open as if she had been just deliver'd of a full-grown Child, she did verily believe one of her wicked Accomplices did then convey into her Womb part of the Monster ... being the Claws and Body of a Cat and the Head of a Rabbet; this put her to much Pain: After that time she believed nothing was ever put into her Womb, but into the Passage only, by the Advice of a Woman Accomplice ... who told her she had now no occasion to work for her Living as formerly, for she would put her in a Way of getting a very good Livelihood, and promised continually to supply her with Rabbets, and should therefore expect part of the Gain.... The Woman told her she must put up her body so many pieces of Rabbets as would make up the Number of Rabbets which a Doe Rabbet usually kindles at one time, otherwise she would be suspected. Mary Toft asked how many that was; the Woman told her, sometimes thirteen.

"From that time Mary Toft did often, by the Assistance of that Woman, convey parts of Rabbets into her Body, till at last she could do it by herself, as she had an Opportunity to do so." [R. Manningham: *An Exact Diary of*

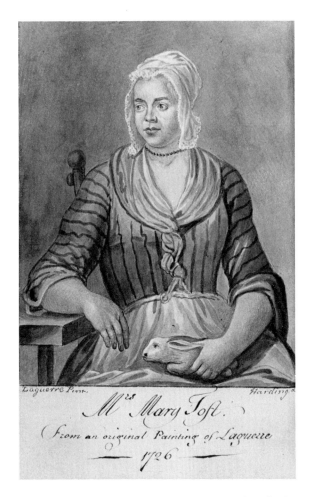

Fig. 4-95. Mary Toft, 1726. Lithograph of the "Rabbet-Breeder of Godalming." The Royal Society of Medicine, London.

What Was Observ'd During a Close Attendance upon Mary Toft, the Pretended Rabbet-Breeder of Godalming in Surrey from Monday Nov. 28, to Wednesday Dec. 7 Following. Together with An Account of Her Confession of the Fraud. London, 1726.]

After the exposure of Mary Toft's fraud, London's cartoonists had a heyday, and to the flood of caricatures that soon appeared were added unnumbered ribald verses. None failed to make capital of the fact that Nathaniel St. André, a hapless victim of the ruse, had formerly been a dancing teacher.

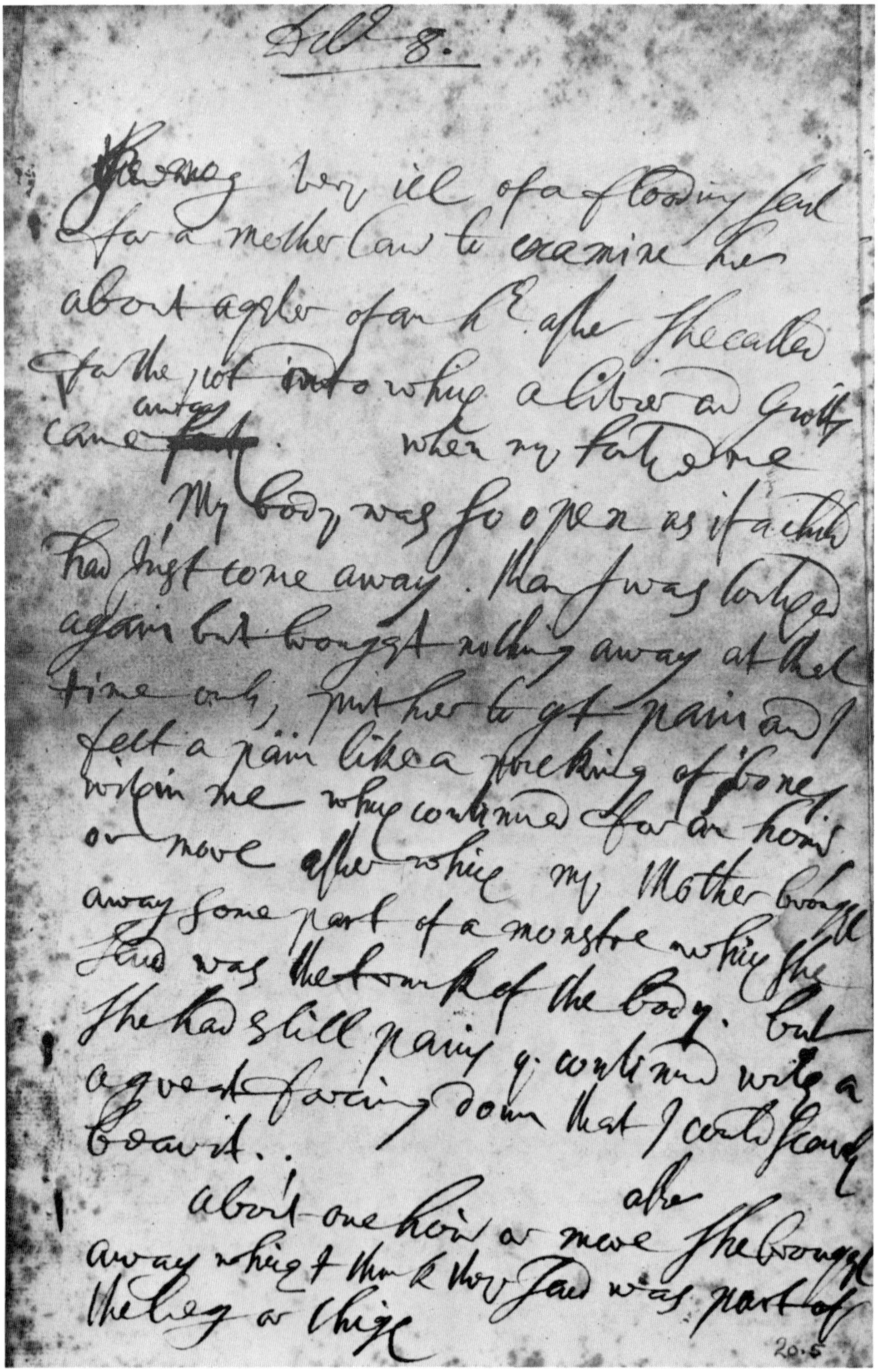
Feb. 8.

She was very ill of a flooding sent for a mother came to examine her about a quarter of an h[ou]r after she called for the pot into which a liver or growth came away when my tooth ... me

My body was so open as if a child had just come away. Mary was touched again but brought nothing away at that time only put her to get pain and I felt a pain like a breaking of bones within me which continued for an hour or more after which my Mother brought away some part of a monster which she said was the trunk of the body. but she had still pains & continued with a great forcing down that I could scarce bear it..

about one hour or more after she brought away which I think they said was part of the leg or thigh

Fig. 4-96. Mary Toft's confession. Written by James Douglas from her dictation. Glasgow University Library, Glasgow, Scotland.

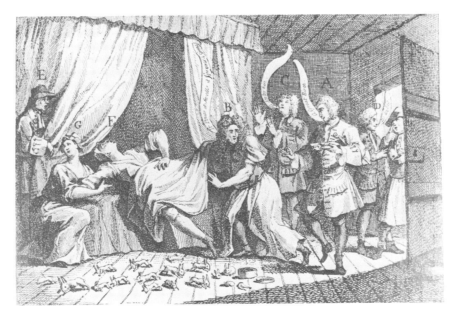

Fig. 4-97. "Cuniculari or the Wise Men of Godalming in Consultation." Engraving by William Hogarth, 1726, bearing the verse, "They hold their Talents most Adroit for any mystical Exploit." Manningham examines Mary Toft while St. André, violin in hand, dances, and John Howard, at the door, dismisses a boy bringing a rabbit with the words, "This one is too big."

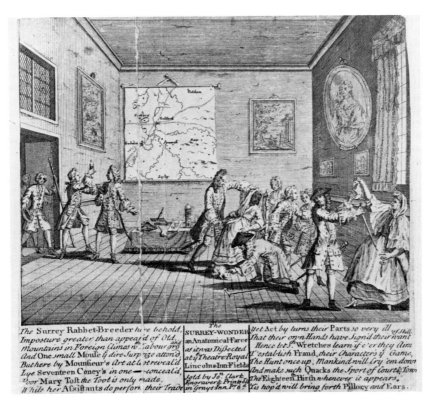

Fig. 4-98. "The Surrey Wonder." Drawing by one of the Vertue brothers, probably George (1684–1756), showing the birth of Mary Toft's rabbits. The Royal College of Medicine, London.

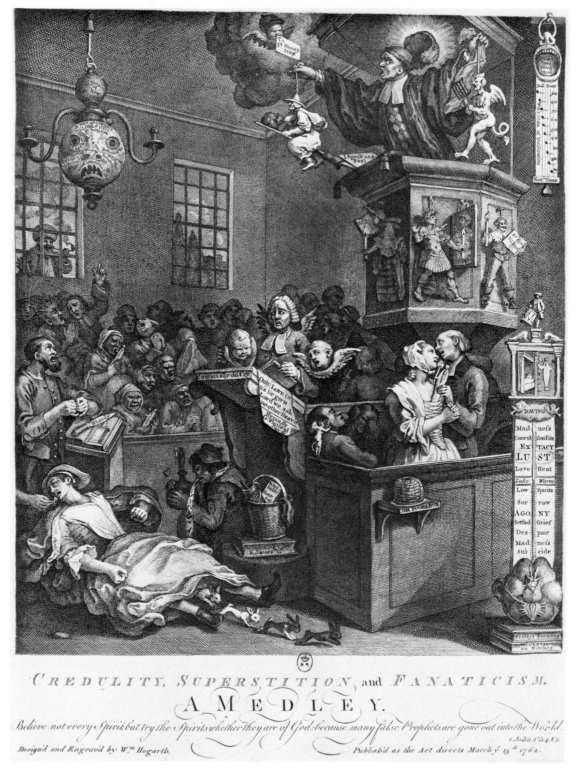

Fig. 4-99. "Credulity, Superstition, and Fanaticism. A Medley." Engraving by William Hogarth, 1762, lampooning the rabbit hoax of Mary Toft. Bibliothèque Nationale, Paris.

BIRTH SCENES 141

JOY AND GRIEF AT BIRTH

Within the birth chamber, cradle of emotion, are ever enacted scenes of joy and grief, humor and pathos, hope and dread—at the arrival of new life, premature death, and offspring either wanted or unwanted, sound or malformed, and of desired or undesired sex.

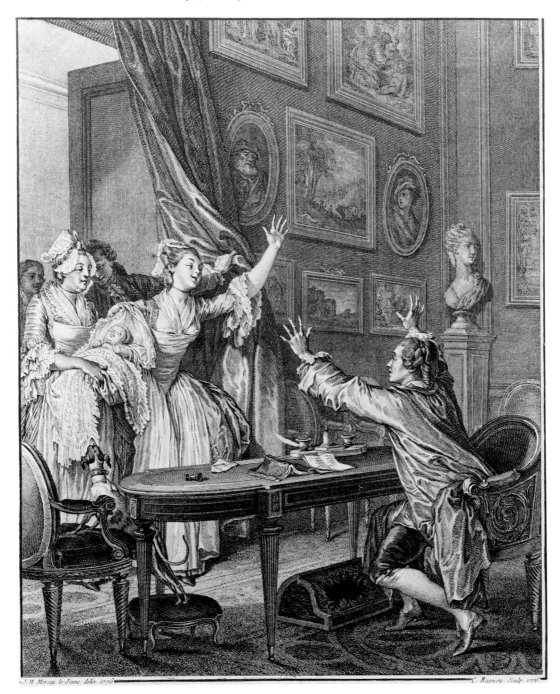

Fig. 4-100. *"C'est un Fils, Monsieur!"* Engraving, 1776, by Jean Charles Baquoy (1721–1777) from a drawing by Jean Michel Moreau, the younger (1741–1814). Bibliothèque Nationale, Paris.

142 ICONOGRAPHIA GYNIATRICA

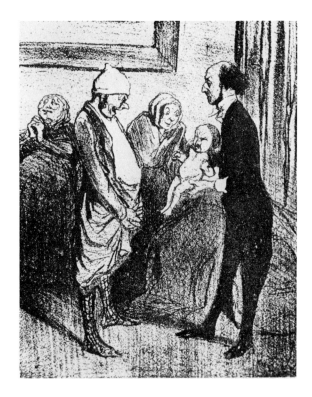

Fig. 4-101. *L'Entrée dans la Vie.* By Honoré Daumier (1808–1869). The accoucheur presents the newborn infant to the proud father, who joyfully exclaims, *"Enfin... en voilà donc un qui me ressemble!"* (At last... here's one who looks like me!)

THE DEATH OF RACHEL

"And they journeyed from Beth-el; and there was but a little way to come to Ephrath: and Rachel travailed, and she had hard labor. And it came to pass, when she was in hard labor, that the midwife said unto her, Fear not; thou shalt have this son also. And it came to pass, as her soul was in departing, (for she died) that she called his name Ben-oni: but his father called him Benjamin. And Rachel died, and was buried in the way to Ephrath, which is Beth-lehem." [Genesis 35:16-19]

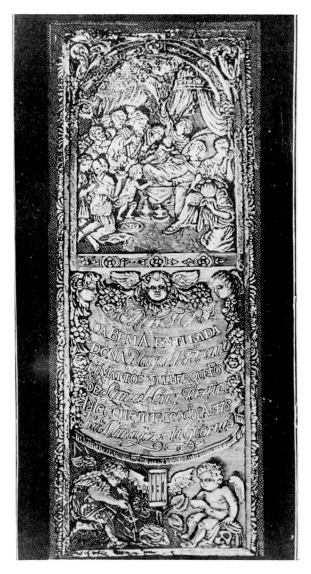

Fig. 4-102. The death of Rachel. Relief on the tombstone of Dona Rachel Teicheira de Mattos who died in 1716, found in the cemetery of Onderkerk an der Amstel, Netherlands, among the old graves of the Portugese Jews. Rachel, on her deathbed in a tent by a tree, is shown her newborn son by the midwife behind whom stands Jacob and his household, weeping.

BIRTH SCENES 143

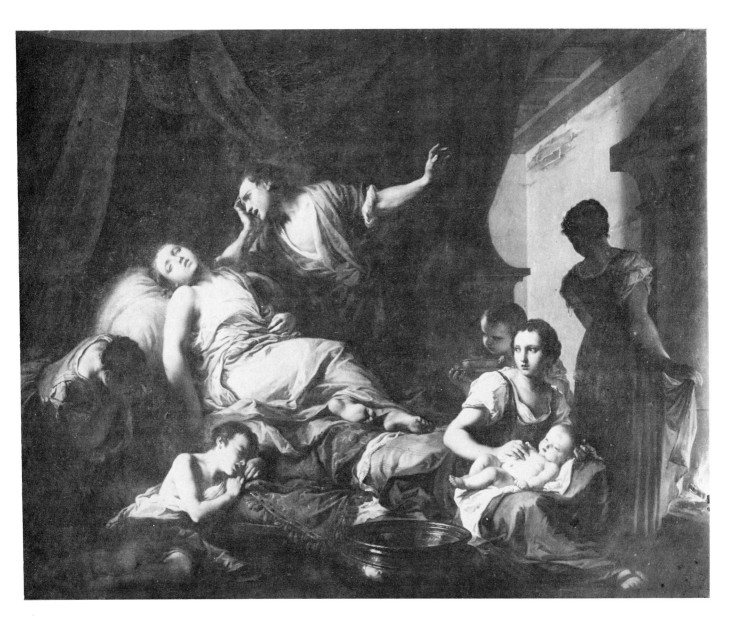

Fig. 4-103. The death of Rachel. By Giovanni Bettino Cignaroli (1706–1770). Although Biblical scholars have put Rachel's age at her death at about 50 years, she appears in Cignaroli's painting as a younger woman.

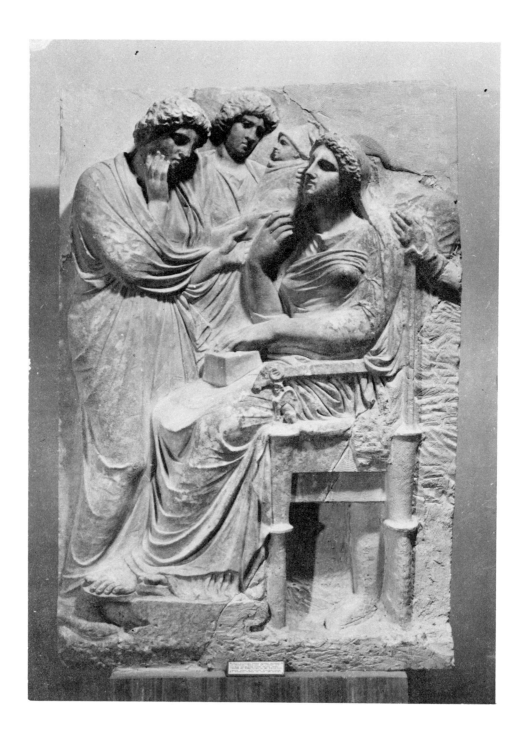

Fig. 4-104. Marble grave stone. Fourth century BC memorial to a young woman who died in childbirth, found in Piraeus, Greece, in 1839. On her lap the parturient holds her jewel box. One of the two standing figures, variously interpreted as men, women, grieving midwives, and servants, holds up to the dying mother her newborn child, in swaddling bands and conical cap. National Archaeological Museum, Athens.

Fig. 4-105. Attic gravestone. Sixth through fourth century BC, found in Oropus, Greece, portraying in relief the last moments of a dying parturient. Two women offer assistance while the grief-stricken bearded husband stands by, head in hand. National Archaeological Museum, Athens.

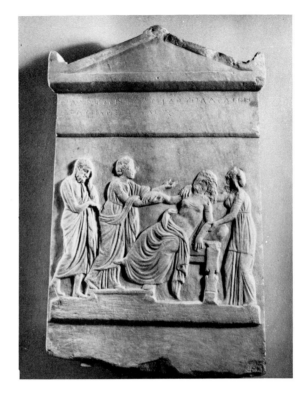

Fig. 4-106. Attic marble vases. Fourth century BC with figures of women dying in childbirth. National Archaeological Museum, Athens.

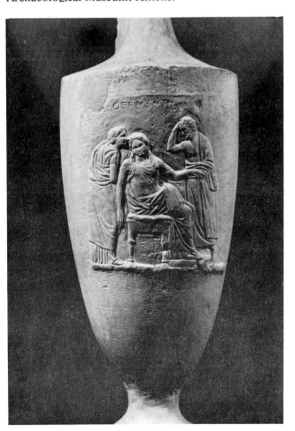
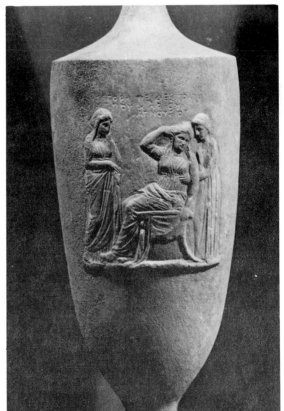

146 ICONOGRAPHIA GYNIATRICA

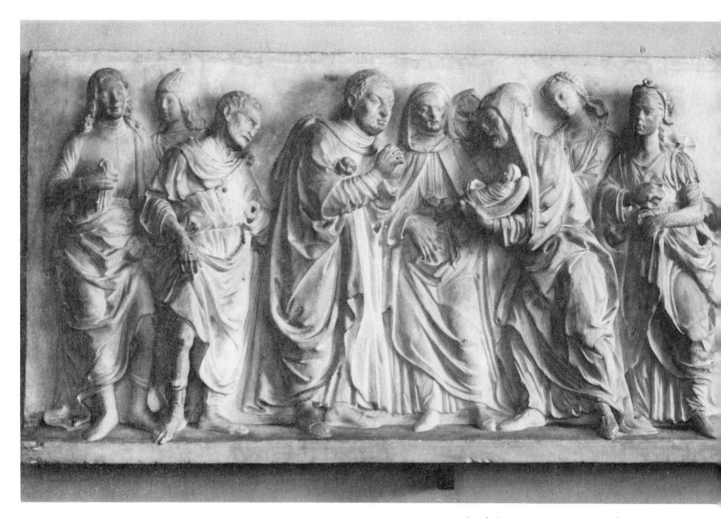

Fig. 4-107. Death of the parturient. Detail of marble bas-relief by Andrea del Verrocchio (1435–1488), originally on grave in Church of Santa Maria sopra

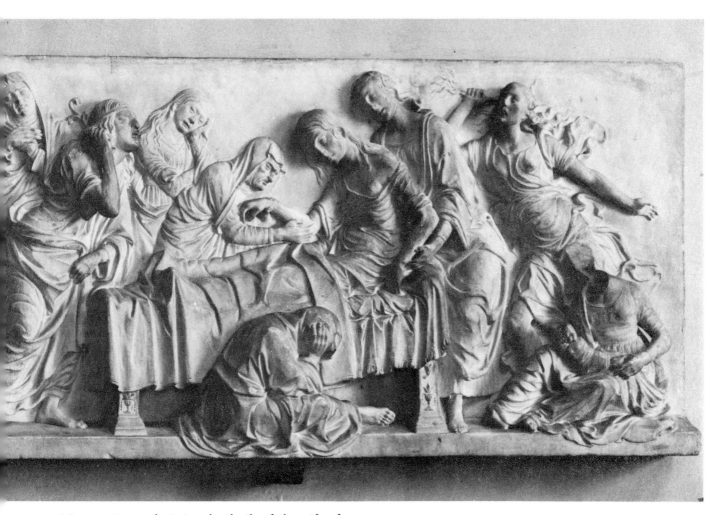

Minerva, Rome, depicting the death of the wife of Giovanni Francesco Tornabuoni in 1477, after delivering twins. Museo Nazionale, Florence.

148 ICONOGRAPHIA GYNIATRICA

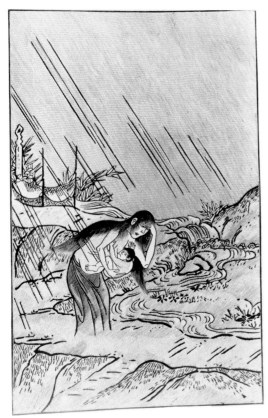

Fig. 4-108. *Ubame* (the parturient). Japanese woodcut by Toriyama Sekiyen. The wandering spirit of a woman who died in childbirth wades through a stream, in the rain, carrying her newborn infant. Bamboo posts on the bank in left background support a cloth for collecting water for the *Nagara-kan-jo*, traditional sacrifice for the dead. Behind stands the *Rei-dai*, wooden grave marker with notched edges.

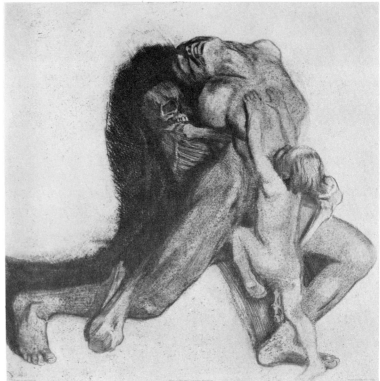

Fig. 4-109. "Woman and Death." Etching and sandpaper aquatint, 1910, by Käthe Kollwitz (1867–1945). The Philadelphia Museum of Art.

THE PUERPERIUM

"If a woman have conceived seed, and born a man child: then she shall be unclean seven days; according to the days of the separation for her infirmity shall she be unclean. . . . And she shall then continue in the blood of her purifying three and thirty days; she shall touch no hallowed thing, nor come into the sanctuary, until the days of her purifying be fulfilled. But if she bear a maid child, then she shall be unclean two weeks, as in her separation: and she shall continue in the blood of her purifying threescore and six days." [Leviticus 12:2, 4, 5]

Like the birth act itself, the puerperium has been endowed with an aura of sanctity and special privilege. In ancient Rome wreaths were hung from the doors of the homes of puerperal women. In Athens criminals who found refuge in the house of a parturient were granted immunity from the law.

Fig. 4-110. Mary in childbed, after giving birth to Jesus. Swabian woodcarving, about 1510. Germanisches Nationalmuseum, Nürnberg.

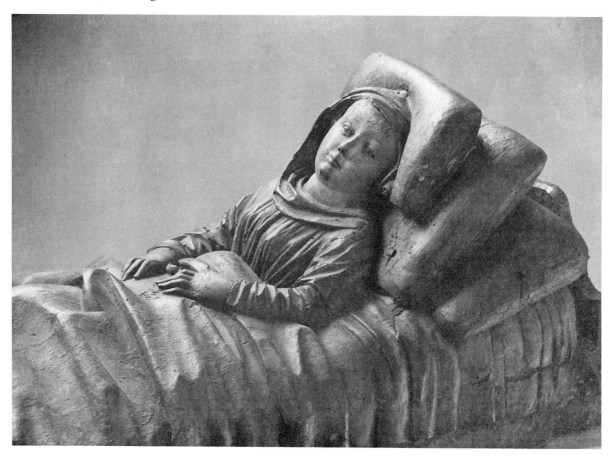

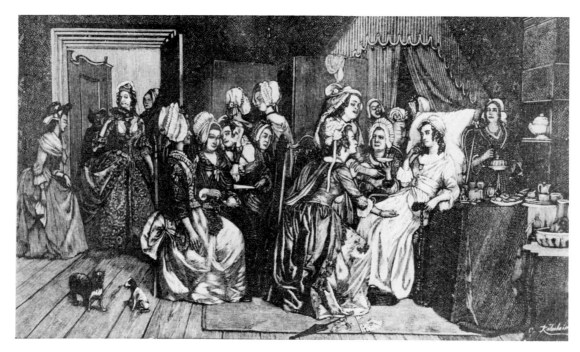

Fig. 4-111. A Danish lying-in room. Oil painting by Wilhelm Nicolai Marstrand (1810–1873). The parturient, having left her bed, is seated in an armchair holding to her nose either a flower or a medicine jar. Surrounding her are the nurse, midwife, friends, and female members of the household. A lady visitor is being received with a curtsy by a young girl, at left.

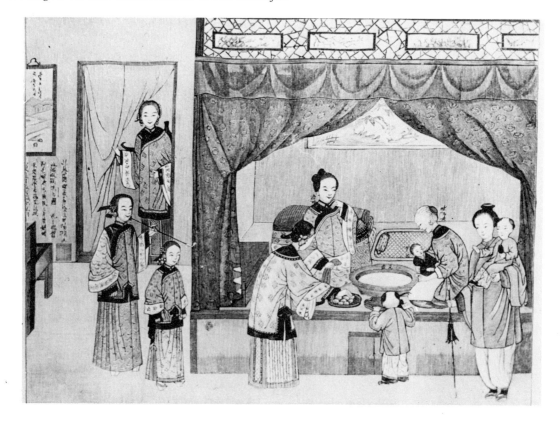

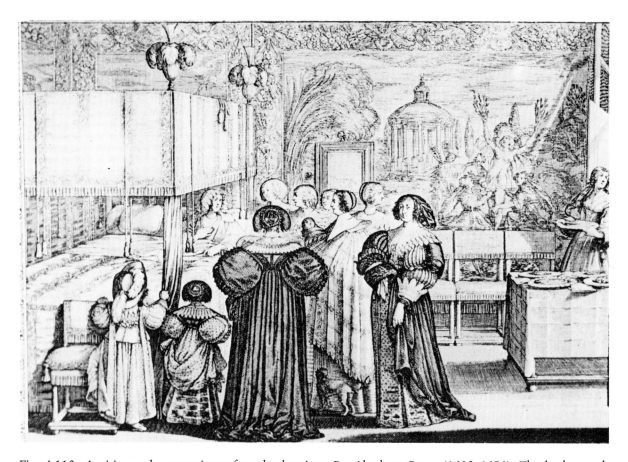

Fig. 4-113. A visit to the parturient after the baptism. By Abraham Bosse (1602–1676). The background painting depicts the birth of Adonis.

Fig. 4-112. Visit to a parturient. Chinese watercolor. The mother, seated on a platform and supported by cushions, is receiving several visitors. The midwife kneels before a basin, holding the newborn infant.

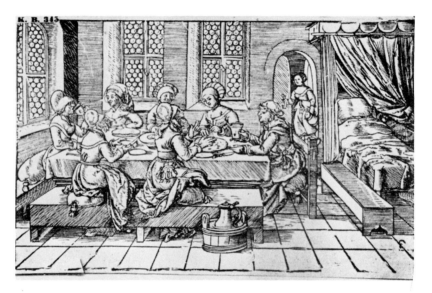

Fig. 4-114. Puerperal feast. Sixteenth century. The entire puerperium of six weeks was a period of celebration, visiting, and feasting. Peter Frank referred to the puerperium as "a constant source of debauchery among womenfolk, and the ruination of midwives." (*System einer vollst-med. Polizei,* Mannheim, 1804) Formerly Germanisches Nationalmuseum, Nürnberg.

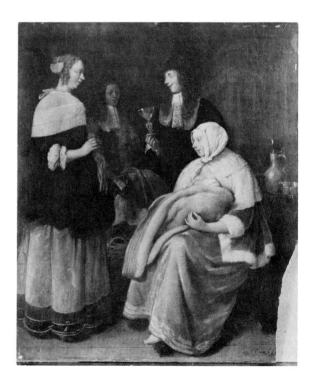

Fig. 4-115. Visit to the Parturient. Painting by Quiringh Gerritsz van Brekelenkam (1620–1668) showing the interior of a Dutch home where well-wishers gathered in large number to drink heavily to the future of the parturient and her offspring.

Chapter 5

THE ANATOMY OF PREGNANCY

The anatomy of pregnancy has been depicted by two general types of illustrations: those of the entire pregnant woman and those of the gravid uterus and its contents. Earliest of the former is found among the *Fünfbilder* or five figures outlining the skeleton, nerves, muscles, veins, and arteries of the human body, and often including a sixth figure revealing the reproductive organs of a pregnant woman. The origin of these diagrammatic figures, all of which show the subject in a semi-squatting posture, has been traced back to the fourteenth century in Persian manuscripts, to the twelfth in European. Some historians believe that both series may be derived from a common source in Hellenistic Alexandria; others ascribe a Mongolian origin to these primitive anatomic drawings.

The earliest known figures of the fetus in utero appear in a ninth century Moschion codex based on Soranus' *Gynecology*. In it the fetus is pictured in 12 different positions, in a flask-shaped uterus. Later manuscripts show 16 positions. These diagrams, copied by Rösslin for his *Rosengarten*, remained the standard illustrations for obstetric texts for 100 years, even after Leonardo da Vinci, from direct personal observation in the early sixteenth century, depicted the fetus in its natural position. Jean-Louis Baudelocque, famous French accoucheur of the eighteenth century, described 94 postures that the intrauterine fetus might assume, in his handbook for midwives (*Principes sur l'art des accouchemens,* Paris, 1775). In the middle of the same century, the beautifully illustrated atlases of William Smellie and William Hunter were published. These contained anatomic representations of the human fetus in utero, faithfully drawn from nature and faultlessly reproduced.

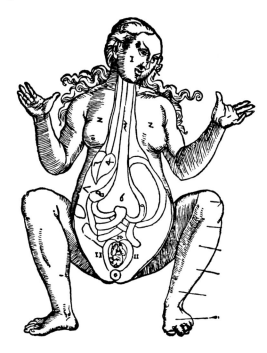

Fig. 5-1. Anatomy of the pregnant woman. From the European prototype of the *Fünfbilder* series, in *Propleumata Aristotelis,* Strassburg, 1543.

154　ICONOGRAPHIA GYNIATRICA

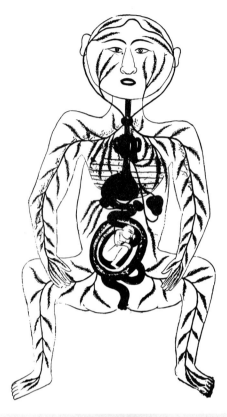

Fig. 5-2. The arterial system of the pregnant woman. From an oriental prototype of the *Fünfbilder* series.

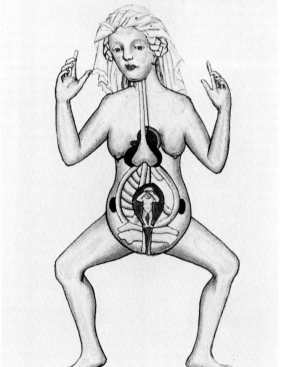

Fig. 5-3. Pregnant woman, miniature, about AD 1400. The woman is pictured without external genitalia. The fetus, in standing position with hands covering eyes, is shown in the traditional flask-shaped uterus. Leipzig Universitätsbibliothek.

THE ANATOMY OF PREGNANCY 155

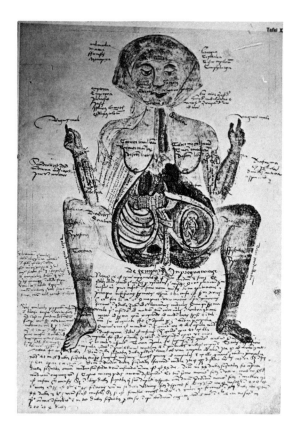

Fig. 5-4. The organs of a pregnant woman. From a manuscript of the late fifteenth century.

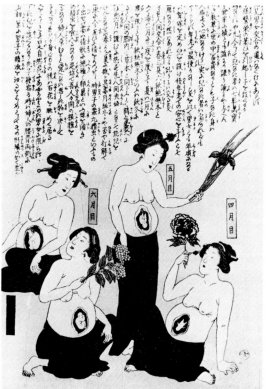

Fig. 5-5. Pregnant women with fetus in utero at various stages of development. Japanese print.

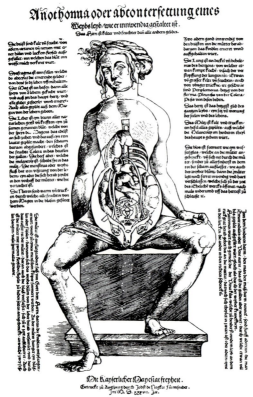

Fig. 5-6. Anatomy of a pregnant woman. Broadside by Jobst de Negker, Augsburg, 1538.

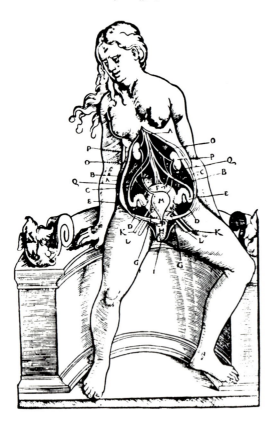

Fig. 5-7. Anatomy of a pregnant woman. From Walther Hermann Ryff's *Description anatomiques de toutes les parties du corps humain,* Paris, 1543. (A Latin edition was also published in Paris the same year.)

THE ANATOMY OF PREGNANCY 157

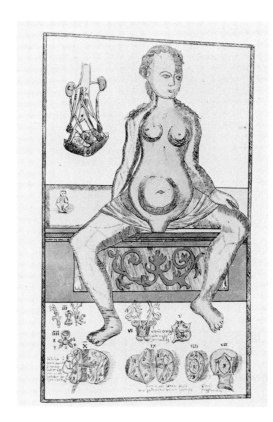

Fig. 5-8. Pregnant woman with figures of her uterus, its contents, and their relations. Broadside from Heinrich Vogtherr, *Tabula foeminae membra demonstrans,* Strassburg, 1539.

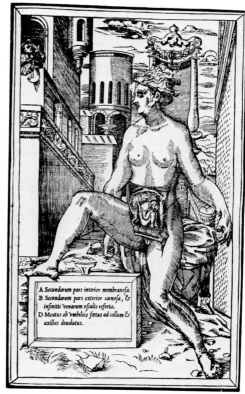

Fig. 5-9. Anatomy of the pregnant woman showing the interior of her uterus. From Charles Estienne's *De dissectione partium corporis humani libri tres,* Paris, 1545, plate XXI. Produced in collaboration with the surgeon Stephanus Riverius, this volume has been hailed as one the finest anatomical works of the sixteenth century.

158 ICONOGRAPHIA GYNIATRICA

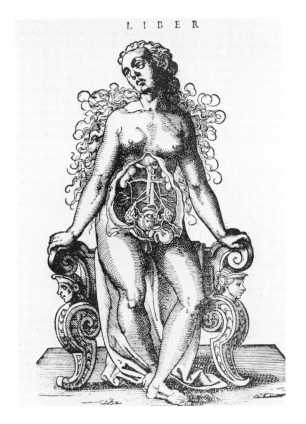

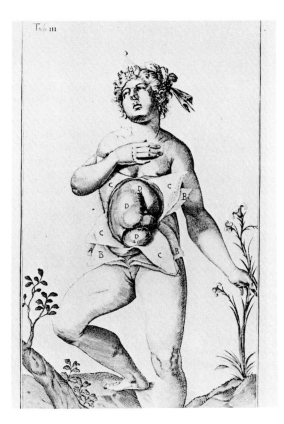

Fig. 5-10. Anatomy of the pregnant woman. From Jacob Rueff's *De conceptu et generatione hominis*, Frankfurt a. M., 1580, p. 11. This edition of Rueff's work was illustrated by Jobst Amman. The anatomical figures were modified from those of Vesalius in the latter's *De humani corporis fabrica*, 1543. Compare this figure with Fig. 1-6.

Fig. 5-11. Gravida at term. From Adrian Spiegel's *De formato foetu*, Padua, 1626.

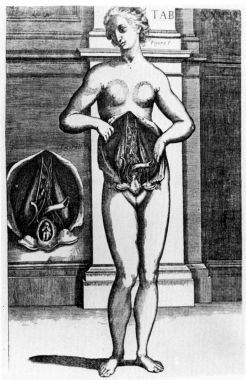

Fig. 5-12. Anatomy of the pregnant woman. An artistic but inaccurate representation from Petro Berrettino's *Tabulae anatomicae*, Rome, 1741.

THE ANATOMY OF PREGNANCY 159

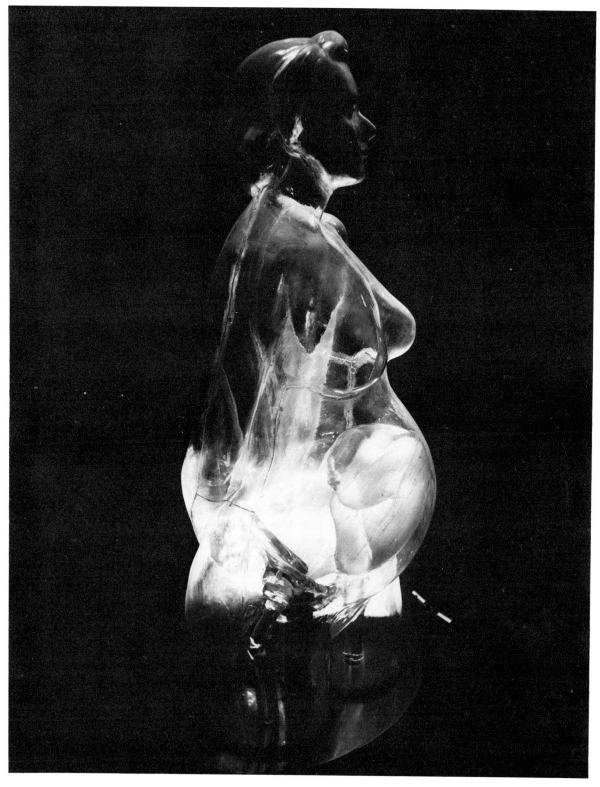

Fig. 5-13. Pregnant woman, transparent plastic model. Museum of Science and Industry, Chicago.

160 ICONOGRAPHIA GYNIATRICA

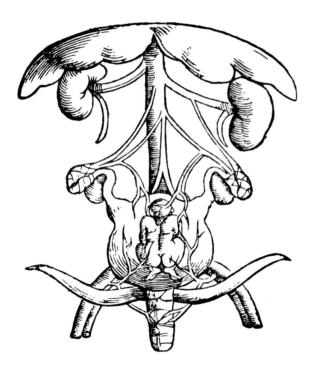

Fig. 5-14. Pregnant uterus, fetus in squatting position. From Walther Hermann Ryff's *Des allerfürtrefflichsten höchsten und adelichsten geschöppffs aller Creaturen*, Strassburg, 1541. (Note similarity of fetal position in next two figures, especially Fig. 5-16.)

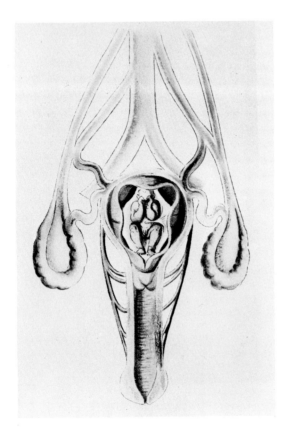

Fig. 5-15. Pregnant uterus and adnexa. From the *Kunstbuch* of Georg Bartisch, 1575.

THE ANATOMY OF PREGNANCY 161

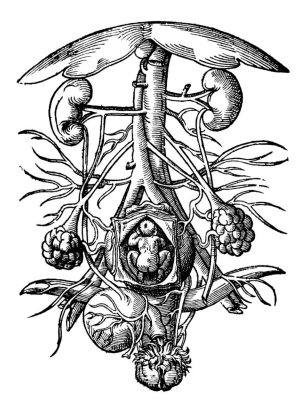

Fig. 5-16. Reproductive tract in pregnancy. From Jacob Rueff's *De conceptu et generatione hominis,* Frankfurt a. M., 1580, p. 16. (Compare with Fig. 5-14.)

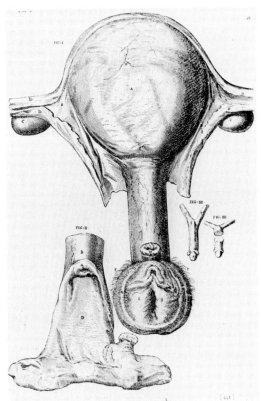

Fig. 5-17. Uterus, about two months pregnant. Schematic drawing from Hieronymus Fabricius' *De formato foetu,* Frankfurt a. M., 1624. Shown also are the ovaries, which Fabricius called *testes penduli.* This major contribution to anatomy and embryology, first published about 1604, contained much new information on the anatomy of the fetus and its membranes and the placenta of many species besides man, including the dog, cat, rabbit, mouse, rat, guinea pig, sheep, cow, goat, deer, horse, pig, and shark.

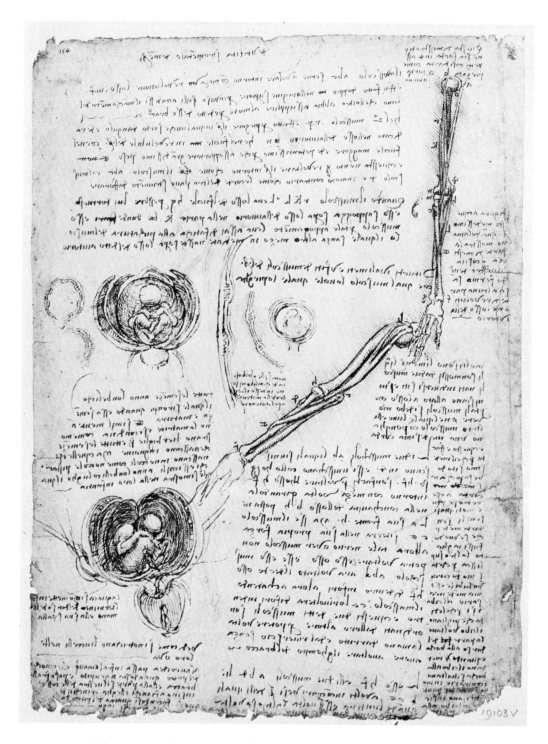

Fig. 5-18. Uterus with fetus. From the notebooks of Leonardo da Vinci, 1510–1512. Leonardo's drawings introduced a new fidelity of detail into medical illustration. Shown here, in contrast to the erroneous drawings that preceded, are the correct relations of cervix and vagina. When William Hunter, about to publish his *The Anatomy of the Human Gravid Uterus* in 1774, witnessed da Vinci's drawings, he stated that the Italian master was 300 years ahead of his time. Windsor Castle.

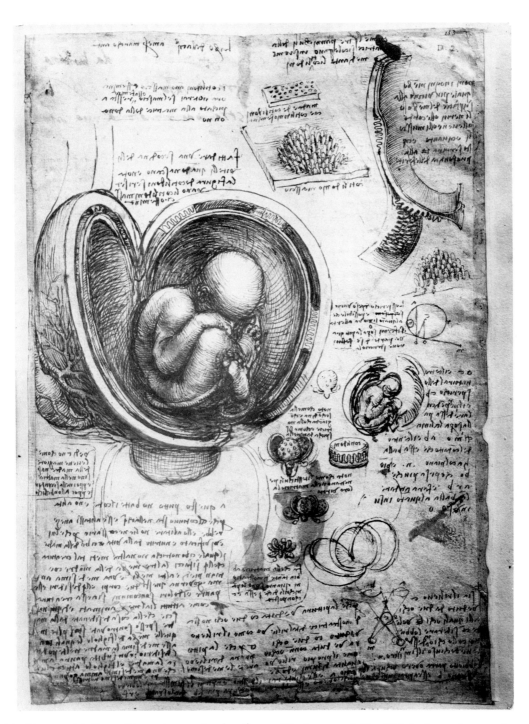

Fig. 5-19. Uterus with fetus. From the notebooks of Leonardo da Vinci, 1510–1512. Clearly shown are the shortened, partially effaced cervix and the dilated adnexal vessels. Noted da Vinci, in his left-handed mirror writing: "See how the great vessels of the mother pass into the uterus..." Of the fetus he commented further, "In the case of this child the heart does not beat and it does not breathe, because it lies continually in water. And if it were to breathe it would be drowned, and breathing is not necessary to it, because it receives life and is nourished from the life and food of the mother." Windsor Castle.

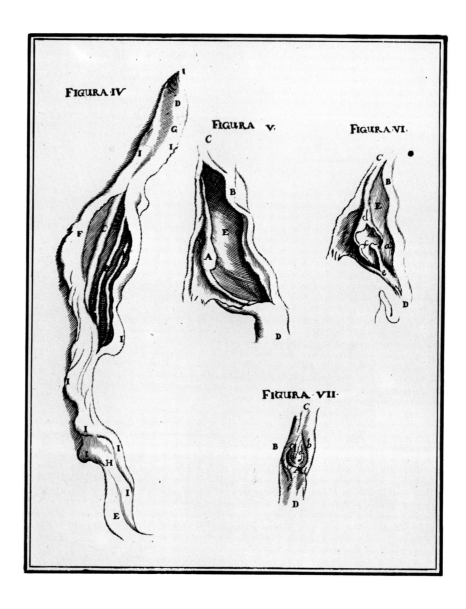

Fig. 5-20. The umbilical vessels and their *folds, valves,* and *nodes.* From Nicolaas Hoboken's *Anatomia secondinae humanae,* Utrecht, 1669. With the publication in 1628 of William Harvey's *Exercitatio anatomica de motu cordis,* the Galenic teaching that the direction of blood flow was the same in both the umbilical vein and the arteries was no longer tenable. Anatomists noted morphologic differences between the umbilical vessels and the blood vessels of the body proper. The umbilical veins, they observed, lacked true valves; but within these vessels, and more noticeably within the umbilical arteries, they saw intraluminal folds or projections to which was ascribed a valvelike function. These structures are best known as the valves or folds of Hoboken, for the Dutch anatomist, physician, mathematician, and philosopher (1632–1678) who gave the first full account of them.

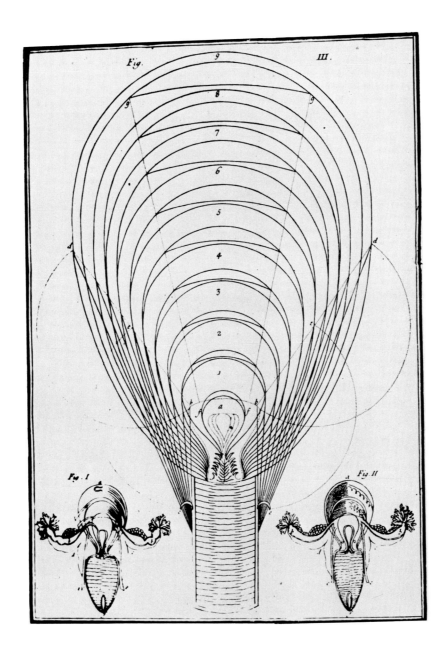

Fig. 5-21. Mechanism of normal pregnancy. Diagrams from André Levret's *L'art des accouchemens*, 2 ed., Paris, 1761, Plate I (1 ed., 1753), schematic coronal sections of the uterus, vagina, and adnexa at progressive stages of pregnancy. Figures I and II, the generative organs at the time of conception and in the first and second months; Figure III, the volumetric relations of the uterus at the various months of gestation, with a geometric representation of the points of insertion of the round ligaments and the fancied sites of attachment of the placenta.

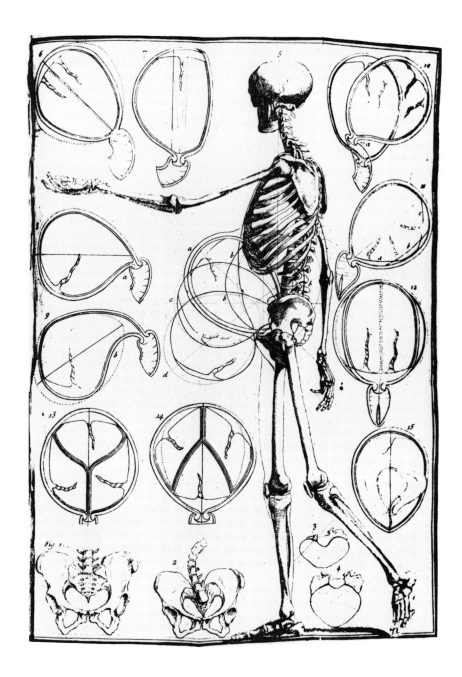

Fig. 5-22. Anatomical variants of pregnancy. Plate from André Levret's *L'art des accouchemens,* 2 ed., Paris, 1761, Plate II, illustrating the normal and rhachitic pelvis, variations in the uterine axis at term, and the forms of placentation in multiple pregnancy.

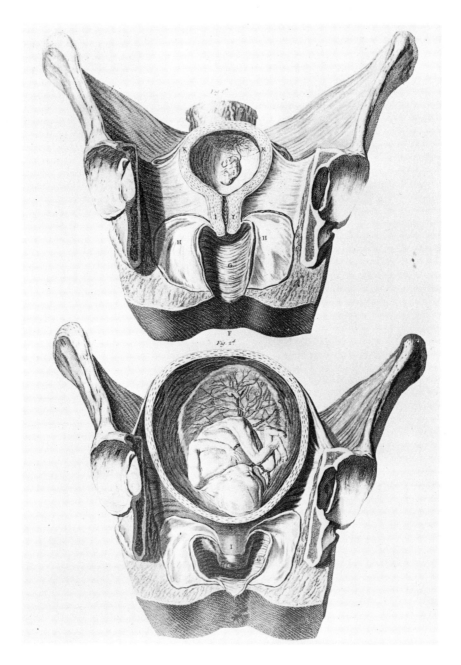

Fig. 5-23. "The *Uterus* as it appears in the second or third month of pregnancy" (upper) and "the *Uterus* in the fourth or fifth month of pregnancy" (lower). From William Smellie's *A Sett of Anatomical Tables*, London, 1754, Plate VI. Of the lower illustration Smellie wrote,

"The *Uterus* now is so largely stretched as to fill all the upper part of the *Pelvis,* and begins also to increase so much as to rest on the brim, and to be supported by the same, the *Fundus* at the same time being raised considerably above the *Pubes*. From the *Abdomen* being now more stretched, the woman is more sensible of her growing bigger, and the *Uterus* also, from the counterpressure of the contents and parietes of the *Abdomen,* is kept down . . ."

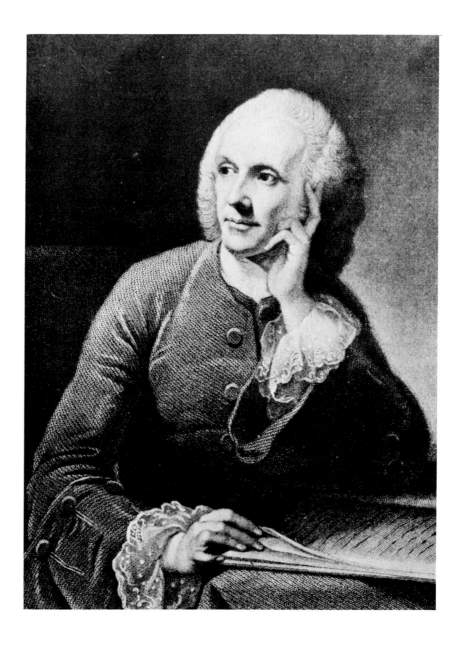

Fig. 5-24. William Hunter (1718–1783). Born at Kilbridge, in Lanarkshire, Scotland, he achieved renown as an obstetrician in London and attended Queen Charlotte in three pregnancies. His brother John attained equal if not greater fame as a surgeon. Before the irreconcilable dispute between them, the two brothers collaborated in anatomic dissections. Best known of William's contributions is his *The Anatomy of the Human Gravid Uterus,* published in 1774. Containing 34 plates with life-size illustrations measuring up to 22 x 16½ in., the majority from drawings by Jan van Rymsdyck, this magnificent folio, representing the labor of nearly a quarter-century, surpassed in both artistic beauty and anatomic accuracy all previous efforts to portray the anatomy of pregnancy. The studies from which this atlas resulted began in 1751, when William obtained the corpse of a woman who died suddenly near the end of pregnancy. Its blood vessels injected with colored wax, the uterus became the subject of the first 10 plates in Hunter's masterpiece. The subsequent plates were based on his dissection of 12 additional pregnant cadavers. The text, in parallel columns of Latin and English, contains only the anatomic description of the illustrations.

THE ANATOMY OF PREGNANCY 169

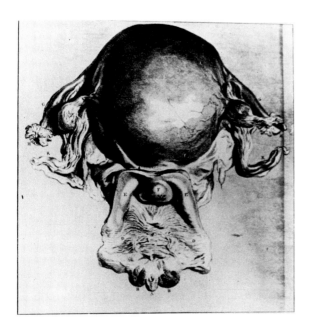

Fig. 5-25. Uterus and adnexa, in the fifth month of pregnancy. From William Hunter's *The Anatomy of the Human Gravid Uterus,* Birmingham, 1774. Shown is the posterior aspect of the uterus, with the vagina slit open to expose the cervix.

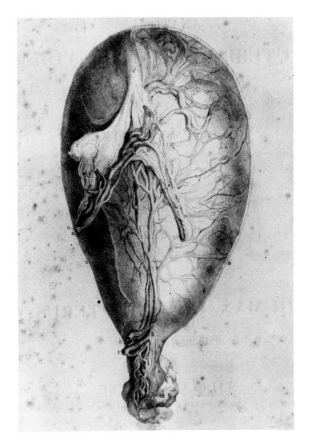

Fig. 5-26. Uterus in the eighth month of pregnancy, viewed from the right side, the blood vessels injected and dissected to show their branching and anastomoses. From William Hunter's *The Anatomy of the Human Gravid Uterus,* Birmingham, 1774, Plate XVI.

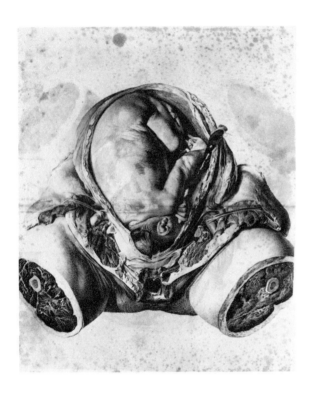

Fig. 5-27. "Child in womb, in its natural situation," anatomical preparation from a woman who died suddenly near the end of pregnancy. From William Hunter's *The Anatomy of the Human Gravid Uterus*, Birmingham, 1774, Plate VI.

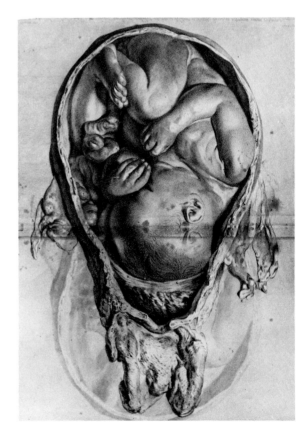

Fig. 5-28. "View of womb and vagina fully opened to show situation of child and placenta at inside of mouth of womb, the occasion of the fatal hemorrhage," anatomical preparation from a woman with placenta previa. From William Hunter's *The Anatomy of the Human Gravid Uterus*, Birmingham, 1774, Plate XII.

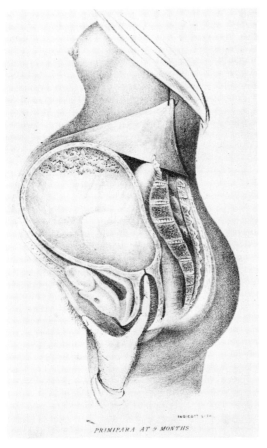
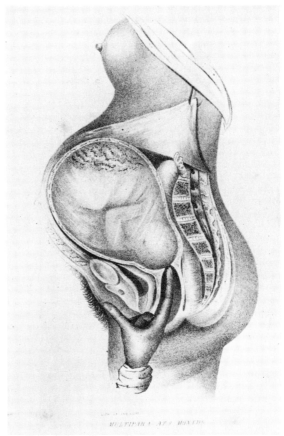

Fig. 5-29. The cervix at term, figures contrasting the uneffaced, closed cervix of the primipara, left, with the effaced, partially dilated cervix of the multipara, right. From Evory Kennedy's *Observations on Obstetric Auscultation with Notes and Additional Illustrations,* by Isaac E. Taylor, J. & H. G. Langley, New York, 1843.

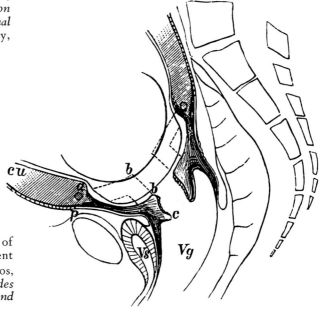

Fig. 5-30. Concept of Ludwig Bandl (1842–1892) of the relations of the cervix and lower uterine segment in late pregnancy and labor, (b) histologic internal os, (a) retraction ring. From his *Über das Verhalten des Uterus und Cervix in der Schwangerschaft und während der Geburt,* Enke, Stuttgart, 1876.

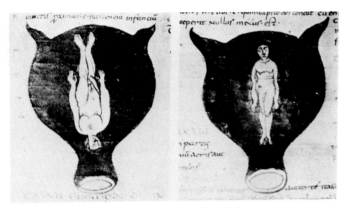

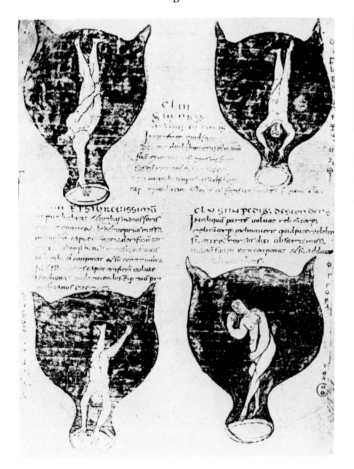

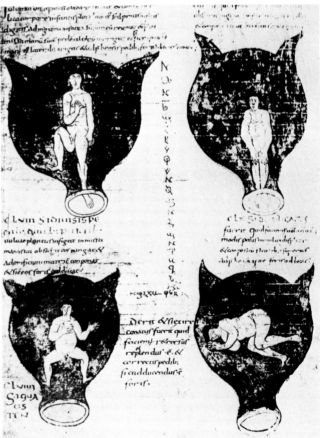

Fig. 5-31. Positions of the fetus in utero. From a ninth century Moschion manuscript. Of unknown place and date of birth or death, Moschion, identified only by this single name, translated the *Gynecology* of Soranus from Greek into Latin, probably about AD 580, in an abridged form consisting of questions and answers, for the instruction of midwives. Copies of Moschion's manuscript, of various dates, are owned by several European libraries. Each manuscript contains slightly different illustrations, reflecting changing concepts of uterine form; all, however, show the fetus in much the same crude, stylized fashion. These figures of the fetus in utero were adopted, with little change, by the major obstetric texts of the sixteenth, seventeenth, and eighteenth centuries. Bibliothèque Royale, Brussels.

A
B C

THE FETAL POSITIONS

"... the foetus in the later months of pregnancy assumes a characteristic posture, which is described as its *attitude* or *habitus;* and, as a general rule, it may be said to form an ovoid mass, which roughly corresponds with the shape of the uterine cavity. Thus, it is folded or bent upon itself in such a way that the back becomes markedly convex, the head is sharply flexed so that the chin is almost in contact with the breast, the thighs are flexed over the abdomen, the legs are bent at the knee-joints, and the arches of the feet rest upon the anterior surfaces of the legs. The arms are usually crossed over the thorax or are parallel to the sides, while the umbilical cord lies in the space between them and the lower extremities.

This attitude is usually retained throughout pregnancy, though it is frequently modified somewhat by the movements of the extremities, and in rare instances the head may become extended, when a totally different posture is assumed. The characteristic attitude results partly from the mode of growth of the foetus, and partly from a process of accommodation between it and the outlines of the uterine cavity." [J. W. Williams: *Obstetrics.* D. Appleton & Co., New York, 1903, p. 180.]

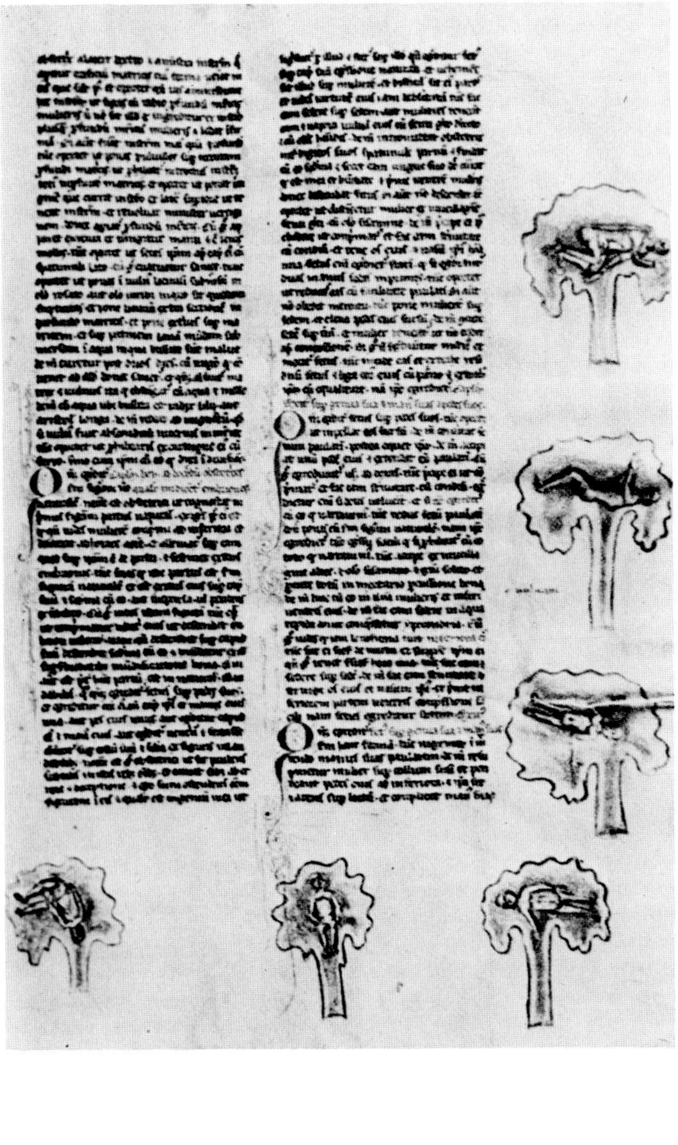

Fig. 5-32. Positions of the fetus in utero. From a manuscript translation by Gerard of Cremona (1114–1187) of the *Surgery* of Abulcasis. Biblioteca Nazionale Marciano, Venice.

174 ICONOGRAPHIA GYNIATRICA

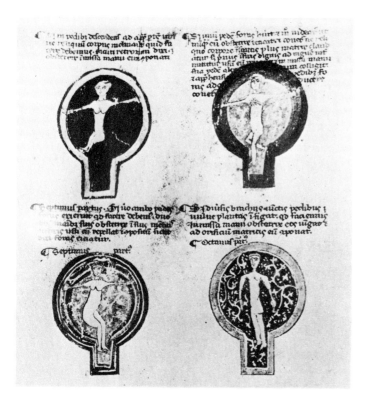

Fig. 5-33. Positions of the fetus in utero. From a thirteenth century manuscript of Moschion. Universitätsbibliothek, Munich.

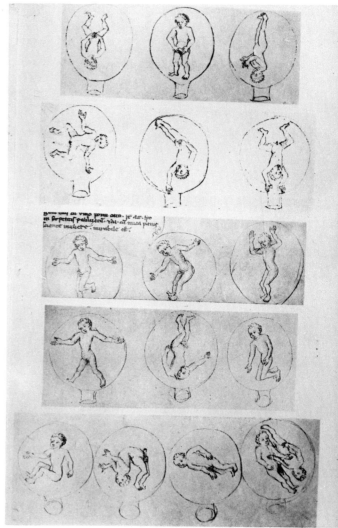

Fig. 5-34. Positions of the fetus in utero. Drawings from another thirteenth century Moschion manuscript. Bibliothèque Nationale, Paris.

THE ANATOMY OF PREGNANCY   175

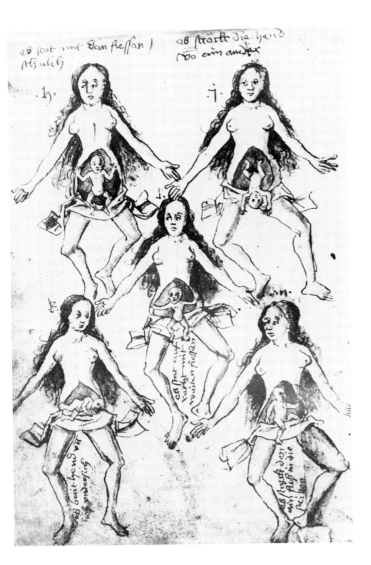

Fig. 5-36. Positions of the fetus in utero. Illustrations from a fifteenth century manuscript of Hermann Heyms, royal physician at Rothenburg ob der Tauber, Bavaria, and rector of the Wiener Hochschule, 1472. Heyms is believed to have written a large part of the codex in his own hand. His illustrations clearly show the Moschion influence. Königliche Öffentliche Bibliothek, Dresden.

Fig. 5-35. Positions of the fetus in utero. Watercolor illustrations from a fifteenth century Moschion manuscript. Universitätsbibliothek, Erlangen, Germany.

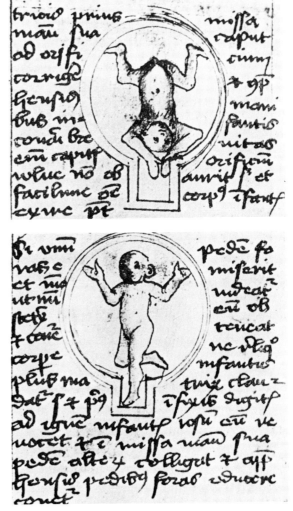

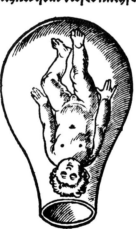

Fig. 5-37. Positions of the fetus in utero. Taken directly from the illustrations in the Moschion manuscript, with but trivial modifications, were these figures from the *Rosengarten* of Eucharius Rösslin, published initially in 1513, the first obstetric text for midwives in the German language. Most of these illustrations were faithfully reproduced in *La Comare*, the Italian counterpart by Scipione Mercurio, first published in 1595.

⁋Zū de tritten/so die zeit d̄ ge
burt hie ist/so soll in natürlicher
g̃ burt d̄ ussgāg des kindes be
hend vn̄ ring sein/on mercklich
verlegerũg Aber das heißt die
vnnatürlich geburt die nit ge
schicht wie yetzundt gesagt ist.
Doch spricht Auicenna/wan
d̄z kindt vß müter leib köpt zū
ersten mit d̄e füesse/vn̄ hat sein
arm/sein hend nebē seine seite
hinab vff die dicke der bein ge
streckt/als in dieser figur be
zeichnet ist das solichs ein vn

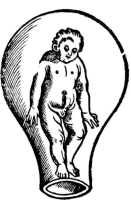

natürlich geburt sie/doch sey sie aller gleichest der natür
lichen geburt/darūb das sie nit gantz als sorglich ist als
ander vnnatürlich geburten.

B

⁋Wo aber d̄z kind erscheynt
vn̄ kompt mit vnnatürlicher
geburt/mit bede füessen/vnd
seind die hend vnnd arm ne
ben den beinē hinab gestreckt
als dise figur anzeygen ist/
so sol die bebam die arm vn̄
hend des kindes schickliche wy
sen/siege vn̄ schybē/mit sal
bē vn̄ anderen dingē die glatt
machē. Also d̄z die hend vnd
arm des kindes gestreckt blei
bē/nebē des kind seitē vnder
sich hinab an die dicke d̄ bein
Vnd darnach sol sie im von
stadt helffen Wo aber es mö
glich wer/das die bebam die
füess des kindes sennftiklichē
vn̄ subtilichē obersich wyse/
also d̄z inwedig in müter leib
die solen des kindes füesslin/
geschybē wurdet gegē d̄ mü
ter nabel/vnd sein heuptlin
gegē seiner müter rucke/vnd
sich gegē dē vssgang gestürtzt
vn̄ gewendet/wer vyl bösser

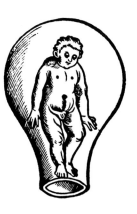

D

ter die frucht nit ring geberē kan. ⁋Zūm vierdē mal d̄z
umb d̄z im affterē seind eyssen/schrūdē/geschwell̄ug d̄
plütadrē die mā nēnet die güldin ader̄/od̄ verstopff̄ug
des hertē vestē stülgangs. Vn̄ auch so die fraw nit wol
mag vnd sich truckē/vō des wege die bermüter gehindert
würt an ire werck. ⁋Zūm fünfften mal darūb d̄z die fraw
blöd ist vn̄ kracker coplexion/od̄ kalter natur/zū iung/zū
alt/zū feißt/zū dürr/zū mager/die vor nit kind gehebt
hat/vnd forchtsam vn̄ vnlydlich ist/Darumb sie auch
vnrüwig würt vnd einer schnellen bewegūg von einem
ort zū dem andern/die sie bringt vnd ursachet zū vnbequē
licher harter geburt. ⁋Zūm sechsten ist zū wissen das ein
knab vyl ringer zū geberē ist dan̄ ein meytlin. ⁋Zūm sy
bēden mal ist die geburt hart vn̄ schwarlich/so d̄z kind zū
vyl groß ist/darūb das
es die schloß seiner mü
ter nit leichtiglich durch
tringē mag. Auch wan̄
d̄z kid zū klein ist v̄.z zū
leicht/darūb d̄z es sich
vnd sich vester münder
wendet vn̄ senckt/vnd
mind mag vß getruckt
werden.
⁋Zūm achten mal/d̄z
umb das der kind mer
dan̄ eins ist/Oder ein
kindt mitt mer glidern
dā natürlich ist/besun
der mit zweyē heuptern
als in disem .xij. iar in
der graffschafft. Wer

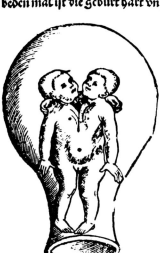

⁋Wo aber d̄z kind erscheint
mit beyden füssen/vnd hatt
die hend nit neben im/vnder
sich hinab gestreckt/als ob
stadt/sonder obersich.

E

F

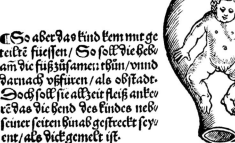

⁋So aber das kind kem mit ge
teilte füessen/So soll die heb
am die füß zūsamen thūn/vnnd
darnach ußfüren/als ob stadt.
Doch soll sie alltzeit fleiß anke
rē das die hend des kindes nebē
seiner seiten hinab gestreckt sey
ent/als dick gemelt ist.

C ij

⁋Wo aber das kind zum
erſten kem mit einem fůß al=
lein/ So ſoll man die můter
do an rucken legen/ die bein
vberſich/ dz haupt vnderſich
vnd den hindern wol erheben
Vñ ſol die hebam mit ir håd
des kindes fůß wider hinder=
ſich ſentffrüklichē ſchybē/ Vñ
ſoll die můter ſich zům dicker
male vmbſchybē vnd waltzē/
ſo lang biß dz kind ſein haupt
vnderſich gekeret/ zů dem vß=
gāg/ Darnach ſoll die můter
widerumb ſitzē vff iren ſtůl
vñ ſol ir die hebam wid helff=
en als obſtat.

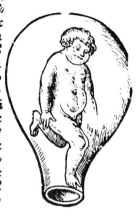

G

⁋Iſt ob das kind ein hand
erzeugte/ So ſol die hebam
das kind mit empfahē/ ſondʒ
ſie ſoll mit yngelaßner håd
die ſchultern des kindes be=
greiffen vnd hinderſich ſchē
vnd die hand neben des kin=
des ſeyten hynab ſtrecke/ dz
haupt begreiffen/ vñ im zů
vßgāg helffen. Wo aber ſo=
lich wyſen vnd ſchicken der
hend nit ein fürgāg wolt ha
ben So iſt aber not dz man
die fraw an ruckē lege/ vnd
mit dē haupt nider vnd mit
dē hindern hoch/ damit das
das kind hinderſich fall/ vñ
als dan wider ſitzē/ vñ dem
kind zů vßgang helffen.

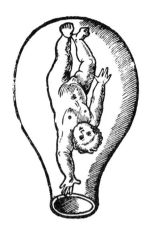

H

J

⁋Wo aber das kind ſich in můter leib nit wolt vmbwen
den damit das das haupt vnderſich keme/ ſo ſoll die hebā
am den andern fůß auch zů der geburt ſchicken/ vnd dem
kind vßhelffen/ doch allwegen das die arm vnd hend ne=
ben ſeiner ſeiten hinaß geſtreckt ſeyent/ als obſtat.

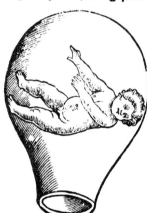

⁋Wo aber das kind ke=
me mit einer ſeitē an die
geburt/ So ſoll aber die
hebam das kind ſchicke/
richten vnd wyſen vber=
ſich/ wie es vorhin in mů
ter leib geſeſſen iſt vñ im
darnach zů bequēlichem
vßgang helffen.

⁋Item ob der kinde mer
dañ eins wer/ als zwiling
vnd ſich gleich erzeugten
mit den höuptern/ So ſol
die hebam eins nach dem
andern vßfůrē/ beſonder
das erſt empfahen/ als ob
ſtadt/ vnd das ander nitt
verlaſſen.

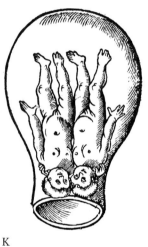

I

K

L

⁋Vnd ſo das kind ſich mit
den kniwen erzeugt/ od mit
einē kni kem an die geburt
So ſoll die hebam dz kind
vberſich heben vnd die fůß
begreiffen/ vñ wie obgeſchri
ben iſt dem kind zů vßgang
helffen

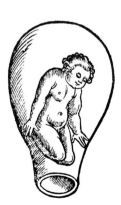

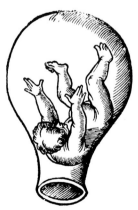

⁋Item ob das kind mit ge=
bognem/ geneygtē od krum
mem haupt erſchyne/ Soll
die hebam das haupt ſchicke
vñ die achſeln leichtlich vber
ſich heben/ vnd vßfůren

THE ANATOMY OF PREGNANCY 179

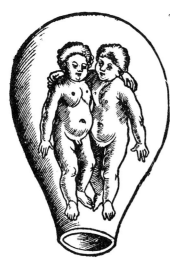

⁋Wo aber die zwiling kommen mitt den füessen/ Sol sie aber mals thün fleiß inkeren/ eins nach dem anderen vß füren/in massen als ob stadt.

M

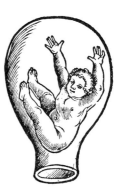

⁋Item ob das kind sich mit de hindern erzeügte/ So soll die hebam mit yngelaßner handt das kind obersich hebe/ vn mit den füssen vßfuren

Wo aber müglich wer das sie das kind schyben möcht/ damit es mit de haupt vndersich kem/ wer vyl besser dan die erst geburt.

P

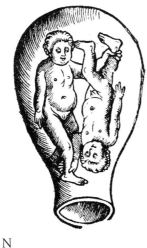

⁋So aber der zwyling einer kompt mit dem haupt der ander mit den füessen Sol abermals die hebam fleiß ankere/ dem nechsten zu ersten helffen/ vnd das ander nit verlassen/ Vnd das soll also geschehe/ on quetzung ir beyder.

N

O

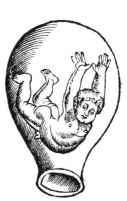

⁋Ite ob das kind geteilt lege oder vff seinem angesicht/ so soll die hebam leichtlich ynlassen ir finger/ vnd dz kind in der seite der muter vmkere/ Oder ob sie ein handt mag ynlassen soll sie dz kind ordnen vn richte also/ Welche theil des lybs de vßgang aller nechst seind/ die selbe soll sie halten vn vß füre/ doch sol sie aller meist dz haupt süche/ halte vn vßfüre.

Q

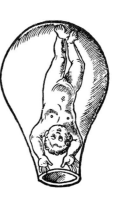

⁋Ob aber das kind mit beiden henden rschyne/ so soll die heb am mit iren hede beid schultern oder achßlen begreiffen/ vn das kind wid hindersich heben/ Vn als oben geschabe stadt/ des kindes hend nebe seinen seiten hynab strecken/ vnd das haupt begreiffen/ vnd im darnach zu vßgang helffen.

R

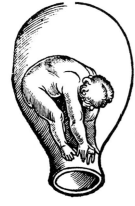

⁋Vnd so das kind keme mit beyden oder einem füß/ vnnd mit dem haupt/ Als dan soll die hebam das haupt begreiffen/ vnd die füeß obersich richten/ vnnd also dem kind zu vßgang helffen.

Æ ij

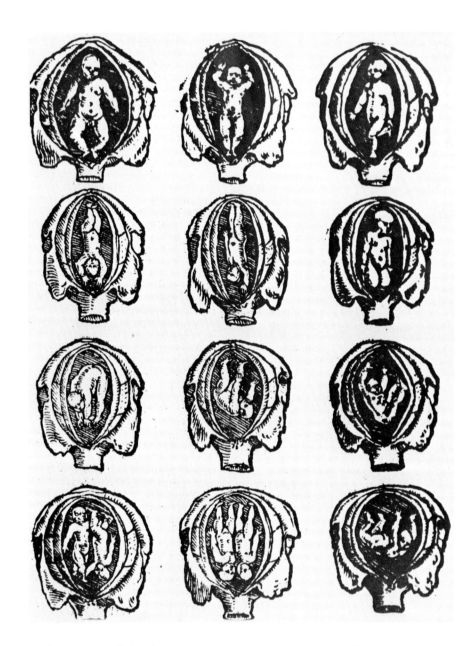

Fig. 5-38. Abnormal positions of the fetus in utero. From Johannes Dryander's *Artzenei Spiegel*, Frankfurt a. M., 1547.

THE ANATOMY OF PREGNANCY 181

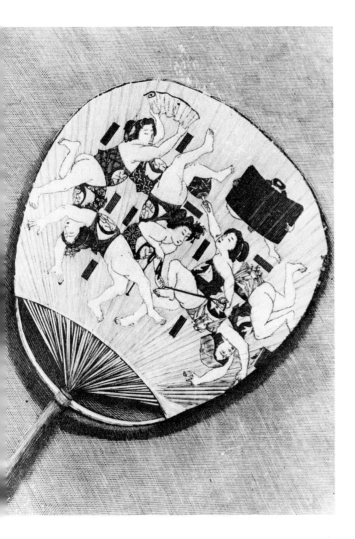

Fig. 5-39. Positions of the fetus in utero. Novelty fan from a Japanese teahouse. The five upper bodies and five lower bodies are cleverly arranged so that they can be combined in nine different ways to form the figures of pregnant women.

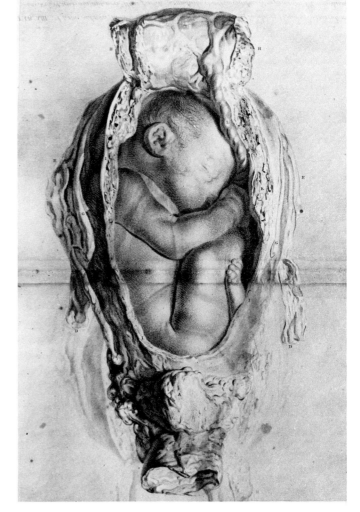

Fig. 5-40. Breech presentation, in a woman who died in the ninth month of pregnancy. Table XIII from William Hunter's *The Anatomy of the Human Gravid Uterus*, Birmingham, 1774.

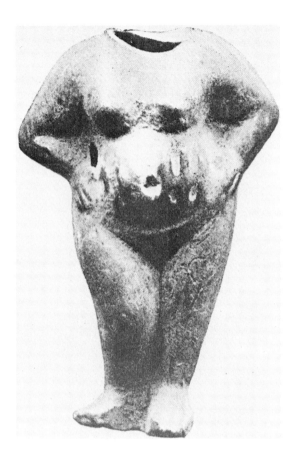

Fig. 5-41. *Striae gravidarum*. During the puerperium, rapid readjustments take place from the pregnant to the nonpregnant state. The *striae gravidarum* or "stretch marks," which develop during pregnancy over the lower abdomen, also on the breasts, thighs, and buttocks, tend to fade, the markings becoming silvery and inconspicuous. In some women, however, the pigmentation in the *striae* persists, bearing permanent testimony to the woman's motherhood. Shown here, with *striae gravidarum,* a figure of a parturient from the third century BC or earlier, discovered near Izmir, on the Gulf of Smyrna, an inlet of the Aegean Sea.

EXTRAUTERINE PREGNANCY

"If the Egg is too big, or if the Diameter of the *Tuba Fallopiana* is too small, the Egg stops, and can get no farther, but shoots forth, and takes root there; and having the same Communication with the Blood-Vessels of the Tuba, that it would have had with those of the Womb, had it fallen into it, is nourished, and grows big to such a degree, that the Membrane of the Tuba being capable of no such Dilatation as that of the Uterus, breaks at last, and the *Foetus* falls into the Cavity of the *Abdomen*; where it sometimes lies dead for many years and at other times occasions the death of the Mother, by breaking open its Prison." [Pierre Dionis: *A General Treatise of Midwifery.* London, 1719, p. 81, translated from his *Traité général des accouchemens.* Paris, 1718.]

The first known reference to extrauterine pregnancy appears in the writings of the famous Arabian physician Abulcasis (936–1013). Confirmation of this complication was late in coming, however, because of the restrictions on human dissection, limited to executed criminals, mostly male. Not until the seventeenth century were autopsies performed in significant number on the bodies of people who died of disease. With the increasing availability of cadavers and the liberalization of anatomic study, extrauterine pregnancy came to light. Jean Riolan, a Parisian surgeon and anatomist, recorded the first authentic case in 1616, fatal tubal rupture in a 31 year old multipara on January 3, 1604.

THE ANATOMY OF PREGNANCY 183

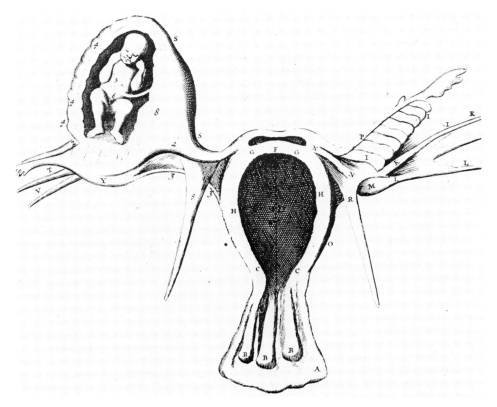

Fig. 5-42. A seventeenth century concept of tubal pregnancy. Illustration from Reinier de Graaf's *De mulierum organis generationi inservientibus,* Leyden, 1672.

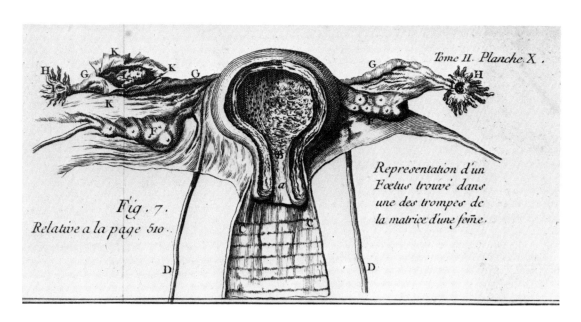

Fig. 5-43. Tubal pregnancy, discovered at autopsy in 1689 on a woman of 23 years and reported by J. G. Duverney in his *Oeuvres anatomiques,* vol. 2, Paris, 1761.

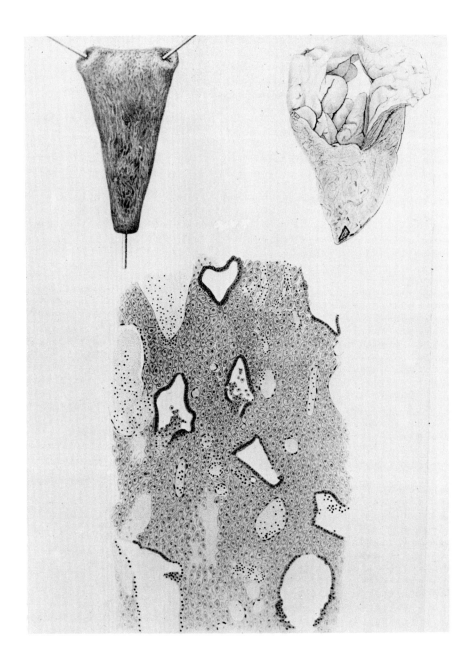

Fig. 5-44. The decidua in ectopic pregnancy. Illustrations from the 1891 monograph of Paul Zweifel showing decidual casts expelled from the uterus in cases of ectopic gestation and a histologic section of the endometrium with its characteristic decidual cells. Describing the genital organs of a woman who died of an ectopic pregnancy, P.A. Boehmer called attention, two centuries ago, to the decidual membrane lining her uterus (*Observationum anatomicarum rariorum,* Halle, 1752–6), an observation confirmed two decades later by John Hunter (*Medical and Philosophical Commentaries,* ed. 2, vol. 1, London, 1774 p. 429). Estimates vary as to the frequency with which uterine decidua is recoverable in cases of early tubal pregnancy. Its frequent absence from curettings is attributed to prior slough, either piecemeal as in menstruation or, rarely, as an intact endometrial cast.

THE ANATOMY OF PREGNANCY 185

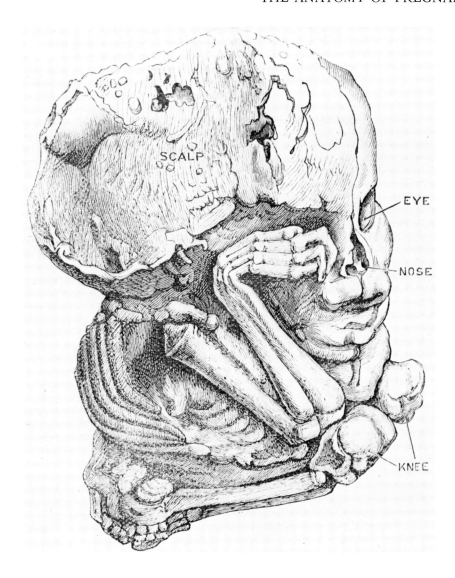

Fig. 5-45. Lithopedion, a compressed, shrivelled, and partly ossified fetus, 4 inches in greatest diameter, excised from the fallopian tube of a woman in whom it had been retained for more than 14 years. The operation was performed successfully in Hamburg, Germany, in the early nineteenth century. The preserved specimen, purchased by the Royal College of Surgeons of England, was destroyed in the bombing of London in 1941.

In modern practice, ectopic pregnancy is treated by surgical removal of the conceptus. Until late in the nineteenth century, however, when laparotomy carried grave risk, surgical intervention was undertaken rarely, and then only as a last resort. The first abdominal operation for ectopic pregnancy was performed in 1759 by John Bard (1716–1799), New York surgeon and father of Samuel Bard (*Medical Observations and Inquiries II*, London, 1762, 369–372). Alexander Hamilton, Scottish obstetrician, in 1784 wrote in his *Outlines of the Theory and Practice of Midwifery*, "When nature points it out, by a local inflammation or abscess, the foetus, or bones of the foetus, may be cut upon and extracted; but otherwise the Surgeon's art will not avail . . ." Some patients were treated by venesection; in many cases efforts were made to destroy the fetus, as by injecting it with morphine or by subjecting it to a galvanic current. Often the condition remained undiagnosed. If the woman survived, the retained extrauterine fetus then underwent absorption, liquefaction, or compression, occasionally calcification. The fetal bones sometimes eroded into the woman's hollow viscera, especially bowel, from which they were eventually extruded. Rarely the calcified fetus, or lithopedion, was retained for years, to be discovered only at autopsy.

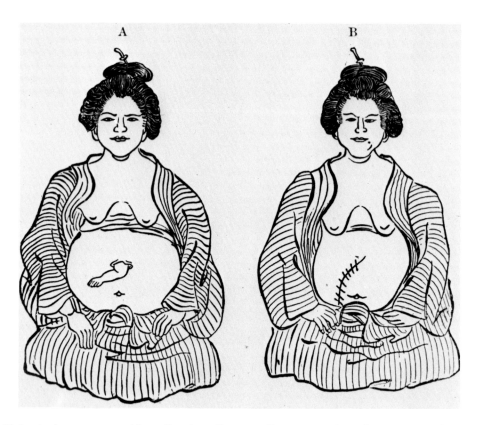

Fig. 5-46. Abdominal pregnancy, with perforation of the maternal abdomen by a fetal arm. Illustrations of a Japanese patient, late nineteenth century, before and after successful operation.

Chapter 6

MAN'S BEGINNINGS
Embryology

Only recently in the history of man has he learned to associate the birth of his children with antecedent sexual union rather than to the intervention of his gods. Some primitive peoples, failing to recognize the relation between coitus and generation, still date pregnancy from the onset of quickening. The Arunta and other Australian aborigines regard the mother as merely an incubator for the developing infant, viewing the relation between parent and child as essentially social rather than physiologic.

Among the earliest evidence of embryologic knowledge and of a recognition of the parental role in the reproductive process is a hymn to the sun god Aton, written in the fourteenth century BC by Amenophis IV (Akhnaton) and translated 34 centuries later by James H. Breasted.

Creator of the germ in woman
Maker of seed in man,
Giving life to the son in the body of his
    mother,
Soothing him that he may not weep,
Nurse (even) in the womb,
Giver of breath to animate everyone that he
    maketh
When he cometh forth from the womb on the
    day of his birth,
Thou openest his mouth in speech,
Thou suppliest his necessity.

Job says, "Hast thou not poured me out as milk, and curdled me like cheese?" (Job 10:10). The Wisdom of Solomon, chapter 7, tells in like vein, "I . . . in my mother's womb was fashioned to be flesh in the time of ten months, being compacted in blood, of the seed of man, and pleasure that came with sleep." (*The Apocrypha,* Authorised Version, 1611). The union of the male and female elements was explained by Aristotle, in the fourth century BC. The mammalian egg, he taught, resulted from the admixture within the uterus of the menstrual blood and the male semen. The female seed gave substance to the embryo; the male, the formative impulse to its growth.

According to the Talmudists, the formation of the embryo required three essentials, provided respectively by the father, the mother, and God. From the father came the white semen, from which the infant's bones, brain, and whites of the eyes originated; from the mother, the red semen, for the formation of the skin, flesh, hair, and iris. Facial expression, vision, hearing, speech, and motion were given by God himself. Almost identical was the teaching of the Indian Ayur-Veda (sixth to seventh century BC) that four factors enter into the formation of the fetus: (1) the father's semen, (2) the mother's blood, (3) the *átman* or subtle body composed of fire, earth, air, and water, and (4) the *manas* or

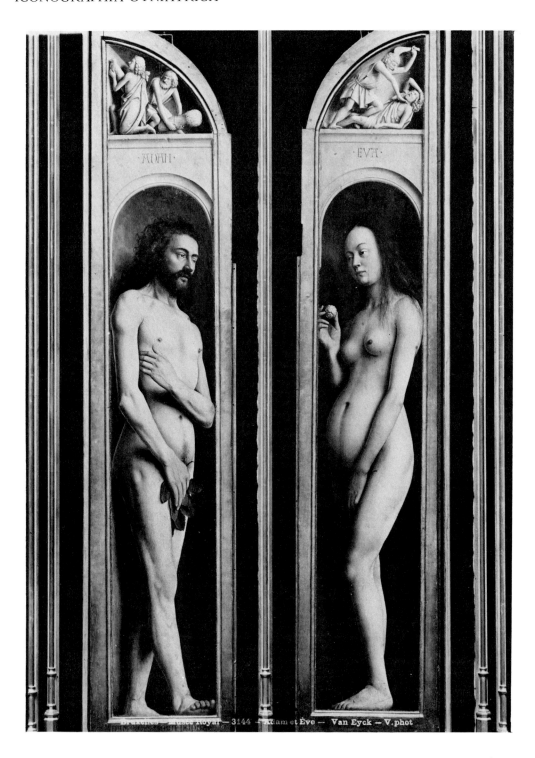

Fig. 6-1. Adam and Eve, end panels of altarpiece completed in 1432 by the van Eyck brothers, Huybrecht (1366?–1426) and Jan (1390?–1440). These figures showed a new appreciation of human form and dignity. Adam, once bowed by shame, symbolizing man's Original Sin, now stands erect, divinely created. In contrast to many medieval representations, the primeval pair are depicted here with navels. Cathedral of St. Bavon, Ghent, Belgium.

mind. The child's sex, added Alcmaeon in the sixth century BC, corresponded to that of the parent contributing the greater quantity of seed.

Somewhat different was the view of generation espoused by the great Galen, in the second century BC. The female semen, he taught, originating in the ovarian vessels, was separated or strained in the *female testes* (ovaries), then passed down the tubes and into the uterus. Union there with the semen produced a frothy coagulum, from which the embryo evolved. Like Hippocrates, Galen believed that male infants were a product of the right ovary; females, of the left.

Virtually unquestioned for more than a millennium was the doctrine of preformation or *emboîtement* which regarded the fetus as the product of the female. Each being in compressed form lay encapsulated within the body of its mother; successive generations resulted from the mere unshelling and subsequent increase in size of the next order of individuals. Seneca wrote (c. 3 BC–AD 65) in his *Quaestiones naturales*,

"In the seed are enclosed all the parts of the body of the man that shall be formed. The infant that is borne in his mother's wombe hath the rootes of the beard and hair that he shall weare one day. In this little masse likewise are all the linements of the bodie and all that which posterity shall discover in him."

After Antoni van Leeuwenhoek (1632–1723), the Dutch draper and lens grinder, published his sensational discovery of spermatozoa in 1678, divergent doctrines developed. The animalculists, or spermists, regarded this newly discovered cell as the real germ of the embryo; and by the end of the seventeenth century Niklaas Hartsoeker and Dalenpatius (pseudonym of François de Plantades, secretary of the Montpellier Academy of Sciences) had published illustrations of the imaginary homunculus, a miniature human being within the sperm.

The ovists or ovulists, on the other hand, insisted that the egg is the "common original of all animals." William Harvey (1578–1657), best known for his discovery of the circulation of the blood, attributed to the sperm an intangible influence, or *aura seminalis,* which explained the resemblance of offspring to father, but he denied the sperm's role in the formation of the embryo.

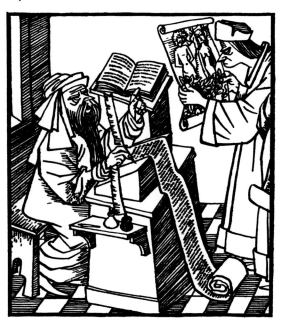

Fig. 6-2. A twentieth century caricature of a medieval woodcut depicting study of the question whether Adam and Eve had navels. In many of the medieval and Renaissance paintings of the first pair the mid-abdomen, as well as the pubic region, was covered with greenery, not for fear that sight of the umbilicus would result in titillation, but to bypass the theological question of the structure's existence in the original sinners. Since Adam was created from dust and Eve from one of Adam's ribs, neither was ever nourished through an umbilical cord. Would the Deity, some asked, who creates nothing superfluous, have endowed the pair with navels? Or, as others held, were Adam and Eve blessed with navels as the archetypes of all humanity?

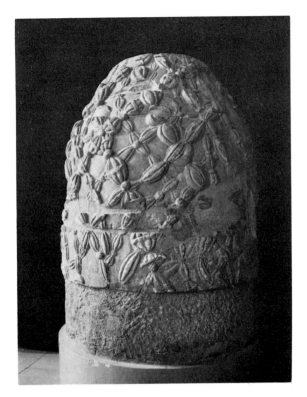

Fig. 6-3. The Omphalos of Delphi, found near the great altar of Delphi. It was regarded by the ancient Greeks as the central point of the Earth. Venerated in Greek mythology the umbilicus was symbolized by this marble omphalic statue. Its ornamental bands in criss-cross relief, intertwined but not knotted, are believed symbolic of the intimate relation of life and death.

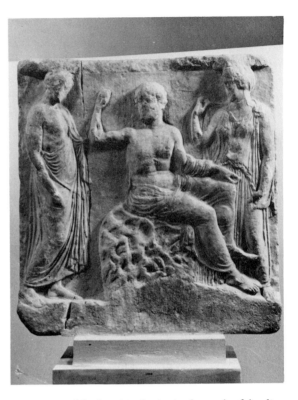

Fig. 6-4. Asklepios (Asclepius), the god of healing, sitting on the Omphalos, symbol of divine intuition, with the goddess Hygeia at his side. Stone relief, fifth century, from the Athens Asklepieion. National Archaeological Museum, Athens.

Resurrected by Harvey in the early seventeenth century was the theory of epigenesis, voiced by Aristotle 1,000 years earlier. Denying the doctrine of preformation, the proponents of epigenesis viewed the embryo's growth as a gradual aggregation and building up of its component parts. Little attention did this radical view receive until the publication in 1759 of Caspar Friedrich Wolff's *Theoria generationis*. Peering through his microscope into the chick embryo, Wolff saw not an expansion of a pre-existing form, but rather a host of minute globules producing the organs of the embryo by growth and multiplication. Thus was stilled forever the teaching of *emboîtement*.

Continuing meanwhile was the quest for the mammalian ovum, a labor that had engaged man's efforts for 2,000 years. Between 1666 and 1672 the Dutch anatomists Jan Van Horne and Jan Swammerdam, working together, their fellow countryman Reinier de Graaf, and the Danish Niels Stensen developed the idea that the human female testes, like the ovaries of birds, produce eggs. Intense rivalry led to bickering over priority; and while the other two quibbled and procrastinated, de Graaf in 1672 published his own observations, in a volume entitled *De mulierum organis generationi inservientibus*, which resulted in the eponymic association of his name with the ovarian follicles. De Graaf

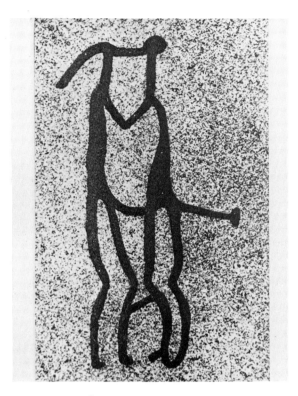

Fig. 6-5. Sexual marriage. Rock carving (c. 1300–500 BC) from a hillside near Vitlycke, province of Bohuslan, Sweden. The tail on one of the partners may represent a garment of animal skin.

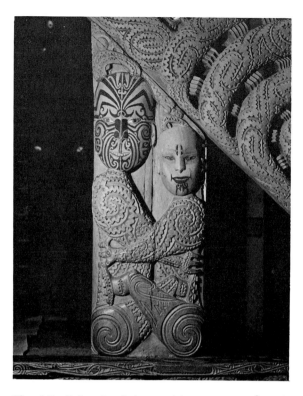

Fig. 6-7. Coitus in sitting position, partners face to face, common among the tribes of West Australia. Maori carved pillar, New Zealand. The Aukland Museum.

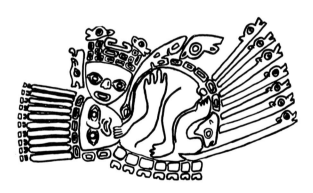

Fig. 6-6. Copulating couple, possibly a sun god and an earth goddess. Decoration on a Chimú pot, from an ancient Indian civilization on the northern coast of Peru, c. 1200. Carrion Cachot de Girard.

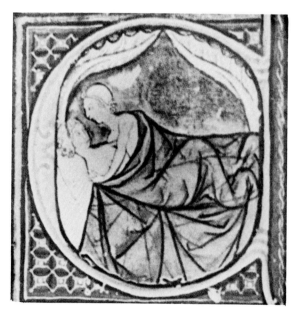

Fig. 6-8. Coitus. Miniature from a thirteenth century manuscript of *Régime du corps* by Aldobrandin of Siena. The British Museum, London.

192   ICONOGRAPHIA GYNIATRICA

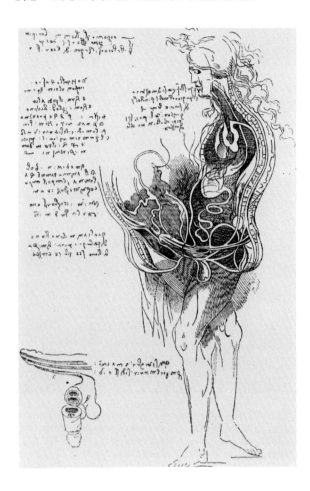
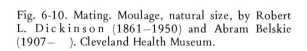

Fig. 6-9. Anatomical drawing by Leonardo da Vinci (1452–1519), subsequently titled *De Coitu* by Gabriel Peillon, 1891. In the man, vessels are shown connecting the lungs with the genitalia, to carry air for erection; in the woman, connecting the uterus and breasts.

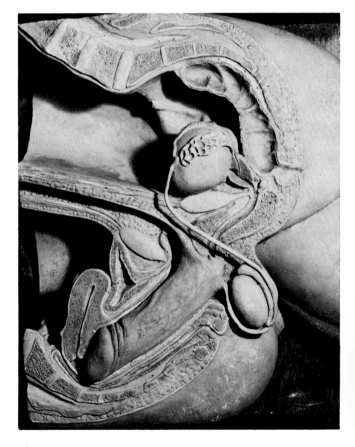

Fig. 6-10. Mating. Moulage, natural size, by Robert L. Dickinson (1861–1950) and Abram Belskie (1907–   ). Cleveland Health Museum.

MAN'S BEGINNINGS   193

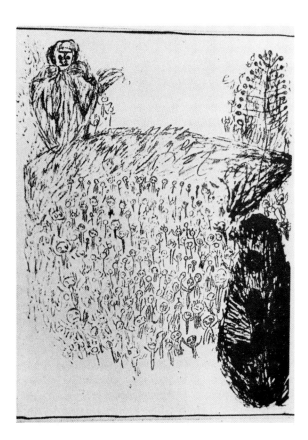

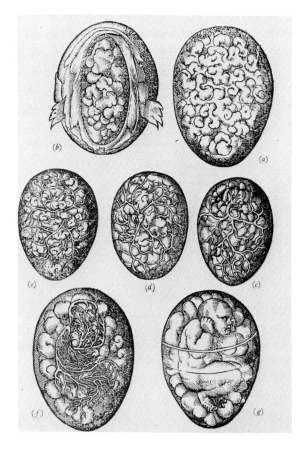

Fig. 6-11. Drawing by an Australian aboriginal woman illustrating the native theory of generation. A swarm of spirit children are leaving the crowded breasts of one of the two ancestral women who live in the sky and in whom all tribal life originates. Some of the spirit children pause to feed on the fruit and blossoms of the gum tree, at right, during their descent to earth, where they will seek suitable mothers in whose wombs to lodge until human development is complete.

Fig. 6-12. Figures from Jacob Rueff's *De conceptu et generatione hominis*, 1554, (arranged by Singer) illustrating Aristotle's concept of human embryogenesis. (a) The coagulum of semen and menstrual blood in the uterus; (b) the same mass, surrounded by the fetal membranes; (c) the origins of the liver, heart, and brain, represented by "three tiny white points not unlike coagulated milk;" (d) the four principal blood vessels, branching peripherally from the heart; (e) a beginning outline of the cranium; (f) the blood vessels outlining the human body; (g) the fully formed fetus.

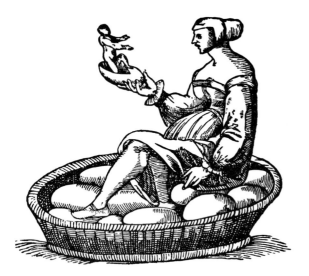

Fig. 6-13. The birth of man. Sixteenth century woodcut depicting in fantasy an infant emerging from an egg. From U. Aldrovandi's *Monstrorum historia,* Bononiae, Tebaldini, 1642, p. 36.

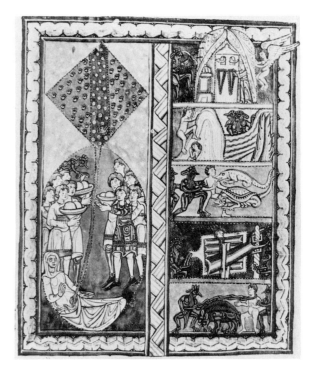

Fig. 6-14. The descent of the soul into the embryo, as illustrated in the *Liber Scivias,* depicting the visions of St. Hildegard (1098–1180). In the panel on the left, the soul is shown descending earthward from Heaven, into the intrauterine fetus. Representing the divine wisdom is the square above, its angles pointing to the earth's four corners. A long tube descends, through which the soul passes into the mother's womb. Königliche Landesbibliothek, Wiesbaden, Germany.

erred, however, in assuming the entire contents of the mammalian follicle to be the ovum; for when he immersed the ovaries of swine or cows in boiling water the contents of the follicle coagulated into a white opaque mass which, when shelled out of the ovary, resembled the boiled albumen of the hen's egg. Another century and one-half was to elapse before the mammalian ovum was actually revealed, about the first of May, 1872.

As early as 1778, William Cumberland Cruikshank, of Edinburgh, had found spherical bodies, considerably smaller than the Graafian follicles, in the oviducts of a rabbit three days after mating, and on the fourth day he found these tiny cystic structures in the uterus.

Studying the embryology of the dog a half-century later, Karl Ernst von Baer departed slightly from the usual procedure of examining the embryos in sequential stages of development and worked backward instead, investigating the later phases first in order to recognize more easily the next earlier. He thus observed embryos of 24 days, next 12 days, then free blastocysts in the uterus, and finally tubal ova. Von Baer recounted,

"It remained for me to ascertain the condition of the ova in the ovary, for it seemed clearer than light that the ova were not the very small Graafian vesicles expelled from the ovary, nor did I consider it likely that such solid little bodies had been coagulated in the

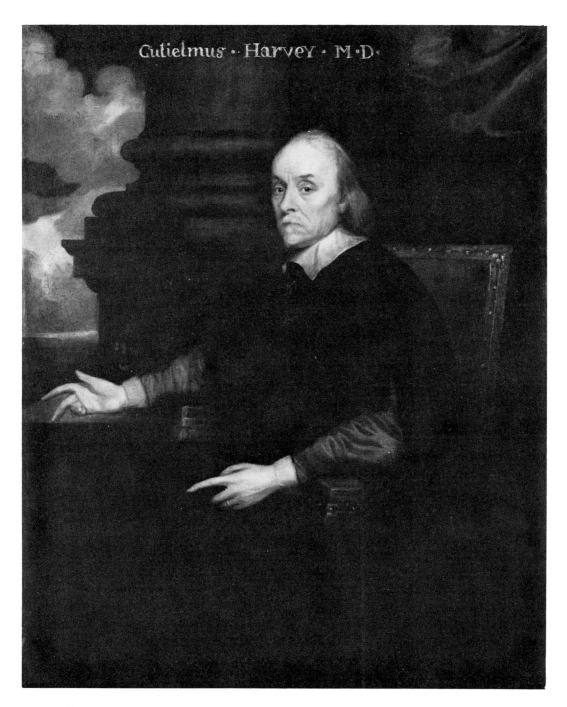

Fig. 6-15. William Harvey (1578–1657). Besides discovering the circulation of the blood, he revived the Aristotelian theory of epigenesis, which viewed embryonic development as a growth process rather than the mere unfolding of a pre-existing form; and made important contributions to mammalian embryology and human obstetrics. Espousing personal observation rather than reliance on authority, Harvey wrote, in the introduction to his *De generatione animalium*, 1651,
"Nature herself is to be addressed; the paths she shows are to be trodden boldly; for thus, and whilst we consult our proper senses, advancing from inferior to superior levels, shall we penetrate at last into the heart of her mystery." Royal College of Physicians of London.

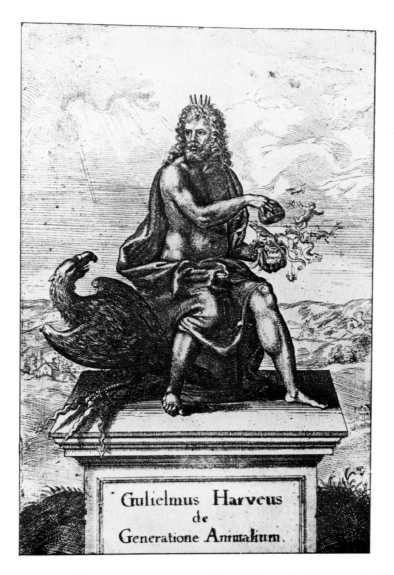

Fig. 6-16. Frontispiece to William Harvey's *De generatione animalium,* 1651. Zeus holds an egg bearing the inscription *Ex ovo omnia* and liberating living beings of various species. From this inscription originated the epigram, often attributed to Harvey, *Omne vivum ex ovo.*

tubes from the fluid of the vesicles. When I examined the ovaries before incising them, I clearly distinguished in almost all the vesicles a whitish-yellow point which was in no way attached to the covering of the vesicle, but as pressure exerted with a probe on the vesicle clearly indicated, swam free in the liquid. Led on more by inquisitiveness than by the hope of seeing the ovules in the ovaries with the naked eye through all the coverings of the Graafian vesicles, I opened a vesicle . . . with the edge of a scalpel . . . and placed it under the microscope. I was astounded when I saw an ovule . . . so plainly that a blind man could scarcely deny it. It is truly remarkable and astonishing that a thing so persistently and constantly sought and in all compendia of physiology considered as inextricable, could

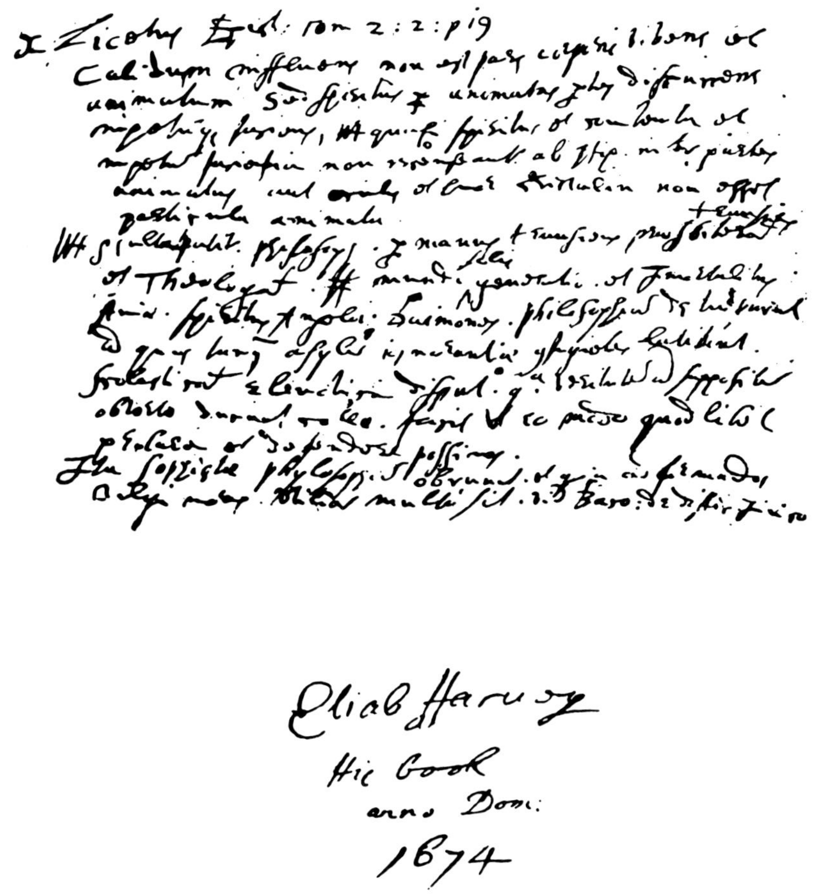

Fig. 6-17. Notes of William Harvey written in a mixture of English and Latin on the fly-leaf of a copy of his *De generatione animalium*, which he gave to his brother Eliab. The symbol ⊃C, in the left margin, was used by Harvey to designate his original ideas.

be put before the eyes with such facility."

Summing up, von Baer concluded, "Every animal which springs from the coitus of male and female is developed from an ovum, and none from a simple, formative liquid. The male semen acts through the membrane of the ovum, which is pervious by no foramen, and in the ovum it acts first on certain innate parts of the ovum."

With the mammalian ovum identified at last, the science of embryology was soon infused with the vigor of fresh discovery. Less than two decades after von Baer's epochal observation, Martin Barry demonstrated a spermatozoon within the egg cell; and 30 years later, in 1875, Oskar Hertwig witnessed the actual union of the nuclei of the male and female gametes.

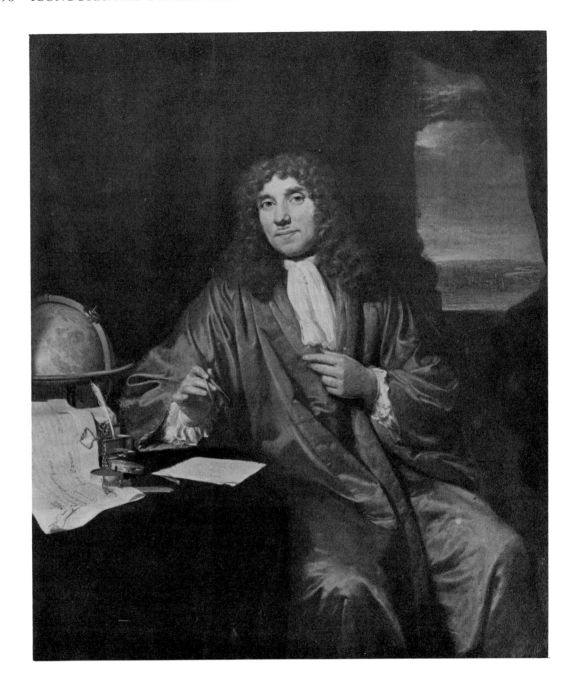

Fig. 6-18. Antoni van Leeuwenhoek (1632–1723). Portrait by Johannès Verkolje, 1668. A shopkeeper and linen draper in the town of Delft, self-taught and with knowledge of no language save his native Dutch, Leeuwenhoek became known as "the father of scientific microscopy." Although not the first to use the microscope, he made 247 such instruments, ground over 400 lenses, examined all sorts of biological tissues and fluids, and reported his observations in more than 300 letters to the Royal Society of London. The first to describe spermatozoa and protozoa, Leeuwenhoek also measured blood corpuscles, discovered the capillary circulation, recorded the anatomic structure of the teeth, demonstrated microorganisms on their surface, and called attention to the laminated structure of the lens and to the fiber bundles in voluntary muscle. Rijksmuseum, Amsterdam.

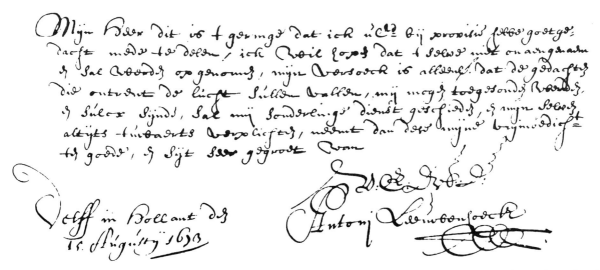

Fig. 6-19. The last few lines of one of Leeuwenhoek's letters to the Royal Society of London, dated August 15, 1673.

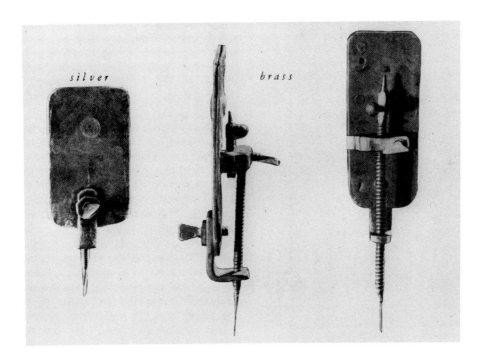

Fig. 6-20. Three of Leeuwenhoek's microscopes. The compound microscope was probably invented by Zacharias Janssen, a Dutch spectacle-maker, about 1590, two decades before Galileo adapted the optical system of his telescope to microscopic use. Leeuwenhoek's instruments were not true microscopes which contain multiple lenses, but rather, as he himself called them, simple *magnifying-glasses,* each consisting of but a single biconvex lens, mounted between two perforated metal plates. In contrast to the modern compound microscope, with adjustable lenses, the mechanical parts of Leeuwenhoek's instruments were so arranged as to move the object under examination into the focus of the lens, which remained in a fixed position. All Leeuwenhoek's microscopes were small; their metal plates, which served as a handle as well as the lens mount, were usually less than 2 inches long and about 1 inch wide. The Smithsonian Institution, Washington, D.C.

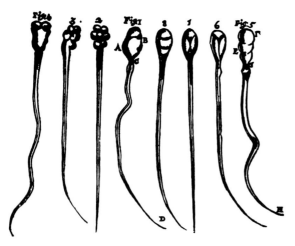

Fig. 6-21. The first published illustrations of mammalian spermatozoa, of dog and rabbit. Drawings accompanying Leeuwenhoek's letter to the Royal Society of London, March 18, 1678. The spermatozoa were so small, Leeuwenhoek wrote, that a "middle-size grain of fine sand would contain at the least ten thousand."

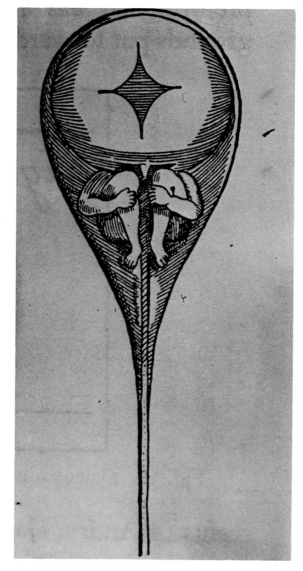

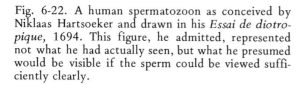

Fig. 6-22. A human spermatozoon as conceived by Niklaas Hartsoeker and drawn in his *Essai de diotropique*, 1694. This figure, he admitted, represented not what he had actually seen, but what he presumed would be visible if the sperm could be viewed sufficiently clearly.

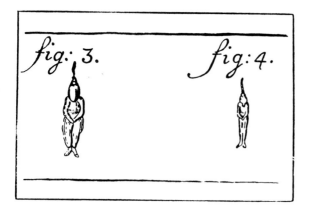

Fig. 6-23. Dalenpatius' drawings of human spermatozoa, 1699, as reproduced by Leeuwenhoek. Some believe that these were a hoax, which Dalenpatius never intended seriously.

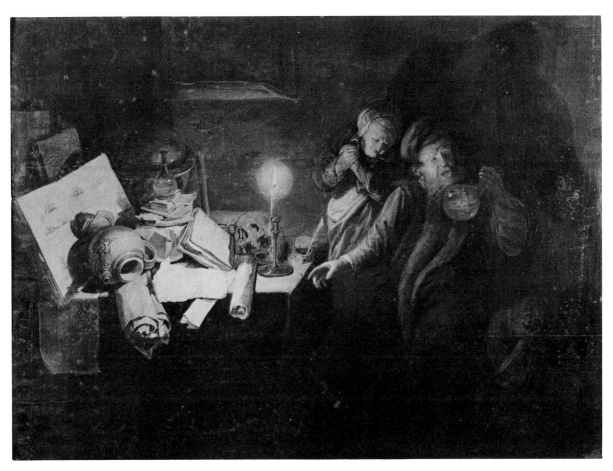

Fig. 6-24. Homunculus. Painting by David Ryckaert III (1612–1661).
"Let the semen of a man putrefy by itself in a cucurbite with the highest putrefaction of the *venter equinus,* for forty days, or until it begins at least to live, move, and be agitated, which can easily be seen. After this time it will be in some degree like a human being, but nevertheless transparent and without body. If now after this, it be every day nourished and fed cautiously and prudently with the arcanum of human blood, and kept for forty weeks in the perpetual and equal heat of a *venter equinus,* it becomes thenceforth a true and living infant, having all the members of a child that is born from a woman, but much smaller. This we call a homunculus..." [Paracelsus: *Treatise Concerning the Nature of Things,* Book I, 1520.] Städtisches Reiss-Museum, Mannheim, Germany.

202 ICONOGRAPHIA GYNIATRICA

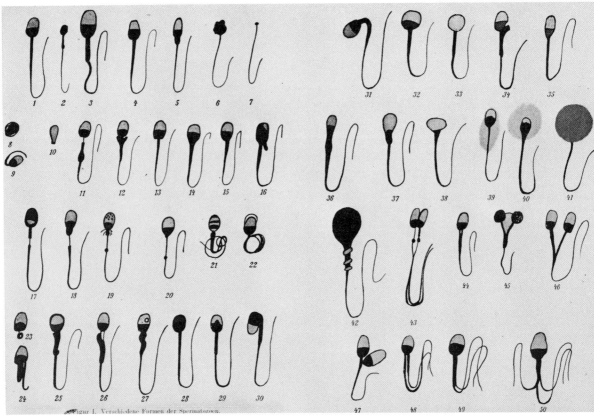

Fig. 6-25. Variants of human spermatozoa. From G.L. Moench, Studien Zur Fertilität, Z. Geburtsh. Gynaek. 99: 1, 1931.

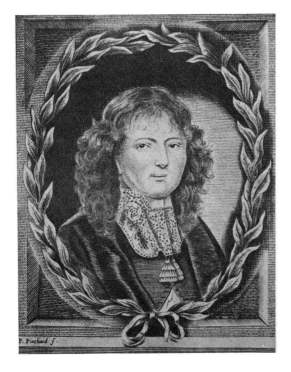

Fig. 6-26. Reinier de Graaf (1641–1673). He described the ovarian follicles, subsequently named for him, but thought them ova.

MAN'S BEGINNINGS 203

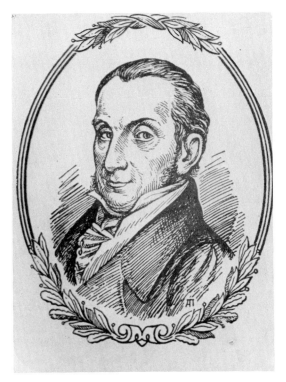

Fig. 6-27. Caspar Friedrich Wolff (1733–1794). He disproved the theory of preformation and sparked the modern study of embryology with his *Theoria generationis,* 1759.

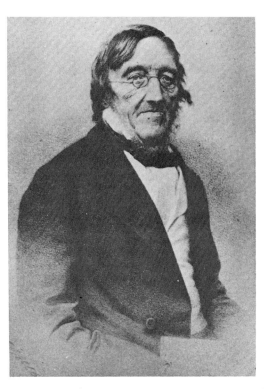

Fig. 6-28. Karl Ernst von Baer (1792–1876), discoverer of the mammalian ovum.

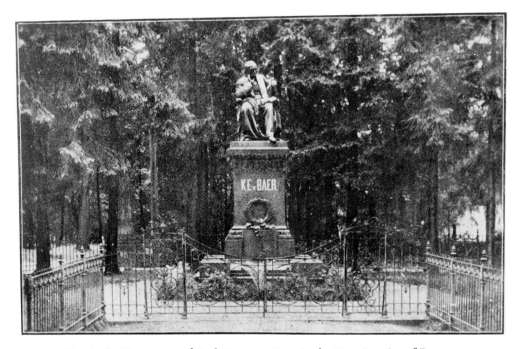

Fig. 6-29. Monument of Karl Ernst von Baer in the Estonian city of Dorpat.

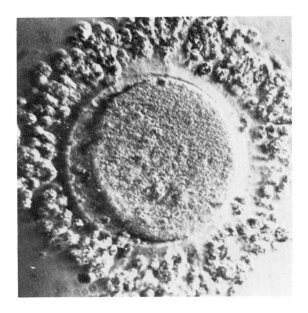

Fig. 6-30. The human ovum freshly ovulated. Recovered from the fallopian tube, the ovum is encased in granulosa cells, the corona radiata.

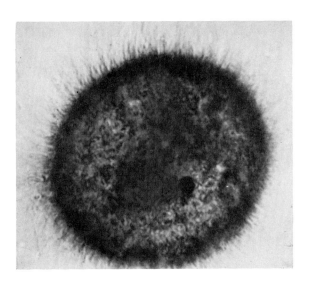

Fig. 6-31. The human ovum surrounded by myriads of spermatozoa. Only one succeeds in penetrating the egg and merging with its nucleus.

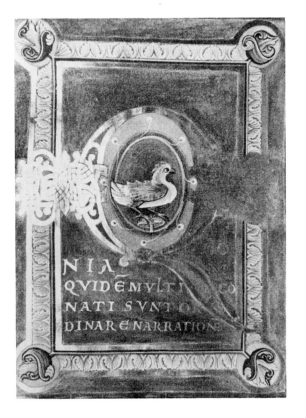

Fig. 6-32. Spermatozoa attached to the egg. Emblem from an illuminated manuscript, about AD 1000, written by the monks of the monastery at Reichenau, Germany. This figure suggests that a knowledge of egg and sperm existed, but was allowed to perish, long before Leeuwenhoek. Library, Cologne Cathedral, Germany.

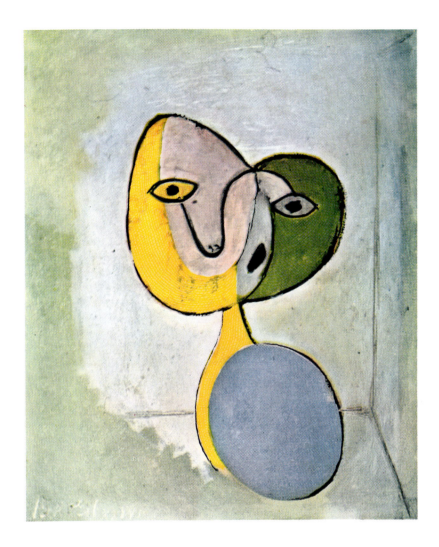

Fig. 6-33. "Splitting of the Cell." Painting by Pablo Picasso (1881–), a dynamic interpretation in modern art of the beginning of life. (Lithofilms courtesy of Abbottempo.)

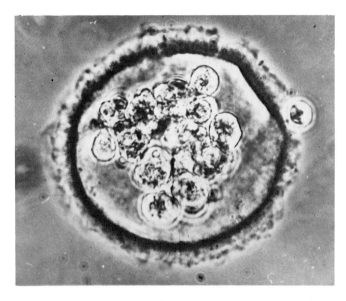

Fig. 6-35. The implanted human ovum at 12 days. Surface view of the endometrium, the ovum showing as the rounded raised area in the center. Carnegie Institution of Washington.

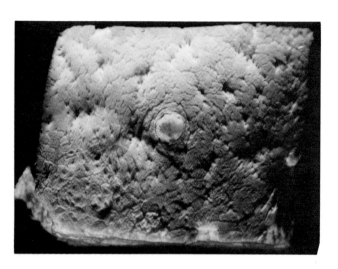

Fig. 6-34. The dividing human ovum. Thirty-two cell stage, beginning formation of blastocyst, 72 hours after fertilization.

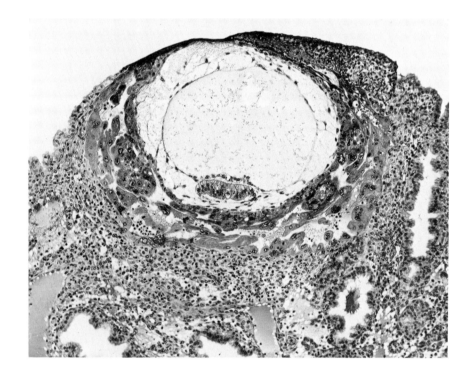

Fig. 6-36. The embedded human ovum at 12 days. Photomicrograph of the endometrium. Carnegie Institution of Washington.

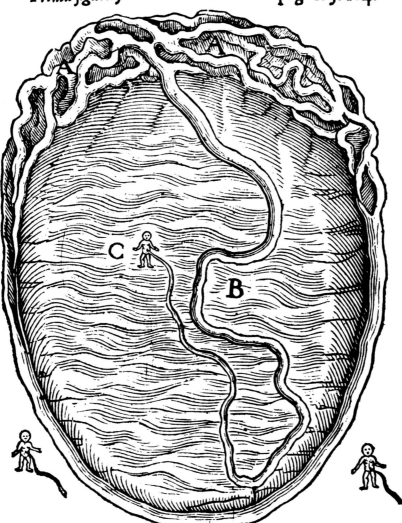

A. A. *Placenta, in qua sunt radices & trunci venæ & arteriæ umbilicalis.* B. *vasa umbilicalia.* C. *fœtus duodecim dierum.*

Fig. 6-37. A seventeenth century concept of the fetus and placenta of 12 days. From S. Pineau's *De integritatis et corruptionis virginum notis*, Leyden, 1641. Prominently pictured are the placental blood vessels More than a century earlier, Leonardo da Vinci, writing on mammalian embryology, had stated in the third volume of his notebooks *(Quaderni d'anatomia),*

"The veins of the child do not ramify in the substance of the uterus of its mother but in the placenta, which takes the place of a shirt in the interior of the uterus, which it coats and to which it is connected but not united . . ."

Leonardo thus asserted in one sentence a fact that, in the words of Joseph Needham, "it took all the ingenuity of the seventeenth century to prove to be true, namely, that the fetal circulation is not continuous with that of the mother. . . ."

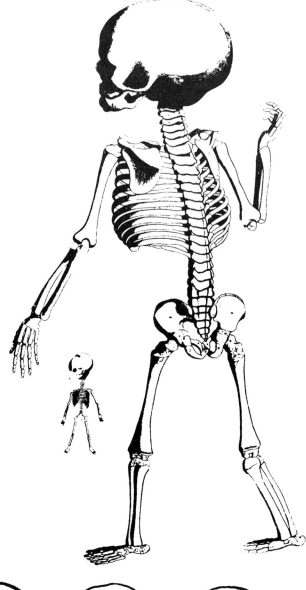

Fig. 6-38. Skeletons of fetuses of three and six months. Drawings by Volcher Coiter for his *Externarum et internarum principalium humani corporis tabulae,* Nürnberg, 1572, which contained the first illustrations of embryologic and pediatric anatomy.

Fig. 6-39. The human fetus from the first to tenth month, as illustrated in a Chinese obstetric text of 1638, *Shê shêng pi p-ón tsang yao* (The most important secret instructions in obstetrics).

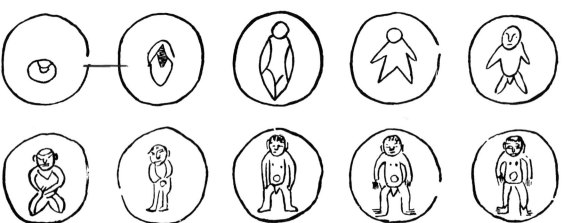

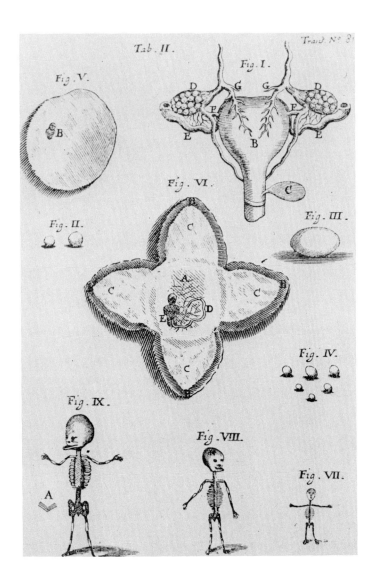

Fig. 6-40. The highly imaginative drawings of Theodore Kerckring, 1670, to illustrate the stages of human development. From *Philosophical Transactions of the Royal Society*, 1672, no. 81. Figures II and III, Eggs [ovarian follicles] of different sizes as found in the testicles [ovaries] of a woman. Figure V, An egg [gestation sac] "3 or 4 days after it was fallen into the Matrix [uterus] of a woman, and in which he saw that little embryon marked B, whereof he found the head begun to be distinguished from the body...." Figure VI, "A bigger egg, opened a fortnight after conception." Figures VII, VIII, and IX, "The sceletons of Infants 3 weeks, 4 weeks and 6 weeks after conception."

According to an untraced story related by Joseph Needham in his *History of Embryology*, 2 ed., Cambridge University Press, 1959, p.65, Cleopatra, the Ptolmaic queen, to satisfy her curiosity concerning fetal development, ordered the dissection of slaves at designated stages of pregnancy, patterning her research after the model established by Hippocrates in his study of the chick's development. A similar story is told of an early Chinese king.

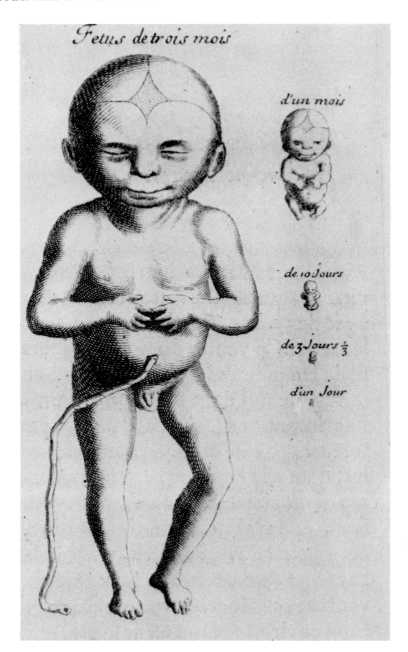

Fig. 6-41. Relative proportions of the human fetus from conception to three months, as illustrated by François Mauriceau in his *Traité des maladies de femmes grosses*, Paris, 1694.

Chapter 7

THE OBSTETRIC PELVIS

The process of birth is an exercise in mechanics involving the diameters and contours of a passage, the maternal pelvis; a passenger, the fetus; and a propulsive force, the uterine contractions of labor. Anathema to parturient and accoucheur alike was the contracted pelvis, until the advent of safe cesarean section, which permitted bypass of the vaginal delivery route. Diminished pelvic capacity, whether constitutionally determined, as by genetic factors, or the result of postnatal processes, such as rickets, tuberculosis, osteomalacia, or trauma, often led to the death of both mother and child. Our concept of the role of the pelvis in labor has undergone marked change over the centuries. Long prevalent was the erroneous belief that the fetus propelled itself during labor through a distensible girdle whose bones separated to permit its tenant's easy egress. The protestations to the contrary by those who insisted on the unyielding character of the bony pelvis were ignored. Perhaps the first precise description of the female pelvis appeared in the texts of the Indian Susruta Samhita, in the early years of the Common Era.

The active role of the fetus in the birth process was questioned by Vesalius, in 1543. Three decades later his pupil Arantius clearly described the effect of pelvic contraction on labor. Arantius wrote, in his *De humano foetu liber,*

"The most important point [in difficult labor] lies in the conformation of the pubic bones themselves as they are first formed in the uterus. For if the bones have been well and properly formed, not too broad, convex on the outside, and if the concave part which is placed under the convex corresponds proportionally, if a semi-circular cavity and a lofty arc are concealed under the pubic bone, if at the same time favorable space is left between the pubic bone and the coccyx, which will allow an easy entrance to the advancing fetus—then, even if, as sometimes happens, the child be doubled up or have a bad position, presenting with a hand or foot, no difficulty will offer itself to the helpfully directing hand of the wise master. If, however, the pubic bones, due to the fault of the formative faculty, have not been favorably arranged, that is to say if they are too broad and in the exterior region so compressed that they become humped rather than concave on the inside, and if they come very near the sacrum and coccyx, then the parts of the parturient become so narrow that the road is not wide enough for the fetus, even if turned upon its head according to nature, especially if it is endowed with a relatively large and solid head. The reason is that the fetus, with its occiput or sinciput gets so stuck to the posterior part of the pubic bone that it can by no means proceed on its own account. And,

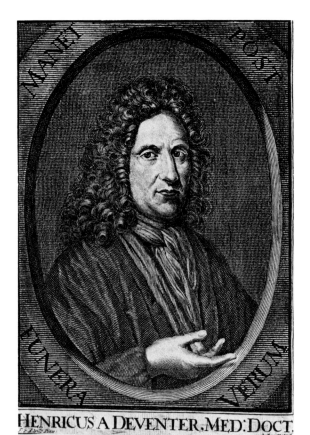

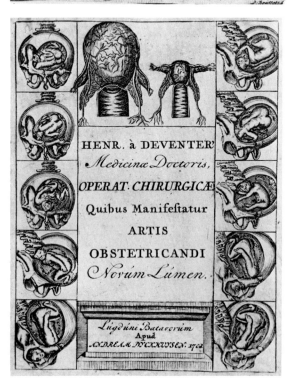

what is worse, the helping hand of the operator which is about to bring aid, cannot reach there because of the narrowness of the parts. Thus it usually happens that not only the fetus but the puerpera herself succumbs...."

Not until 1701, however, with the publication of Hendrik van Deventer's *Novum lumen*, did the concept of the pelvic inlet as a rigid ring achieve credence.

Pelvic mensuration was introduced in 1753 by André Levret with his complex system of pelvic planes and axes. Pelvimetry gained clinical application the following year when William Smellie proposed the diagonal conjugate as a simple and reliable index of the inlet's capacity. To this day, the diagonal conjugate remains the obstetrician's most valuable single measurement in his clinical evaluation of pelvic adequacy.

Popularization of clinical pelvimetry followed the publication of Jean-Louis Baudelocque's *L'art des accouchemens,* in 1781; but this, Baudelocque's best known contribution, embodied an error that was to hinder obstetric practice for the next century and one-half. The anteroposterior diameter of the pelvic inlet, Baudelocque taught, could be estimated reliably by subtracting 3 inches from the external conjugate, measured from the middle of the pubis to the tip of the spine of the last lumbar vertebra. Baudelocque's diameter, as this measurement soon came to be known, which could be obtained with greater ease to the examiner and less discomfort to the patient than could the internal

Fig. 7-1. Hendrik van Deventer (1651–1724). Dutch obstetrician whose *Novum lumen* lit the way toward an understanding of the bony pelvis.

Fig. 7-2. Title page of the first edition (1701) of van Deventer's *Novum lumen*. It was published simultaneously in Dutch and Latin, *Operationes chirurgicae novum lumen exhibentes obstetricantibus.*

THE OBSTETRIC PELVIS   213

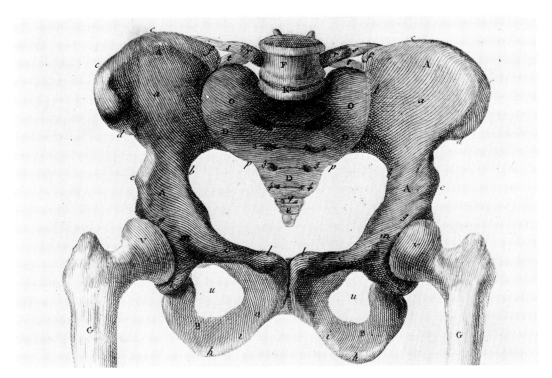

Fig. 7-3. The well-formed female pelvis. From Jean-Louis Baudelocque's *L'art des accouchemens,* ed. 4, Paris, 1807.

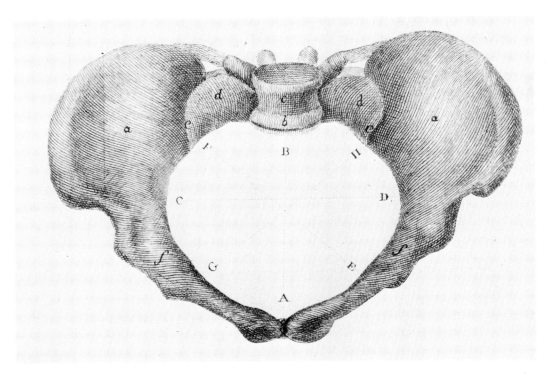

Fig. 7-4. The inlet of the well-formed female pelvis. From Jean-Louis Baudelocque's *L'art des accouchemens,* ed. 4, Paris, 1807.

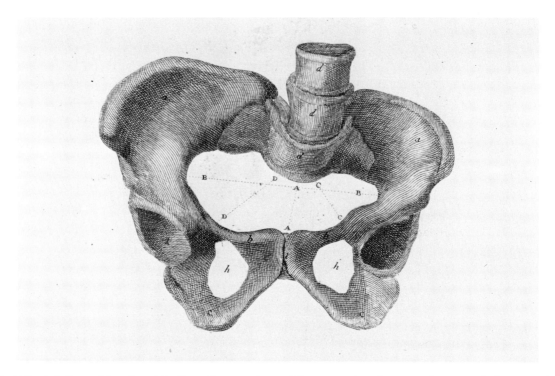

Fig. 7-5. A deformed female pelvis. From Jean-Louis Baudelocque's *L'art des accouchemens,* ed. 4, Paris, 1807.

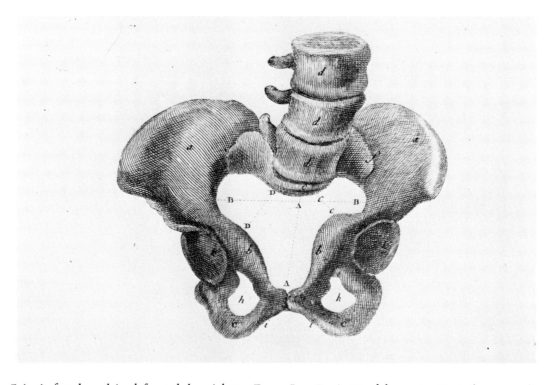

Fig. 7-6. A female pelvis deformed by rickets. From Jean-Louis Baudelocque's *L'art des accouchemens,* ed. 4, Paris, 1807.

THE OBSTETRIC PELVIS 215

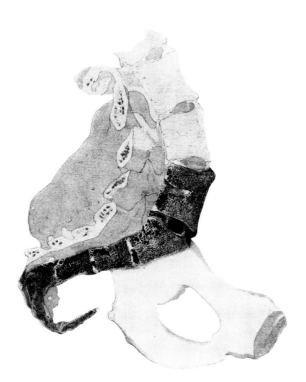

Fig. 7-7. A rhachitic female pelvis, sagittal section. From Carl Conrad Litzmann's *Die Formen des Beckens*, Berlin, 1861.

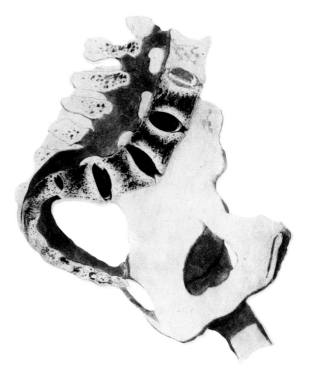

Fig. 7-8. A female pelvis deformed by osteomalacia, sagittal section. From Carl Conrad Litzmann's *Die Formen des Beckens*, Berlin, 1861.

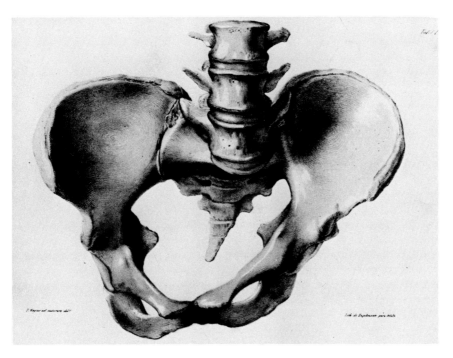

Fig. 7-9. The obliquely contracted pelvis (Naegele pelvis), a rare type of distortion. From Franz Carl Naegele's *Das Schräg Verengte Becken*, Mainz, 1839.

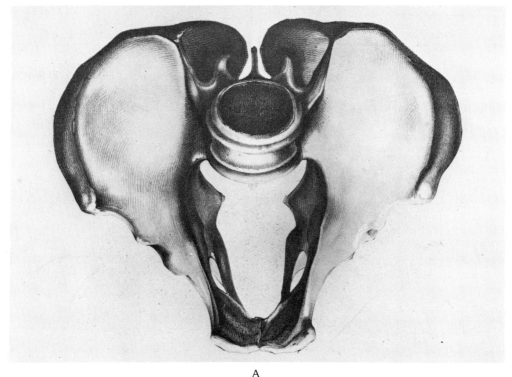

A

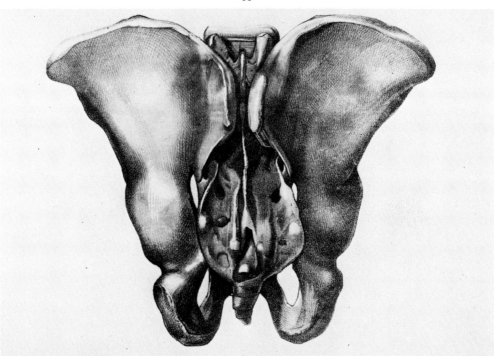

B

Fig. 7-10. The Robert pelvis. Perhaps the rarest of all types of contracted, pelvis characterized by extreme transverse narrowing due to bilateral, probably congenital, absence of the sacral alae. From Heinrich Ludwig Robert's *Beschreibung eines im höchsten Grade Querverengten Beckens,* Carlsruhe & Freiberg, 1842.

conjugate, rapidly eclipsed the latter and for many years virtually supplanted it. The obstetric unreliability of external pelvimetry was demonstrated later, but so great was the appeal of Baudelocque's simple measurement that obstetricians finally renounced it only toward the middle of the twentieth century. Since the time of Baudelocque, scores of calipers have been devised for measuring the diameters of woman's pelvis.

Among the first to emphasize the inadequacy of the external conjugate for pelvic mensuration was the German Gustav Adolf Michaelis (1798–1848) in his *Das Enge Becken*. A product of the study of 1,000 patients, this work provided the basis of modern clinical knowledge of the bony pelvis. Edited by Carl Conrad Litzmann (1815–1890) and published in 1851, three years after Michaelis' death, *Das Enge Becken* attracted little attention, its importance remaining unrecognized for several years. Having succeeded in selling only a few copies, the publisher destroyed the remainder, considered unsalable. Not until 1865 had the book generated enough interest to warrant its reprinting.

Extending the work of his friend Michaelis, Litzmann contributed another classic to the obstetric literature in 1861 with *Die Formen des Beckens*. Its first paragraph succinctly interpreted the female pelvis. Litzmann wrote,

"The pelvis fulfills more extensive functions in the female body than in the male. In the female it forms not merely the bony founda-

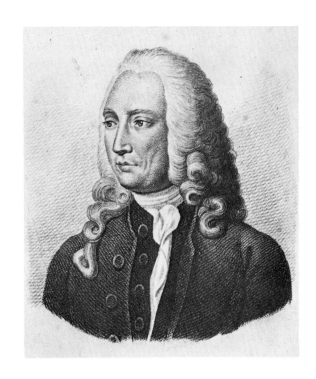

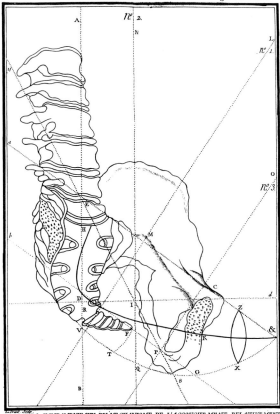

Fig. 7-11. André Levret (1703–1780). The leading French obstetrician of his day, one of the early students of pelvic mensuration and the mechanism of labor, designer of the long French forceps. The New York Academy of Medicine.

Fig. 7-12. Levret's concept of the pelvic planes and axes including the first curvilinear representation of the axis of parturition. From the second edition of his *L'art des accouchemens*, Paris, 1761.

tion of the trunk... to which strong and numerous muscles are attached, but also shelters the largest part of the sexual apparatus in addition to the distal end of the intestinal canal and urinary passages, and thereby assumes great importance in reproduction. In addition to admitting the male organ during coitus, it has to provide space for the whole uterus at the beginning of pregnancy, and later for expansion of the lower uterine segment at least, and at birth a passageway into the outer world for the mature fetus together with its membranes. Nature has understood how to satisfy, in an amazing manner, the diverse and to some degree contradictory demands with which she is thus confronted. She has imparted the necessary firmness to the pelvis with maximal economy in bony substance by giving it an annular shape and supporting its joints with powerful ligaments, but amassing larger concentrations of bone only in the regions exposed directly to pressure. She has placed the canal that opens at the lowermost part of the trunk in such a position that the pelvis can maintain the burden of the abdominal viscera and provide support and purchase for the enclosed organs, by inclining the pelvis anteriorly at a sharp angle to the horizon, bending its axis in a curve convex posteriorly, and covering and finishing its walls with contractile and elastic soft parts; and in this way also achieving adequate capacity and dilatability for the act of birth. However, the space is so proportioned that even a relatively slight deviation from

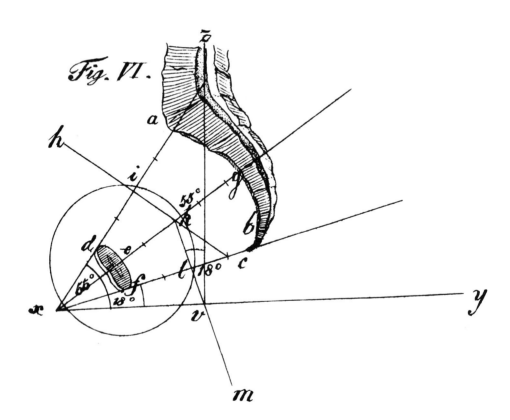

Fig. 7-13. The *curve of Carus*. A simplified concept of the birth axis from Carl Gustav Carus' *Lehrbuch der Gynäkologie*, Leipzig, 1820.

its normal size can interfere with delivery, insofar as a correspondingly more favorable condition in the remaining birth factors does not compensate for the difficulties."

Roentgen pelvimetry, the ultimate in precise pelvic mensuration in the living woman, was introduced toward the close of the nineteenth century, by W. Albert in Germany and Pierre-Constant Budin and Henri-Victor Varnier in France. Subsequent technical refinements coupled with twentieth century studies of pelvic morphology, principally those of William E. Caldwell and Howard C. Moloy, have provided the obstetrician with a great boon, an objective method for predicting and observing the course of labor and for guiding him in his management of feto-pelvic disproportion.

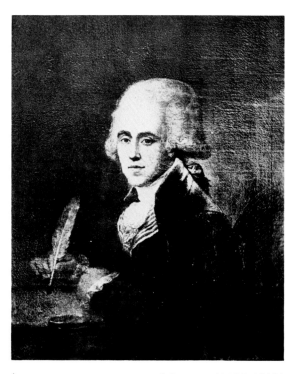

Fig. 7-14. Jean-Louis Baudelocque (1746–1810). Master French accoucheur, he authored a famous textbook for midwives, redesigned the obstetric forceps, and popularized pelvimetry. The New York Academy of Medicine.

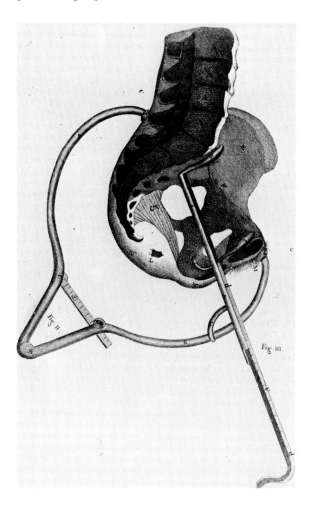

Fig. 7-15. Early pelvimeters. The caliper of Baudelocque (Fig. II) for measuring the external conjugate *(Baudelocque's diameter)* and the pelvimeter of Coutouli (Fig. III) for measuring the internal conjugate. From Baudelocque's *L'art des accouchemens*, ed. 4, Paris, 1807.

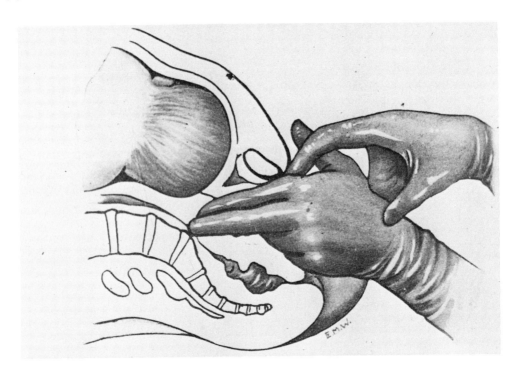

Fig. 7-16. Measuring the diagonal conjugate manually.

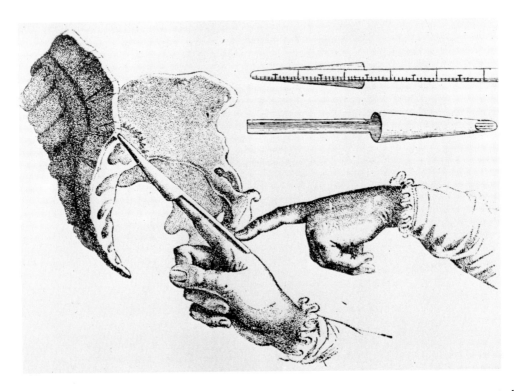

Fig. 7-17. The *thimble of Asdrubali*. An aid for measuring the diagonal conjugate. From F. Asdrubali, *Elementi di Ostetricia*, 1795.

THE OBSTETRIC PELVIS 221

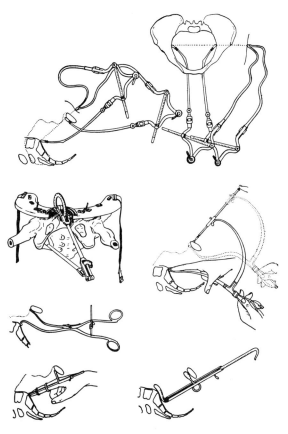

Fig. 7-18. A few of many nineteenth century internal pelvimeters. From F. Skutsch, *Die Beckenmessung an der lebenden Frau*, 1887.

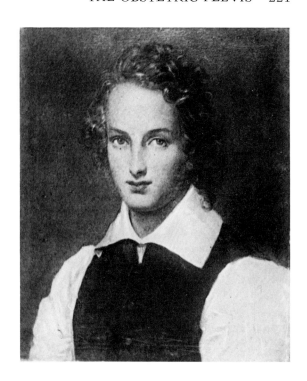

Fig. 7-19. Gustav Adolf Michaelis (1798–1848). His book *Das Enge Becken* was perhaps the greatest single contribution to the study of pelvic contraction until the advent of roentgen pelvimetry.

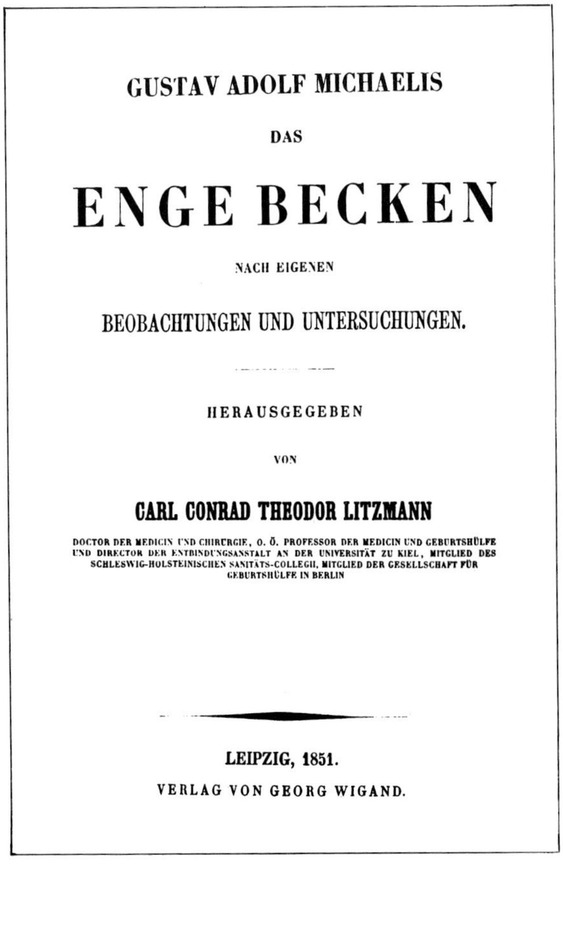

Fig. 7-20. Title page of *Das Enge Becken*. Only a few copies of the first edition could be sold, so little was the interest in contracted pelves and so little recognized the importance of Michaelis' work.

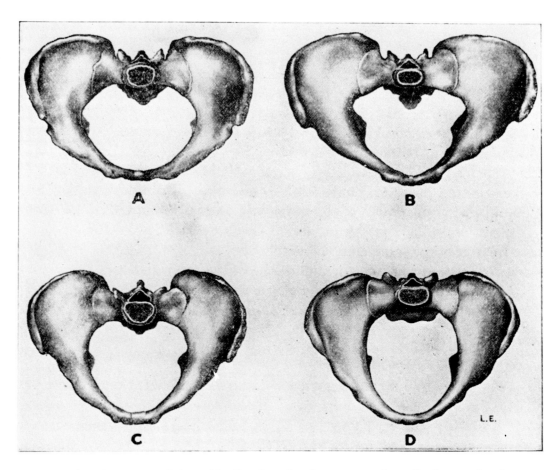

Fig. 7-21. Female pelvic types of the Caldwell-Moloy classification. A. platypelloid, B. android, C. gynecoid, D. anthropoid.

Chapter 8

LABOR AND ITS COMPLICATIONS

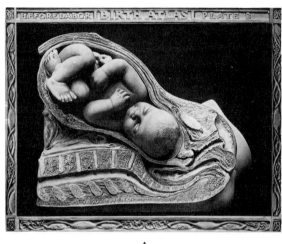

A

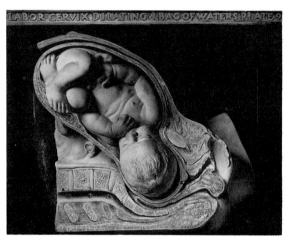

B

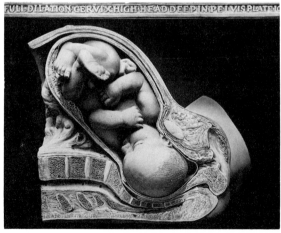

C

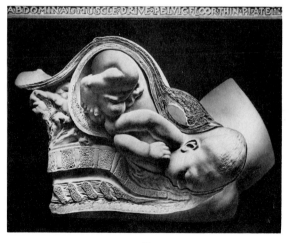

D

Fig. 8-1. Labor and birth. Moulages by Robert L. Dickinson (1861–1950) and Abram Belskie (1907–). (A) Onset of labor, (B) A uterine contraction, (C) Beginning of the second stage, (D) Crowning, (E) Extension of the head, (F) Delivery of the anterior shoulder.

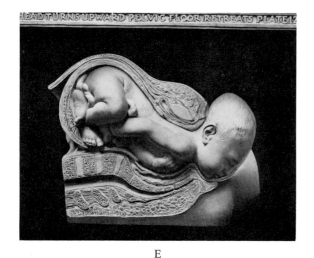

E

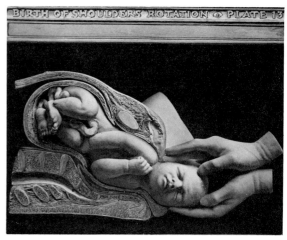

F

"For I have heard a voice as of a woman in travail . . ." (Jeremiah 4:31)

The act of birth remains one of Nature's mysteries. Subject of countless theories, the cause of labor's onset is yet to be learned. Hippocrates wrote, in his *On Generation,*

"I say it is the lack of food which leads to birth, unless any violence has been done. . . . The bird grows inside the egg and articulates itself exactly like the child. . . . When there is no more food for the young one in the egg and it has nothing on which to live, it makes violent movements, searches for food, and breaks the membranes. . . . When the mother breaks the shell there is only an insignificant quantity of liquid in it. All has been consumed by the fetus. In just the same way, when the child has grown big and the mother cannot continue to provide him with enough nourishment, he becomes agitated, breaks through the membranes, and incontinently passes out into the external world. . . ."

Still prevalent 2000 years later and endorsed by William Harvey in his *De genera-* *tione animalium* (1651) was the concept that the efforts of the fetus aided its birth. In the English translation from his Latin, Harvey stated,

"The assistance of the foetus is chiefly required in the birth, is evident, not in Birds onely, which do by their own industry without the help of their Parent break up the shell; but also in other Animals; for all Flies, and Butterflies, doe perforate the little membranes (in which they did lurk when they were the Worme Aurelia) and likewise the Silk-worm doth at his appointed time mollifie and erode the little Silken Bagge, which he had weaved for his defence and security, and so gets out without any forraign aide." [*Anatomical Exercitations,* London, 1653]

PROTECTORS OF THE PARTURIENT

Associated with grave risks of death as well as pain, birth required protective dieties. Every primitive culture had its own; some had several. Prayers to them for a safe delivery were often accompanied by the offering of articles of dress: a veil, sandals, robe, or breast band.

LABOR AND ITS COMPLICATIONS 225

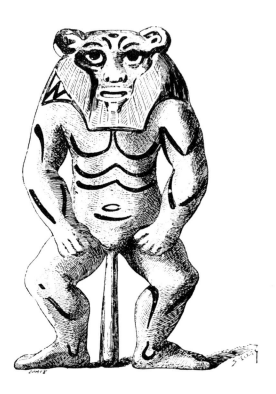

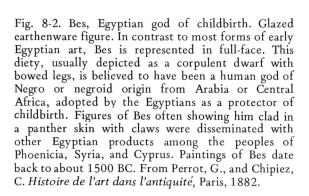

Fig. 8-2. Bes, Egyptian god of childbirth. Glazed earthenware figure. In contrast to most forms of early Egyptian art, Bes is represented in full-face. This diety, usually depicted as a corpulent dwarf with bowed legs, is believed to have been a human god of Negro or negroid origin from Arabia or Central Africa, adopted by the Egyptians as a protector of childbirth. Figures of Bes often showing him clad in a panther skin with claws were disseminated with other Egyptian products among the peoples of Phoenicia, Syria, and Cyprus. Paintings of Bes date back to about 1500 BC. From Perrot, G., and Chipiez, C. *Histoire de l'art dans l'antiquité*, Paris, 1882.

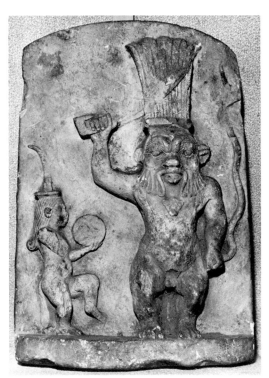

Fig. 8-3. The god Bes and his wife. Bas-relief. Musée du Louvre, Paris.

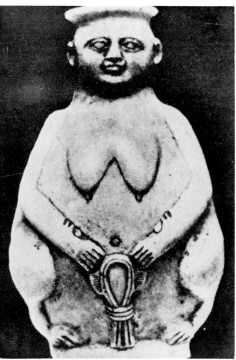

Fig. 8-4. Taurt, an Egyptian birth goddess. In the form of a hollow vessel. Shown between her legs, the uterus, symbolizing birth. From A. A. Barb, *Diva Matrix*, J. Warburg and Courtauld Inst., 1953.

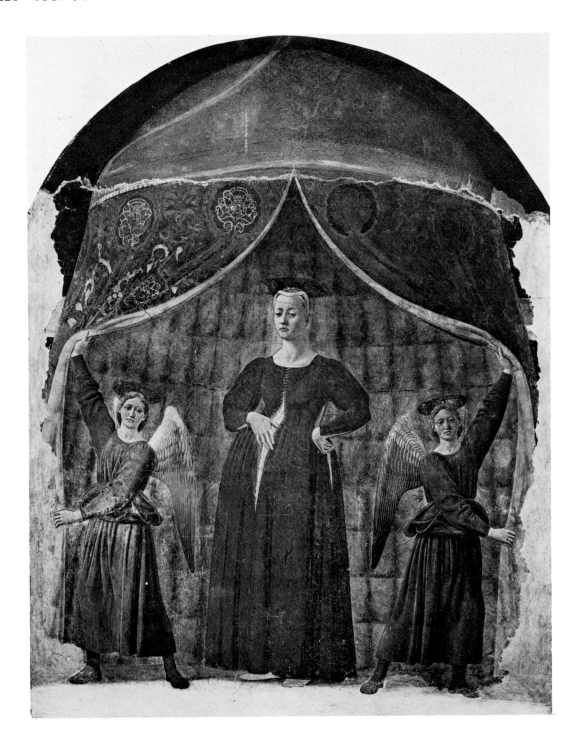

Fig. 8-5. *Madonna del Parto*. Fresco by Piero della Francesca (real name Franceschi), (1420?–1492). Mary has been regarded by some Christians as a source of strength and help in childbirth. Her image appears in special altars in some churches where expectant mothers bring offerings and invoke her help. The Virgin is shown in this painting at the onset of labor, her face filled with pain and calm resignation. Chapel of Monterchi, Arezzo, Italy.

LABOR AND ITS COMPLICATIONS 227

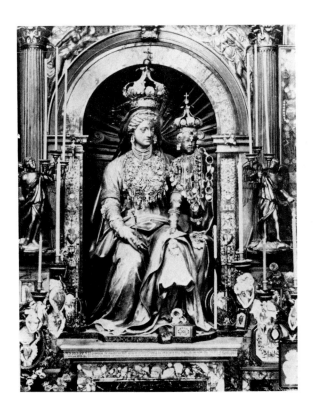

Fig. 8-6. *Madonna del Parto.* Marble figure by Jacopo Sansovino (real name Tatti), (1477–1570). Created in the sixteenth century, this statue of Mary and the Christ Child, in Rome, is still visited by expectant mothers praying for help in childbirth who continue to adorn both figues with offerings of many sorts, especially jewelry and watches. Chapel of San Agostino, Rome.

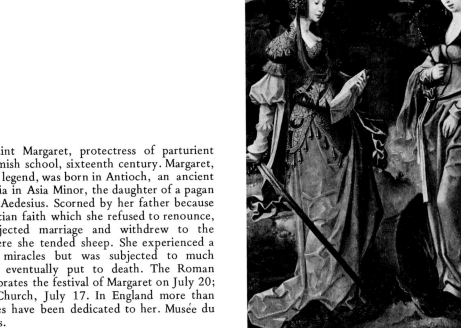

Fig. 8-7. Saint Margaret, protectress of parturient women. Flemish school, sixteenth century. Margaret, according to legend, was born in Antioch, an ancient city of Pisidia in Asia Minor, the daughter of a pagan priest name Aedesius. Scorned by her father because of her Christian faith which she refused to renounce, Margaret rejected marriage and withdrew to the country where she tended sheep. She experienced a number of miracles but was subjected to much torture and eventually put to death. The Roman Church celebrates the festival of Margaret on July 20; the Greek Church, July 17. In England more than 250 churches have been dedicated to her. Musée du Louvre, Paris.

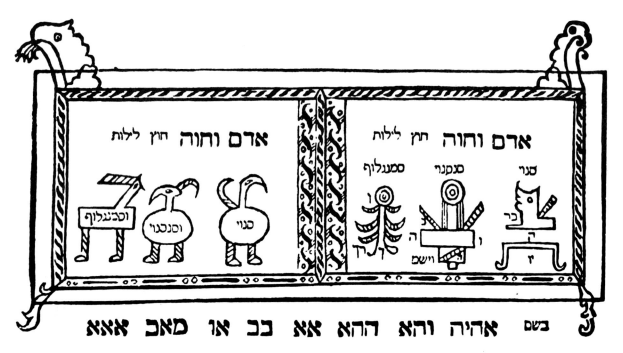

Fig. 8-8. Hebrew childbirth amulet. For protection of the parturient against Lilith, the embodiment of the devil. Prominent are the three protective angels, Senoi, San-Senori, and Sammangelof.

BIRTH AMULETS

Persistent from ancient Jewish folklore even into the twentieth century was the legend of mischievous Lilith, demon to women in childbirth. Lilith, according to belief, bound Adam to herself after his separation from Eve, but soon wearied of this connection and forsook him. At Jehovah's command the three angels Senoi, San-Senori, and Sammangelof sought Lilith out and commanded her to return to Adam on pain of losing 100 of her own children daily. Adamant, Lilith strove to avenge the death of her offspring by strangling other newborn infants wherever found. Only the names of the three angels could avert her attacks.

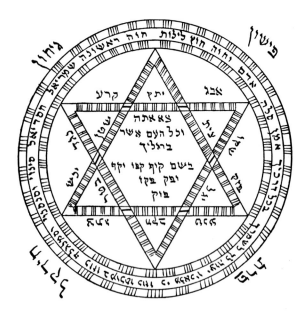

Fig. 8-9. Hebrew amulet. To protect the parturient and her newborn infant from the evil Lilith.

LABOR AND ITS COMPLICATIONS 229

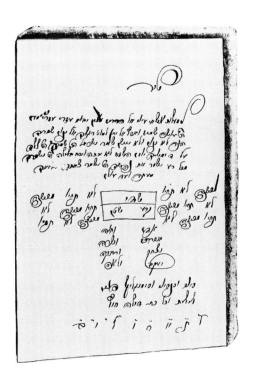

Fig. 8-10. Amulet *(childbirth card)* against Lilith. Used among the South Russian Jews in Elisabethgrad for protection in childbirth.

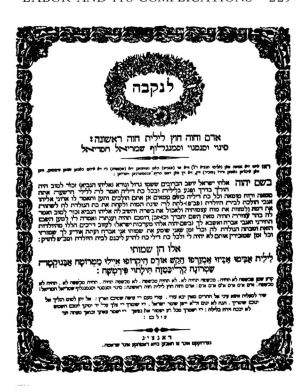

Fig. 8-11. Amulet. Sheet 19 x 25 cm, fitted with ribbon for hanging. Used by the Jews in Northern Russia, nineteenth century, for parturient women and their children. A prayer invoking God's protection and exorcising Lilith ended with Psalm 121.

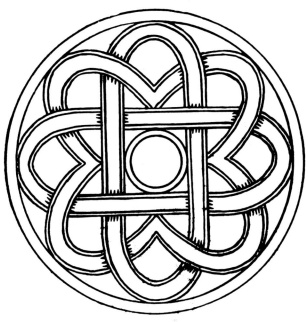

Fig. 8-12. Woodcarving, early nineteenth century, of a *sigurlykkja,* or victory loop, a band tied over Icelandic women to expedite labor and ease its pain.

230   ICONOGRAPHIA GYNIATRICA

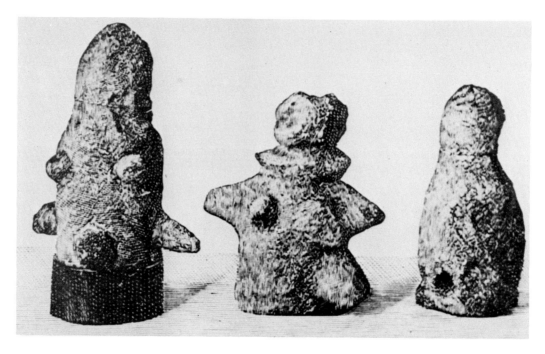

Fig. 8-13. Clay figures from Agitome, Togoland. Erected in the villages of women in labor as sentinels against demons or as offerings to them to spare the parturient. Museum für Völkerkunde, West Berlin.

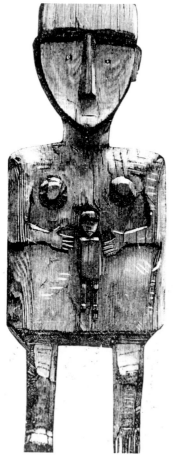

Fig. 8-14. Wooden figure, in the form of a woman with child (73 cm, 9.5 Kg). Placed on the abdomen by the Goldi of Siberia in cases of difficult labor. Museum für Völkerkunde, West Berlin.

BIRTH POSTURES

When ent'ring Delos, she, that is so dear
To dames in labor, made Latono straight
Prone to delivery, and to wield the weight
Of her dear burden with a world of ease,
When, with her fair hand, she a palm did
  seize,
And, staying her by it, stuck her tender knees
Amidst the soft mead, that did smile beneath
Her sacred labor; and the child did breathe
The air the instant. All the Goddesses
Brake in kind tears and shrieks for her quick
  ease.

[Homer: "Hymn to Apollo,"
Chapman's translation]

The positions assumed by women in labor and at delivery, usually prescribed by local or tribal custom, have varied greatly, their relative merits much disputed. Engelmann observed,

"According to their build, to the shape of the pelvis, [the parturients of different peoples] stand, squat, kneel or lie upon the belly; so do they vary their position in various stages of labor according to the position of the child's head in the pelvis.... Primitive peoples have solved this problem by virtue of their instinct." [*Labor among Primitive Peoples,* ed. 2. J. H. Chambers & Co., St. Louis, 1833].

Engelmann enumerated 16 different postures for parturition among various races, and Ploss and Bartels in their *Das Weib* (ed. 8, 1905), expanded this list to 40. In an effort to learn *the* natural position, F. C. Naegele surreptitiously observed a young primigravida, left alone during labor in a room containing a bed, chair, couch, and obstetric stool. She assumed every possible position on each, finally giving birth while tossing about on the bed.

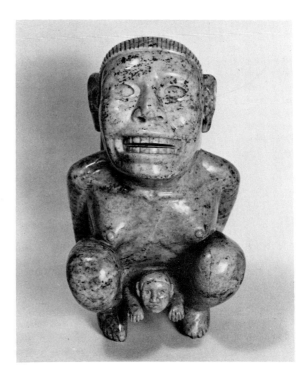

Fig. 8-15. Tlazoltéotl. Aztec fertility deity and mother of gods giving birth in squatting position to Centeotl, goddess of agriculture. Mexican stone figure, 8½ inches, studded with garnets. This posture, used by ancient Mexicans in childbirth, was also assumed by the priests, attired in female garb, in the harvest ritual. Dumbarton Oaks, Washington, D.C.

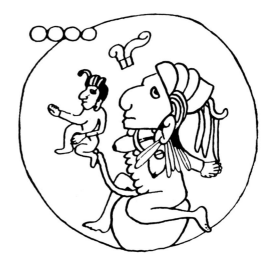

Fig. 8-16. Parturition. Sixteenth century Mexican pen drawing. In early Mexican art forms, the birth act was usually depicted in the squatting position. From Ann. Med. Hist., 1932.

232   ICONOGRAPHIA GYNIATRICA

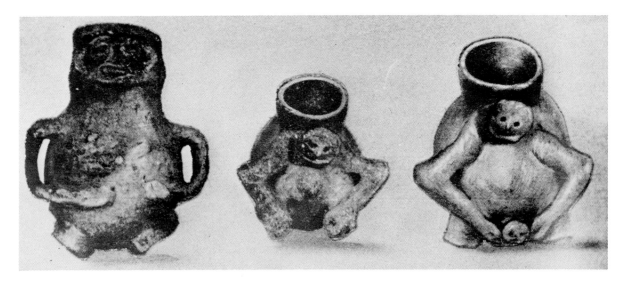

Fig. 8-17. Obstetric effigies. Relics of the Mound Builders of Eastern Arkansas, a prehistoric culture of unknown date. Their osseous remains together with pottery, stone weapons, and primitive agricultural implements showing no evidence of European influence have been recovered from shallow graves. The ceramic urn on the left represents a pregnant woman, with protuberant abdomen and prominent breasts; the central figure, a pregnant woman squatting with hands on thighs, vulva protruding; the urn on the right, a mother assisting the birth of her child whose head is emerging from the vulva.

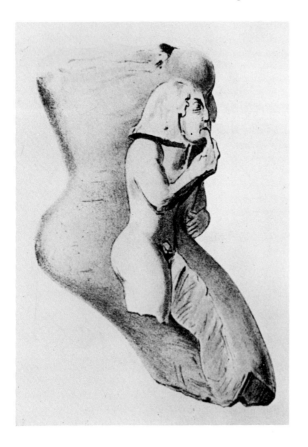

In the early days of Greece and Rome, the standard for parturition was a semi-recumbent position with the woman either in bed or on a low stool. Adapted from the latter was the obstetric stool or birth chair which enjoyed popularity during the Middle Ages, but later fell into dususe with the widespread acceptance of the dorsal decubitus as the preferred position for delivery in most continental European countries and the lateral decubitus in the British Isles.

Fig. 8-18. Birth in kneeling position. Marble figure, Sparta, about 500 BC. From Marx, F., Marmogruppa aus Sparta, 1885.

LABOR AND ITS COMPLICATIONS 233

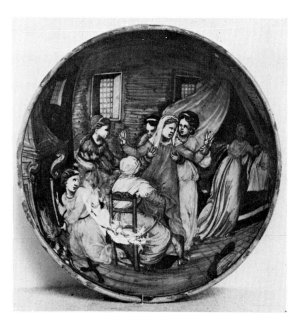

Fig. 8-20. Parturition in standing position. Sixteenth century majolica bowl from Urbino, Italy. The parturient is supported from behind by two women; on a chair before her sits the midwife waiting to receive the child. This unusual birth posture was once common in Central Africa, on the eastern coast of India, in the Antilles, and among the Negritos of the Philippines. Formerly in Kunstgewerbemuseum, Berlin. Destroyed in W.W. II.

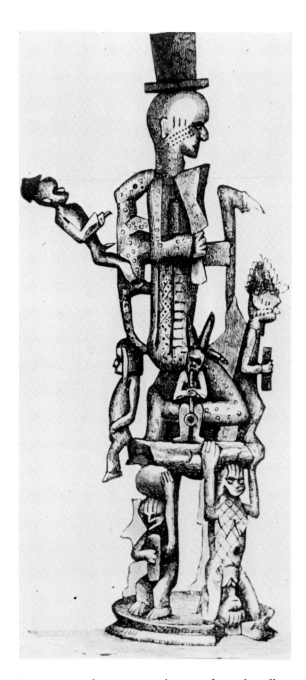

Fig. 8-19. Birth scene. Woodcarving from the village of Uitsha, Republic of the Niger, West Africa. At the lower right of the group, a woman kneels for the birth of her child whose head and neck appear between her legs.

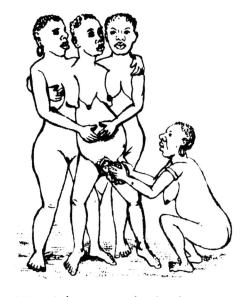

Fig. 8-21. Birth scene. Wakamba district, western part of Central Africa, late nineteenth century. Supported on either side by women, the natives of this and neighboring tribes usually gave birth in the semi-erect position.

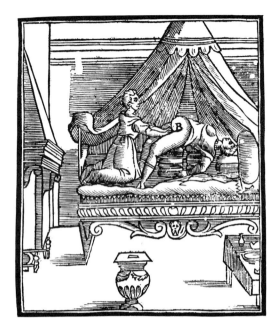

Fig. 8-22. The hanging-legs position. First described by Abulcasis (936–1013) and advocated by Avicenna (c. 979–1037) for the delivery of obese patients, to facilitate exposure of the vulva. This position, a woodcut of which is reproduced here from Scipione Mercurio's famous Italian textbook of obstetrics *La Comare o Raccoglitrice* first published in 1595, bears the caption, "Position essential in every abnormal delivery, in which all pregnant women must be placed who give birth with difficulty from any cause whatsoever." Sebastiano Melli, professor of surgery in Venice, redescribed the same position in his *La Comare*, 1721, more than a century after Mercurio. Proposed by Gustav Adolf Walcher (1856–1935) in 1889 as a method of enlarging the pelvic inlet in cases of cephalopelvic disproportion, the hanging-legs position has since been known as the Walcher position.

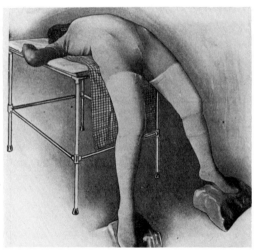

Fig. 8-23. At mid 20th century, a few European texts still recommended the Walcher position in selected cases of inlet disproportion. In America, however, the hanging-legs position was completely abandoned. Joseph B. DeLee taught it, but without enthusiasm, in the early editions of his textbook *The Principles and Practice of Obstetrics,* W.B. Saunders, Philadelphia, 1913, from which this figure is taken. "In a few cases," he wrote, "I have gotten the head to enter the pelvis by this procedure, but it is very painful and few women can be compelled to keep it up over twenty to forty minutes." Later editions denied the position's value altogether.

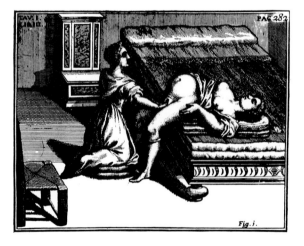

Fig. 8-24. Position for delivery of very fat women. From Melli's *La Comare,* Venice, 1721. Melli explained,

"The midwife takes two or three cushions or bolsters, arranging them in such manner that only the back of the patient is supported when placed upon it, so that the abdomen protrudes and the head hangs downward to the floor. The patient being placed firmly upon the bolsters, she will bend her feet inward toward the pelvis, a posture that tends to enlarge the vagina, rendering it possible for women, however fat, to be delivered with ease, because the corpulency of the abdomen in this posture ... does not interfere with the child's normal birth."

BIRTH PRACTICES

Labor scenes and birth postures among African Tribes were observed and sketched by Robert W. Felkin, a medically educated British anthropologist, during two journeys to various parts of the African continent between 1878 and 1881.

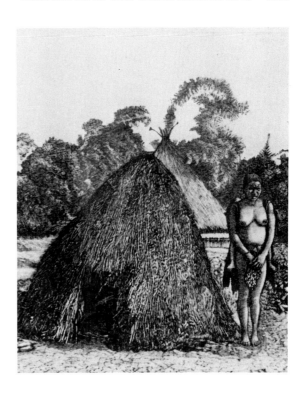

Fig. 8-25. Parturition hut, Ukinga, Lake Nyasa, Southeast Africa. A conical grass shelter, about 6 ft. high and 5 ft. in diameter, furnished with only a crude couch for the parturient. Long-standing custom required that the husband build such a hut for his wife toward the end of pregnancy. In some African tribes the hut was used only for parturition; in others, the expectant mother remained secluded in it for days or weeks before and after labor, visited only by her mother and the midwife, for the parturient was considered unclean.

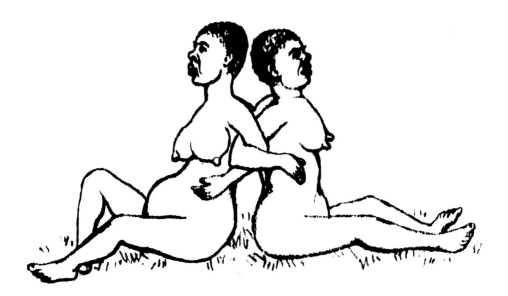

Fig. 8-26. Labor scene, Bari district, Central Africa. The parturient, her arms interfolded with those of another tribeswoman to expedite delivery, was said to have been in labor for two days, a victim of uterine inertia. Felkin succeeded in delivering her with forceps.

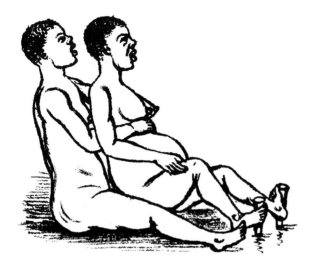

Fig. 8-27. The native women of Central Africa, according to Felkin, underwent labor in seclusion. In the Madi district the parturient paced in her hut while her friends prepared a layer of sand outside, sloping down to two stout stakes firmly driven into the ground. The laboring woman then seated herself upon the sand, her feet propped against the stakes and her back supported by a friend, who rubbed and pressed against her abdomen. Another woman, seated before the parturient, received the child, cut the cord with a stone knife or bit it but did not tie it. If hemorrhage from the cord ensued, the assistant clamped its stump between her teeth until all bleeding ceased. The placenta was buried outside; that of boys on one side of the hut, that of girls on the other.

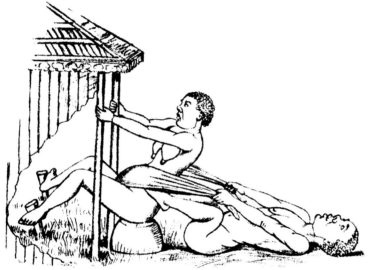

Fig. 8-28. A case of dystocia at Kerrie, on the White Nile. The parturient, seated on an inverted bowl at the entrance to her hut, grasped its posts while pressing with her feet against two stakes in the ground. A man assisted by pulling against the woman's abdomen with a strap of bark, his feet exerting counterpressure against her pelvis.

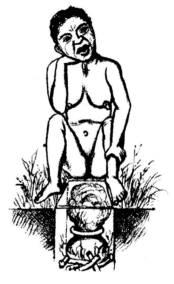

Fig. 8-29. A method for easing labor practiced at Kerrie in Central Africa. The parturient is shown squatting over a steaming kettle of herbs, placed in a hole in the ground. The warm, moist emanations were believed to soften the birth passage and facilitate delivery.

LABOR AND ITS COMPLICATIONS 237

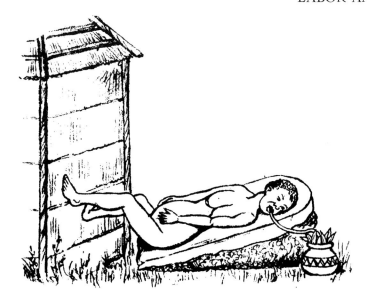

Fig. 8-30. Labor scene, Moru district, Central Africa. The parturient reclined upon a mat, her feet propped against the side of a hut. For pain relief she sucked through a drinking tube from a jug of native beer, made from millet seed.

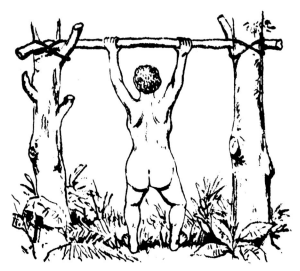

Fig. 8-31. Labor scene, Bongo district, Central Africa. With the onset of a labor pain the parturient grasped a post supported horizontally by two trees and bore down. Between pains the woman walked about.

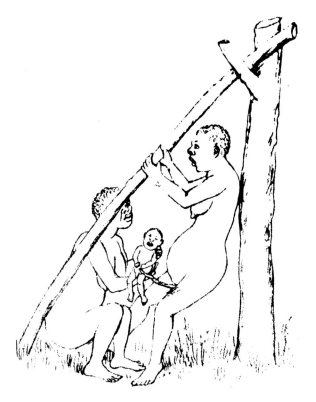

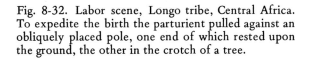

Fig. 8-32. Labor scene, Longo tribe, Central Africa. To expedite the birth the parturient pulled against an obliquely placed pole, one end of which rested upon the ground, the other in the crotch of a tree.

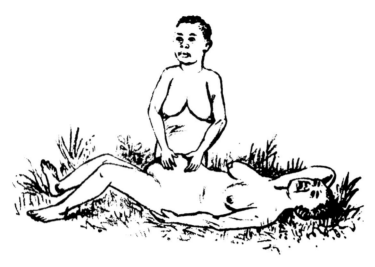

Fig. 8-33. Labor scene, Longo tribe, Central Africa. In cases of prolonged labor or retained placenta, an attendant or friend kneaded the abdomen of the recumbent parturient.

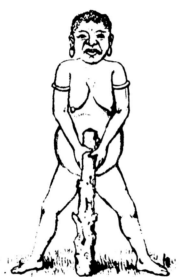

Fig. 8-34. When the placenta failed to come away promptly after childbirth, women of the Unyoro district kneaded their abdomen with the end of a broad pole or log.

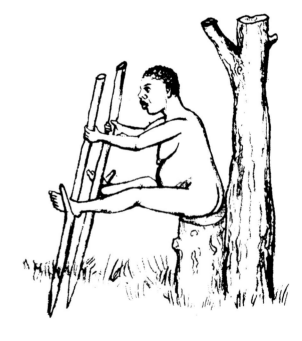

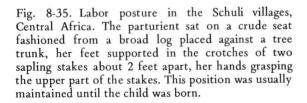

Fig. 8-35. Labor posture in the Schuli villages, Central Africa. The parturient sat on a crude seat fashioned from a broad log placed against a tree trunk, her feet supported in the crotches of two sapling stakes about 2 feet apart, her hands grasping the upper part of the stakes. This position was usually maintained until the child was born.

LABOR AND ITS COMPLICATIONS 239

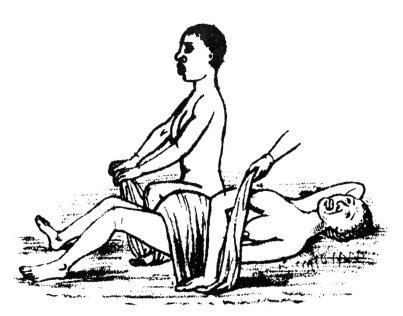

Fig. 8-36. Expression of the retained placenta, Darfour district, East Africa. Across the abdomen of the supine parturient was placed a cloth, its ends held by a woman on either side. By standing on the cloth's folds they then applied pressure against the subject's uterus.

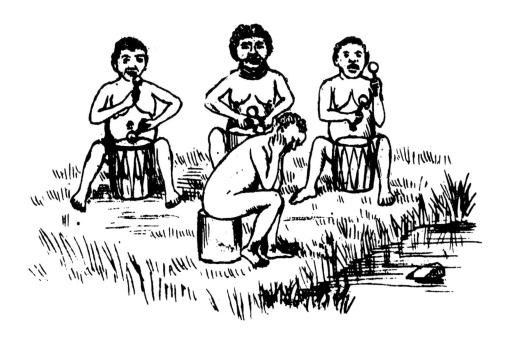

Fig. 8-37. Labor scene among the Nyam-Nyam tribe, cannibals of East Africa. At the onset of labor the parturient was accompanied by other tribeswomen to a secluded spot, by a stream if possible. The expectant mother sat on a log, while her friends beat the tom-toms or blew horns. After the delivery, the umbilical cord was bitten rather than cut. The mother then bathed the child and herself in the stream.

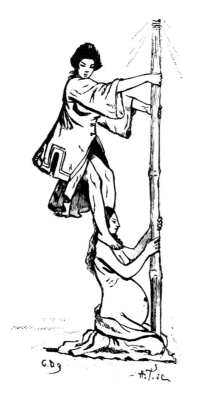

Fig. 8-38. Induction of labor in Cochin China, which became part of Vietnam in 1949. The accoucheur held fast to an upright pole to maintain his balance, while standing on the shoulders of the kneeling parturient.

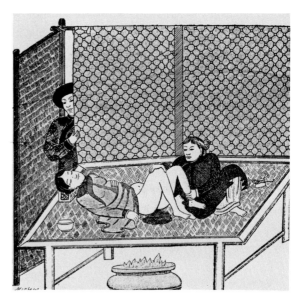

Fig. 8-39. Delivery of an Annamite woman over a brazier in French Indo-China, now Vietnam. Oriental water color.

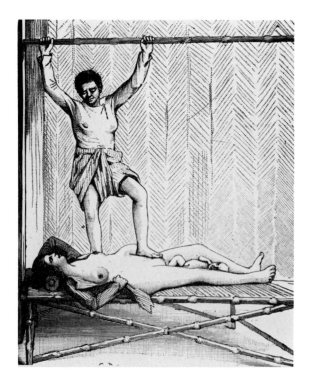

Fig. 8-40. Aid in delivery of the placenta, Annam, formerly coastal French Indo-China, since World War II part of Vietnam. After the birth of the child, seen between the parturient's legs, the accoucheur, supporting himself from an overhead beam, massaged the woman's abdomen with his feet to speed expulsion of the placenta.

LABOR AND ITS COMPLICATIONS   241

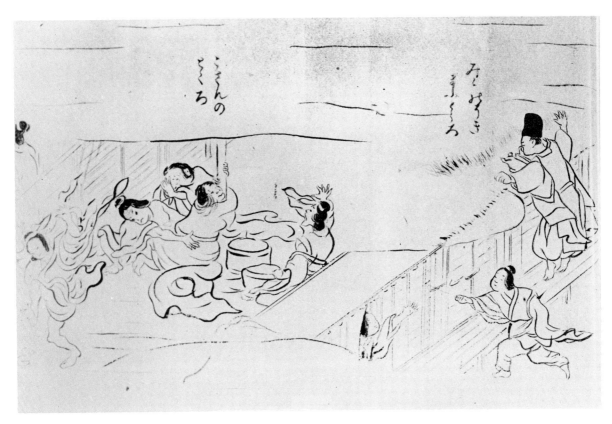

Fig. 8-41. Japanese labor scene. From an old medical text. The laboring woman in a *parturition house* is surrounded by female attendants. Peering in through the thatched roof, a curious prince observes the goings-on.

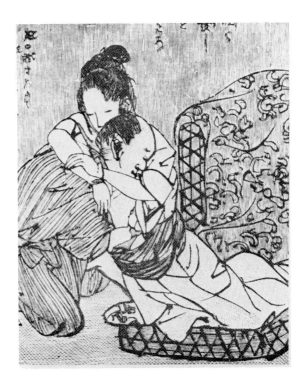

Fig. 8-42. Labor scene. Old Japanese woodcut. The accoucheur massages the parturient's abdomen to expedite delivery. Museum für Völkerkunde, West Berlin.

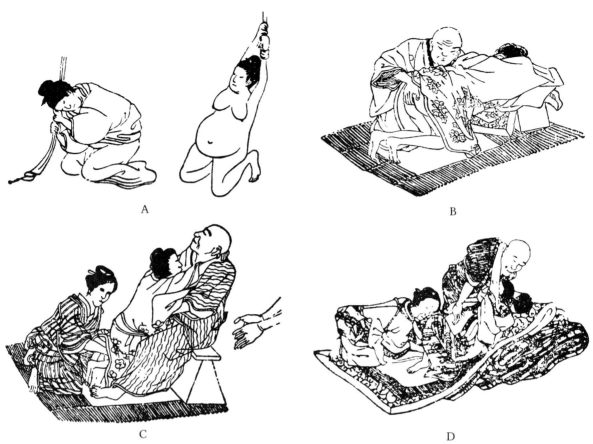

Fig. 8-43. Labor postures. From early nineteenth century Japanese medical texts. (A) The parturient augments her explusive efforts by pulling on a rope suspended from the rafters. (B) Delivery in the knee-chest position. A male midwife or physician attended difficult cases. (C) The kneeling parturient supports herself against her seated husband, as the midwife conducts the delivery. (D) Delivery in a semi-recumbent position, on a folded mattress, assisted by a midwife and a male attendant.

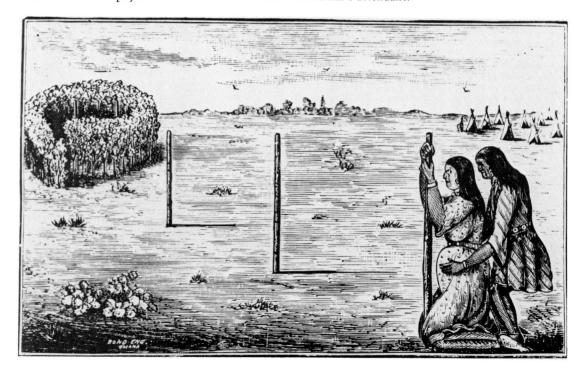

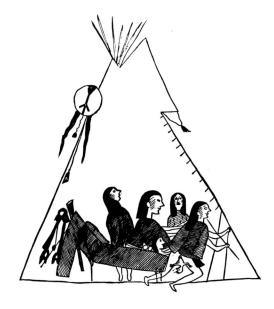

Fig. 8-45. Labor scene, Kiowa Indians. Native drawing. Most common among the squaws of this tribe was the kneeling position.

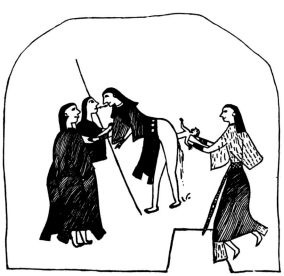

Fig. 8-46. A difficult labor among the Kiowa Indians. Native drawing. To strengthen the parturient's expulsive efforts, the midwife blows an emetic into her mouth.

Fig. 8-44. Parturition hut and labor scene among the Comanche Indians. As observed and sketched by Major W. H. Forwood, Surgeon, U.S.A., mid nineteenth century.

"Inside the shelter were two rectangular excavations in the grass-covered soil, about twelve by sixteen inches ... in one of these holes was a hot stone, and in the other a little loose earth to receive any discharge that might take place from the bladder or bowels; the ground about was strewn with a few aromatic herbs.... I found my patient walking with her assistant, a female relative, up and down the line of stakes outside the shelter, stooping now and then to kneel at the nearest stake and grasping it with both hands during a pain ... occasionally she would enter to kneel over the hot stones.... During each pain ... the assistant stood behind, astride of or between the patient's feet, and stooping over, passed her arms around the body ... in this position she performed several manipulations ... while the pain lasted, such as rubbing, kneading, etc., but most frequently a quick jerking or shaking upward movement, something like that of shaking a pillow into its case. The patient never assumed a recumbent position...."

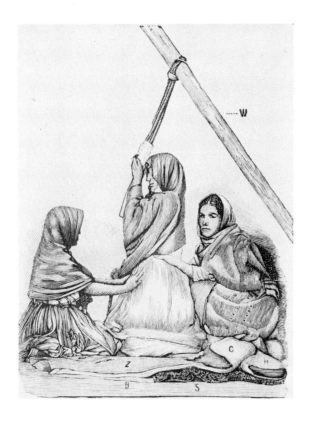

Fig. 8-47. Mexican labor scene. The kneeling parturient, pulling on a rope suspended from a beam, is assisted by two women—the older and more experienced *partera* in front and the younger *tenadora* behind. The partera kneels and presses against the parturient's abdomen and rubs her genitalia to make them more supple. The tenadora supporting her knees against the parturient's hips, presses downward on her fundus. In difficult labors the tenadora would lift the parturient in her arms, shake her, and let her fall, repeating the maneuver as the patient came down on the mat.

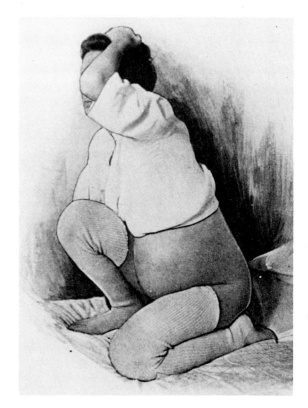

Fig. 8-48. Crouching or Indian attitude. Illustrated in an early twentieth century American textbook, showing how "a head which has slid off the inlet into one iliac fossa may be led back over the inlet."

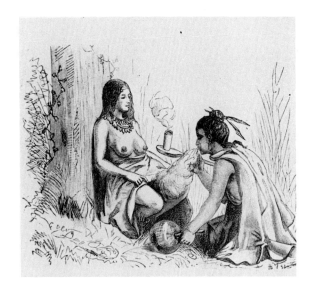

Fig. 8-49. Labor scene, Pawnee Indians, North American plains. To assist delivery by magical powers, a shaman blows smoke against the parturient's vulva.

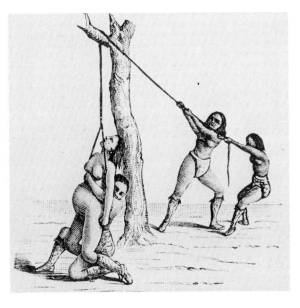

Fig. 8-50. A difficult labor among the Coyotero Indians, a division of the Apaches. Squatting was the customary posture for parturition in this tribe. When delivery from this position failed, wrote U.S.A. Surgeon Walter Reed,

"a rope or lariat is tied around the woman's chest just beneath her arms, and the other end thrown over a stout limb of an adjacent tree, while two or three squaws draw upon this until the woman's knees barely touch the ground; others . . . encircle the body with their arms, and 'strip' down with considerable force. . . ."

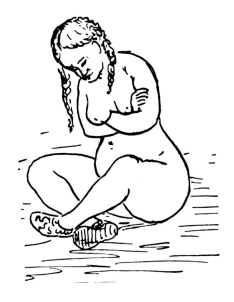

Fig. 8-51. Birth posture. Observed by U.S.A. Surgeon B. B. Taylor in the mid nineteenth century of a Sioux squaw who retired to the bank of a stream at the onset of labor. There he watched her sitting cross-legged, thighs widely separated, arms folded, and head bowed, especially during labor pains, until birth occurred, 40 minutes later. Almost identical is the posture shown in an Egyptian hieroglyph, found on several ancient monuments, believed to represent a woman in the act of parturition.

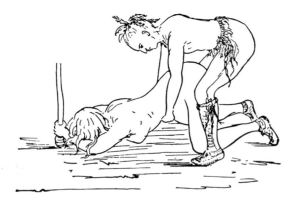

Fig. 8-52. The squaws of some American Indian tribes who normally gave birth stooping or squatting assumed a knee-chest or prone position in difficult labors. The Nez-Percé and Gros-Ventre Indians placed a broad band, known as a squaw-belt, against the parturient's abdomen and with each labor pain assistants on either side applied force backward and downward by pulling on the belt's ends. In lieu of the squaw-belt the Kootenai Indians resorted to the encircling arms of an assistant who straddled the legs of the parturient, as shown here, to provide abdominal pressure.

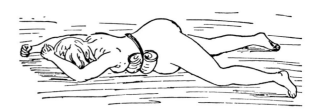

Fig. 8-53. Labor posture of the Creek Indians. Mid nineteenth century, as described by Dr. M. P. Pomeroy of the Crow-Creek Agency.
"When the fetus is about to be expelled the mother straps the belt across her chest, allowing it to extend somewhat on to the abdomen. As the labor proceeds the strap is buckled tighter and tighter, until the expulsion is accomplished; meantime the position assumed by the mother is prone upon her face, her chest and abdomen across a pillow; in this position she remains until the expulsion. She then stands up . . . with the feet spread wide apart. This is to let the blood flow more freely, and . . . to allow the placenta to be more rapidly and easily delivered."

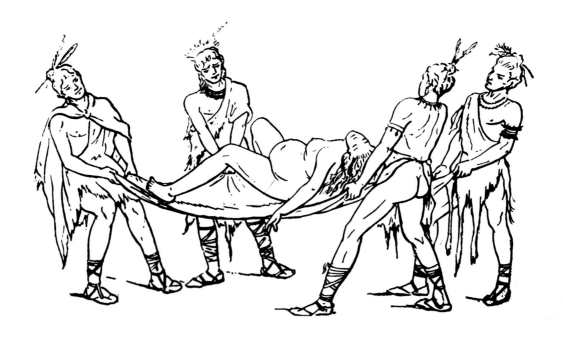

Fig. 8-54. Induction of labor by the Indians of the Canadian Plains. The parturient was tossed in a blanket, held at each corner by a brave.

LABOR AND ITS COMPLICATIONS 247

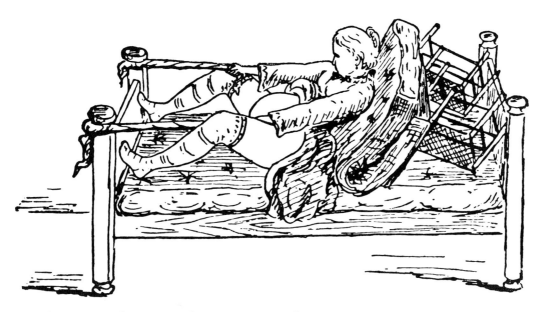

Fig. 8-55. Labor scene, early Virginia. The parturient is maintained in a semi-recumbent position by a doubled mattress, held against her back by an inverted chair. With each labor pain she pressed with her feet against the footboard and pulled on ropes fastened to the bedposts.

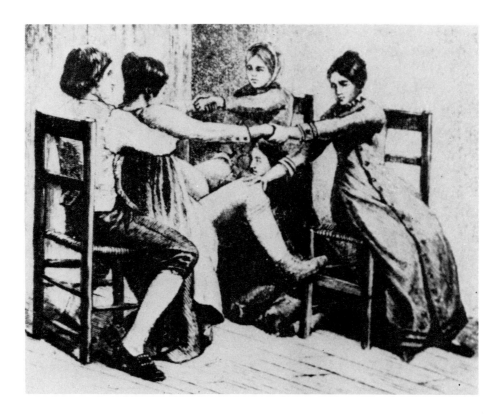

Fig. 8-56. Labor scene, early Virginia. Supported from behind in a semi-recumbent position by her husband, the parturient grasps the hands of two other women. Kneeling before her, the midwife observes the progress of labor. From G. J. Engelmann, *Die Geburt bei den Urvölkern,* Vienna, 1884.

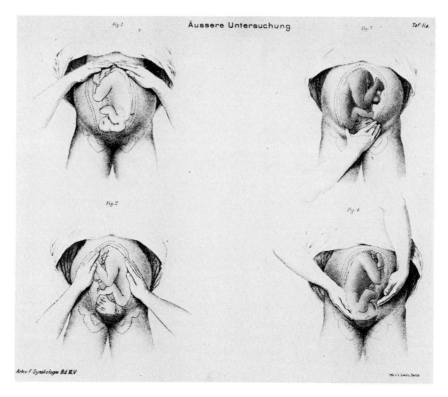

Fig. 8-57. The Leopold maneuvers. Recognizing the hazards of indiscriminate vaginal examination during labor, Gerhard Leopold (1846–1912) and his distinguished father-in-law Carl Credé (1819–1892) urged abdominal palpation as a substitute for the internal examinations routinely practiced by German midwives and physicians during the nineteenth century. In a paper with M. E. C. Pantzer (Arch. Gynaek. 38:330, 1890) Leopold outlined four steps in abdominal palpation, subsequently known as the *Leopold maneuvers,* for ascertaining the position of the fetus and the progress of labor.

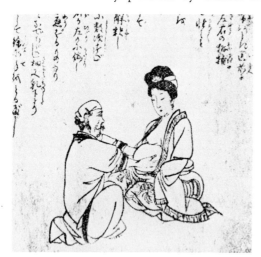

Fig. 8-58. Abdominal palpation of a kneeling gravida. Old Japanese broadside. In ancient Japan and China women customarily gave birth in this position on a straw mat. Institut für Geschichte der Medizin, Leipzig.

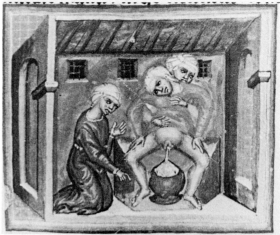

Fig. 8-59. The placenta and membranes are being extruded as two midwives attend the parturient. From a fourteenth century Latin manuscript of Abulcasis' "Surgery." Nationalbibliothek, Vienna.

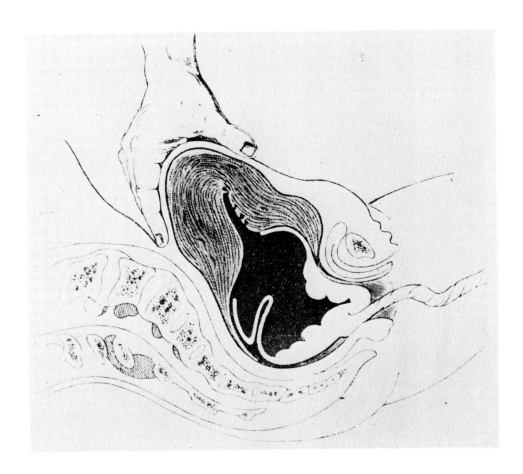

Fig. 8-60. The Credé maneuver. Delivery of the placenta, like the birth act itself, varies from a simple, rapid process to a tedious, delayed effort, often associated with excessive bleeding from the uterus. To expedite the afterbirth's expulsion while avoiding the hazards of internal manipulation, a technique of external pressure or massage of the uterus was advocated by John Harvie in 1767, and by Samuel Bard in 1807. Unaware of these earlier teachings, Carl Credé in 1854 outlined a method of placental expression known since by his name. Credé wrote,

"In most cases the placenta is expressed from the uterus by spontaneous postpartum contractions after about a quarter hour.... However, hemorrhage can occur at any moment; and the longer the time elapsed after birth of the child the more difficult is artificial removal of the placenta from the uterine cavity, should this become necessary.... The simplest and most natural method of artificial delivery of the placenta consists in stimulation and augmentation of the lazy uterine contractions. A single vigorous contraction of the uterus brings the whole process to a speedy termination.... As soon as it reached the peak of its contraction, I grasped the whole uterus with my entire hand, so that the fundus lay in my palm with my five fingers surrounding the corpus and then exerted gentle pressure. Under my fingers I always felt the placenta glide out of the uterus, and indeed this usually occurred with such force that the placenta appeared immediately at the external genitalia, or at least in the lower vagina." [*Klinische Vorträge über Geburtshilfe,* Hirschwald, Berlin, 1854.]

PLACENTAL SEPARATION

"When the *placenta* is delivered by nature alone... it comes away inverted; that is, the side which was in contact with the child, comes first; and the side which adhered to the *uterus,* is covered by the membranes; thus the lobular side is rendered smooth.... If the *placenta* be separated with force... the reverse takes place; that is, the lobular side comes away first...."

Thus wrote John Harvie two centuries ago (*Practical Directions, Shewing a Method of Preserving the Perinaeum in Birth, and Delivering the Placenta Without Violence,* London, 1767). Later obstetricians embraced the teaching that the presenting surface of the placenta indicated the mechanism of the organ's detachment from the uterine wall.

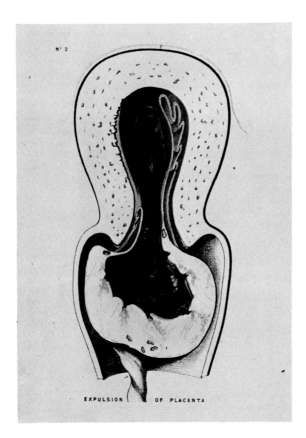

Fig. 8-61. The Schultze mechanism. An atlas of obstetric wall charts published in 1865 by Bernhard Schultze (1827–1919) (*Wandtafeln zur Schwangerschafts-und Geburtskunde,* Leipzig) illustrated his conception of the normal mechanism, since associated with his name, of placental separation and expulsion. Emphasizing the role of the retroplacental hemorrhage from the uterine sinuses in the completion of the placenta's separation, Schultze pictured its egress through the same rent in the membranes from which the fetus emerged, the placenta pulling its attached membranes along, inner surface showing, like a sock turned inside out.

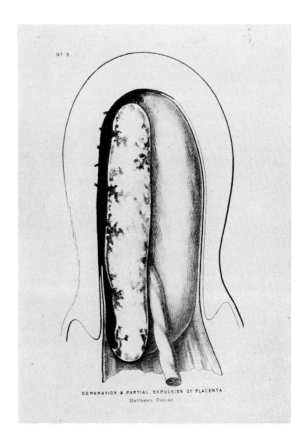

Fig. 8-62. The Duncan mechanism. Contrary to Schultze's teaching was the view of James Matthews Duncan (1826–1890), distinguished Scotch obstetrician who reported to the Obstetrical Society of Edinburgh in 1871 that

"inversion of the placenta, or its folding upon itself transversely to the passage, or the presentation of the foetal surface... is a very rare occurrence.... The placenta is folded upon itself during the process... but the folds are according to the length of the passage, not transverse to it, as inversion or presentation of the foetal surface imply."

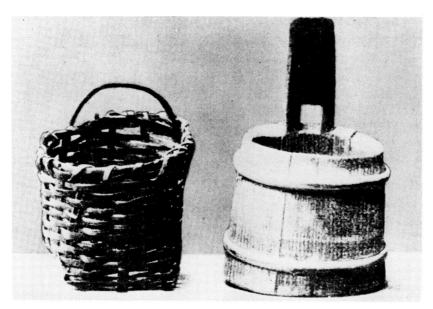

Fig. 8-63. Placental baskets. Methods of disposing of the placenta have varied among different cultures. In Upper Austria and the Province of Salzburg, for example, it was customary to bury the placenta under a green tree to ensure the woman's continuing fertility. In the Serbo-Croation province of Dalmatia on the Adriatic coast, the placenta was buried under a rose bush, thus might the child always have rosy cheeks. Some groups buried the placenta to prevent the harm that would come to the mother or child if an animal touched the organ. Special burial vessels were used. The Alaskan Indians often cremated the placenta, preserving the ashes for ultimate burial with those of the child after its death. Shown are two baskets as once used in Bosnia and Herzegovina, now provinces of Yugoslavia, for burial of the placenta.

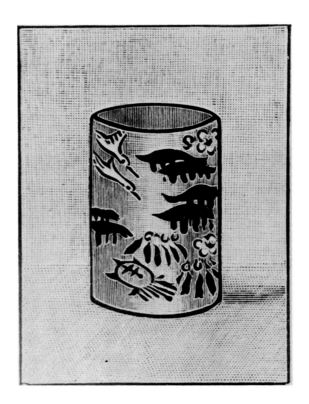

Fig. 8-64. Japanese cedarwood box for the placenta. The organ was usually buried at a depth of 7 feet at a site selected by the Shinto priest from his interpretation of signs. The ritual varied according to the sex of the child. The placenta of a boy was buried with India ink and a writing brush; that of a girl, with a needle and thread.

SOME COMPLICATIONS OF LABOR

"The mother may suffer difficult labor through psychic influences... as well as from physical reasons... too fat a condition and excessive size of the body, broad shoulders and narrow hips and narrow pelvis; the child can be too big in general or in particular parts... there may be several children present; the embryo may have died and then does not assist delivery; and finally it may have a faulty presentation." [Soranus]

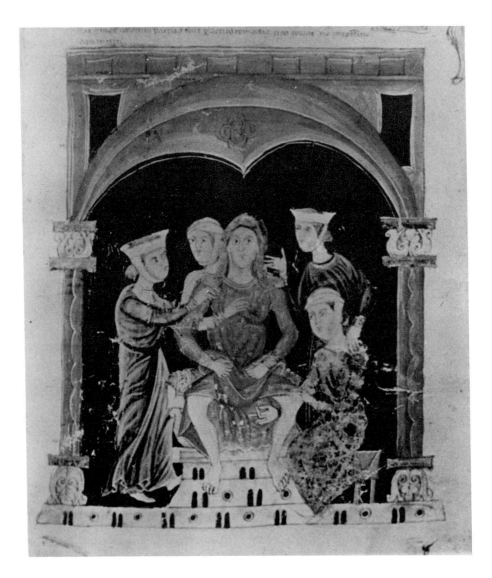

Fig. 8-65. Uterine inertia treated with coriander seed. Miniature of a sixth century figure from the thirteenth century handbook of Apulejus, *De medicaminibus herbarum*. The midwife, kneeling on the right, applies the coriander seed to the parturient's vulva. The text contains the admonition that the seed be removed promptly lest the patient's intestines be brought forth with the fetus. Six centuries later in an editorial note in its December 26, 1891 issue, the *Journal of the American Medical Association* advised, "for a tardy delivery: Sneezing favors the expulsion of the child in a case of labor, hence the use of tobacco, snuff or pepper, or other substances that will bring on the paroxysm by irritating the Schneiderian membrane, will hasten a tardy delivery." Nationalbibliothek, Vienna.

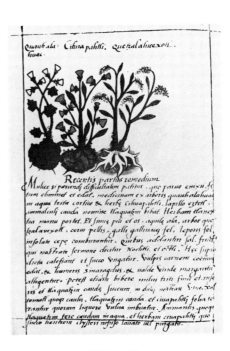

Fig. 8-66. Drugs used in labor by the Aztecs, pre-Columbian Mexico. Obtained from the middle plant was *cihuapatli* (*cihuatl*, woman; *patli*, drug) which has been shown by modern experiment to have oxytocic properties. In addition to herbals the Badianus codex recommended parturitional aids of dubious pharmacologic value such as *tlacuatzin,* a potion made from opossum tail. The Badianus codex, the work of an Indian physician Martin de la Cruz has been named erroneously after the Mexican scribe, Juan Badiano who translated the medical parts of the codex into Latin in 1552 under the title *Libellus de medicinalibus Indorum Herbis.*

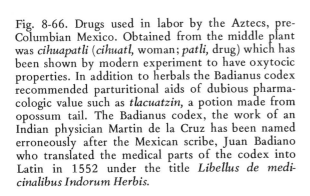

Fig. 8-67. The first mention of the use of ergot as an oxytocic. In the 1582 edition of Adam Lonicer's *Kreuterbuch.* The "long black hard narrow corn pegs, white on the inside, often protruding like long nails from among the greens in the ear," were prescribed in a dose of three sclerotia (about 0.5 Gm) repeated several times, for stimulating uterine contractions. European midwives used ergot for its oxytocic effects during the eighteenth century, but the drug achieved its first formal medical recognition in 1808 in the United States in the form of a letter published in the *Medical Repository of New York* from Dr. John Stearns of Saratoga County to a Mr. S. Akerly. "*Pulvis parturiens,*" as Stearns called his ergot preparation,

"I have been in the habit of using for several years, with the most complete success. It expedites lingering parturition, and saves to the accoucheur a considerable portion of time.... Previous to its exhibition it is of the utmost consequence to ascertain the presentation... as the violent and almost incessant action which it induces in the uterus precludes the possibility of *turning....* If the dose is large it will produce nausea and vomiting. In most cases you will be surprised with the suddenness of its operation; it is, therefore, necessary to be completely ready before you give the medicine.... Since I have adopted the use of this powder I have seldom found a case that detained me more than three hours."

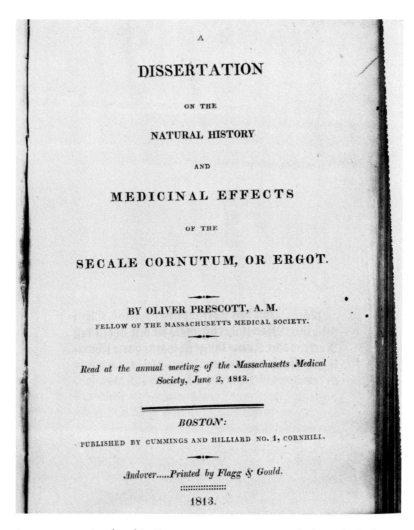

Fig. 8-68. Interest in ergot was stimulated in Europe by "A Dissertation on the Natural History and Medicinal Effects of the Secale Cornutum, or Ergot." Read by Oliver Prescott before the Massachusetts Medical Society on June 2, 1813 and published in pamphlet form later that year. Subsequently reprinted in Philadelphia and London, Prescott's dissertation was also translated into French and German.

Echoing Stearns' enthusiasm W. Michell, a Cornish physician, wrote in his book *On Difficult Cases of Parturition and the use of Ergot of Rye,* published in London in 1828, "I am of the opinion that as soon as it is generally known in female practice, it will supersede the necessity for male practitioners, except in a very few cases." George Barger, who published a monograph on ergot in 1931 (*Ergot and Ergotism,* Gurney and Jackson, London) even suggested that "had the action of ergot been known earlier, lever and forceps would never have been invented...."

The rumblings of dissent were soon heard, however. David Hosack of New York wrote in a letter dated June 2, 1822 to James Hamilton, Professor of Obstetrics in the University of Edinburgh, that an inquiry had already been begun by New York's medical society because of the great increase in the number of stillborn infants since the introduction of ergot. "The ergot has been called," continued Hosack, "*pulvis ad partum;* as it regards the child, it may with almost equal truth be denominated the *pulvis ad mortem.*" Nonetheless Hosack approved the use of ergot for the control of postpartum hemorrhage. Thus restricted, ergot has proved an inestimable boon to subsequent generations.

LABOR AND ITS COMPLICATIONS 255

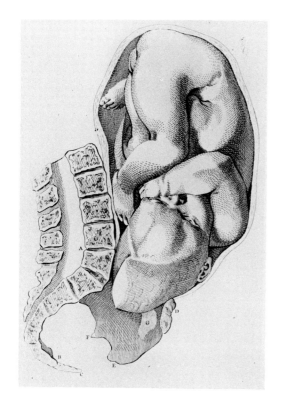

Fig. 8-69. Cephalopelvic disproportion. Plate 28 from William Smellie's *A Sett of Anatomical Tables,* London, 1754, showing "a side view of a distorted *Pelvis* . . . with the head of a full grown *Foetus* squeezed into the brim, the *Parietal* bones decussating each other, and compressed into a conical form."

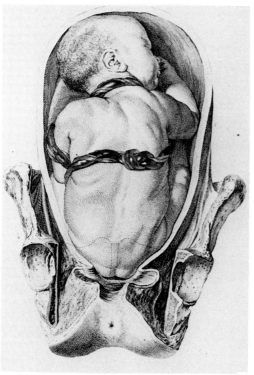
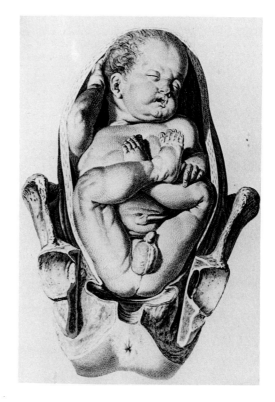

Fig. 8-70. Breech presentation. From William Smellie's *A Sett of Anatomical Tables,* London, 1754.

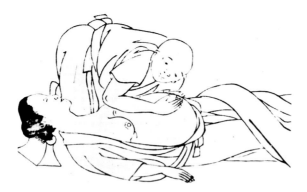

Fig. 8-71. The infant loss with breech delivery greatly exceeds that associated with the more common cephalic presentation. This disparity results, in part, from the higher proportion of breech presentation in premature than in term labors, and in part from asphyxia due to cord compression and mechanical injuries caused by breech delivery itself. In some cultures breech birth was considered an evil omen. In nineteenth century Uganda, for example, it was believed that children born feet first, if allowed to live, would cause the death of their parents. These ill-fated offspring were therefore killed soon after birth and buried at a cross-roads. To reduce the hazards of breech delivery to the infant, some obstetricians attempt external version in late pregnancy, changing the polarity of the fetus by turning it within the uterus. This procedure is here illustrated, as practiced by Japanese accoucheurs during the nineteenth century, from a treatise on obstetric maneuvers by Gaksiu Kondo published in 1864.

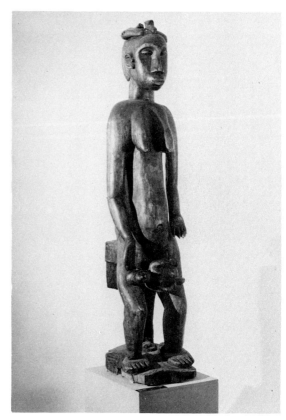

Fig. 8-72. Cameroon woodcarving, 1.95 meters. Believed to symbolize a transverse lie of the fetus, least favorable for spontaneous delivery.

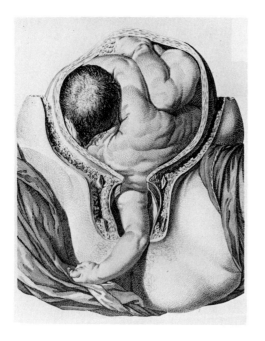

Fig. 8-73. Transverse lie with prolapse of arm. From William Smellie's obstetric atlas, 1754,

"the breech and fore parts being towards the *Fundus Uteri,* the left arm in the *Vagina,* and fore arm without the *Os Externum,* the shoulder being likewise forced into the *Os Uteri.*"

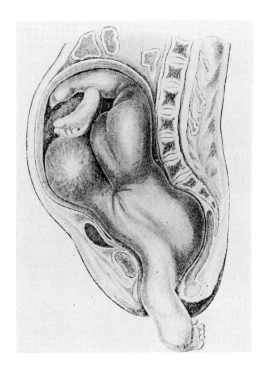

Fig. 8-74. Without obstetric intervention the fetus in transverse lie has little chance of live birth, and in neglected cases the mother too may perish. Rarely, if the maternal pelvis is large and the fetus small, unassisted delivery may be accomplished by a remarkable mechanism known as spontaneous evolution. First described by Thomas Denman (1733–1815) in 1783, spontaneous evolution has since been associated with his name. A variant of this complex labor mechanism, recorded by John C. Douglas (1778–1850) in 1811, has been identified with the name of the latter. Illustrated here in sagittal section is the pelvis of a woman who died in labor, the fetus in an arrested stage of spontaneous evolution, preparation by Domenico Chiara, Milanese obstetrician, 1878. An arm and the cord prolapsed after the midwife ruptured the membranes. Repeated attempts at version, by a surgeon, were unsuccessful. The shoulder is fixed under the pubic arch, the neck elongated, and the head in the process of rotating around the pubis. From D. Chiara, *La Evoluzione Spontanea*, Milan, 1878.

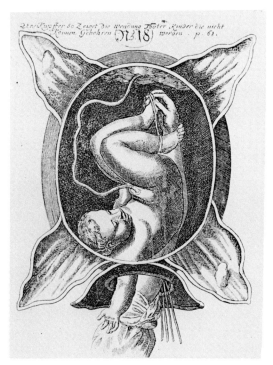

A

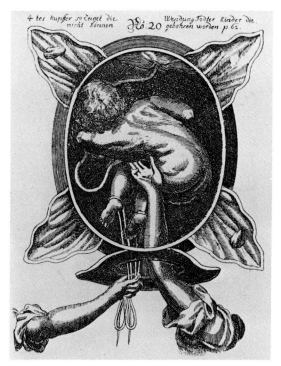

B

Fig. 8-75. Version and extraction. For oblique or transverse lie, as practiced by Justine Siegemundin, famous German midwife of the late seventeenth and early eighteenth century. With one hand the midwife pulled on the fillets applied to the ankles of the fetus, while assisting version by intrauterine manipulation with her other hand. From J. Siegemundin, *Die Chur-Brandenburgische Hoff-Wehe-Mutter*, 1690.

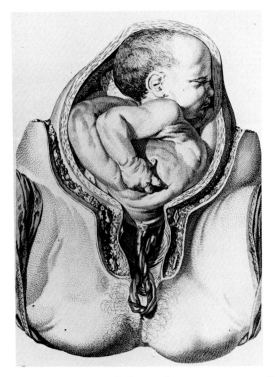

Fig. 8-76. Prolapse of the cord, a common complication of transverse lie. From Smellie's obstetric atlas, 1754.

Fig. 8-78. Uterine retraction ring. In normal labor dominance of the musculature of the uterine fundus over that of the relatively passive lower uterine segment coupled with the myometrial tendency to retract results in a progressive disparity between the two zones of the uterine wall, the upper thickening at the expense of the lower. In obstructed labor as from fetopelvic disproportion or fetal malpresentation, the retraction ring between the upper and lower uterine segments rises increasingly higher even to the level of the umbilicus while the lower segment continues to thin, in neglected cases to the point of rupture. Reproduced here from Ludwig Bandl's monograph of 1875 on uterine rupture is his plate showing (1) normal and (2-6) pathologic retraction rings. Bandl, a Viennese physician who made important contributions to our knowledge of the mechanics of the uterus in labor, was appointed to the chair of obstetrics and gynecology in the University of Prague in 1886, but retired after a few months because of the anxiety he experienced at lecturing. He died in 1892 in a psychiatric institution.

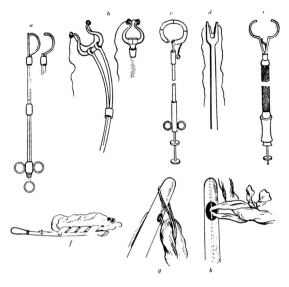

Fig. 8-77. Cord repositors. In common use during the nineteenth and early twentieth centuries in management of prolapse of the umbilical cord. Rarely successful, attempts at reposition of the cord as well as its traumatic alternative, version and extraction, have given way to cesarean section in the treatment of this fetal emergency.

Fig. 8-79. Fetal death in utero.

"In many instances it would be highly important, could we determine with certainty, that the child was dead while in utero—it would serve to abridge the sufferings of the mother, and sometimes would spare the accoucheur a deep drawn sigh; but this is a matter of great difficulty, as well as oftentimes of great moment to decide. All the commonly enumerated signs have been known to fail, and even when many of the strongest were united."

Thus wrote Dewees in 1830 in his *A Compendious System of Midwifery*. In 1921 D. A. Horner and Alfred B. Spalding independently discovered pathognomonic roentgenographic evidence of fetal death in utero—overriding of the skull bones distinct from the overlapping produced by molding. Illustrated here from Spalding's report of three cases, this skull change has since been known as *Spalding's sign*.

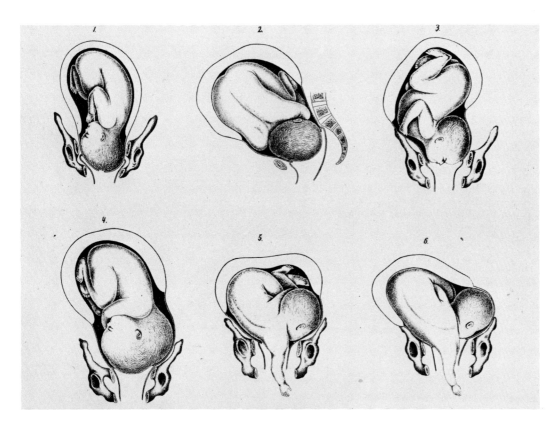

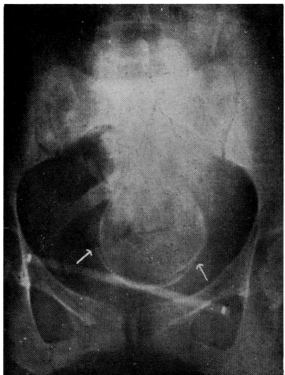

Fig. 8-80. Placenta previa. Palpation *per vaginam*, a time-honored method of diagnosis.

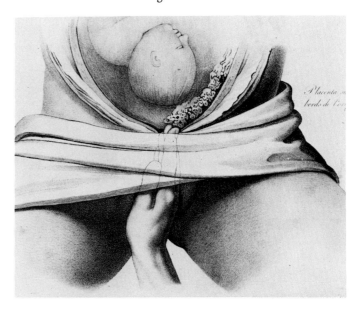

Fig. 8-81. Bipolar version, a nineteenth century method of management of placenta previa. Illustrations from a paper of John Braxton Hicks, "On a new method of version in abnormal labour." Lancet 2:28, 1860. Hicks wrote,

"Anything which gave the practitioner some power of action was to be earnestly welcomed; anything better than to stand with folded arms, incapable of rendering assistance for hours and even days, every moment of which might be carrying the sinking and suffering patient nearer to the grave. . . . Turn, and if you employ the child as a plug the danger is over. Then wait for the pains, rally the powers in the interval and let nature, gently assisted, complete the delivery."

THE LANCET,] DR. J. B. HICKS ON A NEW METHOD OF VERSION IN ABNORMAL LABOUR. [JULY 14, 1860.

men downwards, the knees of the fœtus are opposite the os uteri; and if the os is large enough to introduce a finger, the knee can be hooked down and the presentation secured. Thus it is evident that it is merely necessary for the fœtus to assume the above position, where delivery by knee or foot is sought for, or where we wish that the delivery may be at our command. I shall defer alluding to version of cephalic into pure breech presentation till I speak of the method of operation.

The next fact to be borne in mind is that, should the fœtus, either naturally or by the method to be described, present by its back to the os uteri, the case would be very rare in which one side or the other was not the more dependent, and consequently one or the other knee be within finger-reach of the os.

The third fact needful to reflect upon is this, that the shape of the cavity of the fully-developed uterus being oval, with the long axis placed vertically, the tendency of the slight pains towards the end of pregnancy is to place the longer axis of the fœtus in a corresponding direction; or, in other terms, to cause it to present by the head or breech: so that if the fœtus be at any time situated transversely, a slight preponderance of force in either direction will be sufficient to determine the ultimate presentation. It will be thus perceived that, the head being heavier than the pelvic extremity, the natural tendency of a spontaneous rectification will be to head presentation; but at the same time it would have taken but little force to have caused it to rise to the fundus.

Having premised these considerations, we will discuss the other facts as they arise in the application of the above principles, taking for granted that it is admitted possible to turn the fœtus in utero from the outside. The method I have found successful, and very easy of application, is conducted thus:—We will suppose the simplest condition, a case where the uterus is passive, membranes unbroken, the liquor amnii plentiful, the os uteri expanded sufficiently to detect the presentation, which is cephalic, and in the first or fourth position (occiput to left side); the patient is in the ordinary position, the trunk curved forwards as much as possible, to relax the abdominal muscles. Introduce the left hand, with the usual precautions, into the vagina, so far as to fairly touch the fœtal head, even should it recede an inch. (This generally requires the whole hand.) Having passed one or two fingers (if only one, let it be the middle finger) within the cervix, and resting them on the head, place the *right* hand on the *left* side of the breech at

FIG. 1.

the fundus uteri, as shown at Fig. 1. Employ gentle pressure and slight impulsive movements on the fundus towards the right side, and simultaneously on the head towards the left iliac fossa. In a very short time it will be found that the head is rising and at the same time the breech is descending. The shoulder is now felt by the hand in place of the head, as in Fig. 2; it in like manner is pushed to the left, and at the same time the breech is depressed to the right iliac fossa. The

FIG. 2.

fœtus is now transverse; the knee will be opposite the os, and, the membranes being ruptured, it can be seized, as at Fig. 3, and brought into the vagina.

Having now the labour at command, the case must be treated according to the circumstances which called for turning. In

FIG. 3.

obedience to the law above stated, when the fœtus is placed transversely, a slight impulse will determine the final position of the head. When the leg is seized, therefore, it is advisable

29

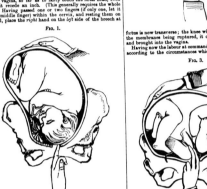

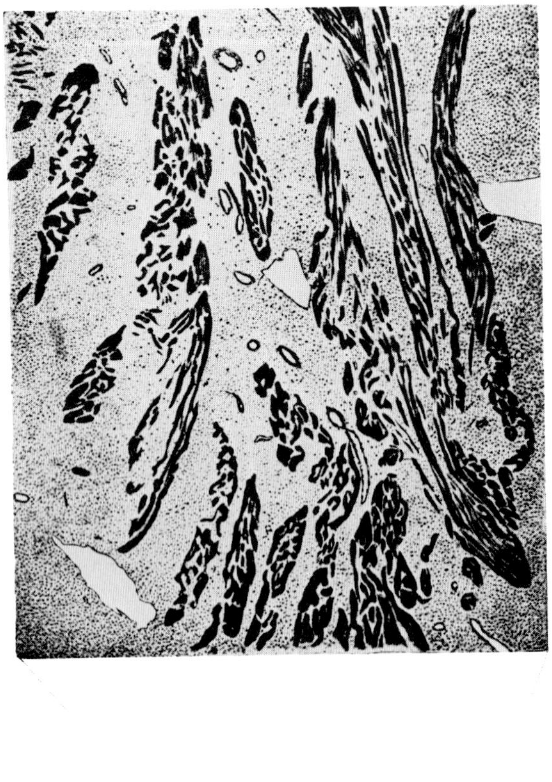

Fig. 8-82. Placental abruption, *Couvelaire uterus.* Section showing dissociation of muscle bundles by hemorrhage into the myometrium. Illustration from Alexandre Couvelaire's paper, 1911, in which he used the term *uteroplacental apoplexy* for the first time. The patient was a 26 year old primigravida with toxemia of pregnancy who suffered placental abruption with shock and fetal death in utero during the eighth month. At laparotomy the uterus and adnexa appeared extensively infiltrated with blood. Recovery of the mother followed cesarean-hysterectomy and bilateral salpingo-oophorectomy.

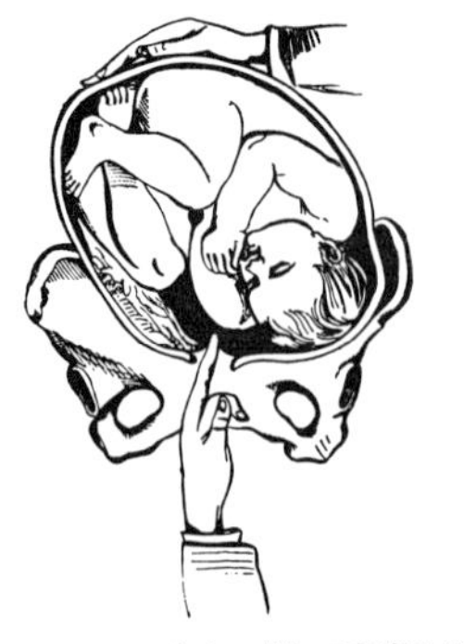

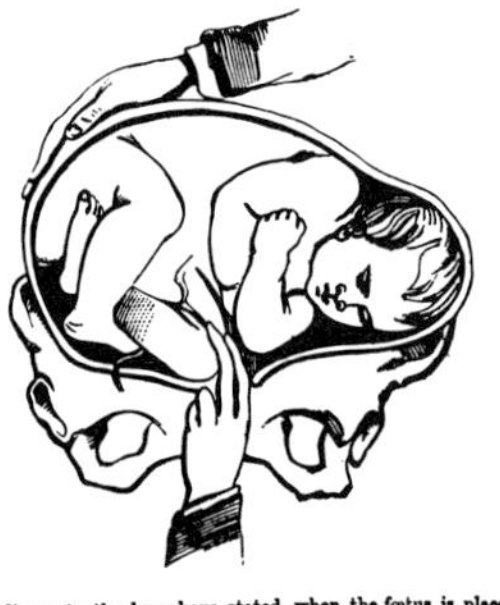

LABOR AND ITS COMPLICATIONS 261

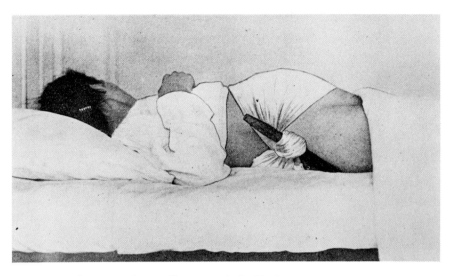

Fig. 8-83. The Spanish windlass. A cloth binder tightened by a stick for uterine compression in cases of placental abruption.

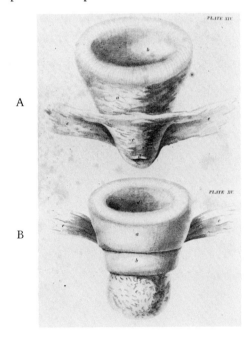

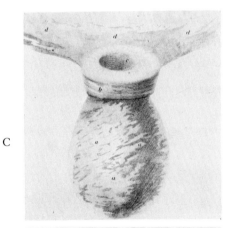

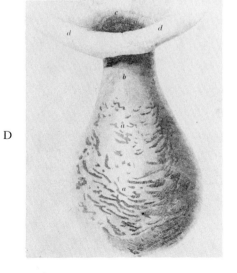

Fig. 8-84. Inversion of the uterus. A cause of postpartum shock as illustrated in an early nineteenth century textbook. (A) The beginning of the process, a depression forms in the uterine fundus. (B) The inverting corpus of the uterus, turned inside out like a sock, protrudes through the cervix, the endometrial surface exposed. (C) As inversion continues, the contracting cervix embraces the protruding corpus. (D) Inversion complete, a flasklike concavity is seen from the abdominal side.

262 ICONOGRAPHIA GYNIATRICA

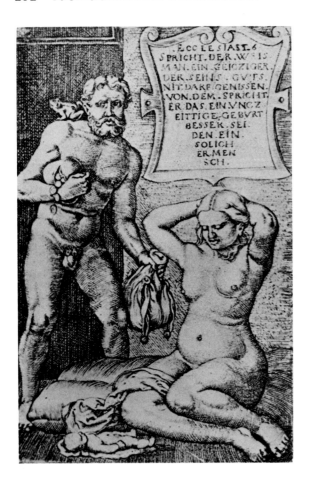

Fig. 8-85. The miscarriage. An allegorical etching by Barthel Beham (1502–1540). The unhappy woman contemplates the half-finished object of her desire as her greedy husband stands by, holding fast to his earthly wealth. Engraved on the tablet above appear the words of the wise man, "Better a miscarriage than such a person."

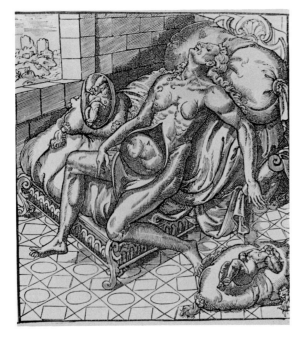

Fig. 8-86. Missed labor with lithopedion. Woodcut, 1582, by Jean Cousin (1501?–1589). The woman, age 28, started into labor at full-term after an uneventful pregnancy. The membranes ruptured with discharge of the fluid and a blood clot, but labor ceased and fetal movement could no longer be felt. After a while the woman's breasts began to shrink, but she continued to have the full abdomen of pregnancy. At age 68 she died, having borne her burden 40 years. Within her uterus was found a female infant with hands and feet like marble, encased in calcified membranes.

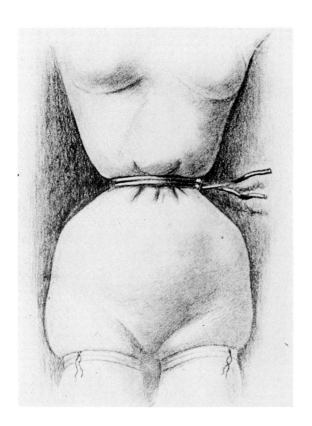

Fig. 8-87. Momburg's tourniquet. Early twentieth century, for the arrest of postpartum hemorrhage. Circular constriction of the waist with a rubber tube to cut off the distal circulation was used initially in surgical cases. This method of treatment was abandoned after several instances were reported of gangrene of the thigh, intestinal hemorrhage, and heart failure on release of the tourniquet.

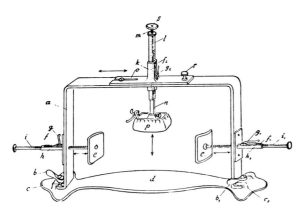

Fig. 8-88. Gauss's aortic compressor. For arresting uterine hemorrhage, early twentieth century. In some regions of Europe as in Styria, a province of Austria, parturient women held tight to the *blood-stone,* a piece of iron ore, to control postpartum blood loss.

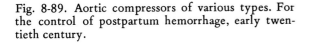

Fig. 8-89. Aortic compressors of various types. For the control of postpartum hemorrhage, early twentieth century.

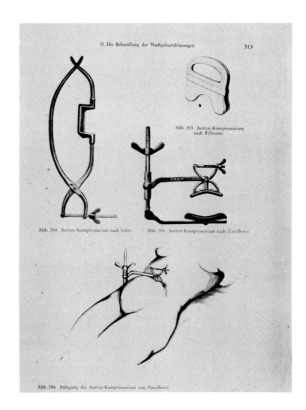

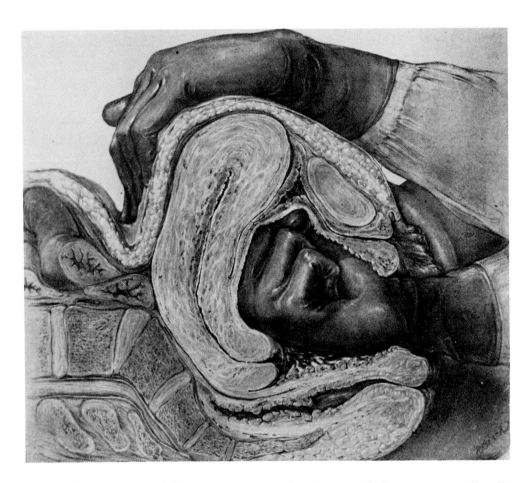

Fig. 8-90. Bimanual compression of the uterus. For the control of postpartum hemorrhage, advocated by G. Hamilton in 1861. Hamilton wrote,

"I have found that usually the most effectual mode of restraining the haemorrhage...is to pass the fingers of the right hand *under* the uterus, which the relaxed state of the parts generally allows being easily done, and then firmly to compress the walls of the uterus between the two hands. This method...has proved completely successful....Clearing out the clots from the interior of the uterus appears to me quite essential, as a preliminary, to successful treatment." [Edinburgh Medical Journal, 7, 315, 1861.]

Chapter 9

ACCOUTERMENTS OF THE BIRTH CHAMBER

BIRTHSTOOLS, CHAIRS, AND TABLES

"When ye do the office of a midwife to the Hebrew women and see them upon the stools..." (Exodus 1:16). Another version of this Biblical passage contains "stones" in lieu of "stools;" the Hebrew word *obnayim* has both meanings. Stones, used by potters as a worktable, were perhaps related to the birth process by the Egyptian ancients in accordance with their belief that God creates and fashions men as a potter does his clay. "To sit on stones" was synonymous in Egyptian hieroglyphics with "to give birth." When two stones or the sides of a stone trough were later connected by a transverse arm, a type of parturition chair resulted, the prototype of the *Kursie el-wilada*, the birth chair still used by some Egyptian women.

The birthstool was recommended for natural labors by Soranus early in the second century AD and by many subsequent writers on obstetrical matters. Moschion, later in the same century, described the obstetric chair "as in form like a barber's chair, but with a crescent-shaped opening in the seat, through which the child may fall." Pictured for the first time in the works of Savonarola in the sixteenth century, the *sella perforata* received the warm endorsement of the illustrious Ambroise Paré (1510–1590). Despite its scorn by François Mauriceau (1637–1709), the lead-

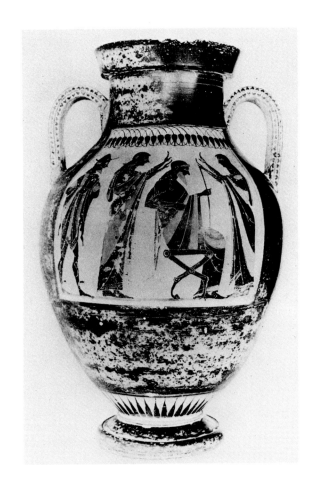

Fig. 9-1. Zeus in labor seated on a birth chair attended by Hermes and two Eileithyiai, goddesses of childbirth. Black-figured amphora from Girgenti, now Agrigento an Italian province.

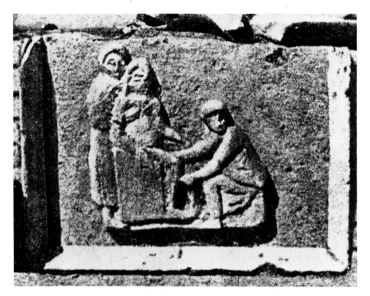

Fig. 9-2. Relief on the gravestone of a Roman midwife. Depicting a labor scene with the parturient on the birthstool. In the practice of her craft the Roman midwife dragged or carried her birthstool along from house to house.

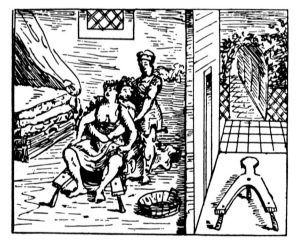

Fig. 9-3. The birthstool and its correct use. Woodcut from the 1547 edition of the works (*Practica major*, Venice) of Giovanni Michele Savonarola (c. 1384–1462). An attendant, sitting on the rounded projection at the apex of the stool, supported the back of the parturient, seated on the forked part.

ing figure in French obstetrics of the seventeenth century, who advocated delivery in bed, the obstetric chair remained indispensable to the equipment of most midwives and accoucheurs to the middle of the eighteenth century. By mid nineteenth century the names of at least 31 different obstetric authorities were associated with chairs of their own design. Each wealthy household had its own; and in Holland, every affluent bride was expected to have a birth chair as part of her trousseau. Among the poor, the obstetric chair was transported from house to house. The birth chairs of the royalty were carved and ornamented with jewels.

As the obstetric forceps gained popularity during the eighteenth century, and accoucheurs gave increasing attention to support of the perineum at delivery, the obstetric chair lost favor. The midwives of Italy were slow to abandon the chair, however, according to Bernardino Ramazzini's account in his *De morbis artificum*, 1713.

"Perhaps in England, France, Germany, and other countries midwives suffer less, because the women give birth to their infants lying in bed instead of sitting on chairs made with hollow seats as they do in Italy, where midwives attend always leaning forward and bent over, with hands stretched out watching for the fetus to appear at the mouth of the womb; they are so fatigued by all this effort and waiting, especially when they attend ladies or there is prolonged labor, that when at last the infant is delivered they go home faint and exhausted, cursing their profession." [Translation by W. C. Wright: *Diseases of Women*. Hafner Publishing Co., New York, 1964.]

By the end of the eighteenth century little more was heard of the birth chair. The judgment of Mauriceau was vindicated; the obstetric chair had given way to the bed and the delivery tables of the nineteenth and twentieth centuries.

ACCOUTERMENTS OF THE BIRTH CHAMBER 267

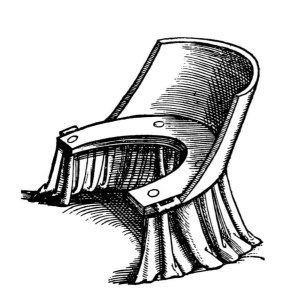

Fig. 9-4. Birth chair. From Jacob Rueff's *De conceptu et generatione hominis,* 1554 edition. More rounded than the angular stool of Savonarola, Rueff's seat with valance added had a back to support the parturient in lieu of an attendant.

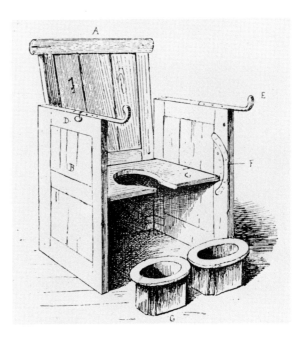

Fig. 9-5. Birth chair of Hendrik van Deventer (1651–1724) with adjustable seat, hand grips, and warming pots.

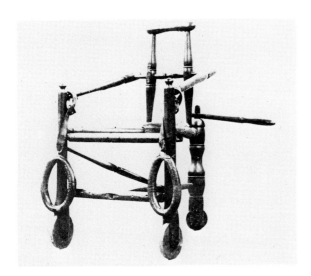

Fig. 9-6. A German birth chair. Seventeenth century.

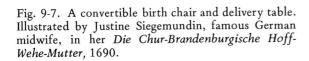

Fig. 9-7. A convertible birth chair and delivery table. Illustrated by Justine Siegemundin, famous German midwife, in her *Die Chur-Brandenburgische Hoff-Wehe-Mutter,* 1690.

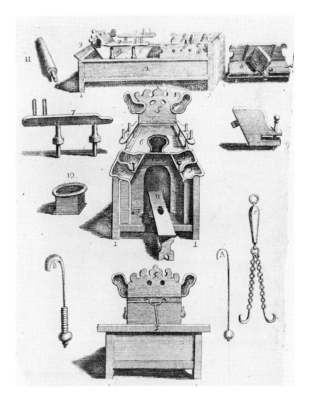

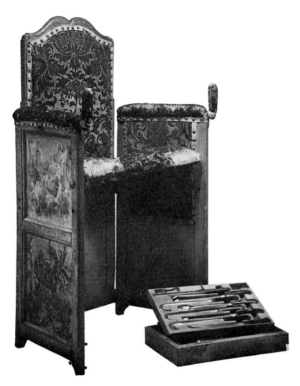

Fig. 9-8. German birth chair. Eighteenth century. Germanisches Nationalmuseum, Nürnberg.

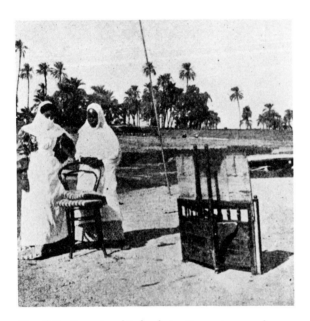

Fig. 9-9. Egyptian birth chair. Late nineteenth century. Folded, the chair was carried to the home of the parturient by the Assuan midwife and her Nubian assistant.

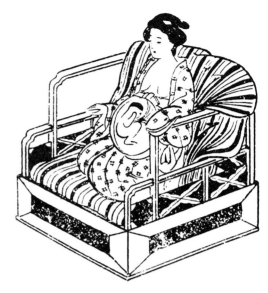

Fig. 9-10. Japanese birth chair. Reproduced from the eighteenth century text *Kagawa-shi San-jitsu Hikki* by Genetsu Shigen Kagawa. If postpartum hemorrhage threatened, the parturient was kept on the chair, her legs clasped tightly together.

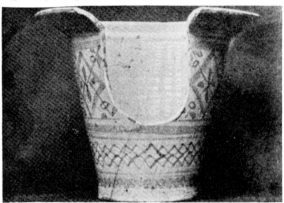

Fig. 9-11. Parturition pan. Nineteenth century from Huelva in southern Spain. A gift, 1894, to Alexander R. Simpson (1835–1916) Professor of Midwifery in the University of Edinburgh from R. Russell Ross a former pupil. Simpson described it thus,
"The vessel is made of strong glazed earthenware, and resembles entirely the pan of a close-stool, except for the excavation on one side through which the hand of the attendant gets access to the patient's pudenda, and through which the child can be guided forward. It is 11-1/2 inches in depth . . . and 6-7/8 inches in width at the bottom. At the brim it measures 10 inches in diameter, extending to 15-1/4 inches at the outer margin of the flange, on which the patient sits. . . . It is spoken of by the natives usually as *Bacin*, the same designation as is given to a large pan or basin which serves as a close-stool or slop-pail."

ACCOUTERMENTS OF THE BIRTH CHAMBER 269

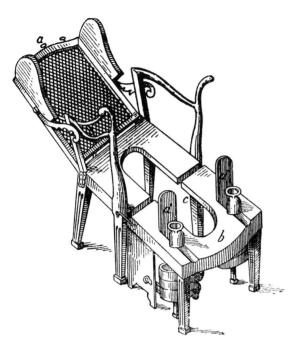

Fig. 9-12. The obstetric chair of Georg Wilhelm Stein (1731–1803). Adjustable foot-stops augmented the parturient's expulsive efforts; the adjustable back permitted sitting or reclining positions.

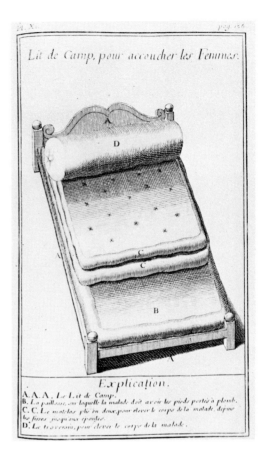

Fig. 9-13. Obstetric cot of Jacques Mesnard (1685–1746). From *Le guide des accoucheurs*, Paris, 1743. A bolster (D) and folded mattress (CC) helped maintain the parturient in a semi-reclining position with her thighs flexed, feet flat against the bed, and head and shoulders above the level of the buttocks which rested at the edges of the folded mattress.

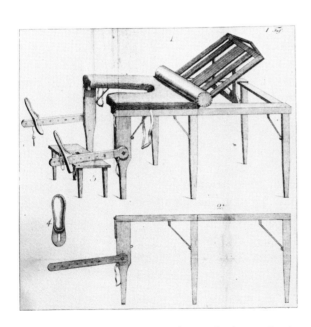

Fig. 9-14. Delivery table of Friedrich Benjamin Osiander (1759–1822). From *Osiander's Geburtsstelle*, 1821.

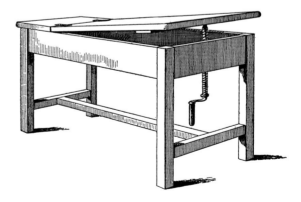

Fig. 9-15. First delivery table in the Sloane Maternity Hospital, New York City, 1887.

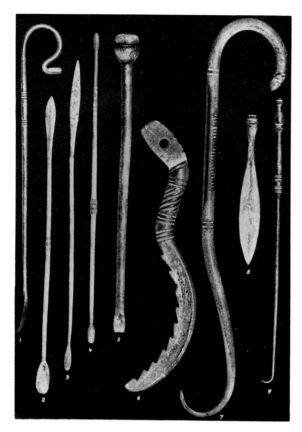

Fig. 9-16. Obstetric and gynecologic instruments. First or second century BC. On the left, curettes, uterine sounds, and a catheter; in the center, half of a cranioclast for crushing the skull; on the right, a blunt hook, embryotome for incising or dismembering the fetus, and a membrane hook. From E. Buchheim, Die Geburtshilflichen Operationen und zuhörigen Instrumente des klassischen Altertums. Jenaer Med. Hist. Beitr. 9, 1916.

OBSTETRIC INSTRUMENTS

Innumerable instruments have been designed to facilitate delivery in cases of labor difficulty resulting from malposition or excessive size of the fetus, contraction of the maternal pelvis, or ineffective uterine contractions. For destruction and extraction of dead infants, hooks, knives, trocars, and prehensile instruments of many descriptions have been fashioned, their origins buried in antiquity—of more recent vintage, to succor the living, the obstetric forceps.

Among the surgical instruments from the Greco-Roman period perhaps as early as the second century BC, cranioclasts, hooks, and other tools for fetal destruction have been found. A serrated device was doubtless used by Arabian physicians in the tenth and eleventh centuries for grasping and extracting the head of the dead fetus; such an instrument is illustrated in a manuscript of Abulcasis (936–1013) who lived at Cyropolis, on the Caspian Sea. The obstetric forceps for the delivery of the living child was probably known as early as the second or third century AD; it is clearly shown in a birth room scene on a marble bas-relief, believed of this era, recently discovered near Rome. Ignored or forgotten, however, the forceps fell into disuse, not to be reintroduced into service until the advent of the colorful Chamberlen family toward the close of the sixteenth century. Since then, in the words of Alfred H. McClintock, "this noble instrument... has done more to abridge human suffering, and to save human life, than any other instrument in the whole range of surgical appliances."

In 1569 William Chamberlen fled with his Huguenot family from Paris to Southampton to escape the religious persecution of Catherine de' Medici. Two of Chamberlen's sons, whom he named Peter the Elder and Peter the Younger, became barber-surgeons; the former invented and with his own hands fashioned the crude instrument from which the many models of the modern obstetric forceps have evolved. Consisting simply of two curved pieces of iron formed in the shape of spoons and joined at a pivot, this invention remained a closely guarded family secret for nearly 100 years, passing from one Chamberlen to another through three generations. In a massive gilt-trimmed chest borne by a special carriage they transported their treasured instrument to the homes of their patients. The parturients were always blindfolded lest the secret of the forceps be discovered.

Having achieved great renown as a surgeon-midwife, Peter the Elder was called into attendance for both Queen Anne and Henrietta Maria, wife of Charles I. A third Peter Chamberlen, son of Peter the Younger, attained a medical degree and was subsequently known as Dr. Peter. After establishing his reputation as an obstetric surgeon, Dr. Peter attempted to organize the midwives of London into a guild. He would teach and license them, he proposed, and in turn would collect a tax for each delivery they conducted. Only through the intercession of the Archbishop of Canterbury were the midwives able to emancipate themselves from their self-styled benefactor.

Hugh Chamberlen, eldest son of Dr. Peter, made the first overt offer to sell the family secret. During a visit to Paris in 1670 he boasted of a device by means of which he could deliver any woman within eight minutes, and proposed its sale to the French government. The illustrious François Mauriceau was summoned to evaluate the Chamberlen claim. Mauriceau had just seen in consultation a rhachitic dwarf whose pelvis was so contracted that even after several days of labor vaginal delivery appeared impossible. Hugh Chamberlen was invited to deliver the hapless patient. Unsuccessful after three hours of violent struggle, Chamberlen emerged exhausted from the room in which he had locked himself with the dwarf, who died the next day, still undelivered, her uterus rup-

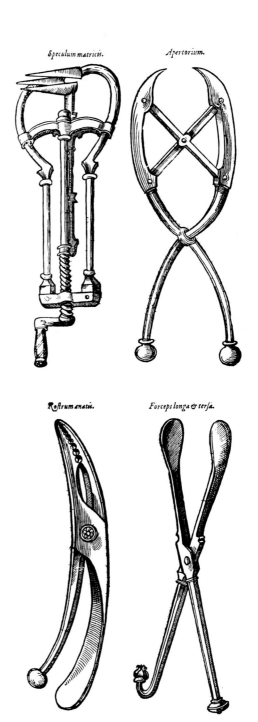

Fig. 9-17. Sixteenth century instruments for extracting a dead fetus. From Jacob Rueff's *De conceptu et generatione hominis,* Frankfurt, 1580. From left to right: vaginal speculum and cervical dilator, pincers, cranioclast, forceps.

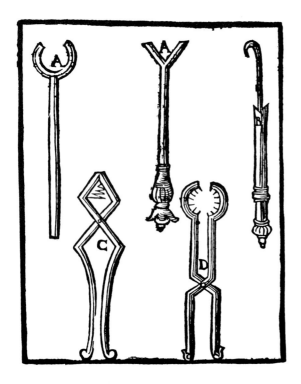

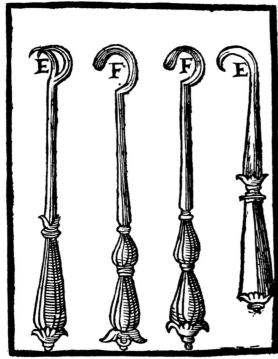

Fig. 9-18. Cervical dilators (A), hooks (B, E, F), and forceps (C, D) for extracting a dead fetus. From Scipione Mercurio's *La Commare*, Venice, 1703. (1 ed., 1596.)

tured. The Chamberlen invention remained unsold.

In Amsterdam Hugh Chamberlen later sold a secret instrument to Rogier van Roonhuyze, a Dutch obstetrician, who then sought passage of a law requiring every practicing physician to purchase it. A sketch of the instrument, which proved to be a curved lever, was released by Roonhuyze's assistant to the Belgian anatomist and surgeon Jean Palfyn (1650–1730). The latter promptly added a second lever for grasping the fetal head and called the resulting instrument the *tire-tête*. Palfyn exhibited this forceps, later known as *les mains de fer* (the iron hands) at a meeting of the French *Academie Royales des Sciences* in 1721.

The design of the obstetric forceps was first made public in 1733 in a book by Edmund Chapman. Since then the instrument has been modified and redesigned probably more times than any other surgical device as knowledge has accrued of pelvic architecture and the mechanism of labor. Hundreds of models have been created, each identified by the name of its inventor. Scarcely a year passes without an

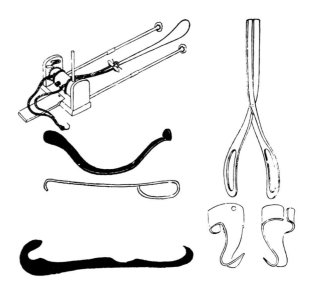

addition to our forceps arsenal.

Hope of recovering the Chamberlens' original instrument, never publicly revealed, had long since been abandoned when in 1813 a later resident of the home of Dr. Peter Chamberlen came upon a trap door while rummaging in the attic. Between the floor boards and ceiling lay a box containing a variety of oddments including letters, fans, trinkets, a Bible of 1695, and several pairs of obstetric forceps, probably including the Chamberlen original. Thus the family secret was first brought to light.

At mid nineteenth century, according to collected European statistics, the obstetric forceps was used in but one out of 167 cases, being reserved for difficult or complicated delivery. In the ensuing 100 years the instrument's place in obstetric practice has undergone great change. Now a commonplace, the forceps is used by many obstetricians in routine or *prophylactic* fashion for the delivery of first infants and for multiparous deliveries as well, if spontaneous birth is not easily accomplished.

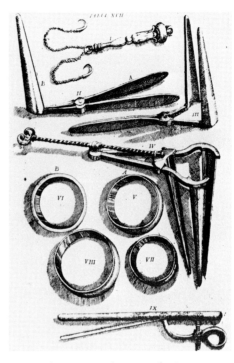

Fig. 9-20. Obstetric and gynecologic instruments. Illustrated by Scultetus (Johann Schultes) in his *Armamentarium chirurgicum,* 1655. (I) Instrument with two chains and hooks, for extracting a dead fetus, either intact or dismembered. (II, III, IV) Speculums. (V, VI, VII, VIII) Ring pessaries of boxwood for supporting a prolapsed uterus. (IX) Cervical dilator.

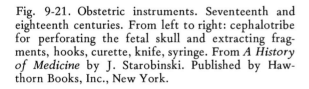

Fig. 9-21. Obstetric instruments. Seventeenth and eighteenth centuries. From left to right: cephalotribe for perforating the fetal skull and extracting fragments, hooks, curette, knife, syringe. From *A History of Medicine* by J. Starobinski. Published by Hawthorn Books, Inc., New York.

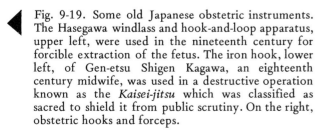

Fig. 9-19. Some old Japanese obstetric instruments. The Hasegawa windlass and hook-and-loop apparatus, upper left, were used in the nineteenth century for forcible extraction of the fetus. The iron hook, lower left, of Gen-etsu Shigen Kagawa, an eighteenth century midwife, was used in a destructive operation known as the *Kaisei-jitsu* which was classified as sacred to shield it from public scrutiny. On the right, obstetric hooks and forceps.

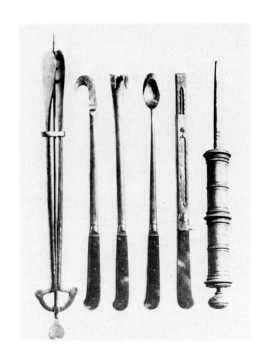

274 ICONOGRAPHIA GYNIATRICA

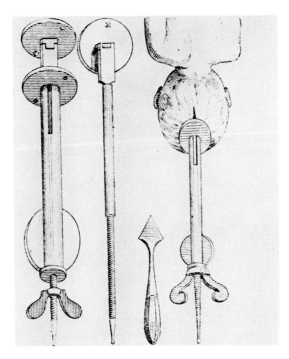

Fig. 9-22. The *perce-crâne* and *tire-tête* of François Mauriceau (1637–1709), instruments for perforating and extracting the fetal head.

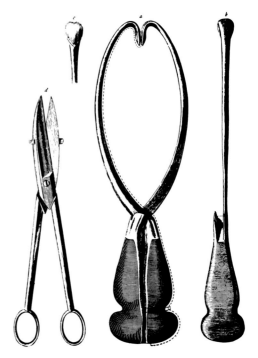

Fig. 9-23. Destructive scissors and double curved crotchet of William Smellie (1697–1763). From his *A Sett of Anatomical Tables,* London, 1754.

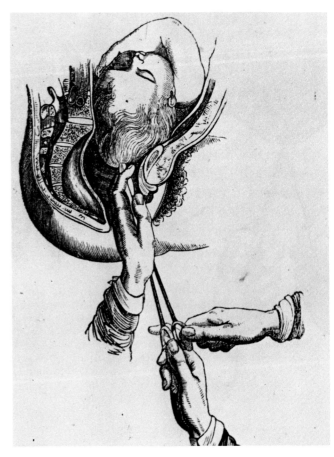

Fig. 9-24. Craniotomy. Mid eighteenth century. Perforation of the skull (A), dilatation of the opening for evacuation of the cranial contents (B), and extraction of the collapsed skull with craniotomy forceps (C).

A

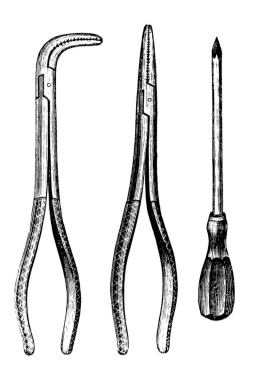

Fig. 9-25. Embryotomy instruments of Charles D. Meigs (1792–1869). Curved and straight pliers, skull perforator.

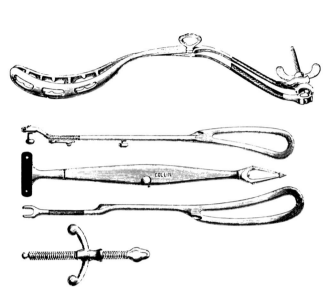

Fig. 9-26. Cephalotribe (above) and basiotribe (below) of Étienne S. Tarnier (1828–1897). For destruction of the fetal skull.

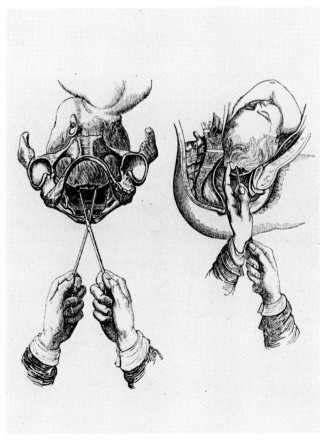

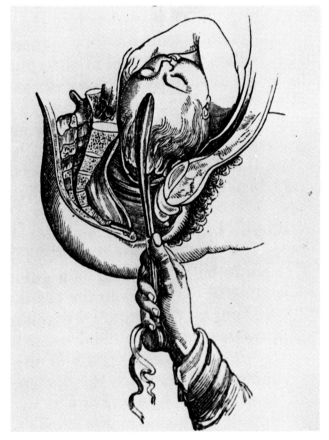

B

C

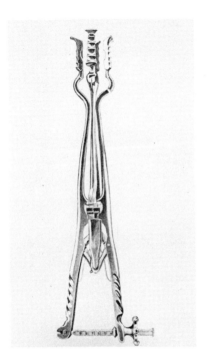

Fig. 9-27. The cervix, when incompletely dilated, precludes vaginal delivery. To overcome this obstacle obstetricians have torn, cut, and stretched the uterine opening using a variety of instruments and techniques to permit egress of the fetus when progress in labor halted or delivery seemed urgent. Tertullian mentioned pronged uterine dilators for this purpose as early as the second century AD. Invented by Luigi Maria Bossi in 1881 was the four-branched dilator shown here. A powerful screw at the bottom produced separation of the blades, placed within the cervix, a scale on the instrument indicating the degree of cervical dilatation thus achieved. Bossi's dilator enjoyed great vogue for a decade, but because of the tissue lacerations it produced fell into disrepute and is no longer used.

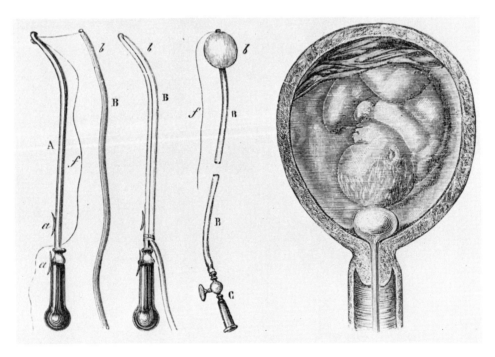

Fig. 9-28. Bags, balloons, and animal bladders have been inserted into the pregnant and puerperal uterus for the induction of labor, the treatment of uterine inertia, cervical dystocia, and placenta previa, and the management of postpartum hemorrhage for over a century. The *ballon excitateur* of Étienne Tarnier, shown here, was introduced in 1862, two decades after Hüter and Busch had used the urinary bladder of the pig and dog to stanch the hemorrhage from placenta previa. A soft rubber bag, Tarnier's balloon was inserted through the cervix on the end of a catheter, then inflated to the size of a hen's egg to dilate the canal.

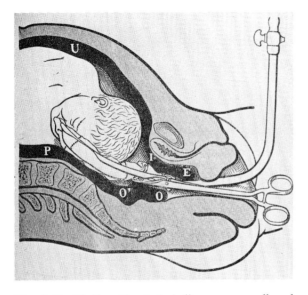

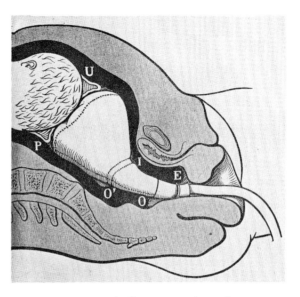

Fig. 9-29. Finding Tarnier's balloon too small and not well shaped for cervical dilatation, Champetier de Ribes devised a larger balloon, conical, of rubber-covered silk which he used for the first time on August 25, 1887. His illustrations show the insertion of the folded balloon and the inflated balloon in position within the uterus.

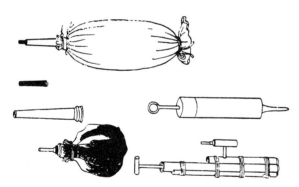

Fig. 9-30. Japanese lubrication syringes. Eighteenth century. Oil was poured through bamboo tubes or metal funnels attached to syringes of various shapes, then injected into the cervix and vagina to facilitate delivery.

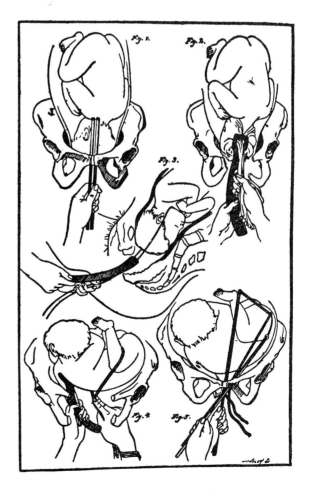

Fig. 9-31. Because of the maternal trauma that commonly resulted from the use of hooks and other metallic instruments, flexible devices of tapes, slings, and nets were designed for fetal extraction. Shown here, the use of a pliable whalebone noose (*tanganki*), introduced in 1775 by Genteki Kagawa of Japan. After being looped over the presenting part or an extremity of the fetus, the sling was connected to a wooden handle, used for traction. The *sei-ochu*, a silk ribbon, and the *tentoken*, a silk cloth, were used in similar fashion to extract the fetus.

278 ICONOGRAPHIA GYNIATRICA

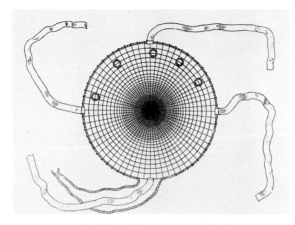
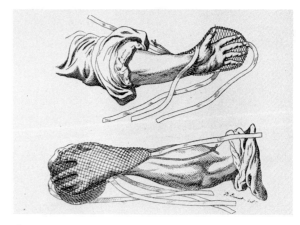

Fig. 9-32. The sling of Pierre Amand (d. 1720) and its application. For extracting the fetal head. Introduced in the early eighteenth century, Amand's device never proved very valuable for its intended purpose.

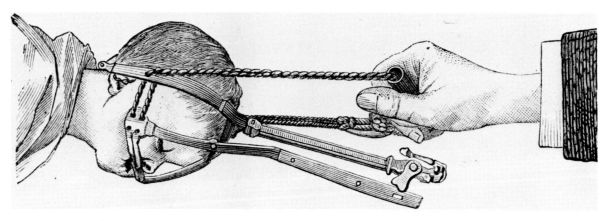

Fig. 9-33. The *sériceps* of Jules Poullet, a short-lived fetal extractor of the mid nineteenth century. Witkowski described the obstetricians of this period as possessed with "an incredible ardor for inventing instruments, sometimes dangerous, often useless, but always ingenious."

Fig. 9-34. The obstetric extractor of Dr. John Evans, Professor of Obstetrics, Rush Medical College, Chicago. Mid nineteenth century. The metallic parts consisted of two parallel steel branches, 14 inches long, with a curve to fit the hollow of the sacrum and a joint permitting limited motion near the end of the curved segment. The bars were held firmly together by a flat clasp on the handles, while the curved ends were introduced into the pelvis. To the curved parts was attached a strong net of silk tape, large enough to embrace the fetal head. After removal of the clasp the branches were separated and one was swept around to the opposite side of the pelvis, to encircle the fetal head in the net. With the long tapes hanging out of the vagina, traction was applied alternately upon their tied ends and upon the steel branches, to produce descent of the fetal head.

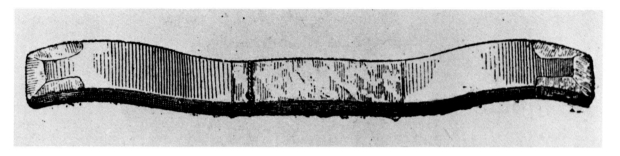

Fig. 9-35. The lever of Rogier van Roonhuyze. Late seventeenth century. A metal strip, slightly curved at each end and covered with leather, was inserted alongside the infant's head to pry it from the pelvis. Dangerous and of little value, the instrument was nonetheless kept secret by Roonhuyze and his associates.

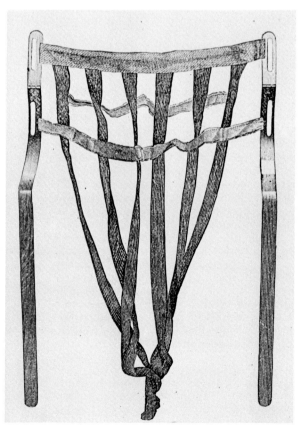 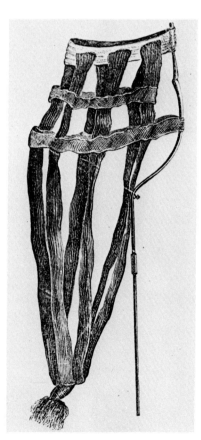 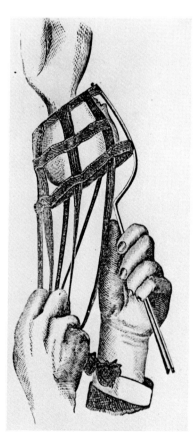

A   B   C

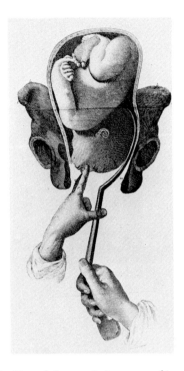

Fig. 9-36. Use of the vectis in a case of brow presentation. Eighteenth century.

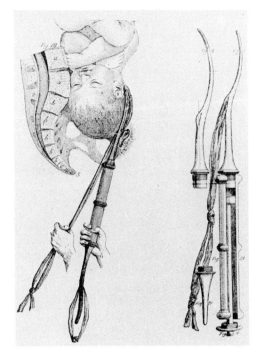

Fig. 9-37. The lever-syringe of Georges Herbiniaux (1740–?) of Brussels. A device for assisting delivery and for baptism in utero in cases of fetal distress.

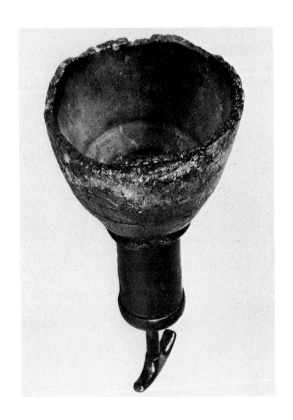

Fig. 9-38. The suction-tractor of James Young Simpson (1811–1870). Rescued from obscurity after having been forgotten for 100 years, the vacuum extractor was reintroduced into obstetric practice in the mid twentieth century. Almost identical with the instrument in current use was Simpson's suction-tractor, a vacuum cup affixed to the presenting part of the fetus to assist its delivery. An air-tractor for this purpose had been suggested even earlier; in 1694 James Yonge recorded a case of prolonged labor in which he had unsuccessfully applied a cupping glass to the fetal scalp to expedite birth. The principle of a pneumatic obstetric tractor was independently suggested later by Saemann of Jena, in 1794, and by Neill Arnott of Scotland, in 1829. The inspiration for his suction-tractor came to Simpson in 1836 when he happened across a group of boys lifting large stones from the street with rough pieces of wetted leather, called "suckers." Simpson demonstrated his tractor in December 1848, a year after his discovery of the anesthetic properties of chloroform. Made from a trumpet-shaped vaginal speculum, the cup was fitted with a piston at its narrow end; the broad end was covered with leather. Withdrawing the piston fixed the cup, greased with lard, to the fetal scalp. Traction on the cup produced descent of the head.

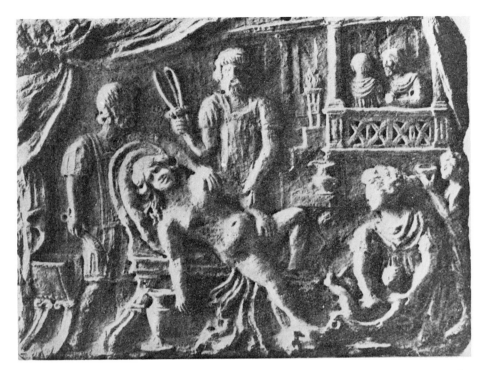

Fig. 9-39. The obstetric forceps. As depicted in an ancient birth scene, second or third century AD. Marble bas-relief, 74 cm x 55 cm, discovered near Rome in the early twentieth century.

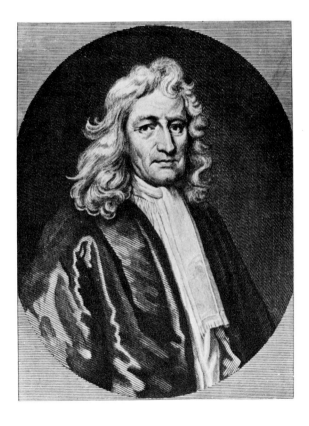

Fig. 9-40. Dr. Peter Chamberlen (1601–1683) at age 57. A member of the colorful clan who kept the secret of the obstetric forceps through three generations for 100 years.

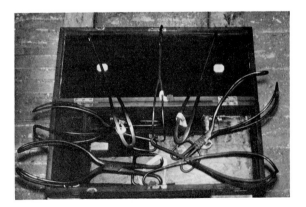

Fig. 9-41. The Chamberlen forceps. The original instruments and their attic repository in the home of Dr. Peter Chamberlen, Woodham Mortimer Hall. The box is not the original.

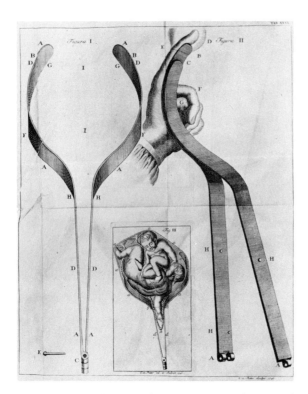

Fig. 9-42. The forceps of Rogier van Roonhuyze and its intrauterine application in a case of twin pregnancy. The presenting fetus in a transverse lie with prolapsed arm and cord.

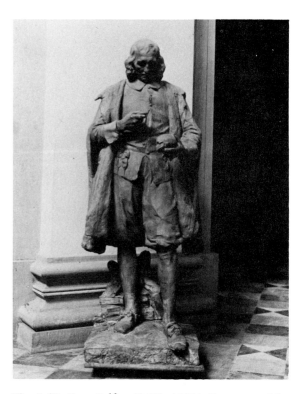

Fig. 9-43. Jean Palfyn (1650–1730). Promoter of *les mains de fer*. Statue installed in the Bÿlokepark, Ghent, June 22, 1952, in the presence of King Baudewijn. Reproduction in the Museum Geschiedenis Wetenschappen.

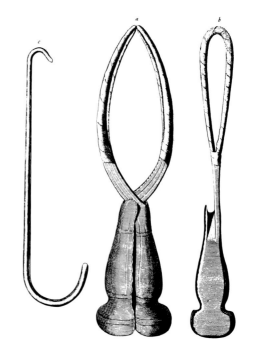

Fig. 9-44. The short straight forceps (*English forceps*) and blunt hook of William Smellie (1697–1763).

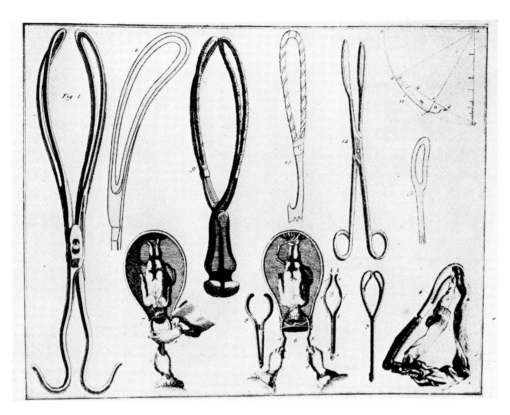

Fig. 9-45. The forceps of André Levret (1703–1780) (*long French forceps*) showing its pelvic curve. From a plate in his *Observations sur les causes et les accidens de plusieurs accouchemens laborieux*, Paris, 1762 (1 ed., 1747). Probably unknown to Levret when he constructed the forceps' pelvic curve in 1751 was a similar but previously unpublished modification of the straight forceps by Benjamin Pugh, fashioned about 1736 to 1740 in England.

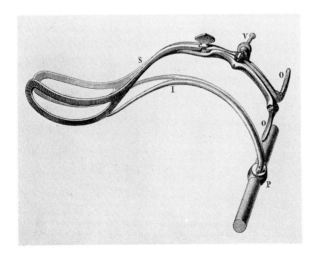

Fig. 9-46. The original axis-traction forceps of Étienne Stéphane Tarnier (1828–1897). Introduced in 1860, this instrument embodied one of the few basic modifications of the obstetric forceps since the introduction of the pelvic curve, for it permitted the application of the traction force in the line of the pelvic axis, even when the fetal head was in the mid or upper pelvis, with minimal trauma to the perineum. In glowing tribute to the Tarnier instrument, Alexander R. Simpson wrote in 1883,

"Let who will continue to use ordinary curved forceps, an obstetrician who has used the Tarnier forceps in a few cases, will no more think of reverting to the other than a man who can afford to keep a carriage will continue to practice as a peripatetic ... in the general run of his work, and in all his difficult cases, the axis-traction forceps becomes for him a valued necessity."

284 ICONOGRAPHIA GYNIATRICA

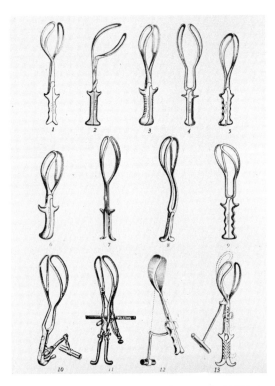

Fig. 9-47. An assortment of obstetric forceps in twentieth century use. (1) Arnold. (2) Barton. (3) Bland. (4) DeLee. (5) Elliott. (6) Hirst-Hale. (7) Kielland. (8) Piper. (9) Simpson. (10) Dewees. (11) Tarnier. (12) Tucker-McLane with traction bar. (13) Zweifel.

Fig. 9-48. A forceps delivery, 1892, by James W. McLane, first Director of New York City's Sloane Maternity Hospital. The Resident Obstetrician Ervin A. Tucker listens to the fetal heart.

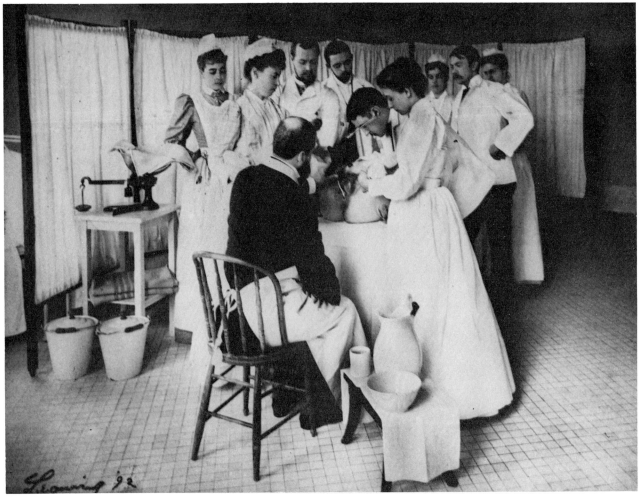

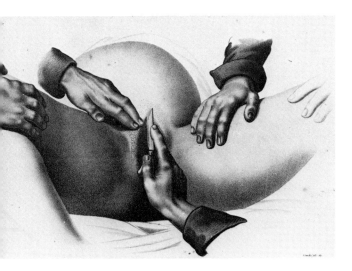

Fig. 9-49. The mistaken notion that progress in labor required a separation of the pelvic bones to permit egress of the fetus was embraced for many generations. Too firm a union at the pubic symphysis was thus regarded as a cause of dystocia. The surgical spreading of the pubes to alleviate this obstruction was accordingly suggested, first by S. Pineau in 1592, and actually performed by J. C. de la Courvée in 1655. But the operation never achieved widespread popularity because of the maternal mutilation it produced. Only in Italy did symphysiotomy enjoy favor. Illustrated here is the beginning of the operation with the symphysiotomy knife of Gennaro Galbiati (1776–1844), Neapolitan surgeon.

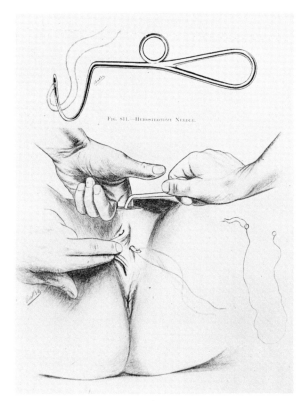

A

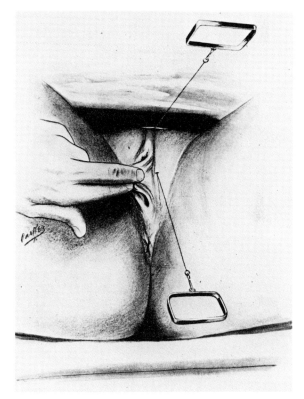

B

Fig. 9-50. Hebosteotomy. (A) Passing the needle for carrying the Gigli saw behind the pubic ramus. (B) The Gigli saw in position. Symphysiotomy was superseded in the late nineteenth century by the operation of dividing the pubic ramus, commonly known as pubiotomy, more properly as hebotomy or hebosteotomy. Suggested by John Aitken of Edinburgh in 1786, this procedure achieved a limited popularity after the invention of a filiform wire saw by Leonardo Gigli (1863–1908) of Florence, Italy, in 1893. With increasing safety of cesarean section, enthusiasm for pubiotomy rapidly waned; the obstetrician abandoned his Gigli saw.

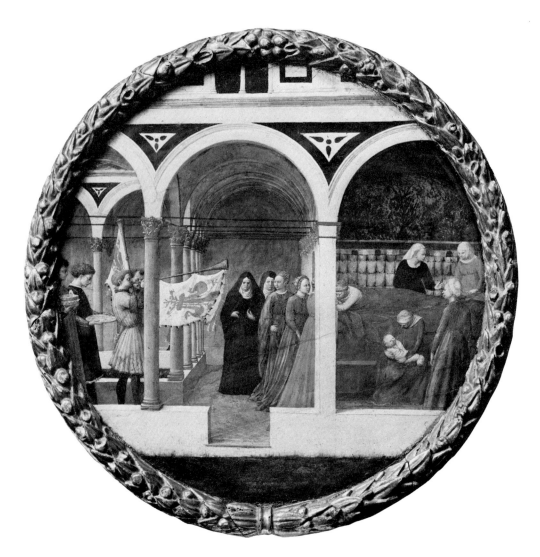

Fig. 9-51. Congratulation of the parturient. A serving platter for the birth chamber painted by Masaccio (real name Tommaso Guidi, 1401–1428). Among the best known of the presentation plates, its scene depicts a palace in Florence with a group of ladies entering through the foyer to visit the distinguished parturient in the room on the right. Staatliche Museen, West Berlin.

DISHES FOR THE PARTURIENT

Of long standing is the tradition of conveying gifts to the parturient. Twentieth century convention calls for flowers, cards, or confections, or perhaps a spoon, trinket, or garment for the newborn. In earlier centuries, friends and neighbors expressed their affection for the new mother by carrying food to her chamber. This custom was particularly popular in Italy, where majolica plates, glazed and richly colored pottery, were specially crafted for the occasion. Decorated with birth scenes and used for serving women in childbed, these plates, known as *deschi da parto*, were also given as wedding presents.

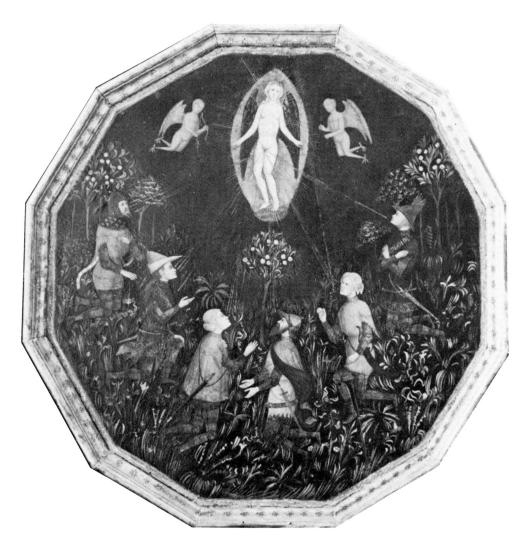

Fig. 9-52. The Triumph of Venus. Anonymous painting on a plate for a parturient, School of Verona, about 1430. This tray of 12 sides is one of the earliest representations of Venus, quasi-Christian goddess of love and beauty, in a pictorial allegory. The nude, winged Venus is flanked by cupids with clawed feet, one holding a bow and quiver, the other an arrow. Below, their faces transfixed by the rays emanating from her vulva, kneel the famed lovers Achilles, Tristan, Lancelot, Samson, Paris, and Troilus. According to Eugene B. Cantelupe (Art Bull. 44:238, 1962.), the meaning of the painting is revealed in its compositional scheme. The mandorla or almond shape in which Venus is framed is reserved in medieval art for the *Maiestas Domini,* the Ascension of Christ, the Last Judgment, and the Assumption of the Virgin. Mother and Son are usually shown with Matthew, Mark, Luke, and John. In the *Triumph of Venus* Christ, Mary, and the Gospel writers are replaced by a crowned Venus and her demonic sons. In scenes of the Annunciation striations extend from the dove to Mary's cheek. Correspondingly here, the golden beams emanate from the genitalia of Venus to the faces of her kneeling knights, arousing in them a procreative rather than a sensual love. "The radiations on the maternity tray," according to Cantelupe,

"bestow upon the six devotees physical beauty, intelligence, and sweetness of temperament—blessings that the planetary Venus visits upon her children. Just as she has tamed and mitigated the contentiousness of Mars, so has she subdued the earthly warriors by love. This astrological image no doubt reminded the matron being served from the birth plate that she too had tempered her husband's fervor, and the imminent child was their reward." Musée du Louvre, Paris.

288 ICONOGRAPHIA GYNIATRICA

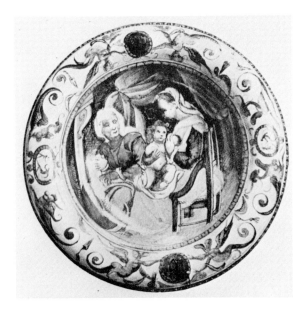

Fig. 9-53. Parturient dish. Italian, sixteenth century. Formerly in Kunstgewerbemuseum, Berlin, destroyed in W.W. II.

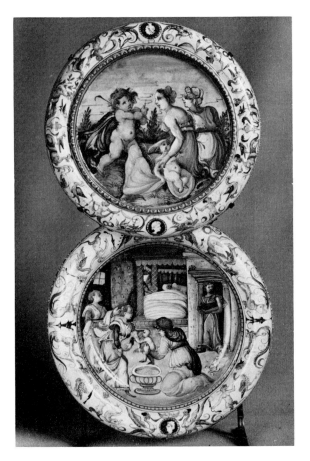

Fig. 9-54. Parturient plate. From Urbino, ceramic center of Italy, 1550. Musée du Louvre, Paris.

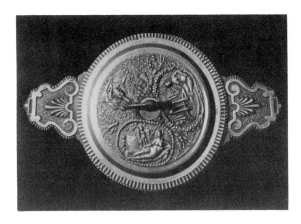

Fig. 9-55. Parturient bowl. By Johann Peter Kamm (1707–1752). Formerly in Germanisches Nationalmuseum, Nürnberg, present whereabouts unknown.

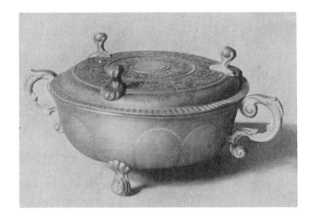

Fig. 9-56. Parturient bowl. Early eighteenth century. The three handles on the cover, serving as legs, permitted its use as a plate when inverted. Formerly in Kunstgewerbemuseum, Berlin, destroyed in W.W. II.

Chapter 10

PUERPERAL FEVER

Recognized for 3000 years as a ruthless killer of women, puerperal infection still commands the wary respect of obstetricians. The *Ayur-Vedas,* books of revealed knowledge of the ancient Hindus which date back to about 1500 BC, mentioned the hazards of childbed fever and prescribed that the midwives keep their fingernails well trimmed. A more detailed reference to this scourge appeared in the Hippocratic tract on the diseases of women, written about 500 BC, ascribing fever in the early puerperium to suppression of the lochia, resulting in turn from an accumulation or imbalance of the humors. One thousand years later Hieronymous Mercurialis (1530–1606), noting the failure of lactation among afflicted women, concluded that the milk, instead of flowing to the breasts, localized in the uterus and produced the purulent discharge from this organ. Thus arose the name *milk fever*. Deaths from infection were infrequent before the establishment of lying-in hospitals and the development of operative obstetrics. With these so-called advances came frequent internal examinations of women in labor, contaminated instruments, dressings, and linens, and crowding of patients. Ignorant of asepsis, physicians and students often proceeded directly from the autopsy room to the birth chamber, their hands unwashed. Spread of infection resulted.

First recorded were the epidemics at the Hôtel Dieu in Paris, in 1646. Later statistics from the Allmänna Barnbördhuset in Stockholm reported one maternal death for every five women delivered there. In Vienna's Allgemeines Krankenhaus, which housed Europe's largest obstetric department, an epidemic that began in 1821 and lasted 20 months took the lives of 829 of 5,139 parturients, a toll of almost 1 in 6. From May 1 to May 10, 1856 death came to 31 of the 32

Fig. 10-1. *La Fièvre de lait* (milk fever). By Lafosse (Jean-Baptiste Adolphe?), 1810–1879.

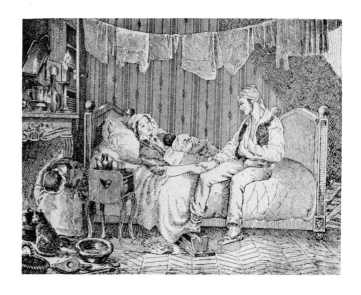

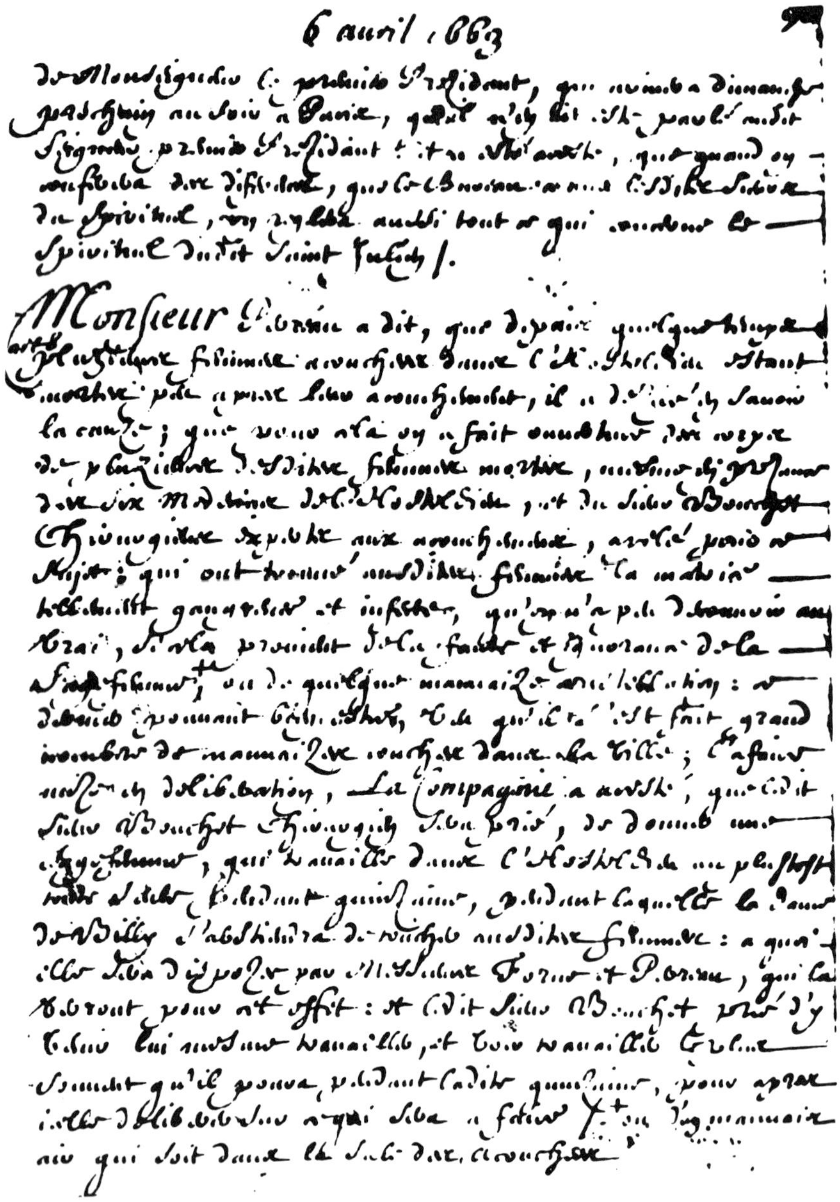
6 auril 1663

Monsieur

Fig. 10-2. Report dated April 6, 1663 of an investigation of an early epidemic of puerperal fever in the Hôtel-Dieu, Paris.

women delivered in the Maternité in Paris. Man's efforts to cope with this killer have produced some of medicine's warmest debates and most colorful prose.

Contagion was first suspected as a factor in childbed fever by certain British physicians. Charles White, of Manchester, England, as early as 1773, associated spread of the disease with uncleanliness. Alexander Gordon of Aberdeen, Scotland in 1795 wrote in his *A Treatise on the Epidemic Puerperal Fever of Aberdeen,*

"This disease seized such women only, as were visited, or delivered, by a practitioner, or taken care of by a nurse, who had previously attended patients affected with the disease.... I arrived at that certainty in the matter, that I could venture to foretell what women would be affected with the disease, upon hearing by what midwife they were to be delivered, or by what nurse they were to be attended, during their lying-in: and almost in every instance, my prediction was verified.... In short I had evident proofs of its infectious nature, and that the infection was as readily communicated as that of the small pox or measles, and operated more speedily than any other infection, with which I am acquainted.... I had evident proofs that every person, who had been with a patient in the Puerperal Fever, became charged with an atmosphere of infection, which was communicated to every pregnant woman, who happened to come within its sphere.... It is a disagreeable declaration for me to mention, that I myself was the means of carrying the infection to a great number of women."

Echoing Gordon's opinions, James Blundell wrote several years later in his lectures on midwifery at Guy's Hospital in London, first published in 1834,

"In my own family, I had rather that those I esteemed the most should be delivered, un-

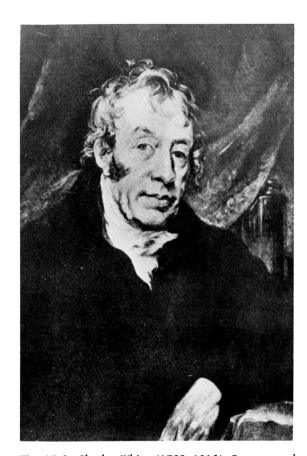

Fig. 10-3. Charles White (1728–1813). Surgeon and obstetrician of Manchester, England who first related puerperal fever to uncleanliness. Mezzotint engraving by W. Ward, 1809, from a portrait by Joseph Allen.

aided, in a stable—by the manger side—than that they should receive the best help in the fairest apartment, but exposed to the vapours of this pitiless disease. Gossiping friends, wet nurses, monthly nurses, the practitioner himself, these are the channels by which, as I suspect, the infection is principally conveyed."

Others took up the cry. Thomas Watson, professor of Medicine in King's College, London, in 1842 voiced

"the dreadful suspicion, that the hand which is relied upon for succour in the painful and perilous hour of child-birth, and which is intended to secure the safety of both mother and child, but especially of the mother, may literally become the innocent cause of her destruction: innocent no longer, however, if, after warning and knowledge of the risk, suitable means are not used to avert a catastrophe so shocking."

In the meantime Robert Collins, Master of Dublin's famed Rotunda Hospital, 1826–1833, had taken positive measures to combat the menace of infection. Collins wrote in his *A Practical Treatise on Midwifery*, 1835, reporting on the 16,654 births under his mastership,

"In February 1829...puerperal fever, which for several months previous had prevailed in the Hospital, now increased in intensity. On consulting the Medical Committee, it was deemed advisable at once to recommend that no patients, except such as were absolutely destitute, should be admitted...until the entire wards of the Hospital should have been thoroughly purified. We then had all the wards in rotation filled with chlorine gas in a very condensed form, for the space of forty-eight hours, during which time the windows, doors and fire-places were closed, so as to prevent its escape as much as possible. The floors and all the wood-work were then covered with chloride of lime [calcium hypochlorite], mixed with water to the consistence of cream, which was left on for forty-eight hours more. The wood-work was then painted, and the walls and ceiling washed with fresh lime. The blankets, etc. were in most instances scoured, and all stoved in a temperature of between 120 and 130 degrees."

Although Collins made no mention of chlorine disinfection of the obstetrician's hands, he recorded the delivery of the next 10,785 women without a single maternal death from puerperal fever, an extraordinary achievement for his time. One century later, in 1927,

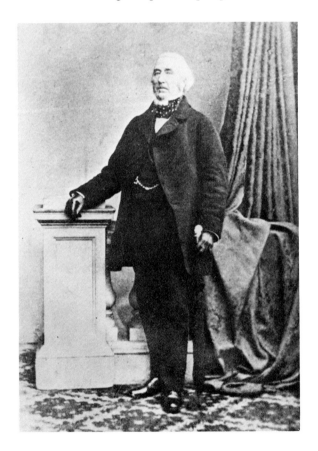

Fig. 10-4. Robert Collins (?–1868), Master of Dublin's Rotunda Hospital, 1826–1833. He demonstrated the effectiveness of quarantine, cleanliness, and chlorination in arresting the spread of puerperal fever.

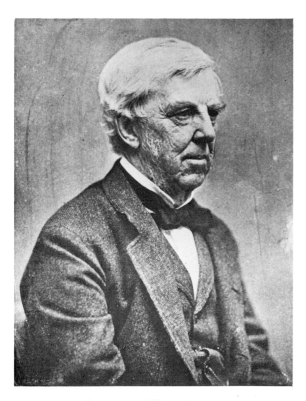

Fig. 10-5. Oliver Wendell Holmes (1809–1894). Physiologist, pathologist, and man of letters, he proposed a set of rules and made an ardent plea for the prevention of puerperal fever. His son and namesake served as Associate Justice on the Supreme Court of the United States, 1902–1923.

virtually identical measures were successfully employed by Benjamin P. Watson in the epidemic of puerperal infection in New York's Sloane Hospital for Women (H. Speert: *The Sloane Hospital Chronicle.* F.A. Davis Company, Philadelphia, 1963, 189-191.)

Stimulated by the challenge of childbed fever and the writings of his British forebears, Oliver Wendell Holmes, who taught physiology and pathology at the Harvard Medical School but did not practice obstetrics, made a critical analysis of the subject's literature, and on February 13, 1843 read before the Boston Society for Medical Improvement his historic essay, "The Contagiousness of Puerperal Fever."

With an eloquence rarely equalled in medical annals Holmes emphasized the physician's role as a carrier of infection and concluded with eight practical prophylactic rules.

"It is as a lesson rather than as a reproach that I call up the memory of these irreparable errors and wrongs. No tongue can tell the heart-breaking calamity they have caused; they have closed the eyes just opened upon a new world of love and happiness; they have bowed the strength of manhood into the dust; they have cast the helplessness of infancy into the stranger's arms, or bequeathed it with less cruelty the death of its dying parent. There is no tone deep enough for regret, and no voice loud enough for warning. The woman about to become a mother, or with her new-born infant upon her bosom, should be the object of trembling care and sympathy wherever she bears her tender burden, or stretches her aching limbs. The very outcast of the streets has pity upon her sister in degradation when the seal of promised maternity is impressed upon her. The remorseless vengeance of the law, brought down upon its victim by a machinery as sure as destiny, is arrested in its fall at a word which reveals her transient claim for mercy. The solemn prayer of the liturgy singles out her sorrows from the multiple trials of life, to plead for her in the hour of peril. God forbid that any member of the profession to which she trusts her life, doubly precious at that eventful period, should hazard it negligently, unadvisedly, or selfishly!"

More dissimilar personalities would be hard to picture than the urbane, cultured, and self-possessed Holmes and his contemporary European counterpart in the conquest of

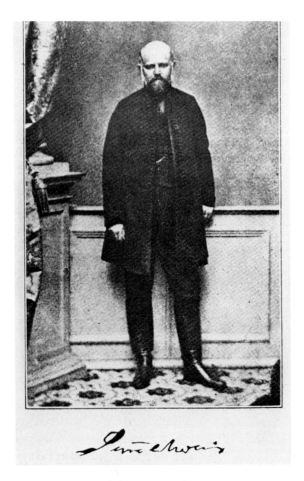

Fig. 10-6. Ignaz Philipp Semmelweis (1818–1865). Magyar obstetrician who proved that puerperal fever could be prevented. Standing in his honor are monuments in Budapest, Hungary in front of the Rokus Hospital and before his tomb at his birthplace in Varhegy, which was established as a museum August 13, 1965, the centenary of his death.

puerperal fever—the irascible and emotionally unstable Ignaz Philipp Semmelweis who served as assistant in the first obstetrical division of Vienna's Allgemeines Krankenhaus. Here, under the direction of Professor Johann Klein, the medical students received their training. In the hospital's second obstetrical division, identical to the first in all other respects, medical students were excluded, all the deliveries being performed by midwives.

During the period from 1841 to 1846, death from puerperal fever had been the lot of one woman of every 11 delivered on the first division; on the second division the corresponding mortality was but one in 29. In 1846 the disparity grew even greater, until the first division's death rate was 10 times that of the second. Simmering in Semmelweis' mind was his observation of the negligible mortality among the women who gave birth before reaching the hospital, at home, or even in the street, and hence without internal examinations during labor. Unschooled in foreign languages, he remained ignorant of the meager British literature on the subject and the teachings of Holmes.

While Semmelweis pondered the problem of puerperal infection, tragedy befell his friend and colleague Jakob Kolletschka, professor of legal medicine in the university, who died from an accidental cut during an autopsy. The pathologic changes in Kolletschka's body, Semmelweis observed, were identical with those in his ill-fated parturients. Semmelweis saw rays of light, quickly concluded that poisons were transmitted from putrid to healthy tissues by the scalpel in the case of Kolletschka and by the examining finger in the case of the woman in labor.

Elated, Semmelweis posted an order in his clinic, May 15, 1847, requiring the students to scrub their hands in a chlorinated lime solution before entering the maternity ward. While they grumbled over this fancied indignity, the maternal mortality in the first obstetric division fell in six months to one-fourth its previous level and bettered the record of the midwives' division. Concluding that examiners might transmit infection from live patients as well as from the dead, Semmelweis then ordered his students to scrub with the chlorine solution before every examination. Like Holmes, whose teachings had met with opposition in America, Semmelweis came under the attack of European authorities, notably Rudolph Virchow, leading pathologist of that era and Friedrich Wilhelm Scanzoni, the continent's outstanding obstetrician. Discredited, Semmelweis was denied reappointment in the Allgemeines Krankenhaus. Two decades later, George Johnston, Master of Dublin's Rotunda, concluded in his "Report" for 1869 that puerperal fever was caused mainly by seduction, remorse, and fretting.

Disillusioned, depressed, and at times irrational, Semmelweis returned to Budapest, was committed to a psychiatric sanitorium in Vienna in 1865 where he died, like his friend Kolletschka, from septicemia resulting from a cut in his finger. His views on puerperal fever were published in 1861 under the title *Die Aetiologie, der Begriff und die Prophylaxis des Kindbettfiebers*. With these pathetic words he concluded his book.

"When I, with my present convictions, look back upon the past, I can only dispel the sadness which falls upon me by gazing at the same time into that happy future when within the lying-in hospitals, and also outside of them, throughout the whole world, only cases of self-infection will occur....

"But if it is not vouchsafed me to look upon that happy time with my own eyes, from which misfortune may God preserve me, the conviction that such a time must inevitably arrive sooner or later after I have passed away will cheer my dying hour."

Not until several years after his death did the doctrine of Semmelweis achieve general

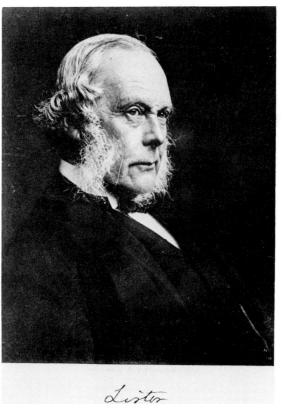

Fig. 10-7. Joseph Lister (1827–1912) at age 69. Professor of Surgery in Glasgow University, the University of Edinburgh, and King's College Hospital, London, and the first physician to be created a peer in Britain. He initiated the era of aseptic surgery and introduced the absorbable ligature.

acceptance in the medical community. In the meantime Louis Pasteur, carrying on his studies in fermentation, demonstrated that decomposition is caused by living organisms, and in 1879 he identified the hemolytic streptococcus, later to be recognized as the foremost villain in puerperal infections. The significance of Pasteur's work associating germs with disease was quickly recognized by Britain's brilliant surgeon, Joseph Lister who devised his famous phenol spray and introduced practical methods of asepsis for the prevention of surgical infection. Aseptic technique was soon introduced into the birth chamber as well as the operating room. As the specter of puerperal fever was laid to rest, hospitals became safe for childbearing; a new era had dawned for obstetrics. Not completely tamed, however, even in the late twentieth century, puerperal infection still shows itself, usually in subdued guise, occasionally in epidemic form, rarely as a killer.

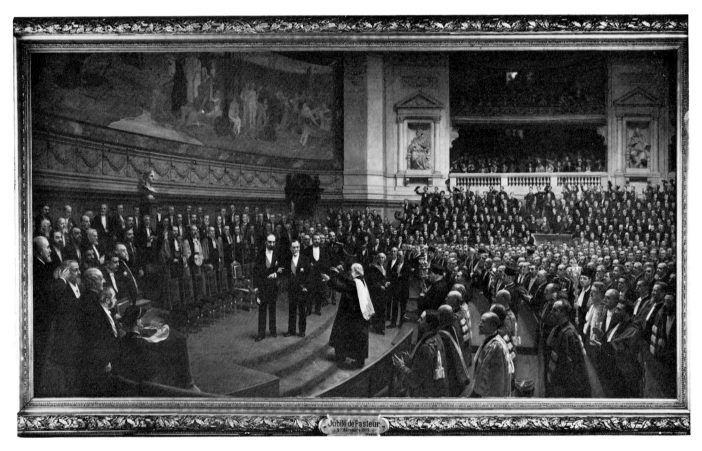

Fig. 10-8. Ovation to Louis Pasteur. December 27, 1892, in the grand amphitheatre of the Sorbonne, on the occasion of his 70th birthday. Painting by Jean André Rixens (1846–1924). Approaching and about to embrace Pasteur, who has just entered the hall on the arm of French President Sadi Carnot, is Lord Lister, who gave an address eulogizing the fraternity of science and medicine, well exemplified by their own work in bacteriology and the development of aseptic surgery.

Chapter 11

CESAREAN SECTION

Obscured by the years are the origins of cesarean section, perhaps the most dramatic of all surgical operations. The Greeks told of abdominal births in their ancient myths. When Apollo learned that his beloved Coronis had been unfaithful, he had her slain, then in compassion removed his unborn son Asklepios from her body on the funeral pyre. Zeus also tore from the belly of the dying Semele the fetal Dionysus, whom he reimplanted in his own thigh and brought to maturity (see chapter 15). Lichas, Virgil tells, was likewise cut out of his dead mother's womb (*Aeneid*, book X, line 315). Brahma, according to ancient belief, emerged from the umbilicus of his mother. Buddha too is said to have been delivered from his mother's flank, in the middle of the sixth century BC.

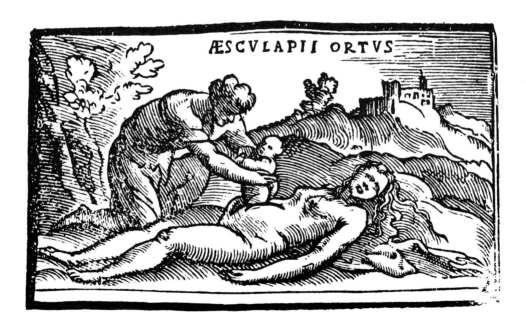

Fig. 11-1. The extraction of Asklepios (Asclepius) from the abdomen of his mother Coronis by his father Apollo. Woodcut from the 1549 edition of Alessandro Benedetti's *De re medica*.

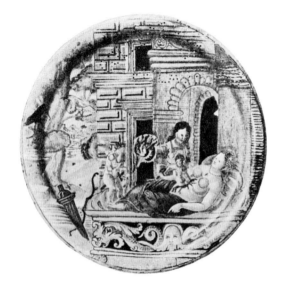

Fig. 11-2. The birth of Asklepios (Asclepius). Majolica plate from Gubbio, Italy, 1534. The slain Coronis lies on a richly decorated bier, to be her funeral pyre, as Apollo extracts Asklepios through her bleeding abdominal wound, and Cupid stands by in tears. The murder weapons, bow and arrow of Artemis, are shown at left.

Abdominal delivery was surely known to the early Jews for the Mishnah, as early as 140 BC, stated that, "in the case of twins, neither the first child which shall be brought into the world by the cut in the abdomen, nor the second, can receive the rights of primogeniture, either as regards the office of priest or succession to property." Children so born were known as *jotze dofan* (Mishnah, Niddah 5:1). The operation may indeed have been performed on living women, for the Talmud prescribes laws of hygiene for survivors. The Niddah, one of its tracts, states that "it is not necessary for women to observe the days of purification after removal of a child through the parietes of the abdomen." Beyond this, however, there is no clear evidence that cesarean section was practiced on the living until the sixteenth century.

The origin of the operation's name probably goes back to the eighth century BC. During the reign of Numa Pompilius

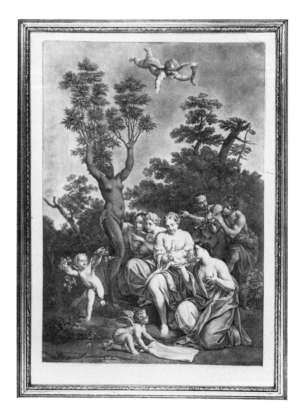

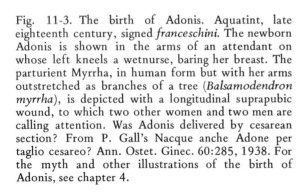

Fig. 11-3. The birth of Adonis. Aquatint, late eighteenth century, signed *franceschini*. The newborn Adonis is shown in the arms of an attendant on whose left kneels a wetnurse, baring her breast. The parturient Myrrha, in human form but with her arms outstretched as branches of a tree (*Balsamodendron myrrha*), is depicted with a longitudinal suprapubic wound, to which two other women and two men are calling attention. Was Adonis delivered by cesarean section? From P. Gall's Nacque anche Adone per taglio cesareo? Ann. Ostet. Ginec. 60:285, 1938. For the myth and other illustrations of the birth of Adonis, see chapter 4.

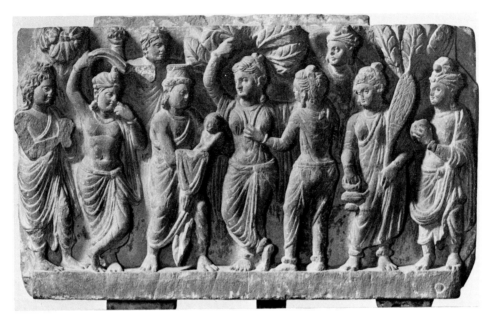

Fig. 11-4. The birth of Buddha from the right flank of his mother Maya. Relief from the Gandhara period (second century BC–fifth century AD). Museum für Indische Kunst, West Berlin.

(715–672 BC), a legendary king of Rome, it was decreed that the child be excised from the womb of any woman who died in late pregnancy. Known initially as the *lex regia* or royal law, the mandate for postmortem section continued under the rule of the emperors or Caesars, when it acquired the name *lex caesarea*.

"*Negat lex regia mulierem quae pregnans mortua sit, humari, antequam partus ei excidatur: qui contra fecerit, spem animantis cum gravida peremisse videtur.* [The *lex regia* forbids the burial of a pregnant woman before the young has been excised: he who does otherwise clearly causes the promise of life to perish with the mother.]" [Justinian's *Digesta*]

Some scholars, on the other hand, have derived the operation's name from the Latin *caedere,* to cut; an abdominal birth was thus termed *partus caesareus*.

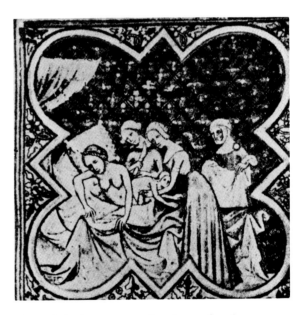

Fig. 11-5. Cesarean section by a female surgeon. Miniature from a fourteenth century *Historie ancienne*.

300   ICONOGRAPHIA GYNIATRICA

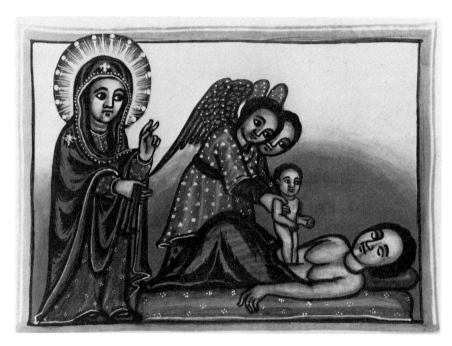

Fig. 11-6. Postmortem cesarean section. Miniature from an Ethiopian manuscript "Lives of Maba Seyon." A priest raises his hand to bless the infant being delivered by the archangels Michael and Gabriel through the abdominal incision of the dead woman. The manuscript makes no further mention of the operation; its purpose was fulfilled with the delivery of a living infant, saved for baptism. The British Museum, London.

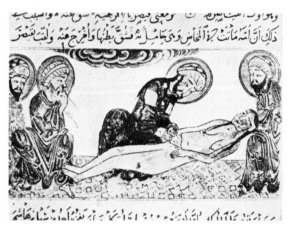

Fig. 11-7. Cesarean section. Miniature from a 1307–1308 Arabian manuscript, *al-Athar al Bagiya*.

Fig. 11-8. The birth of Rustan, legendary Persian hero, by cesarean section. Miniature from Firdausi's (Abul Kasim's) *Book of Kings*, 1010. The patient, surrounded by attendants in oriental garb, lies on an ottoman, her arms held by a woman kneeling behind her. The turbaned operator incises her abdomen with his right hand, extracts the infant with his left. Biblioteca Nazionale, Naples.

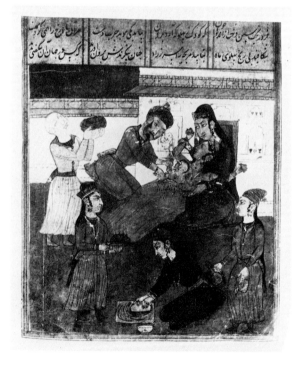

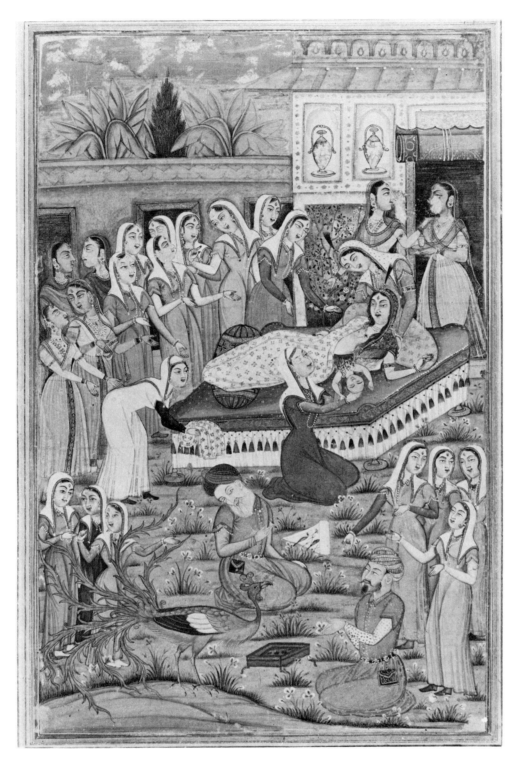

Fig. 11-9. The birth of Rustan. Sixteenth century miniature. A midwife receives the child from the abdomen of the queen Rudabe, surrounded by her happy attendants, while the bird Simurgh, credited with performing the cesarean section, struts proudly in the foreground.

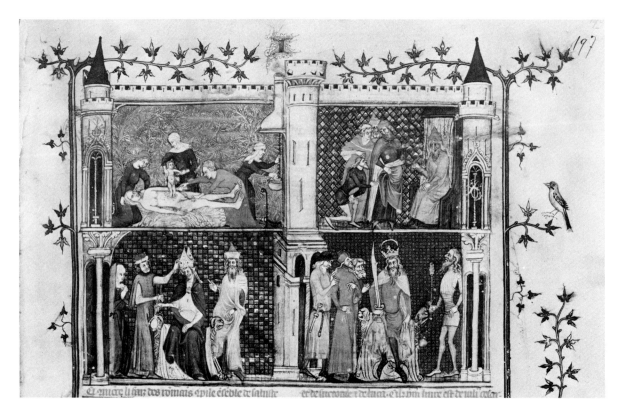

Fig. 11-10. The birth of Caesar. French miniature, fourteenth century. The infant, just being extracted from the abdomen of its dead or dying mother, is shown without an umbilical cord and with its umbilicus already healed. Bibliothèque Nationale, Paris.

It is certain that Julius Caesar, who was born about 100 BC, was not so delivered, and that contrary to widely held belief the operation was not named for him. In Rome abdominal delivery was then practiced only on the dead or dying, and for many centuries thereafter was uniformly fatal when attempted on the living woman. Caesar's mother survived his birth by many years, as attested by his letters to her while he was engaged in his foreign wars. Moreover, others of identical or similar name antedated the great emperor. According to Professor Dyre Trolle of the Department of Obstetrics and Gynecology, University of Copenhagen, the dying queen Dagmar was delivered by cesarean section on May 24, 1212, in the town of Ribe, Jutland.

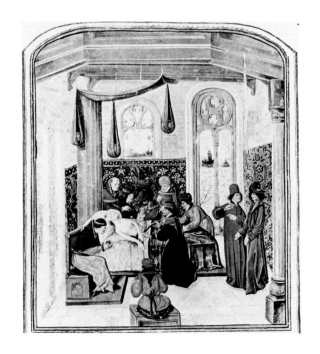

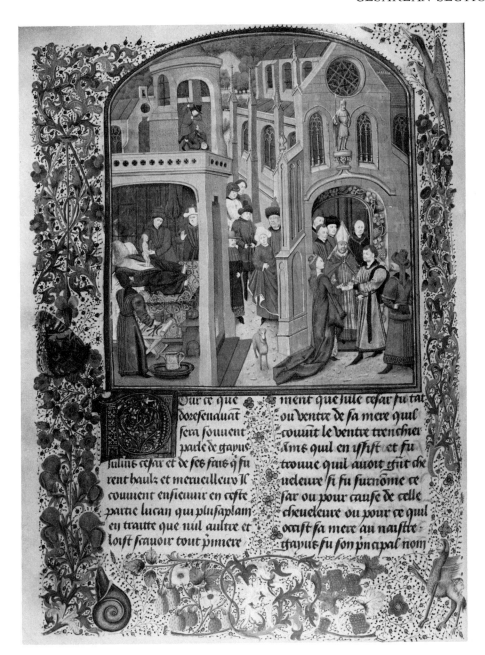

Fig. 11-11. The birth, marriage, and death of Julius Caesar. Miniature by the Flemish artist Loyset Lyedet (*Les histoires romains de Jean Mansel*, 1454–1460). The small surgical chamber on the left is overshadowed by the grand, ornate church buildings. The operator is shown with two assistants, one of whom stands at a small table bearing the surgical instruments. Bibliothèque de l'Arsenal, Paris.

Fig. 11-12. The birth of Caesar. Miniature from a French manuscript of the late fifteenth century. Shown is the interior of a richly furnished palace with Gothic marble pillars. The dead mother, pale and limp, lies on a large bed surrounded by 10 brilliantly robed men, one of whom, the bearded surgeon, is withdrawing his knife from the woman's bleeding abdomen, as another extracts the infant. In most representations of Caesar's birth, in contrast to this one, the attendants are shown as women. Bibliothèque Nationale, Paris.

304 ICONOGRAPHIA GYNIATRICA

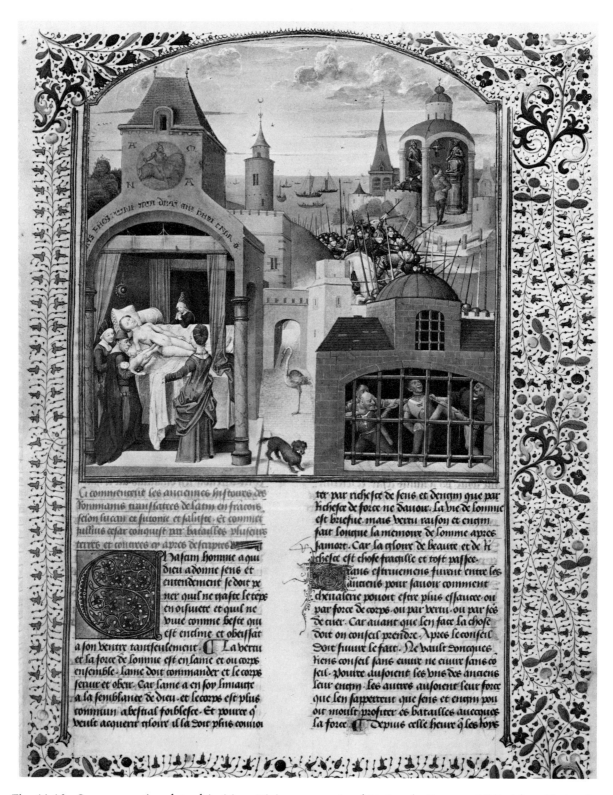

Fig. 11-13. Cesarean section, lateral incision. Miniature from a fifteenth century French manuscript, *Les anciens histoires des Romans*. Bibliothèque Nationale, Paris.

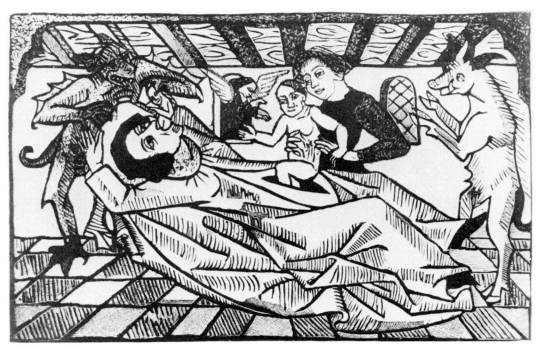

Fig. 11-14. Postmortem cesarean section. Fifteenth century woodcut. As interpreted by Kelchner, this scene depicts the birth of the anti-christ, the product of incestuous intercourse of his mother with her own father. In a low-ceilinged room the fully clad woman lies on a couch, her head elevated. Through her gaping garment protrudes her incised abdomen from which the anti-christ is being lifted. At the foot of the couch stands the devil, represented as a horned pig standing on its hind legs, who is thought to have performed the operation. From the woman's mouth emerges another devil, in the form of an even smaller child taking possession of her soul. An angel tries to enter through the window.

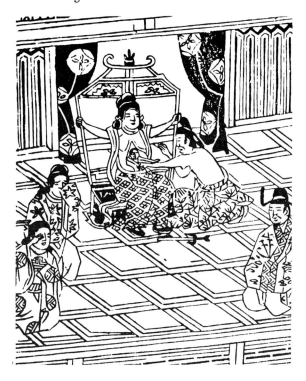

Fig. 11-15. Cesarean section. Japanese woodcut, sixteenth century.

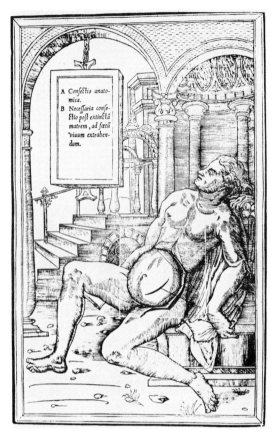

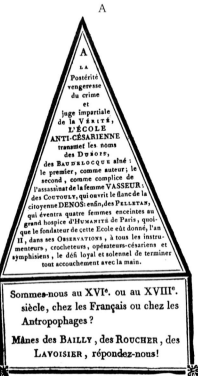

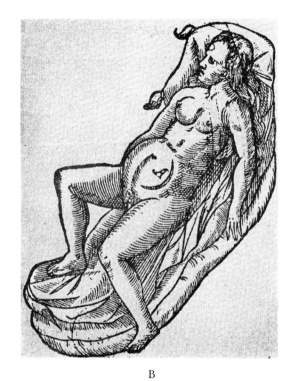

Fig. 11-16. Incision for postmortem cesarean section. (A) Woodcut from Charles Estienne's *De dissectione partium corporis humani libri tres*, Paris, 1545. (B) Woodcut from Boudewijn Ronsee's *Miscellanea, seu epistolae medicinales*, Leyden, 1590.

Fig. 11-17. First issue of the journal of the anticesarean society, founded in 1797 by Jean Sacombe, attacking the proponents of cesarean section on the living.

The first documented cesarean section on a viable patient was performed on April 21, 1610 by Jeremias Trautmann, a surgeon of Wittenberg, Saxony. The abdominal wall was sutured, but not the uterus. The mother survived 25 days, longer than most of the hapless women who underwent this operation during the next two centuries. Many died promptly of hemorrhage; others, within a week from infection. Rarely did the mother recover. In Paris, for example, cesarean section was carried out in 24 cases in the half century from 1750 to 1800 without a single maternal survival. So high did feeling against cesarean section run among some groups in that city that they organized an anti-cesarean society in 1797 under the leadership of Jean Sacombe, and published a journal to help combat the efforts of the operation's advocates.

The first successful cesarean section in the United States was performed in 1794 in a cabin near Staunton, Virginia by Dr. Jesse Bennett on his own wife. By 1878 the operation had been carried out but 80 times in this country with a maternal mortality of 53 per cent. It was noted then that the maternal results were better among nine women whose uteri had been gored open by a bull, or who had incised their own abdomens in desperation, five of whom survived, than among those who had been operated upon by physicians in New York City, of whom one out of 11 recovered.

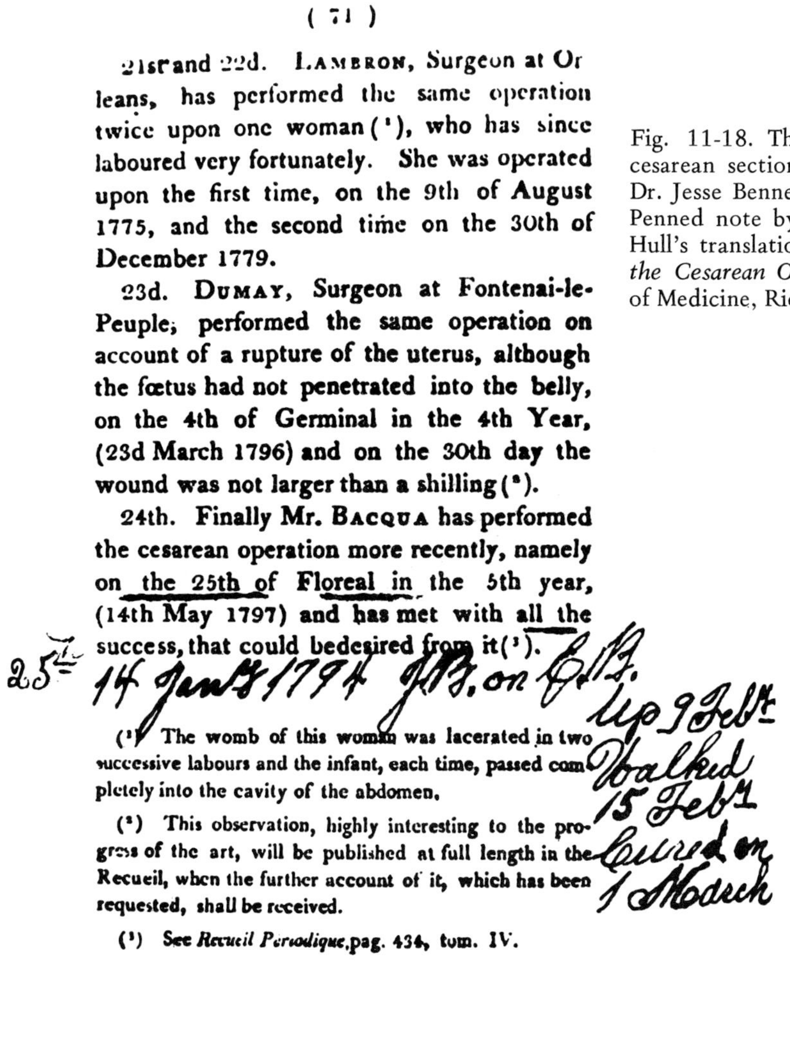
(71)

21st and 22d. LAMBRON, Surgeon at Orleans, has performed the same operation twice upon one woman (¹), who has since laboured very fortunately. She was operated upon the first time, on the 9th of August 1775, and the second time on the 30th of December 1779.

23d. DUMAY, Surgeon at Fontenai-le-Peuple, performed the same operation on account of a rupture of the uterus, although the fœtus had not penetrated into the belly, on the 4th of Germinal in the 4th Year, (23d March 1796) and on the 30th day the wound was not larger than a shilling (²).

24th. Finally Mr. BACQUA has performed the cesarean operation more recently, namely on the 25th of Floreal in the 5th year, (14th May 1797) and has met with all the success, that could be desired from it (³).

25th 14 Jan'y 1794 J.B. on E.B. up 9 Febr Walked 15 Febr Cured on 1 March

(¹) The womb of this woman was lacerated in two successive labours and the infant, each time, passed completely into the cavity of the abdomen.

(²) This observation, highly interesting to the progress of the art, will be published at full length in the Recueil, when the further account of it, which has been requested, shall be received.

(³) See *Recueil Periodique*, pag. 434, tom. IV.

Fig. 11-18. The only written record of the first cesarean section in the United States, performed by Dr. Jesse Bennett on his own wife, January 14, 1794. Penned note by Dr. Bennett in the margins of John Hull's translation of Baudeloque's *Two Memoirs on the Cesarean Operation,* 1801. Richmond Academy of Medicine, Richmond, Va.

308   ICONOGRAPHIA GYNIATRICA

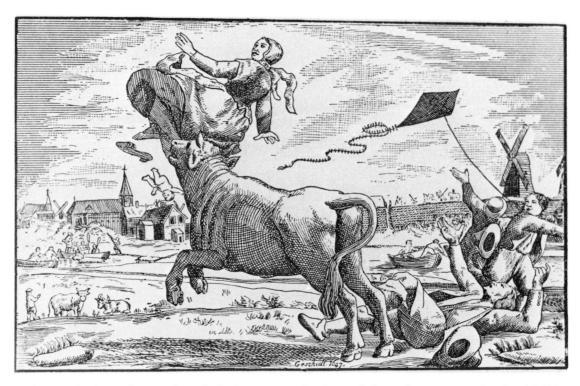

Fig. 11-19. Accouchement by a bull. Cesarean section by cattle-horn, from an engraving dated 1647.

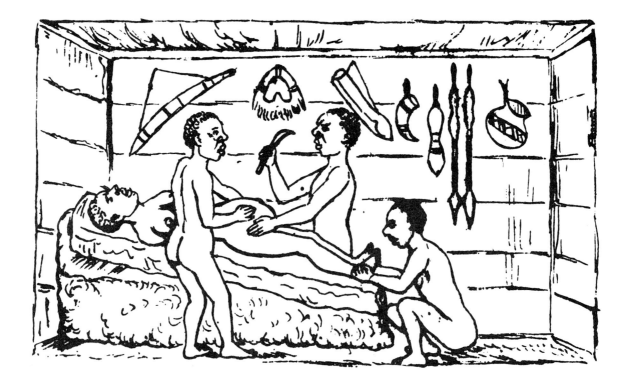

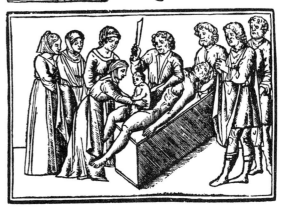

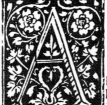

Fig. 11-21. One of the earliest printed illustrations of cesarean section. From Suetonius' lives of the 12 Caesars (C. Suetonius Tranquillus: *Commentaria Philippi Beroaldi necnon Marci Antonii Sabellici in Suetonium Tranquillum foeliciter Venetiis exacta*, 1506).

Fig. 11-20. Cesarean section in Kahura, Uganda, as observed by R. W. Felkin in 1879.

"The woman [a 20-year-old primigravida] lay upon an inclined bed.... She was liberally supplied with banana wine, and was in a state of semi-intoxication. She was perfectly naked. A band of mbugu or bark cloth fastened her thorax to the bed, another band of cloth fastened down her thighs, and a man held her ankles. Another man, standing on her right side, steadied her abdomen. The operator stood ... on her left side ... holding his knife aloft ... and muttering an incantation.... He washed his hands and the patient's abdomen, first with banana wine and then with water. Then, having uttered a shrill cry, which was taken up by a small crowd assembled outside the hut, he proceeded to make a rapid cut in the middle line.... The whole abdominal wall and part of the uterine wall were severed by this incision, and the liquor amnii escaped; a few bleeding-points in the abdominal wall were touched with a red-hot iron by an assistant.... The child was next rapidly removed ... after the cord had been cut ... the operator ... seized the contracting uterus with both hands and gave it a squeeze or two. He next put his right hand into the uterine cavity ... and with two or three fingers dilated the cervix uteri from within outwards. He then cleared the uterus of clots ... removing [the placenta] through the abdominal wound. His assistant endeavoured, but not very successfully, to prevent the escape of the intestines through the wound.... No sutures were put into the uterine wall ... A porous grass mat was placed over the wound and secured there ... she was gently turned to the edge of the bed ... so that the fluid in the abdominal cavity could drain away onto the floor. She was then replaced in her former position ... the edges of the wound ... were brought into close apposition, seven thin iron spikes ... being used for the purpose, and fastened by string made from bark cloth. A paste prepared by chewing two different roots and spitting the pulp into a bowl was then thickly plastered over the wound, a banana leaf warmed over the fire being placed on the top of that, and finally a firm bandage of mbugu cloth.... Eleven days after the operation the wound was entirely healed."

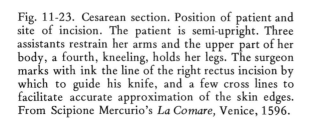

Fig. 11-22. Title page of the first monograph on cesarean section, by François Rousset. Published in Paris, 1581.

A monograph on cesarean section, the first on the subject, was published in Paris in 1581 by François Rousset, although he himself had never performed the operation. Nor had Scipione Mercurio. Yet this Italian physician, who had spent a number of years in monasteries, braved the opposition of the Church by devoting two chapters of his celebrated textbook *La Comare O Ricoglitrice*, 1596 (later spelled *La Commare O'Raccoglitrice*) to the subject. Thus he stood, almost alone, against the authority of his illustrious contemporaries also, such as Ambroise Paré and the latter's accomplished son-in-law, Jacques Guillemeau, who repudiated cesarean section because of its high mortality. Wrote Mercurio, "When the fetus is extraordinarily strong, the passage narrow, the pubic bone flat, it is more than necessary to perform this operation because there is no other way out." Anesthesia and asepsis were yet to be introduced into surgical practice.

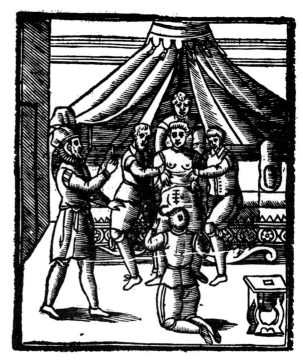

Fig. 11-23. Cesarean section. Position of patient and site of incision. The patient is semi-upright. Three assistants restrain her arms and the upper part of her body, a fourth, kneeling, holds her legs. The surgeon marks with ink the line of the right rectus incision by which to guide his knife, and a few cross lines to facilitate accurate approximation of the skin edges. From Scipione Mercurio's *La Comare*, Venice, 1596.

CESAREAN SECTION 311

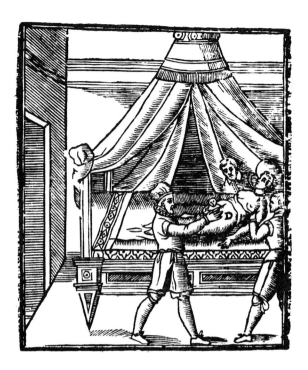

Fig. 11-24. Cesarean section for the woman who is weak. Mercurio directed, "The patient is put to bed with cushions under her so that she is in a half-sitting position. This position is also good for those who are afraid of blood." From Scipione Mercurio's *La Comare*, Venice, 1596.

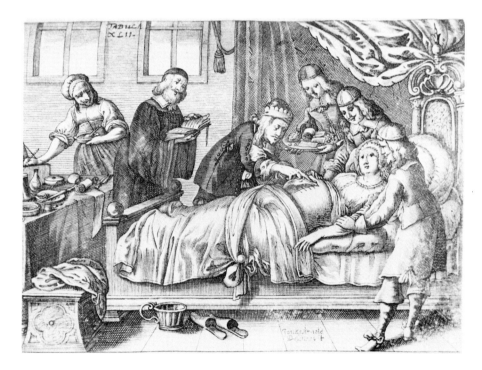

Fig. 11-25. Cesarean section. From Scultetus' *Auctarium ad armamentarium chirurgicum,* published posthumously in Leyden, 1653. The patient, with gown pulled up to expose her abdomen, lies in bed propped up by pillows, her arms restrained by two assistants. A third holds a tray of bandages as the surgeon makes a left rectus incision through the previously marked abdominal wall. At the foot of the bed stands a minister, reciting prayers.

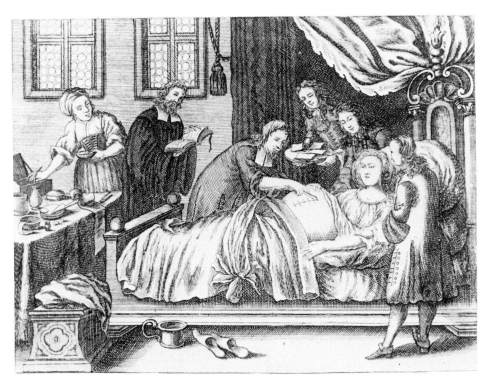

Fig. 11-26. Cesarean section, 1722. So rarely was the operation performed on the living in the seventeenth and eighteenth centuries, and so little was the operation improved during these years, that the same illustration as the preceding (11–25) was reproduced in an obstetric text seven decades later, altered only in the garb of the attendants. From C. Völter's *Neueröffnete Hebammenschule,* Stuttgart, 1722.

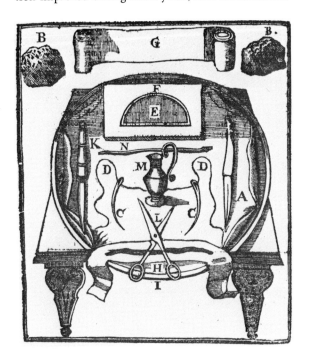

Fig. 11-27. Instruments for cesarean section. From Pierre Adonis' *Cours d'opérations de chirurgie,* Paris, 1708.

CESAREAN SECTION   313

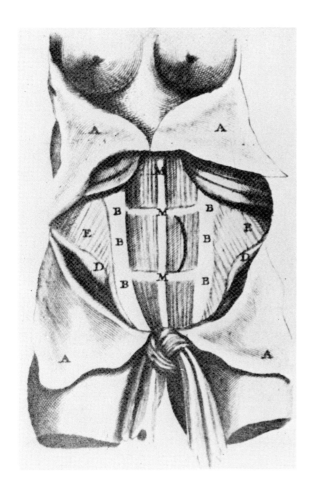

Fig. 11-28. Incision for cesarean section. From Hendrik van Roonhuyze's *Heelkonstige Aanmerkkingen*, Amsterdam, 1663.

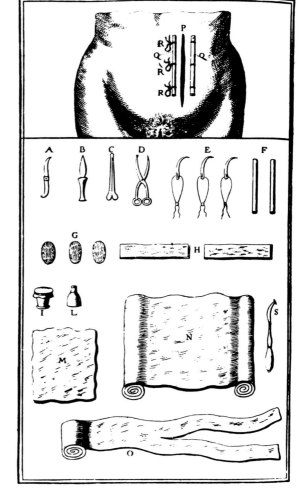

Fig. 11-29. Incision, instruments, sutures, and dressings for cesarean section. From Jacques Mesnard's *Le guide des accoucheurs*, Paris, 1743.

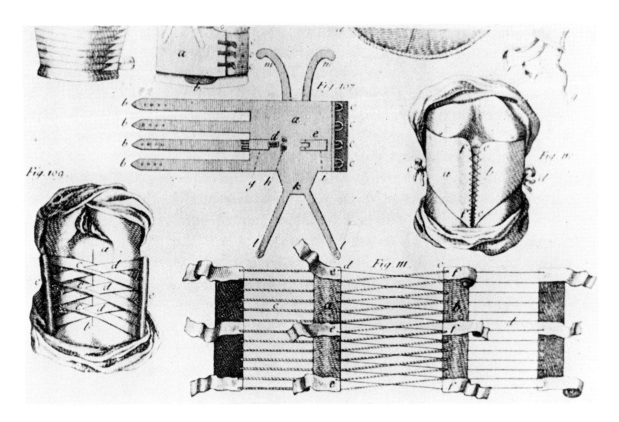

Fig. 11-30. Abdominal binders for use after cesarean section. From J. C. Stark's *Anleitung zum Chirurgischen Verbande,* Berlin, 1802.

To the mid nineteenth century, surgeons labored under the mistaken notion that the uterine wound at cesarean section required no treatment except cleansing. Sutures were regarded as dangerous, preventing retraction of the myometrium and leading to infection. From 1769, when Lebas closed a uterine incision with three silk threads, several additional attempts at uterine suture were made, unsuccessfully, with other nonabsorbable materials. Left long and protruding from the wound, to facilitate ultimate removal, they almost invariably led to the feared result, peritonitis. If unsutured, however, especially after prolonged labor, the uterine musculature retracted poorly and often bled profusely. A safe technique of uterine wound closure was urgently needed.

Silver wire was first used for this purpose with success in 1852 by Frank E. Polin, a surgeon of Springfield, Kentucky. By 1880 uterine sutures had been used in at least 16 cesarean sections in the United States. But only from 1882, with the publication of Max Sänger's widely heralded monograph, did coaptation of the wound edges receive full recognition as an essential part of the cesarean operation. Sänger's technique, of longitudinal

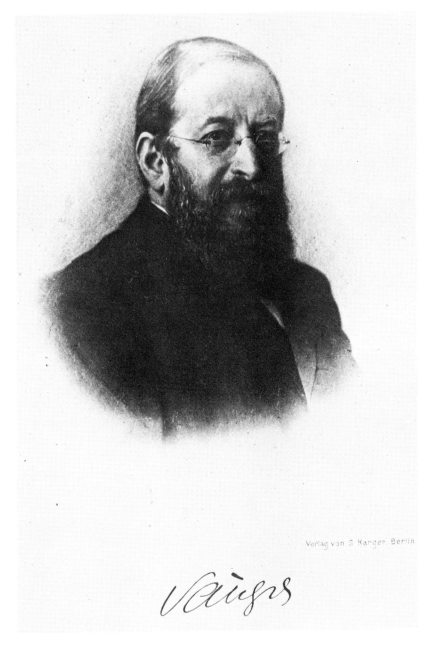

Fig. 11-31. Max Sänger (1853–1903). He emphasized the importance of sutures in cesarean section and popularized the *classical operation*.

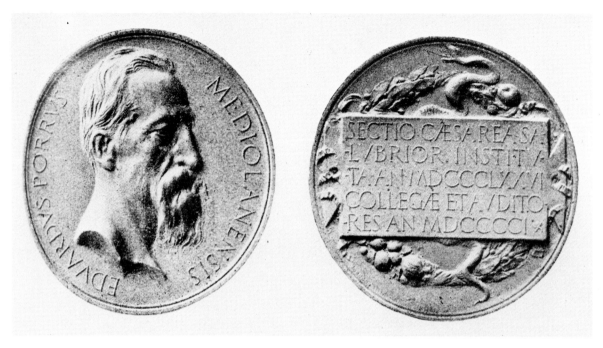

Fig. 11-32. Edoardo Porro (1842–1902). Bronze medal struck in 1901 to commemorate the 25th anniversary of his successfully performed cesarean-hysterectomy (1876).

incision and suture of the uterine fundus, has since been known as the classical cesarean section.

Thus the hazard of hemorrhage was reduced, but the problem of infection remained. Even before the publication of Sänger's report, Edoardo Porro in 1876 demonstrated a method of reducing both dangers of abdominal delivery by removing the uterus at the time of section. No woman had ever survived a cesarean section in Pavia, Italy. Further, abdominal hysterectomy had proved fatal in seven-eighths of the patients on whom it was attempted. On the morning of May 21, 1876, Julia Cavallini, a rhachitic dwarf, fell into labor. Her pelvis was so distorted and contracted, with a diagonal conjugate of only 7 cm, that vaginal delivery was out of the question. Seeing no alternative, Porro performed cesarean section, delivering a normal female infant of 3300 grams. Unable to control the bleeding from the cut edges of the uterus, Porro promptly proceeded with hysterectomy, placing a wire snare around the uterus, drawing it tight at the level of the internal os, and rapidly amputating the organ. The patient made a complete recovery. Thus was cesarean-hysterectomy, subsequently known as the Porro operation, proved feasible.

With the surgical refinements of the twentieth century, cesarean section has been shorn of its erstwhile terror. It carries little more risk now than a natural birth.

Chapter 12

THE NEWBORN
Resuscitation, Swaddling, Circumcision, and Baptism

"And the Lord God formed man of the dust of the ground, and breathed into his nostrils the breath of life; and man became a living soul." [Genesis 2:7]

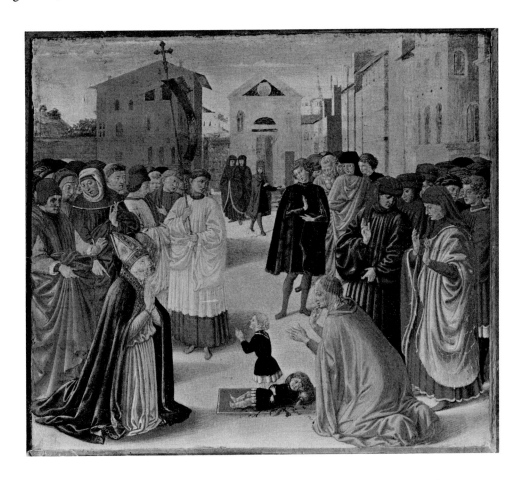

Fig. 12-1. Saint Zenobius Resuscitating a Dead Child. By Benozzo Gozzoli (1420–1497), one of four panels painted for the Alessandri Chapel, San Pier Maggiore, Florence, Italy. The Metropolitan Museum of Art, New York.

RESUSCITATION

"And when Elisha was come into the house, behold, the child was dead, and laid upon his bed.

"He went in therefore, and shut the door upon them twain, and prayed unto the Lord.

"And he went up, and lay upon the child, and put his mouth upon his mouth, and his eyes upon his eyes, and his hands upon his hands: and he stretched himself upon the child; and the flesh of the child waxed warm.

"Then he returned, and walked in the house to and fro; and went up, and stretched himself upon him: and the child sneezed seven times, and the child opened his eyes." [II Kings 4:32-35]

So runs the first description of mouth-to-mouth resuscitation, effective and still used in the absence of special equipment. Post-biblical techniques for restoring life to the limp and apneic newborn have included swinging, spanking, dipping the infant alternately into tubs of hot and cold water, and the administration of stimulant drugs. All have been superseded during the twentieth century by gentle handling, maintenance of a clear airway, and supplementary oxygenation.

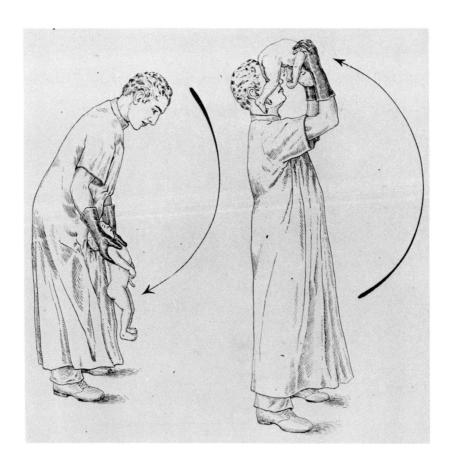

Fig. 12-2. Schultze's method of resuscitation (Bernhard Sigmund Schultze, 1827–1919). The infant was grasped by the shoulders and upper arms and swung upward, above the operator's head. The weight of the viscera, pressing against the diaphragm, helped expel fluid from the air passages. After being held in this position while the operator counted to 5, the infant was swung down again between the former's knees, where the drag upon the diaphragm aided inspiration.

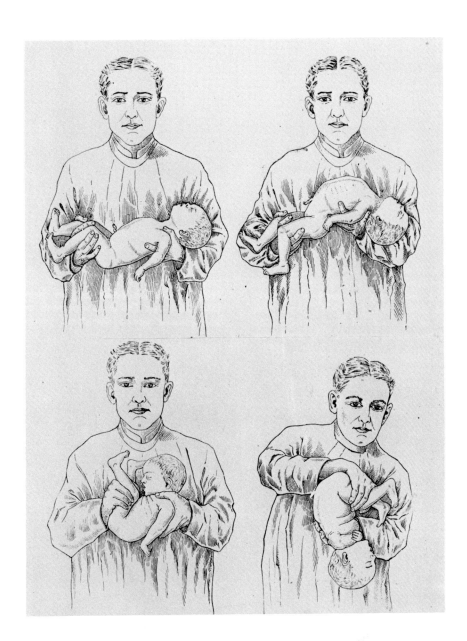

Fig. 12-3. Dew's method of resuscitation. J. Harvie Dew: Establishing a new method of artificial respiration in asphyxia neonatorum. Med. Rec. 43:289, 1893.

"Grasp the infant with the left hand, allowing the neck to rest between the thumb and forefinger, the head falling far over backward.... Then with the right hand... grasp the knees.... This position will allow the back of the thighs to rest in the palm of the operator's hand.... The next step is to depress the pelvis and lower extremities so as to allow the abdominal organs to drag the diaphragm downward, and with the left hand to gently bend the dorsal region of the spine backward. This enlarges the thoracic cavity and produces inspiration. Then, to excite expiration, reverse the movement.... At the same moment bring forward the thighs, resting them upon the abdomen. This movement... so bends the child upon itself as to crowd together the contents of the thoracic and abdominal cavities, bringing about a most complete and forcible expiration."

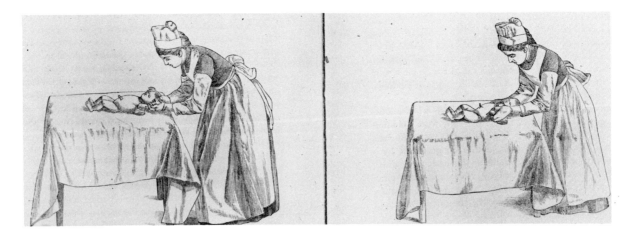

Fig. 12-4. Silvester's method of resuscitation. Henry R. Silvester: A new method of resuscitating still-born children, and of restoring persons apparently drowned or dead. Brit. Med. J. 2:576, 1858. The infant was placed on its back, its shoulders elevated by a rolled towel, extending the neck. The arms were extended slowly over the head and held in this position through the count of 5. This maneuver elevated the ribs, expanding the chest and drawing air into the lungs. The arms were then carried back down and pressed against the chest, producing expiration.

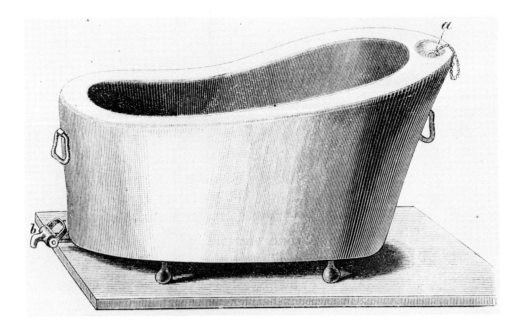

Fig. 12-5. Credé's incubator. The mechanism for regulating body temperature is poorly developed among prematurely born infants. A multitude of devices of varying complexity commonly known as incubators have been designed to compensate for heat loss by the premature or feeble infant and to help it maintain a constant body temperature. Among the simplest was Credé's apparatus (Carl Siegmund Credé, 1819–1892), a copper tub of double walls, the compartment between which had a capacity of 35 pints, for warm water, which was added at (a) and drained at (b).

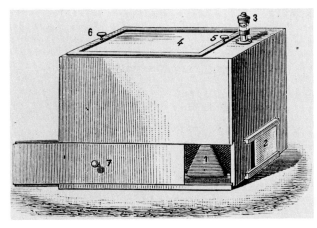
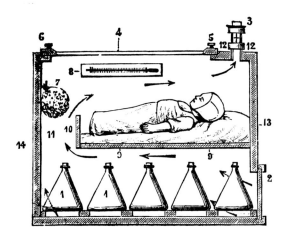

Fig. 12-6. Tarnier's incubator (Etienne Stéphane Tarnier, 1828–1897). A wooden box with a removable glass lid and a ventilating tube containing a small rotary fan. Beneath the infant were placed a number of cans filled with hot water. The interior of the box also contained a thermometer and a sponge, which was saturated with water to humidify the chamber. Popularized anew by Pierre Victor Alfred Auvard (1855–1941), this device became known also as the Auvard incubator.

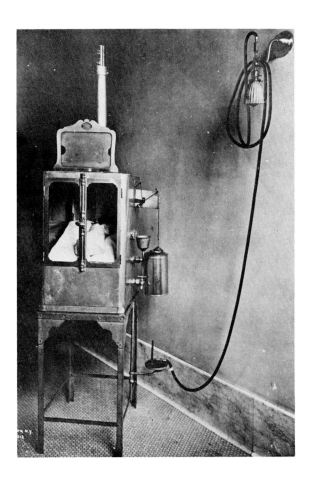

Fig. 12-7. Incubator for premature infants. Sloane Maternity Hospital, New York City, about 1900. Connected to a wall gas-outlet, a Bunsen burner was used to heat the water in the boiler outside the infant's compartment.

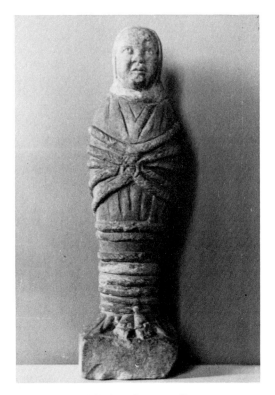

Fig. 12-8. Swaddled infant. Gallic-Roman votive figurine from the ruins of a temple at Sainte-Sabine, France. Musée des Beaux-Arts, Beaune, France.

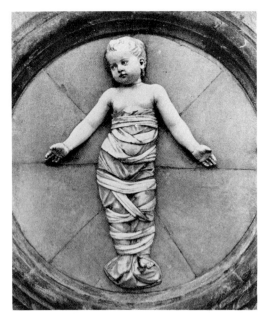

Fig. 12-9. Swaddled infant. Glazed terra cotta relief, by Andrea della Robbia (1435–1525). Loggia Spedale degli Innocenti, Florence.

SWADDLING

"And she brought forth her first born son, and wrapped him in swaddling clothes, and laid him in a manger..." [St. Luke 2:7]

An ancient custom of the early Greeks and Romans, later practiced more widely but long since abandoned by all except a few small communities in Asia Minor, was the ritual of swaddling, the tight wrapping of newborn infants in cloth bindings. Soranus (AD 98–138) valued swaddling as a means of pressing the limbs and body into good shape, removing any deformities caused by birth, and of protecting the newborn against injury.

Galen, who lived immediately after Soranus in the second century, likewise endorsed the bandaging of infants. He wrote,

"The newborn infant... should be powdered moderately and wrapped in swaddling clothes, in order that his skin may be made thicker and firmer than the parts within. For during pregnancy everything was equally soft, since nothing of a harder nature touched it from without, and no cold air came in contact with it, whereby the skin would be contracted and thickened, and would become tougher and denser than it was before and than the other parts of the body. But when the baby is born, it is necessarily going to come in contact with cold and heat and with many bodies harder than itself. Therefore it is appropriate that his natural covering should be best prepared by us for exposure." [R. M. Greene: *A Translation of Galen's Hygiene.* Charles C Thomas, Springfield, Ill., 1951.]

The binding of boys was uniformly tight, but girls were usually wrapped more loosely about the hips. Freedom of movement was markedly restricted, except between reapplications of the bandages. Not uncommonly the wrappings were left undisturbed for days at a time, not being removed even for a change of

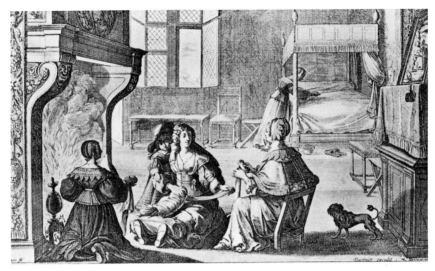

Fig. 12-10. Swaddling the newborn. The puerperal chamber of a French lady of the upper middle class, mid seventeenth century, by Abraham Bosse (1602–1676). The midwife, pillow on lap, swaddles the infant while the puerpera on a stool beside her looks on. In Tavernier's engraving of this scene (*L'Emaillattement*), the following four verses appear, the mother speaking of her labor, the wetnurse asking adequate remuneration for her services, and the two maids stating that the enthusiasm with which they perform their duties will depend on the generosity of their reward.

> La Mine de cette accouchee
> me semble si fort en bon poinct
> que voluntiers pour mon pourpoinct
> je voudrais l'avoir empeschee.
>
> A cette gentile Nourrice
> coiffee de son bauolet
> quand on deburoit troubler son laict
> seroit bon luy rendre seruice.
>
> Et pour cette jeune seruente
> qui chauffe la couche a L'enfant
> qui luy vouldroit en faire autant
> Je croy quelle seroit contente.
>
> J'entens à faire le mesnage
> et sur tout a dresser un lict.
> mais, pour y prendre son desduict
> je fais mieux encor cet ouvrage.

diapers. Physicians began to condemn swaddling as unhygienic during the sixteenth century. William Cadogan, an English physician and social reformer, made an ardent plea for its abolishment in 1748 in his *Essay upon Nursing,* and by the beginning of the nineteenth century swaddling had virtually been abandoned in all enlightened communities. William Heberden (1710–1801), English physician and scholar, urged,

"Let then art take example from nature, and follow in her steps. Let all tight bandages be removed . . . that the play and growth of the limbs be unrestrained. . . . What distortion of the limbs, what bad shapes have we to deplore from the former of these causes!"

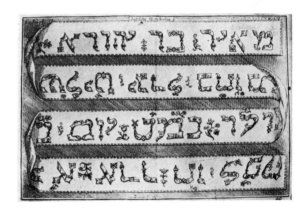

Fig. 12-11. A Jewish swaddling band with the infant's name and date of birth embroidered in Hebrew characters.

CIRCUMCISION

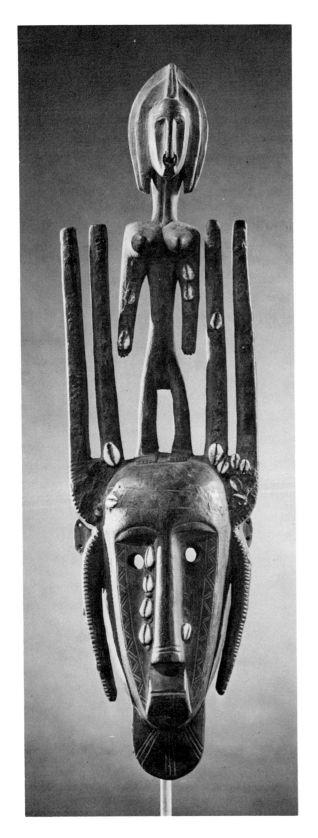

"This is my covenant, which ye shall keep, between me and you and thy seed after thee; Every man child among you shall be circumcised.... And ye shall circumcise the flesh of your foreskin; and it shall be a token of the covenant betwixt me and you.... And he that is eight days old shall be circumcised among you, every man child in your generations, he that is born in the house, or bought with money of any stranger, which is not of thy seed.... And Abraham took Ishmael his son, and all that were born in his house, and all that were bought with his money, every male among the men of Abraham's house; and circumcised the flesh of their foreskin in the selfsame day, as God had said unto him.... And Abraham was ninety years old and nine, when he was circumcised in the flesh of his foreskin.... And Ishmael his son was thirteen years old, when he was circumcised in the flesh of his foreskin.... In the selfsame day was Abraham circumcised, and Ishmael his son.... And all the men of his house, born in the house, and bought with money of the stranger, were circumcised with him." [Genesis 17:10-12, 23-27]

Biblical scholars have computed the circumcision date of Abraham and his household as the year 2047 (1713 BC). Herodotus and several later historians concluded that circumcision was practiced even earlier, by the ancient Egyptians, as evidenced in their

Fig. 12-12. Mask worn at circumcision rite by young men of the Bambara Tribe, Mali, Africa, nineteenth and twentieth centuries. The symbolic female figure and antelope horns were believed to endow the mask with protective powers against illness. In the Brooklyn Museum Collection, Brooklyn, N.Y.

mummies, their bas-reliefs, and in a Biblical reference to the Pharaoh (Ezekiel 31:18). The Semites, it is believed, who migrated from Babylon into northern Mesopotamia, circumcised their males as early as 3200–2700 BC. Practiced originally as a religious, cultural, or fertility rite (*rite de passage*), circumcision has been adopted in widening circles as its hygienic value has become increasingly recognized. Although medical authorities are still not in complete agreement concerning the merits of routine circumcision, most acknowledge its value in preventing phimosis, penile cancer in later life, and possibly in reducing the risk of cervical cancer in the conjugal partner. With the exception of omphalotomy or cutting of the umbilical cord, circumcision is now the most widespread and frequent of all surgical operations.

In many primitive societies, as in certain tribes of South Africa, circumcision remains purely ritualistic even today, and in some such groups it is carried out only at puberty or in anticipation of marriage. The rite is often accompanied by elaborate tribal ceremonies, variously featured by feasting, fasting, dancing, prayer, and symbolic dress. Orthodox Jews still perform circumcision of the newborn on the eighth day, usually employing a professional circumciser or *mohel*. Most non-ritual circumcisions in civilized cultures of the twentieth century are done by a physician, usually the obstetrician, at any convenient time in the neonatal period.

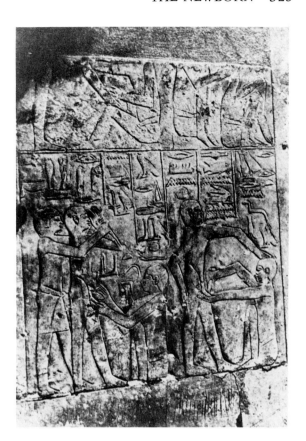

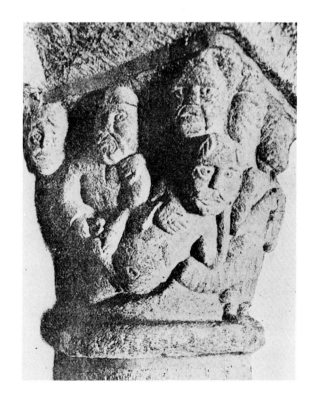

Fig. 12-13. Egyptian circumcision scene, about 2500 BC. Relief on the tomb of Ankhmahor at Saqqara, Egypt, sixth Dynasty. The priest, sitting, circumcises a 13 year old youth with a flint knife. An assistant, on the left, holds the subject. For ritual circumcision, flint knives continued in use long after the introduction of metal instruments.

Fig. 12-14. Circumcision scene. Eleventh century stone carving. Reproduction from a postcard showing the head of a column in the dome of the church at Chambon, France.

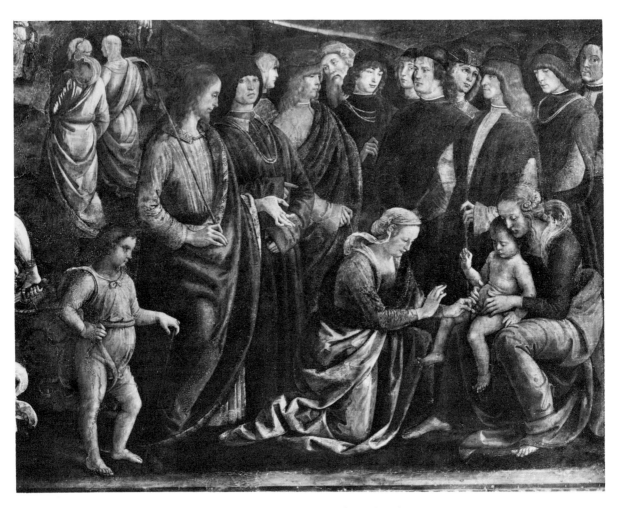

Fig. 12-15. The circumcision of Eleazar, son of Moses. Painting by Pietro Perugino (1450–1524). "Then Zipporah took a sharp stone, and cut off the foreskin of her son, and cast it at his feet, and said, Surely a bloody bridegroom art thou to me" (Exodus 4:25). Biblical commentaries differ in their interpretation of Zipporah's remark. According to Rashi, *bridegroom* refers to Moses who had angered God by his failure to circumcise Eleazar. Zipporah therefore performed the rite for her husband and thus saved his life. Ibn Ezra, on the other hand, believed that Zipporah's remark was directed to her son, the near cause of Moses' death. In this view *bridegroom* was used symbolically, as a title of honor for the newly circumcised child. Sistine Chapel, Vatican.

THE NEWBORN 327

The circumcision of Jesus, a favorite subject for artists, has been depicted in a variety of media. Holding the Infant is Simeon, who has been assured by the Holy Spirit that he would not die until he had seen the Lord's Christ. The immortal words of the *Nunc Dimittis* Simeon uttered soon after, "Lord, now lettest thou thy servant to depart in peace...." The operator is shown drawing forward the Infant's foreskin in his left hand, preparatory to cutting it with the knife, held in his right. In the background or to one side stand the Virgin and the high priest. Commonly included are a wash basin, a bowl to receive the foreskin, and a flask of wine.

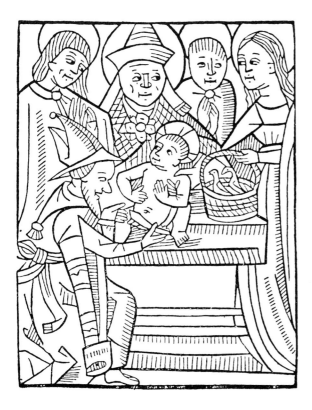

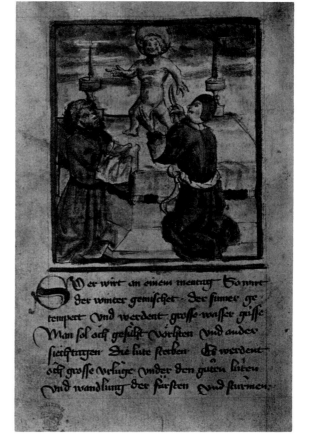

Fig. 12-16. The circumcision of Jesus. Woodcut, fifteenth(?) century.

Fig. 12-17. The circumcision of Christ. Miniature from an anonymous German manuscript, about 1440. The Infant stands between two candles on an altar-like table. The external genitalia, although not shown, do not appear to have been erased. Kneeling before the Infant are the operator and an assistant, who holds an open napkin to receive the foreskin. The British Museum, London.

328 ICONOGRAPHIA GYNIATRICA

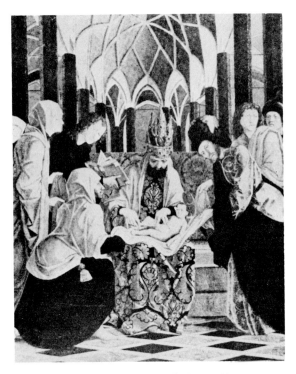

Fig. 12-18. The circumcision of Christ. Altar painting by Michael Pacher (1467–1498). In a setting suggesting a Gothic church, the Infant lies on a cloth held by two assistants while the robed, bearded priest wearing a jeweled miter performs the circumcision. St. Wolfgang's parish church, Salzkammergut, Austria.

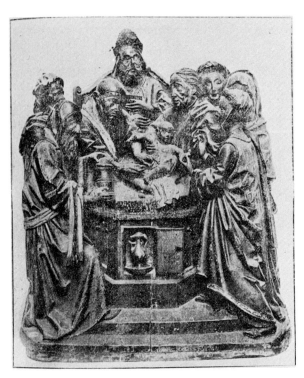

Fig. 12-19. The circumcision of Jesus. Woodcut, late fifteenth century. Oeuvre Notre Dame, Strasbourg.

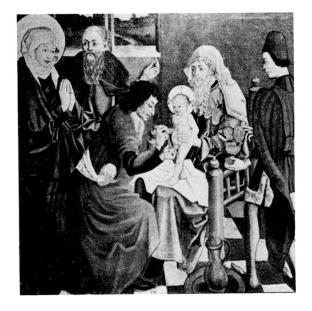

Fig. 12-20. The circumcision. By an artist of the Upper Rhein School, late fifteenth century. On the extreme right an attendant in Florentine garb holds a small bowl to receive the foreskin.

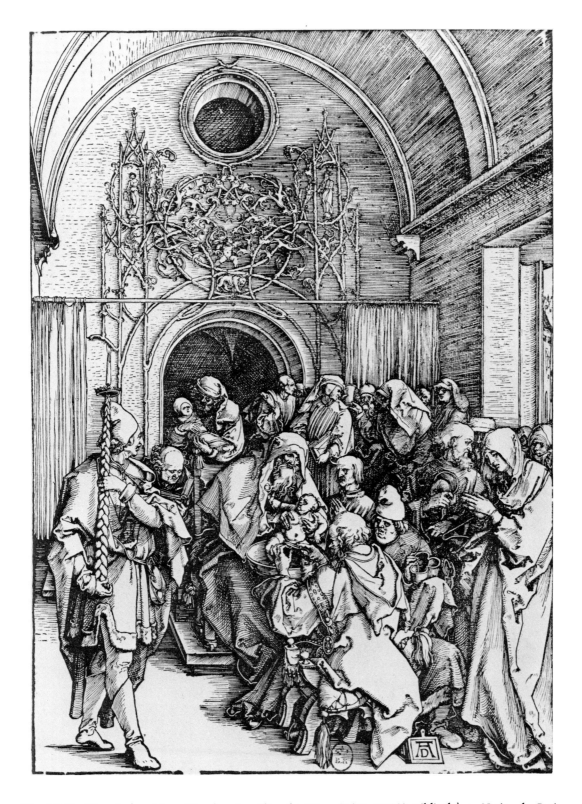

Fig. 12-21. The circumcision. Woodcut by Albrecht Dürer (1471–1528). Bibliothèque Nationale, Paris.

330 ICONOGRAPHIA GYNIATRICA

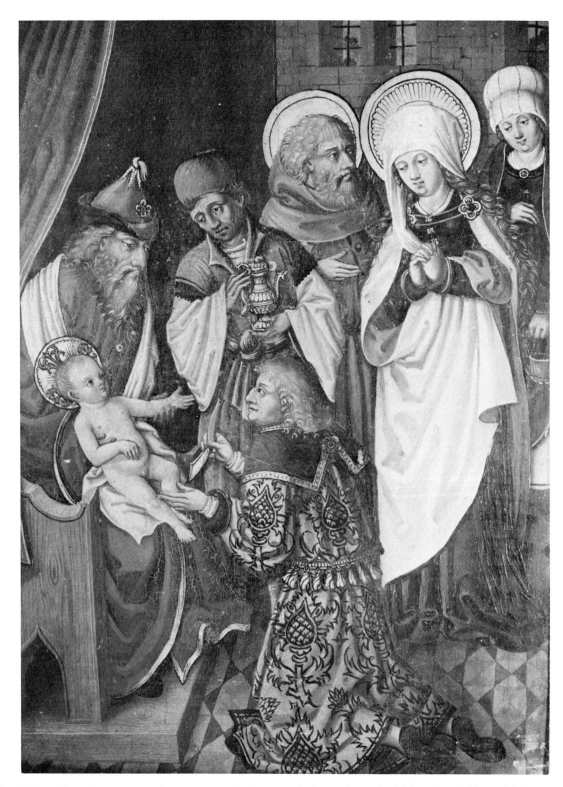

Fig. 12-22. The circumcision. Anonymous painting, 1505. The *mohel*, knife in hand, kneels before the infant whom the high priest holds on his lap. Musée d'Unterlinden, Colmar, France.

THE NEWBORN 331

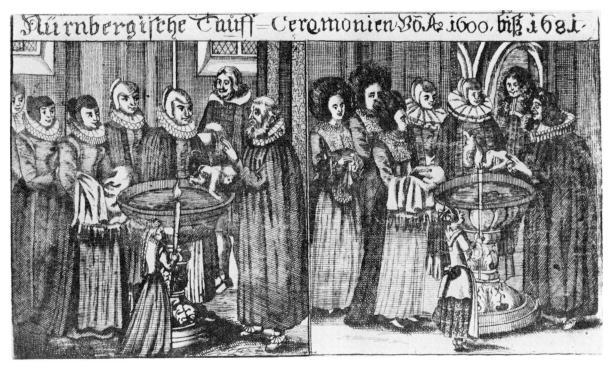

Fig. 12-23. Baptismal ceremony, Nürnberg, 1600. Germanisches Nationalmuseum, Nürnberg.

BAPTISM

"Go ye therefore, and teach all nations, baptizing them in the name of the Father, and of the Son, and of the Holy Ghost." [St. Matthew 28:19]

"And there went out unto him all the land of Judaea, and they of Jerusalem, and were all baptized of him in the river of Jordan, confessing their sins." [St. Mark 1:5]

"Now when all the people were baptized, it came to pass, that Jesus also being baptized, and praying, the heaven was opened,
"And the Holy Ghost descended in a bodily shape like a dove upon him, and a voice came from heaven, which said, Thou art my beloved Son; in thee I am well pleased." [St. Luke 3:21-22]

A symbol of regeneration, the Christian ritual of baptism by immersion or sprinkling with water represents the grace by which the soul is cleansed of the taint of previous sin. Only through this sacrament, according to the doctrine of Original Sin, can salvation be achieved. Special pitchers and bowls, often ornate, serve as vehicles for the holy water used in baptism which is conferred during early infancy by most Christian groups, not until maturity by some.

"Where there is ground to fear that it is dead, we should say, *'Child, I baptize thee, etc. if thou art living';* and where there is reason to suspect it of being a monster, we substitute for *if thou art living,* the words *if thou art worthy of being baptized.* In order to baptize, some part of the naked surface of the child should be touched, if not with the fingers, at least with the water of christening...."
[A. L. M. Velpeau: *Traité élémentaire de l'art des accouchemens.* J.B. Baillière, Paris, 1829.]

332   ICONOGRAPHIA GYNIATRICA

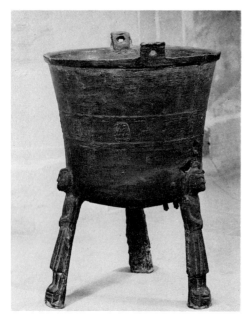

Fig. 12-24. Bronze baptismal font, thirteenth century, from the Cathedral of Liège, Belgium. Germanisches Nationalmuseum, Nürnberg.

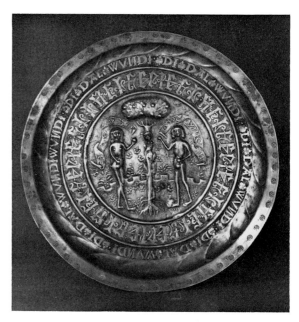

Fig. 12-25. Baptismal bowl, fifteenth century. Germanisches Nationalmuseum, Nürnberg.

Fig. 12-26. Baptismal font from the Hildesheimer Cathedral, Germany.

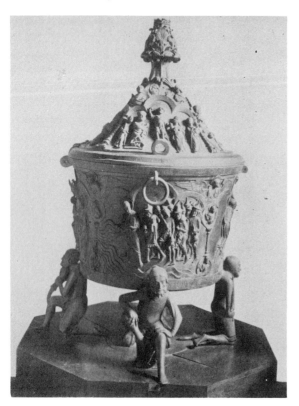

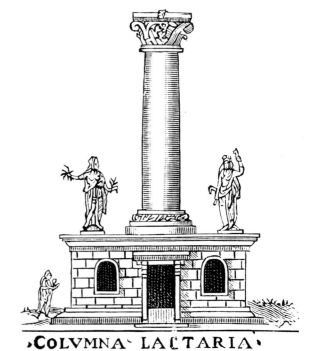

Fig. 12-27. *Columna Lactaria*, a popular repository for abandoned infants in ancient Rome. Here babies were left at night in baskets to be claimed as slaves, until Trajan (Roman Emperor, AD 98–117) decreed their freedom, and Julius Paulus in AD 160 prohibited the abandonment of infants altogether.

Chapter 13

NURSING

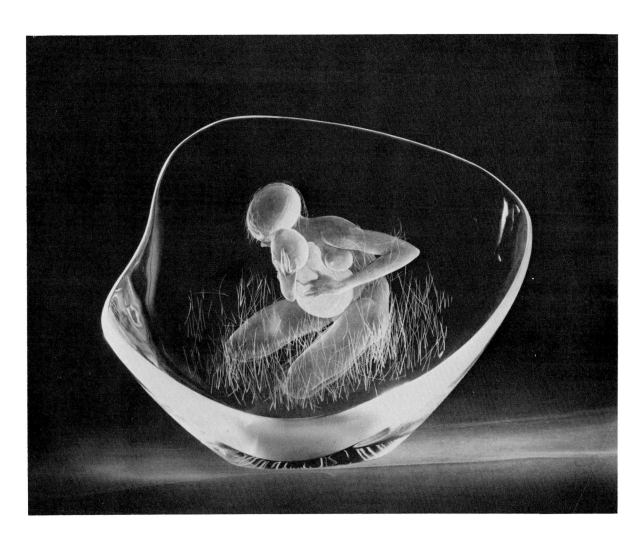

Fig. 13-1. Mother and Child. Crystal bowl, width 12 inches, glass design, George Thompson (1913–   ); engraving, Tom Vincent (1930–   ). Kneeling in a patch of grass, her attitude expressing the tenderness and protection of motherhood, a young woman cradles her nursling.

334 ICONOGRAPHIA GYNIATRICA

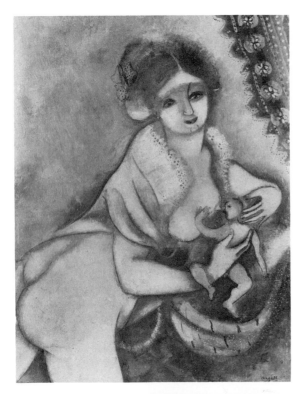

Fig. 13-2. *Maternité*, 1914, by Marc Chagall (1889–   ). Collection Hans Schröder, Saarbruck, Germany.

Fig. 13-3. The Origin of the Milky Way. Painting, about 1577, by Il Tintoretto (real name, Jacopo Robusti) 1518–1594. Illustrated, perhaps for the first time, is the milk-ejection reflex: the spurting of milk from both nipples produced by the sucking stimulus applied to one. The National Gallery, London.

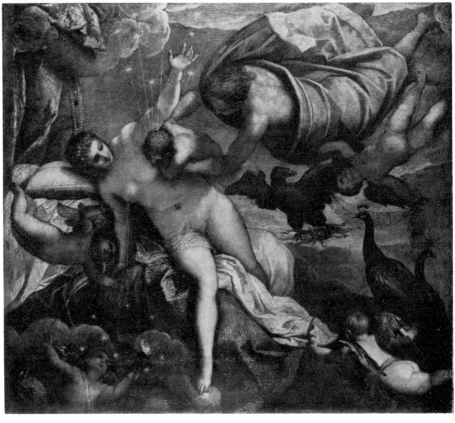

"When the fetus in a pregnant woman begins to grow bigger, the uterus presses on the intestines, stomach, diaphragm, and all the upper parts of the body and forces them into a narrow compass; at the same time it propels the chyle toward the breasts along the lacteals of the abdomen and the thoracic ducts, and thus it is easily carried by the chyliferous ducts to the breasts, the tissues of which are soft and relaxed, or if these ducts are not yet fully open, at any rate it flows through the mammary arteries ... and it needs no other agency to start it than that pressure, though this may be reinforced by the movements of the fetus.... For the first signs of milk appear in the breasts when the child begins to move in the womb....

"We must certainly believe that the Divine Architect fashioned the uterus and the breasts with some structure, some contrivance that so far escapes us, so designed that by an established routine conception in the uterus is followed by the generation of milk in the breasts, on the analogy of what we now know happens when the fetus breaks out of its prison, and its lungs, which for nine months had nothing to do, thereupon enter on their function as the outer air begins to enter the mouth and to inflate them by its elastic force; so that simultaneously the *foramen ovale* falls into disuse and the blood circulates by other channels. We must therefore concede that a marvellous sympathy between the breasts and the uterus does exist, but so far it has not been explained by the sagacity of man or come under the eye of the anatomist." [Bernardino Ramazzi: *Diseases of Workers,* 1713. Trans. by W. C. Wright, Hafner Publishing Co., 1964, pp. 183, 189.]

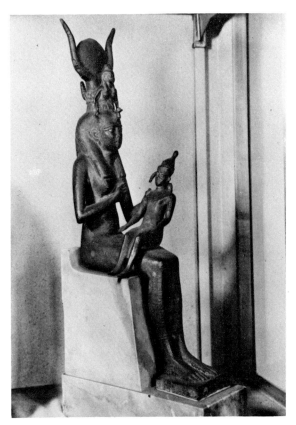

Fig. 13-4. Isis nursing Horus. Egyptian bronze. The goddess was often depicted with a headdress of horns. Musée du Louvre, Paris.

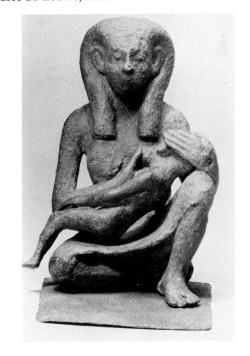

Fig. 13-5. Isis, universal mother, nursing her son Horus. Egyptian copper figure. The worship of Isis originated under the New Empire (about 1700–1100 BC), spread throughout Egypt and into other lands of the Mediterranean world. Staatliche Museen, West Berlin.

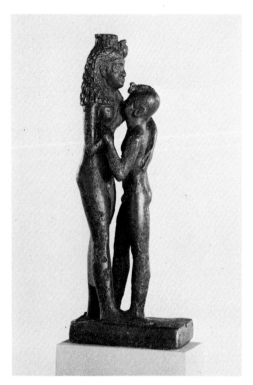

Fig. 13-6. Isis nursing Horus. In this Egyptian figure the young god is shown almost as tall as his mother. Staatliche Museen, West Berlin.

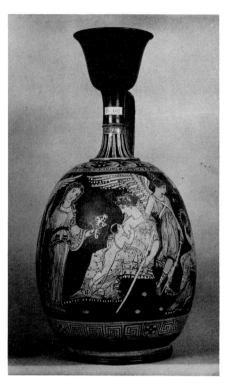

Fig. 13-7. Heracles (Hercules) suckled by Hera. Apulian vase. The sons of Zeus, it was taught, could not qualify for divine worship until they had fed at Hera's breast. The act of suckling thus came to symbolize adoption. Heracles is shown here as a boy, without his traditional club and lion skin, drinking from the right breast of Hera. At the left stands his patroness Athene offering Hera a lily, her favorite flower. Behind Hera stands winged Iris. The British Museum, London.

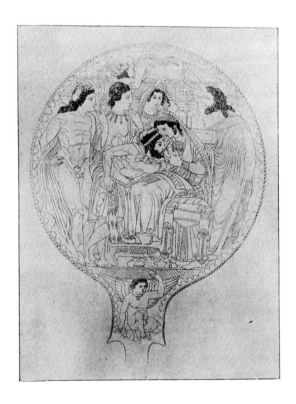

Fig. 13-8. Heracles suckled by Hera. Engraving on an Etruscan mirror, found in Volterra, Italy. The ancient tale states that Hera gave the breast to Heracles, the hated son of her rival Alcmene, after mistaking his identity. But this version is not supported by Etruscan art scenes which show Heracles as a bearded man. This Etruscan representation probably denotes Hera's later adoption of Heracles. On the right stands Zeus, father of Heracles, gesticulating to Apollo on the extreme left. Museo Archeologico, Florence.

NURSING 337

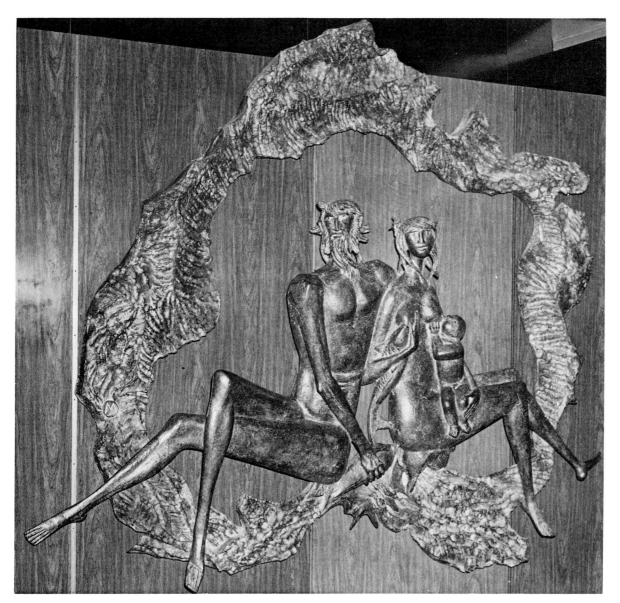

Fig. 13-9. Oceanus, Titan lord of the great river that was believed to encircle the earth, and his wife Tethys. Bronze sculpture, 10 ft. high, 8 ft. wide, by Marcello Mascherini (1906–   ). Tethys is shown nursing a fish as well as a child, symbolizing her gift of life to the creatures of both sea and earth.

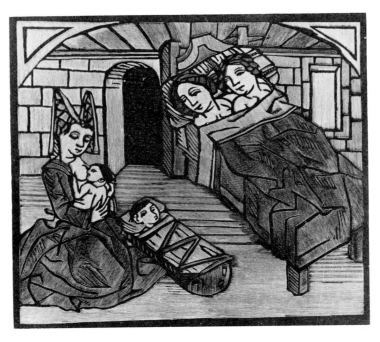

Fig. 13-10. The nymph Melusine nursing her twin children. Woodcut from a German folk-book printed by Heinrich Knoblochtzer, Strassburg, 1483. Widespread at that time was the belief that a woman who died in childbirth, finding no peace in the grave, had to return home every night to nurse her child. The story of Melusine of French mythology was recorded by Jean D'Arras in 1387. Daughter of Helmas, King of Albania, and the fairy Persine, the beautiful Melusine was transformed every Saturday into a serpent from the hips down and was permitted to marry only if she could find a husband who would agree never to see her on Saturdays. Raymond of Poitiers accepted this condition of marriage, but yielding ultimately to his curiosity, he witnessed his wife in her Saturday bath. Discovered, Melusine flew away in serpentine form. According to French folklore, she is to be seen at times on the tower of Lusignan, ancient French town that was her home, clad in mourning garb and uttering lamentations, believed to herald the death of a villager. *Pousser des cris de Mélusine* (To utter the cries of Melusine) is still a popular expression in parts of France. The woodcut shows Melusine, seated on a low seat in her castle chamber, nursing one of her twins, to whom she returned each night. Lying in bed are the twins' two wet nurses.

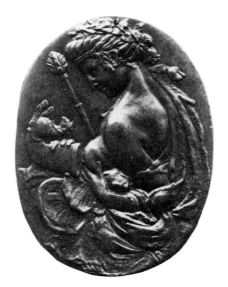

Fig. 13-11. A bacchanal, devotee of Bacchus, expressing milk into a horn. Bronze plaque by the Italian sculptor Donatello (1386–1466). Victoria and Albert Museum, London, Crown Copyright.

MARY AND JESUS

Notable among nursing scenes both for their number and artistic quality are the figures of the Virgin Mary and the Infant Jesus depicted in countless paintings, sculptures, and woodcarvings. In contrast to many early Renaissance representations of the Nativity in which the Infant was painted as a diminutive adult, the nursing scenes show Jesus in the true proportions of a normal child.

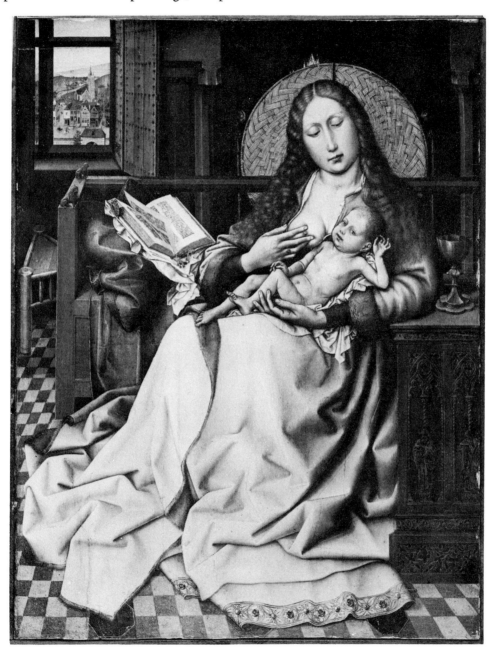

Fig. 13-12. The Virgin and Child before a Fire Screen. By the Master of Flémalle (Robert Campin?, c. 1375–1444). The circular fire screen in the background, behind the Virgin's head, serves as her halo. The National Gallery, London.

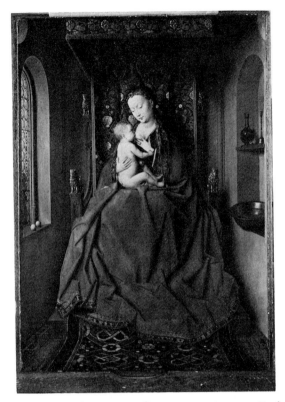

Fig. 13-13. The Virgin of Lucca. By Jan van Eyck (1390?–1440). Städelsches Kunstinstitut, Frankfort a. M.

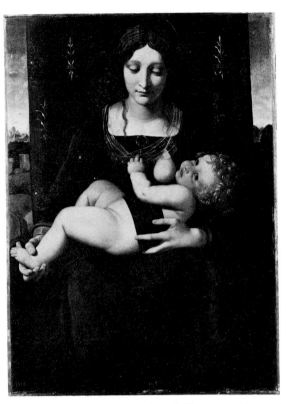

Fig. 13-14. Madonna and Child. By Giovanni Antonio Boltraffio (1467–1516). The Infant is shown in a swaddling band, the Virgin in contemporary garb with slit in upper part of dress especially designed for nursing. The National Gallery, London.

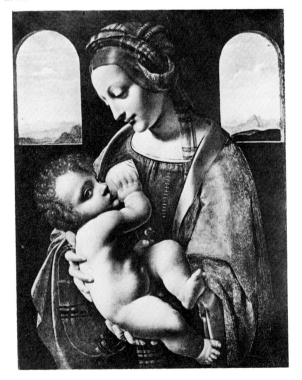

Fig. 13-15. Madonna Litta. From the workshop of Leonardo da Vinci, painted possibly by Ambrogio de Predis, about 1485–1490. Named after Conte Litta, Milan, in whose collection it remained until 1865 when it was acquired by the Hermitage, Leningrad. Shown here is the lacing device by which the maternal dresses of the fifteenth and sixteenth centuries could be opened and closed for nursing. Note similarity to Figure 13-16 by de' Conti. The Hermitage, Leningrad.

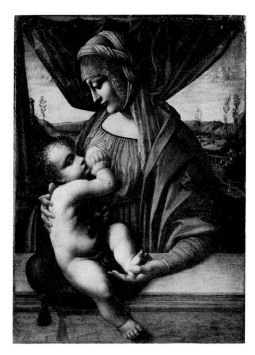

Fig. 13-16. Madonna with Child. By Bernardo de' Conti (1499–1522). Compare with the Madonna Litta, from da Vinci's workshop, Figure 13-15. Museo Poldi-Pezzoli, Milan.

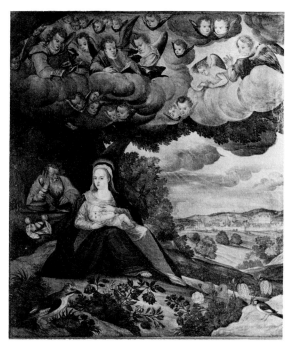

Fig. 13-17. *Vierge nourrice* (The nursing Virgin). Painting attributed to Frédéric Brentel (c. 1580–1651). Joseph brings fruit to Mary. Musée d'Unterlinden, Colmar, France.

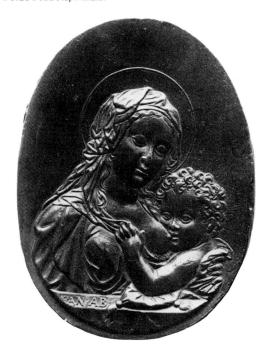

Fig. 13-18. The Virgin nursing Jesus. Bronze plaque by the Milanese sculptor Antonio Abondio (1538–1591). Victoria and Albert Museum, London, Crown Copyright.

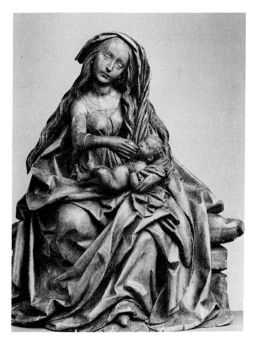

Fig. 13-19. Mary feeding Jesus. Woodcarving by Tilman Riemenschneider (1468?–1531). The naked Infant takes his nourishment from a leather-covered nursing bottle. Staatliche Museen, East Berlin.

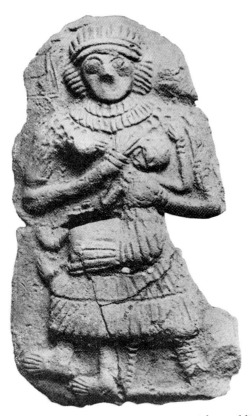

Fig. 13-20. Mesopotamian woman with suckling child. Terra cotta plaque from Lagash, ancient Sumerian city, a center of sculpture and literature which flourished about 3000 BC to 2300 BC. Musée du Louvre, Paris.

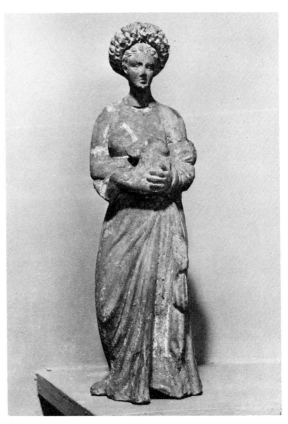

Fig. 13-21. Woman nursing infant. Terra cotta statue from Cirenaica, a region of E. Libya, second century BC. Musée du Louvre, Paris.

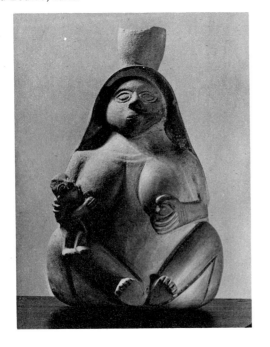

Fig. 13-22. Ancient Peruvian vase. A clay burial urn representing a woman with massive breasts holding a suckling infant at one and manually squirting milk from the other. Museum für Völkerkunde, West Berlin.

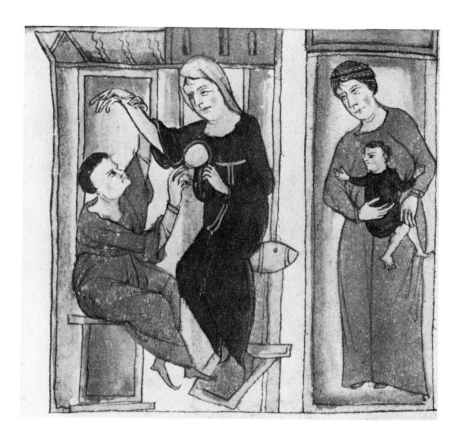

Fig. 13-23. A physician examines the swollen breast of a lactating mother while a nurse holds the wriggling infant, pictured as a child of several years. Miniature from a thirteenth century Latin manuscript of the popular prescription book of Pseudo-Apuleius. Biblioteca Medicea-Laurenziana, Florence.

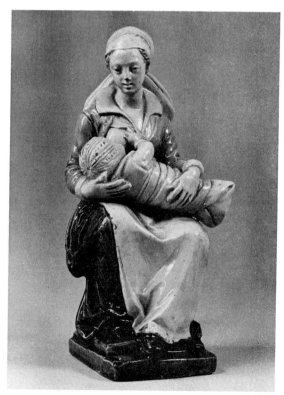

Fig. 13-24. Mother nursing child. Glazed clay statuette by the French potter Bernard Palissy (c. 1510–1590). Note the opening in the mother's dress for nursing. Musée du Louvre, Paris.

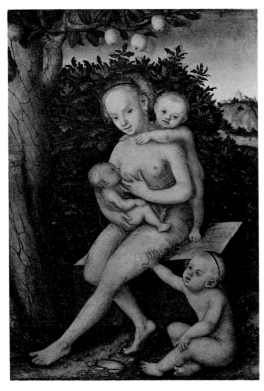

Fig. 13-25. *Caritas*. Painting by Lucas Cranach, the Elder (1472–1553). Koninklijk Museum voor Schone Kunsten, Antwerp.

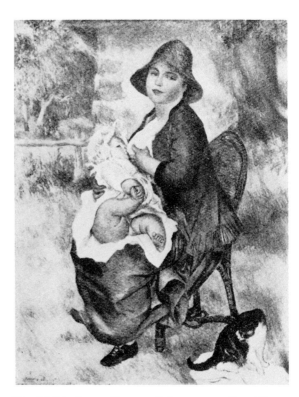

Fig. 13-26. *Jeune femme allaitant son enfant* (Young woman nursing her child). Painting by Pierre Auguste Renoir (1841–1919).

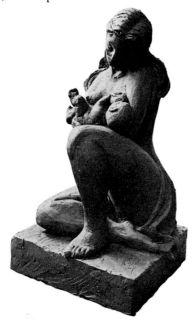

Fig. 13-27. Mother and child. Bronze figure, about 3 feet tall, sculptured in 1960 by George Koras 1925–   ).

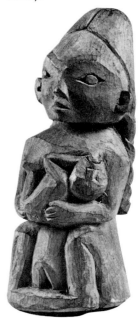

Fig. 13-28. Carved wooden figure of nursing mother and infant. By the Kwakiutl Indians, Vancouver Island, British Columbia, Canada. Museum für Völkerkunde, West Berlin.

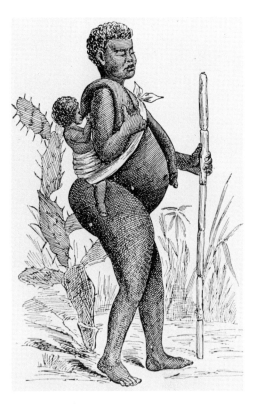

Fig. 13-29. A Bushwoman of the South African tribe of aborigines, with one of her pendulous breasts thrown over her shoulder, nurses her infant strapped to her back.

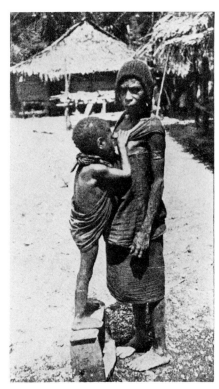

Fig. 13-30. A Kai woman in New Guinea suckling her child. Photograph by Richard Gustav Neuhauss, M.D., early twentieth century. Among primitive peoples in warm regions a woman's breasts, not associated with sentiments of modesty, are usually left bare. In some cultures, as among the Zulus of South Africa, women cover their breasts only during pregnancy; in others, as among the Shortland Islanders in the Solomons, only while lactating, as a protection against evil influences.

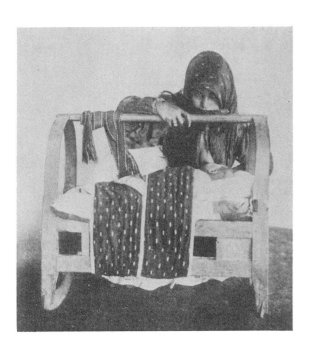

Fig. 13-31. Among several peoples of Western Asia, including the Georgians, the Armenians, and the Maronites, the mother nursed her infant while leaning over the child in its cradle and supporting herself against a transverse bar.

346 ICONOGRAPHIA GYNIATRICA

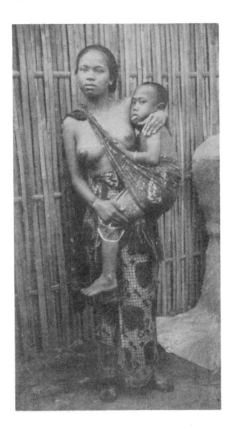

Fig. 13-32. Central Javanese woman with suckling child of four years who smokes a cigarette. Photograph by Fedor Schulze, late nineteenth century. The duration of nursing varies greatly among different cultures. In most civilized communities weaning is usually begun by the eighth month, is completed within the year. Some of the Eskimos of King William Island, Northwest Territories, Canada, on the other hand, are said to suckle their children up to age 14 and 15. In some cultures lactation is prolonged as a means of contraception. Wrote Shakespeare on the weaning of Juliet,

On Lammas-eve at night shall she be fourteen;
That shall she, marry; I remember it well.
'Tis since the earthquake now eleven years;
And she was wean'd, — I never shall forget it, —
Of all the days of the year, upon that day.
For I had then laid wormwood to my dug...
         [Romeo and Juliet: Act I, Scene iii]

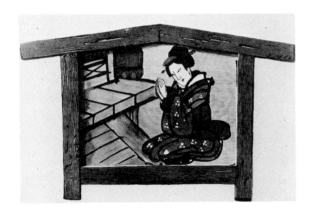

A   B

Fig. 13-33. (A) Japanese woman praying for a bountiful milk supply and (B) the fulfilment of her prayers. Votive paintings on wood. Japanese votive pictures were usually made in pairs and hung together in the temple, the first expressing the supplicant's desire, the second its fulfilment.

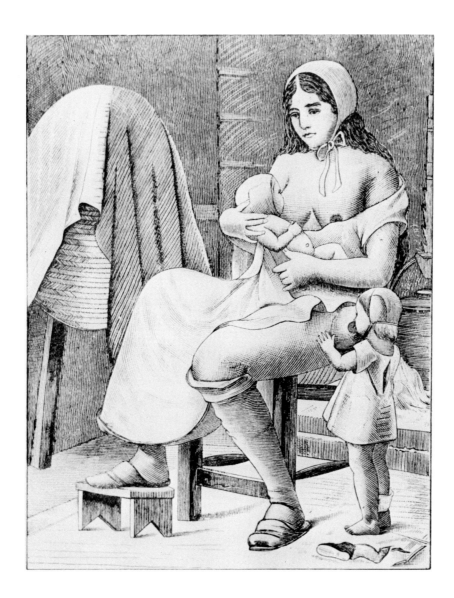

Fig. 13-34. Nursing from an ectopic mamma. The child standing at her mother's side nursed from the supernumerary mammary gland on her mother's thigh for 23 months, while another infant suckled her pectoral breasts. The woman's mother also had three mammae. Patient of a Dr. Robert, Marseille, France, late nineteenth century.

In the human as in other mammals, the mammary apparatus develops from a paired epithelial thickening that extends along the ventral surface of the embryo, from anterior to posterior limb bud. Localized elevations in this milk line develop into the mammary glands while the intervening segments atrophy and disappear. Most supernumerary mammae, which are to be found between the axilla and groin, may be ascribed to persistant embryonic foci in the milk line.

Unexplained are ectopic mammary glands in other locations, as on the face, ear, neck, arm, thigh, and buttock.

Symbolizing fertility, supernumerary mammae adorn ancient figures of the goddess Astarte and Diana of Ephesus whose statue resides in the Vatican Museum. Viewed later as having malign significance, ectopic mammary glands have been referred to as *Teufelswerk, opus mirabile naturae ludentis,* and *une sorte de caprice ou de bizarrerie.* According to at least one account, it was because of her axillary breast that Anne Boleyn was put to death by Henry VIII. Among the Pilgrims in Colonial America, axillary breasts were viewed as a manifestation of witchcraft, and unfortunate possessors of these supernumerary glands were burned at the stake.

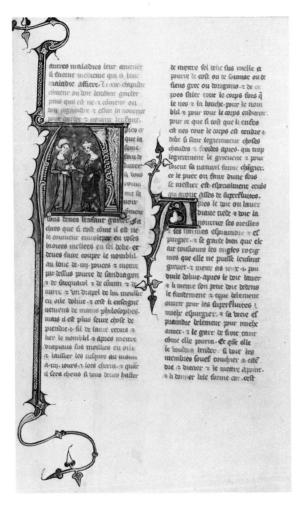

Fig. 13-35. Selection of a wet nurse. Miniature from a fourteenth century manuscript of Aldobrandin's *Régime du corps*. Early medical treatises specified the requirements of a good wet nurse: age, experience, disposition, and character of the breasts. Wet nurses were employed because of maternal ill health, inability or lack of desire to nurse, or to provide a substitute in the early puerperium for maternal colostrum, considered ill-suited for the newborn. Bibliothèque Nationale, Paris.

WET NURSES AND ARTIFICIAL FEEDING

Arguments for and against maternal nursing have raged for centuries. Papyri of the Ptolemaic period (c. 323–30 BC) tell that infants were generally fed at the breast for six months, often by wet nurses, then nourished with animal milk. Soranus (AD 98–138) taught that mothers should not begin to nurse until about three weeks after giving birth; later authorities counseled a waiting period varying from two to ten days. Earlier attempts at nursing were considered harmful because of the mother's delicate condition after parturition and because the newborn was believed incapable of digesting colostrum, precursor of milk. During the early puerperium, before nursing was begun, the breasts were milked manually, to prevent their drying up, or the mother was given an older child to nurse who could digest colostrum. The hazards of artificial feeding, associated with a high infant mortality rate, were widely recognized.

Wet nurses were thus essential to the rearing of the newborn. Many wet nurses were unmarried mothers who allowed their own infants to run the risk of artificial feeding. Others were impecunious women endowed with an abundant milk supply that exceeded the needs of their own child, or women whose children had died soon after birth. Wet nurse agencies, formed in Paris during the twelfth century, later came under strict regulation with medical and police supervision and standardization of pay. As the employment of wet nurses spread, physicians in the fifteenth century began to question the advisability of maternal nursing altogether, and views were expressed that nursing led to debilitation and even sterility.

Attitudes toward breast feeding were profoundly influenced in the mid eighteenth century, especially in France, by the Swiss philosopher and author Jean Jacques

Rousseau (1712-1778), whose views, highly respected by the aristocracy of his adopted country, exerted their impact far beyond its borders. Rousseau's *Émile* (1762), reflecting his advocacy of maternal nursing, appealed to the womanly emotions of his female readers. Almost overnight nursing became fashionable, and mothers began to suckle their infants even at social gatherings.

In the early nineteenth century, by contrast, Conrad Anton Zwierlin (1755-1825), a German physician, took the ultimate step in deprecating nursing. No child, he declared, need be suckled, even by a wet nurse, for the same function could be performed better and more cheaply by a goat. Pointing out the gentle nature of this animal and the tractability of its nipples, Zwierlin proposed that the infant be permitted to suck directly from the goat's udder.

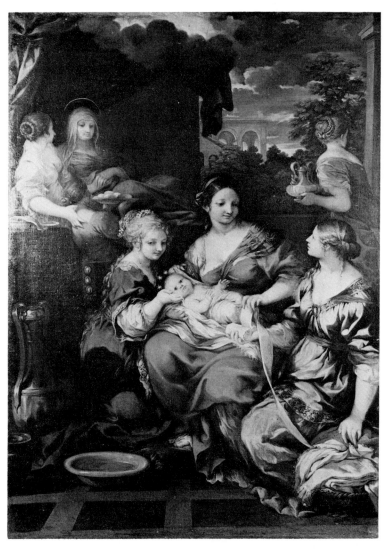

Fig. 13-36. Birth of the Virgin. By Pietro Berettini da Cortona (1596–1669). The wet nurse is shown with open blouse holding the infant Mary on her lap. The artist has depicted Anne, in the left background, as an elderly woman poorly suited for nursing and hence requiring a wet nurse. Although the scriptures fail to indicate Anne's age at Mary's birth, the Gospel of Pseudo-Matthew states that Anne lived 20 childless years with Joachim before conceiving the Virgin. Musée du Louvre, Paris.

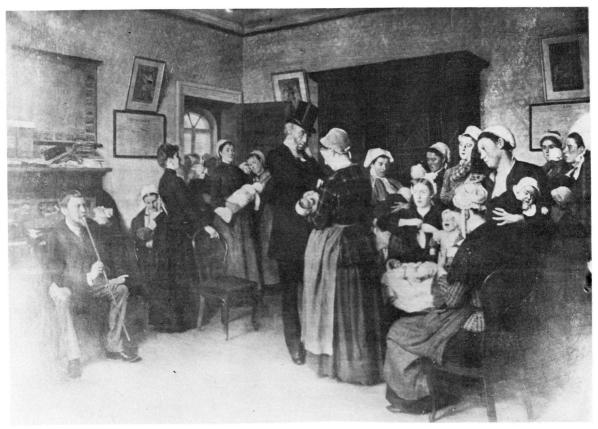

Fig. 13-37. *Le bureau des nourrices.* Painting by José Frappa (1854–1904) depicting the medical examination of wet nurses in Paris. Musée de l'Assistance Publique, Paris.

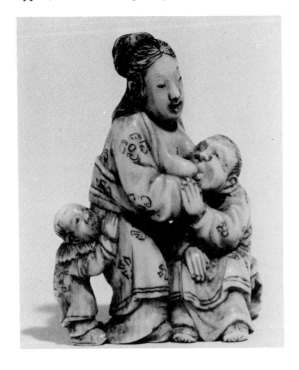

Fig. 13-38. A lactating woman, her child standing beside her, nurses an elderly relative. Japanese ivory figure known as *netsuke* illustrating an old Chinese story in which a woman nurses her toothless great-grand-aunt to keep her from starving. *Netsuke,* small devices up to 3 inches in height carved from wood, ivory, metal, or stone, date back to the late sixteenth century when the Japanese wore them to stabilize the boxes and pouches that hung from their sashes before their kimonos were fitted with pockets. Staatliches Museum für Völkerkunde, Berlin.

BREAST FEEDING OF ADULTS

Human milk has long been considered an ideal food for adults as well as for infants. Gabriele Zerbi (1468–1505), Renaissance anatomist, teacher, and clinician, in his *Gerontocomia* (1489), advised that the elderly patient take his nourishment directly from the breast and prescribed the proper attributes of the wet nurse. Breast feeding of the aged has persisted into the twentieth century. John Steinbeck, modern novelist, in his *The Grapes of Wrath* (1939), pictures a dying old man being nursed by a young mother who has just lost her baby. Subject of legends and works of art, breast feeding of adults has been designated as *Roman charity*.

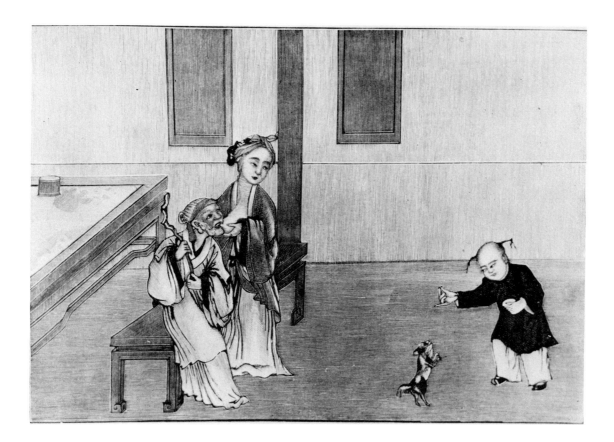

Fig. 13-39. A Chinese woman suckling her mother-in-law. Painting on a banner used in a funeral procession. Illustrated is the following old tale of filial devotion as told in *Urhsheihsze Heaou* and cited by Ploss, Bartels, and Bartels (*Woman*, E. J. Dingwell, ed. Heinemann, London, 1935).

"During the Tang dynasty, the grandmother of Tsuy Shannan, Mrs. Tang, lived with her mother-in-law Changsun, who was so old that she had lost all her teeth. This honorable woman carefully made her toilet every day and betook herself to the room of her aged relative and gave her the breast, by which means the life and health of the old woman were prolonged for many years, as she was no longer able to eat even a little grain of rice. One day she fell ill and summoned all her descendants about her and said: 'Listen, I have no means of rewarding the virtue of my daughter-in-law. I request that the wives of all my children serve her with the same love and respect as she has shown me.'" [Formerly in Museum für Völkerkunde, Berlin, destroyed in W.W. II.]

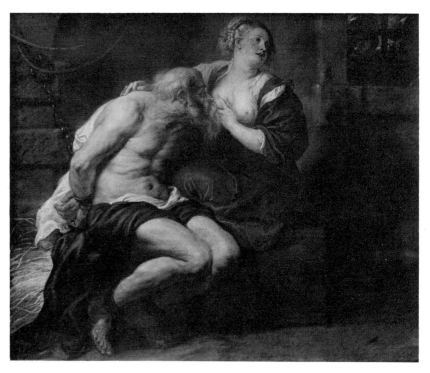

Fig. 13-40. Cimon and Pero. Painting by Peter Paul Rubens (1577–1640) depicting the legendary story of the elderly Greek general who was nursed by his daughter during his imprisonment. Rubens made more than one painting of this theme; another is in the Hermitage in Leningrad. Rijksmuseum, Amsterdam, on loan to Rubenshuis, Antwerp.

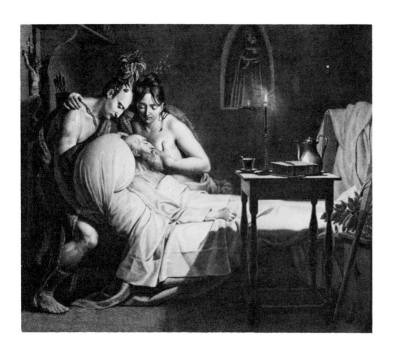

Fig. 13-41. The Illness of Las Casas. Lithograph by Adam Pierre after the painting by Louis Hersent (1777–1860). Born in Seville in 1774, Bartolomé de las Casas sailed with Columbus to the West Indies at age 18, returned to Spain five years later and entered the priesthood. He again accompanied Columbus on his second voyage to Hispaniola, and after the conquest of Cuba settled there and took up the cause of the oppressed natives. Known as *Protector of the Indians,* he strove without success to achieve their liberation, moved to Chiapas, Mexico in 1554 where he served as bishop, died in Madrid in 1566. In addition to several tracts arguing against the *repartimiento,* a system for consigning the Indians to forced labor, he wrote *Historia de las Indias,* a history of Spanish discoveries from 1492 to 1520 and a criticism of the Catholic Church, a work which was suppressed for more than 300 years and not published until 1875–76. Hersent's painting depicts an episode, perhaps apocryphal, in the colorful life of Las Casas when he was nursed from a serious illness back to health at the breast of an Indian woman of Chiapas. Bibliothèque Nationale, Paris.

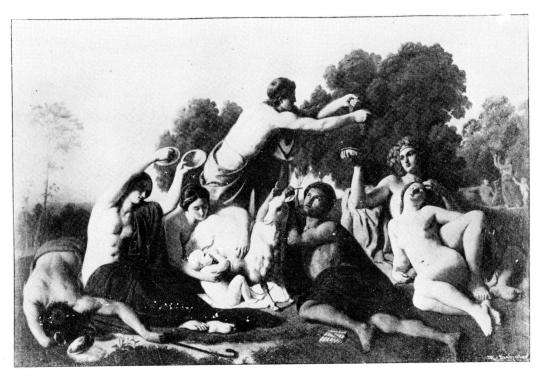

Fig. 13-42. *Erziehung des Jupiter* (Bringing up Zeus). Painting by Hermann Steinfurth (1823–1880). The infant Zeus is shown drinking from the udder of the goat Amalthea. According to legend, Amalthea had a *cornucopia* or horn of plenty which was always full of whatever food or drink anyone wished. In the pastoral populations of Greece and Italy children probably did quench their thirst directly at the teats of lactating goats. On the Canary Islands when a mother died in childbirth, the infant was commonly fed by goats or sheep. Formerly in Wallraf-Richartz Museum, Cologne, Germany, lost or destroyed in W.W. II.

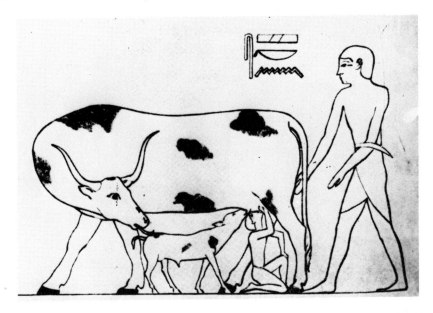

Fig. 13-43. Calf and child nursing from cow's udder. Egyptian, second century BC. Among early civilizations, it is said, cattle permitted milking only after or while suckling their own calf.

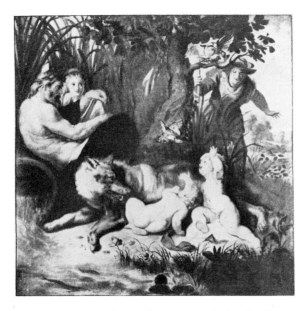

Fig. 13-44. Romulus and Remus. Painting by Peter Paul Rubens (1577–1640). Perhaps most famous of all infants nursed by animals were the legendary twins, suckled by a she-wolf. Mentioned also in Greek mythology was Telephus, son of Heracles, abandoned at birth and nursed by a hind.

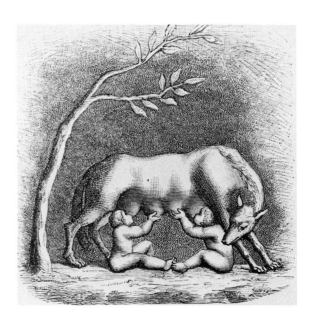

Fig. 13-45. Romulus and Remus. From an antique cameo.

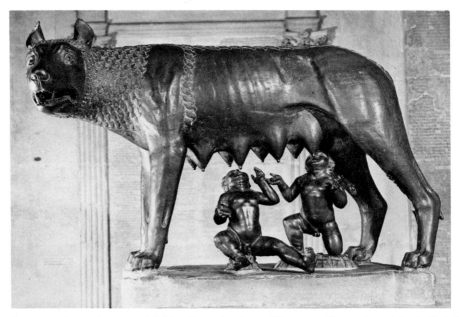

Fig. 13-46. Romulus and Remus drinking from the she-wolf. Bronze figure. Musei Capitolini, Rome.

Fig. 13-47. Bear mother, legendary creature who wed a grizzly, shown with Russian-style cap and cloak, nursing. Black stone carving of *kwawhlhal* (argillite) by members of the Haida tribe of Indians, Queen Charlotte Islands, British Columbia. Many tales originated during the Middle Ages of children, abandoned or lost in the woods, being suckled by bears. A thick growth of body hair was believed to result. These victims of hypertrichosis, some doubtless suffering from disordered adrenal function or tumor, were known as bear men or women.

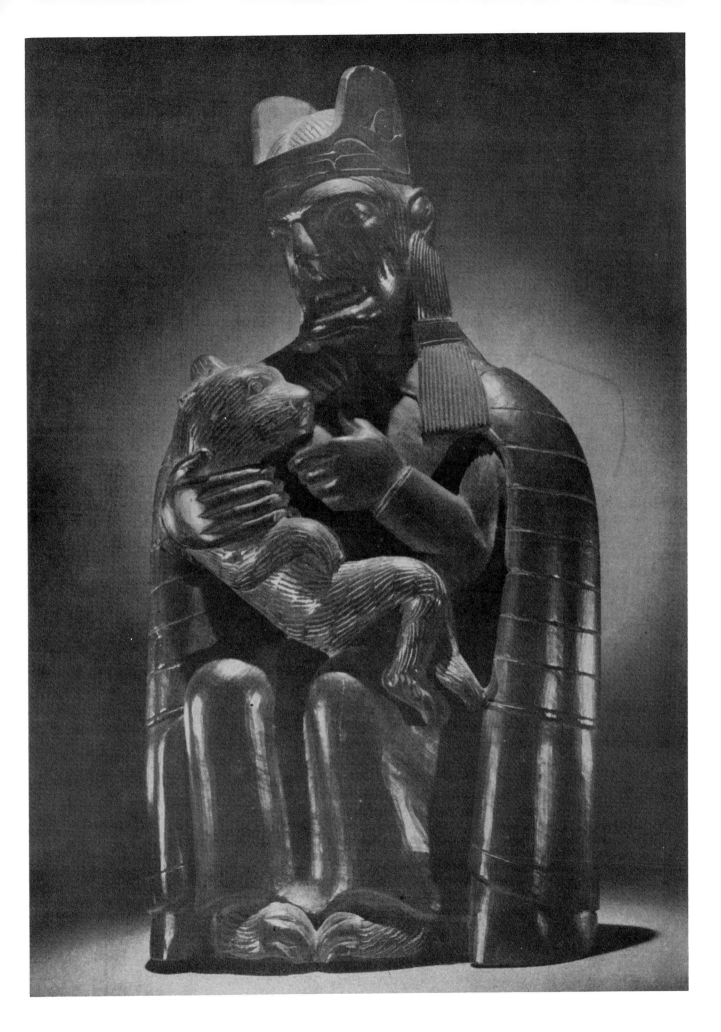

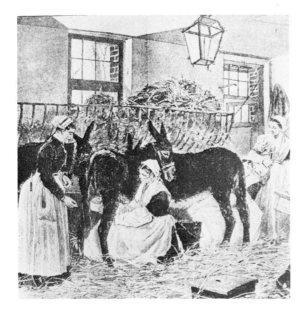

Fig. 13-48. Feeding infants at the udder of an ass. Hôpital des Enfants Assistés, Paris, 1880s. Animal milk for infants became popular during the eighteenth century, but the use of cow's milk for this purpose did not become widespread until the following century. At the Paris Foundling and Children's Hospital, infants suspected of having an infectious disease were not fed by wet nurses, but were allowed to suck directly from the udder of an ass instead. Adjoining the children's ward were three stalls, each accommodating four animals.

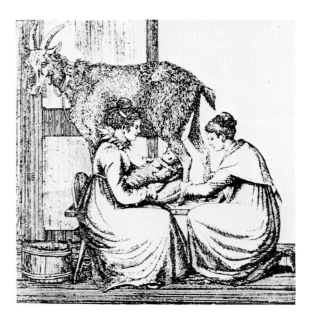

Fig. 13-49. The goat as wet nurse. The animal was placed standing on a wooden table against the wall. It was important that the table's surface not be smooth; otherwise the hooves might slide off. The goat's neck was held fast by a leather collar attached to the wall. One woman supported the sucking child on a pillow under the goat, while a second woman held the animal's hind legs to prevent injury to the infant.

Fig. 13-50. A Japanese newborn receiving the elixir *jumi gokoto* from the midwife, as the parturient looks on. This elixir, made from a variety of roots and herbs, was traditionally fed to the newborn for the first three days after which breast feeding was begun. The ingredients of the *jumi gokoto* were determined by caste—that fed to the highborn had ten components; to the infants of the poor, only five.

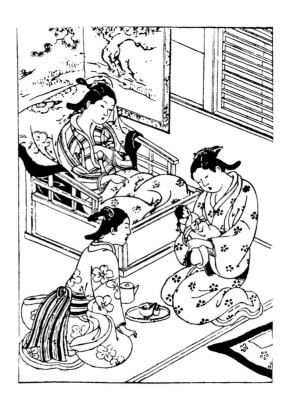

NURSING PARAPHERNALIA

"A pair of substantial mammary glands has the advantage over the two hemispheres of the most learned Professor's brain, in the art of compounding a nutritious fluid for infants." So wrote Oliver Wendell Holmes in his introductory lecture to the medical class of Harvard University, November 6, 1867. Needed, however, in cases of sore or inverted nipples, of ineffective suckling efforts by the infant, or of temporary suspension of nursing by the mother, were mechanical aids for delivering the milk from the breast or for protecting the nipple. A variety of breast pumps and nipple shields came into use.

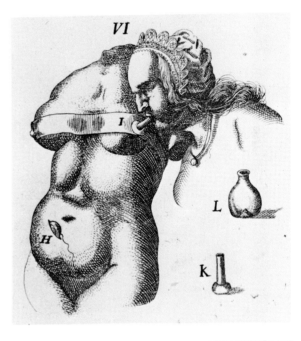

Fig. 13-51. Methods for drawing out inverted nipples. Figure from Table 37 of Scultetus' *Armamentarium chirurgicum*, 1655. The legend in the English translation (*The Chyrurgeons Store-House*, London, 1674) explained that,

"the nipples of those that give suck (I) are oftentimes so hid within the breasts, that the Child new born can neither take hold of them with its mouth, nor suck any milk out of them. In such a case let either the childs nurse set either the bottom of the glass . . . to the nipple that lies hid, and lay hold of the mouth of the pipe with her mouth, and draw forth the nipple by sucking; or one that is of years shall set the long glass (K) to the nipple, and with a band shall bind it fast to the breast; and when this is done, let her take the narrower end of the glass between her lips, and drawing as before, let her suck forth the nipple that lieth hid. *Amatus Lusitanus* filleth a glass with a narrow mouth L with scalding water, which he poureth forth again when the glass is made very hot with it, and he presently claps the mouth of the glass to the nipple; for this presently sticks fast to the nipple, and draws it out so forcibly, that the Child may easily lay hold of it with its mouth. Moreover these instruments not only draw out the nipples, but milk also. But if there be no need to draw forth milk with the nipple, a thumb-stall made of Ivy-wood, is most safely set on to draw forth the nipples."

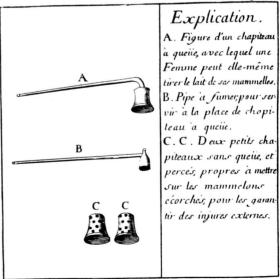

Fig. 13-52. French breast pumps (pipes) (A and B) and nipple shields (C). Mid eighteenth century. From J. Mesnard, *Le guide des accoucheurs*. Paris, 1743.

NURSING VESSELS

Artificial feeding of infants was initially accomplished from pottery, later metal, and ultimately glass nursing vessels, each equipped with a nipple or spout of the same material, or of parchment, sponge, wood, cork, or ivory. Rubber nipples were introduced in 1868. In frontier America nursing bottles were also fashioned from wood, gourds, and bovine horns. Some of the extant nursers date back to about 500 BC.

These feeding vessels were used for both milk and pap, a thick gruel of flour or bread cooked with water or milk. Fed from a boat or a spoon, pap came into use in the mid sixteenth century first as a supplementary food for infants, later as their sole nutriment, even from birth, as a substitute for mother's milk.

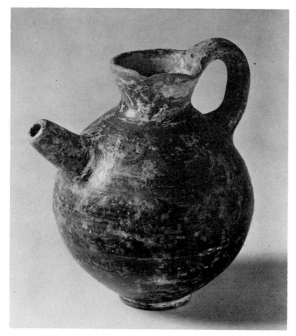

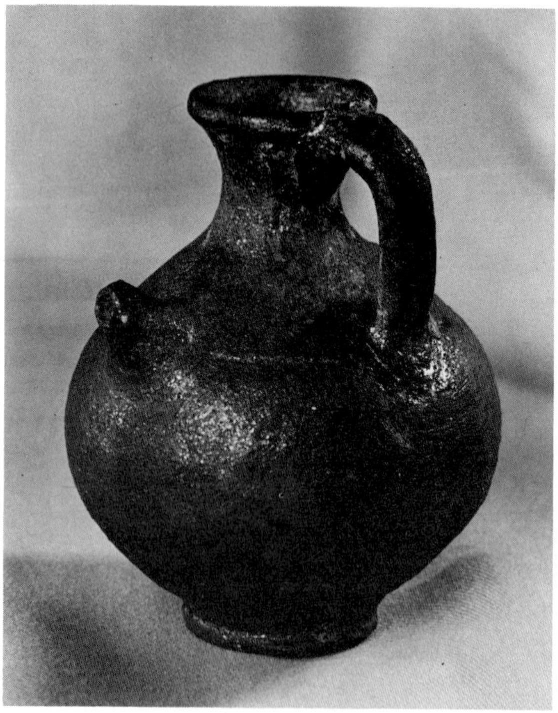

Fig. 13-53. Grecian pottery feeding bottle. About 300 BC.

Fig. 13-54. Roman feeding vessel. Excavated in London from the time of the Roman occupation.

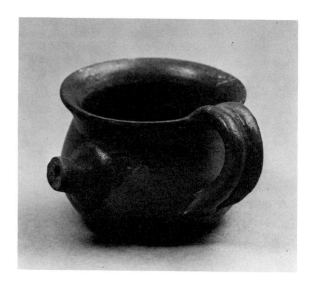

Fig. 13-55. Roman pottery feeding bowl. About 200 BC. The wide mouth permitted easy mixing.

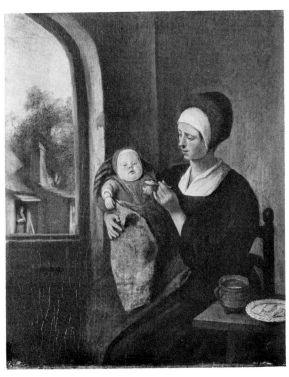

Fig. 13-56. *L'enfant à la bouillie* (Feeding the infant its pap). Painting by Jan Steen (1626–1679). Dresden Gemäldegalerie.

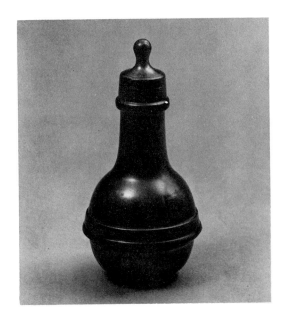

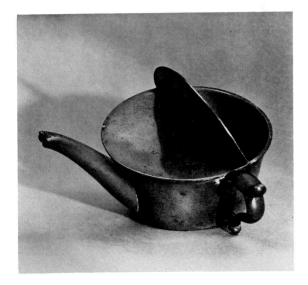

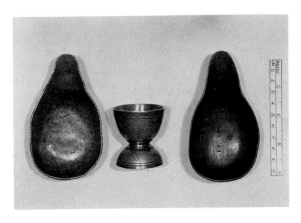

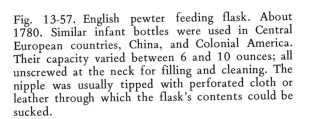

Fig. 13-57. English pewter feeding flask. About 1780. Similar infant bottles were used in Central European countries, China, and Colonial America. Their capacity varied between 6 and 10 ounces; all unscrewed at the neck for filling and cleaning. The nipple was usually tipped with perforated cloth or leather through which the flask's contents could be sucked.

Fig. 13-58. English pewter feeding pot. About 1780. A nipple fashioned of cloth, chamois, or sponge was usually attached to the end of the spout.

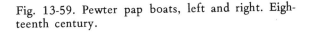

Fig. 13-59. Pewter pap boats, left and right. Eighteenth century.

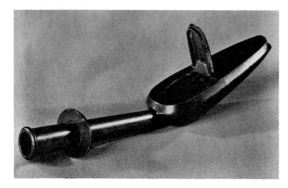

Fig. 13-60. English pewter pap spoon. About 1800. The flow of pap through the end of the spoon into the infant's mouth was controlled by a finger over the end of the hollow handle. The flow could be speeded up by blowing down the handle.

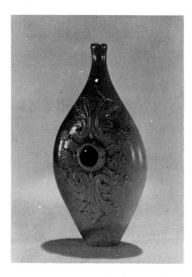

Fig. 13-61. Ornate pottery feeding bottle. The opposite side bears a bas-relief of Queen Victoria. Sponge or chamois was used as a nipple.

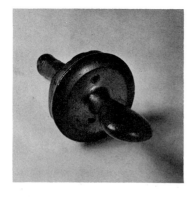

Fig. 13-62. Pewter nipple. About 1800. By 1900 rubber had replaced other materials.

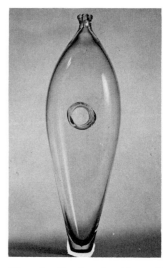

Fig. 13-63. Glass feeding bottle. About 1850. During the nineteenth century when cleanliness received increasing emphasis, glass nursers gradually replaced vessels of pottery and metal.

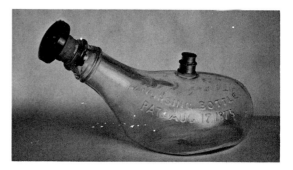

Fig. 13-64. Glass nursing bottle. Patented 1875. Hundreds of glass feeding bottles were patented in the United States, some in the shape of nursery rhyme characters.

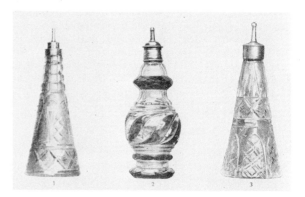

Fig. 13-65. European nursing bottles of thick cut glass. Through clear glass the contents could be observed, but this advantage was lost when opaque glass was used.

Chapter 14

MONSTERS AND MYTHS

Are God and Nature then at strife,
That Nature lends such evil dreams?
So careful of the type she seems,
So careless of the single life.
    [Alfred Tennyson: *In Memoriam*]

Deviations from the normal human form at birth, the subject of intensive scientific study in the twentieth century, have alternately bewildered, guided, frightened, and inspired man, and supplied him with many of his dieties, from earliest recorded time. Long regarded as resulting from the positions of the stars at the moment of birth, monsters forecast the future with the same surety as did the astral bodies themselves. The tablets of the Chaldeans, known as the founders of astrology, tell

When a hermaphrodite is born, the son of the palace shall rule the land.
When a woman gives birth to an infant that has the ears of a lion, there will be a powerful king in the Country....
That has a bird's beak, the Country will be peaceful....
That has no mouth, the mistress of the house will die....
That has no feet, the canals of the Country will be cut and the house ruined.
That has no nose, affliction will seize upon the Country and the master of the house will die.
Whose anus is closed, the Country will suffer from want of nourishment.

Comets and eclipses were considered particularly potent in their teratogenic powers.

Among the Greeks before Aristotle, and for long after, some believed that certain monsters, like the centaur, resulted from sexual union between man and beast. Many malformations, clear evidence of witchcraft or of adultery with the devil, brought to both mother and child death by burning.

Or were the gods merely playing, as Pliny the Elder suggested? *Ludibria sibi, nobis miracula, ingeniosa fecit natura* (Nature made variations as marvels for us and toys for herself) (*Natural History*, book VII, chap. 2). This view is reflected in the lexicons of many languages, for example *sport* and *freak of nature* (English), *lusus naturae* (Latin), *Spielart* and *Naturspiel* (German), and *jeu de nature* (French).

The origin of the term monster remains conjectural. Some would trace it to *monere*, to warn. Others link it to another Latin verb, *monstrare*, to intimate or show. Cicero wrote, "*Quia enim ostendunt, portendunt, monstrant, praedicunt, ostenta, portenta, monstra, prodigia dicuntar* (Because they make manifest, portend, intimate, predict, they are called manifestations, portents, intimations, and prodigies)" (*De divinatione* I, vlii).

Systematic writings on congenital malformations go back at least to the fourth century, when Julius Obsequens tabulated the known miraculous births from the time of Caesar Augustus, linking them with various astronomical phenomena. Better known is the collection of the French surgeon Ambroise Paré, who catalogued all such cases to the sixteenth century in his *Of Monsters and Prodigies*. Pictorial records of malformations were made long before man could write, having been found in the carvings and rock drawings of the stone age, 2000 BC. The illustrations of monsters in the early published works, mostly crude woodcuts, are largely anonymous. Human monstrosities rarely attracted the master artists.

Several of the characters of Greek mythology, such as the one-eyed Cyclops, the sympodial Sirens, and the two-faced Janus, were probably inspired by actual congenital malformations. The legendary names have been incorporated into teratologic terminology, the myths themselves recorded in various art forms.

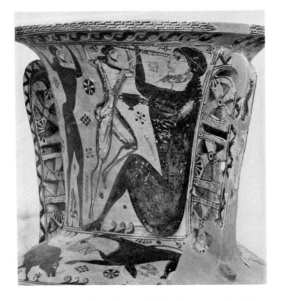

Fig. 14-1. The blinding of Polyphemus. Greek vase painting.

CYCLOPS

On the coast of Sicily dwelt the giant Polyphemus, of the once banished race of Cyclopes, tending his flocks and forging thunderbolts for Zeus. Of this man-eating monster, Homer wrote,

A form enormous; far unlike the race
Of human birth, in stature or in face
As some lone mountain's monstrous growth
  he stood,
Crown'd with rough thickets and a nodding
  wood.

Returning home after the destruction of Troy, Odysseus and twelve men took shelter in the empty cave of Polyphemus. Later, finding the uninvited guests, the giant blocked the exit from his cave with a ponderous boulder, which only he could move, then killed and devoured two of the men. Trapped, Odysseus came upon the cyclops' club.

The monster's club within the cave I spy'd,
A tree of stateliest growth and yet undryed,
Green from the wood; of height and bulk
  so vast,
The largest ship might claim it for a mast.

Next day, during Polyphemus' absence, Odysseus and his remaining men sharpened one end of the cyclops' club. Returning, the giant feasted on another victim, drank freely of Odysseus' wine, fell into a deep sleep. The men then drew their improvised spear from its hiding place, heated its point in the fire, and plunged the glowing tip of the huge spike into the cyclops' eye. The blinded Polyphemus, hoping to catch the men in their attempted escape, pushed aside the boulder and stood guard at the cave's mouth. But Odysseus and his men tied themselves to the underbellies of the fleeing rams, thus outwitting the cyclops.

The oldest known version of the cyclops myth goes back at least as far as 800 BC;

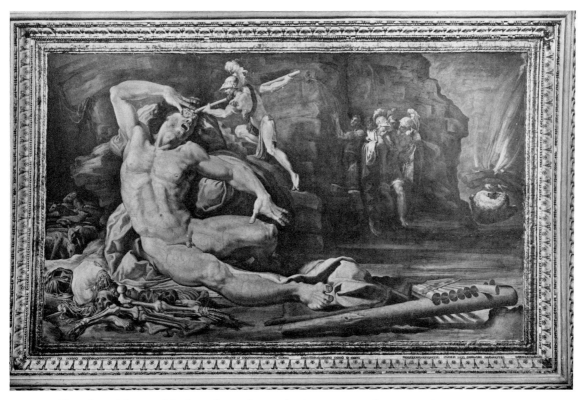

Fig. 14-2. Odysseus blinding the cyclops Polyphemus. By Pellegrino Tibaldi (1527–1598). Palazzo dell' Università, Bologna.

some classical scholars would date the original several centuries earlier. D. Muelder has reconstituted the passage telling of the blinding of Polyphemus.

This to my thinking seemed the best advice.
Beside the fold the Kyklops' great club lay
Of olive-wood yet green, which he had felled
To bear when dry. We, looking on the same,
Likened its size to the mast of a black ship,
Some merchantman broad-beamed and
   twenty-oared
That goes to harbour far across the main,
So huge its length, so huge its girth to view.
Therefrom I, standing close, cut off a fathom,
Gave to my men, and bade them fine it down.
They smoothed it: I stood by and pointed it,
And took and turned it in the blazing fire.
Then 'neath the heap of embers I thrust in
The bar to heat it; and my comrades all
I heartened, lest in terror they should fail me.

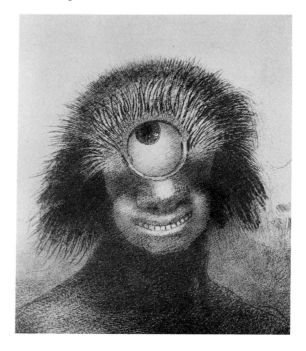

Fig. 14-3. Cyclops. Lithograph, 1883, by Odilon Redon (1840–1916).

364 ICONOGRAPHIA GYNIATRICA

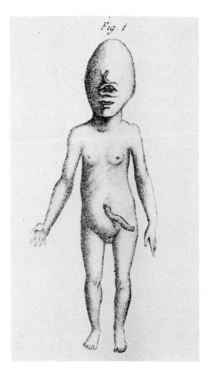

Fig. 14-4. A human cyclops. Illustration from Geoffroy Saint-Hilaire's atlas of congenital malformations, 1857.

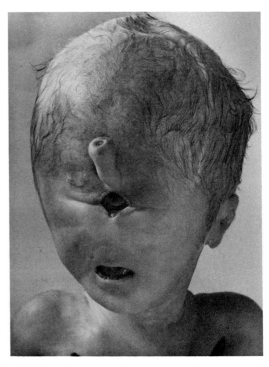

Fig. 14-5. A human cyclops. From E. Potter's *Pathology of the Fetus and the Newborn.* Year Book Publishers, Chicago, 1952, p. 493, fig. 507A.

But, when the olive-bar was like to catch,
Green as it was, and glowed with dreadful
   light,
I fetched it from the fire, while they stood
   round.
And some god breathed great courage into us.
They took the olive-bar, so sharp at the point,
And full in his eyeball plunged it. I uplifted
Twirled it above, as a man drills with a drill
A timber for ship-building, while below
His fellows spin their strap and hold amain
Its either end, and still the drill runs on.
Just so we took the fiery-pointed bar,
And twirled it in his eye: the blood flowed
   round
Its hot end, and the blast singed all about
His lids and eyebrows, as the ball was burnt
Till even its roots were crackling in the fire.
And, as a man that is a coppersmith
Dips a great axe or adze all hissing hot
In water cold to temper it, for this

Is the strength of steel, so hissed the Kyklops'
   eye
About that bar of olive; and he groaned
A ghastly groan—yea, round us rang the rock—
And we in a panic fled, while he from his eye
Plucked out the bar dedabbled with much
   blood.
   [Muelder: Das Kyklopengedicht in der
      Odysee. *Hermes* 38:414, 1903.]

The cyclops deformity consists of a single, central orbital fossa in which varying amounts of global tissue may be found. The nose, when present, appears as a tubular proboscis above the diamond-shaped palpebral fissure. Extensive malformations of the skull and brain coexist. More common in lower forms than in the human, the cyclops malformation occurs with particular frequency in the pig. It can be produced in experimental animals by a variety of techniques.

SYMPODIA

Continuing homeward, Odysseus had to sail his ship past the island of Anthemoëssa in the western sea, the abode of the mysterious Sirens. No man, it was said, had listened to the voices of these two enchanting creatures and lived to tell of his experience; to hear their song was to be lured to certain death. Odysseus knew, for the nymph Kirke had described the Sirens to him thus:

"To the Sirens first shalt thou come, who bewitch all men whosoever come to them. Whoso draws nigh them unwittingly and hears the sound of the Sirens' voice never doth he see wife or babes stand by him on his return, nor have they joy at his coming; but the Sirens enchant him with their clear song, sitting in the meadow, and all about is a great heap of bones of men, corrupt in death, and round the bones the skin is wasting."

To this description Kirke, daughter of Zeus, added counsel, that Odysseus might resist the Sirens' witchery:

"But do thou drive thy ship past and knead honey-sweet wax, and anoint therewith the ears of thy company, lest any of the rest hear the song; but if thou thyself are minded to hear, let them bind thee in the swift ship hand and foot, upright in the mast head, and from the mast let rope-ends be tied that with delight thou mayest hear the voice of the Sirens. And if thou shalt beseech thy company and bid them to loose thee, then let them bind thee with yet more bonds." [Homer: *The Odyssey*, xii, 39–54.]

Fig. 14-6. Odysseus and the Sirens. Vase painting, third century BC. Odysseus stands on tiptoe, lashed to the mast, while his companions, with ears plugged, work at the oars and gaze upon the Sirens. The singing creatures appear perched on branches; one accompanies herself with a tympanon, the other with a zither.

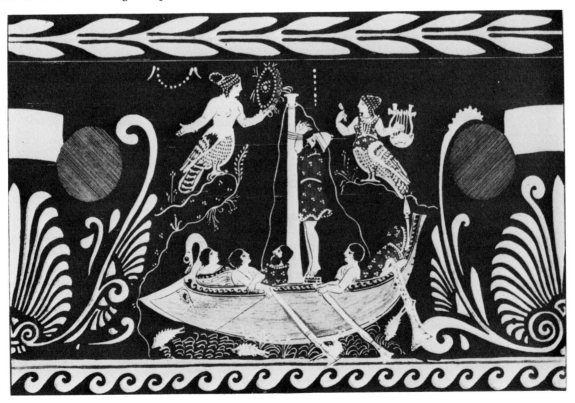

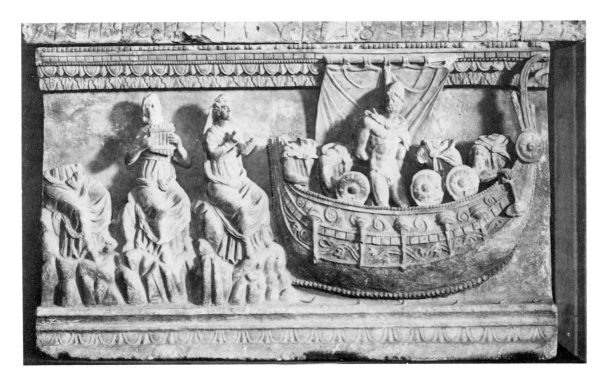

Fig. 14-7. Odysseus and the Sirens. Scene on an Etruscan cinerary urn. The Sirens here, three in number, are depicted as women, with unfused lower extremities. Museo Nazionale, Volterra, Italy.

Heeding Kirke's admonition, Odysseus ordered his men to stop their ears with wax as they approached the island. Determined to hear the Sirens himself, however, the bold leader bade the crew bind him fast to the ship's mast, as Kirke had instructed, so that he could not be enticed into the sea. As the ship sailed past the island of the Sirens, only Odysseus heard their beautiful cadences, calling him to them. His heart ached with longing, but the rope held him secure until the ship had sailed out of danger.

The sireniform malformation is known by a variety of names: sympodia, monopodia, sirenia, sirenomelia, symelia, cuspidate fetus, and mermaid fetus. Its essential feature con-

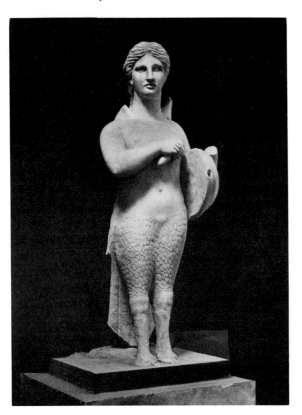

Fig. 14-8. Statue of a Siren. On a tomb in the Dipylon cemetery, Athens, fourth century BC. The thighs, covered with scales, present a fishlike appearance; the knees and legs have a birdlike form; but as in Figure 14-7, the limbs are separate, not fused.

sists of fusion of the lower limbs, which are, in addition, rotated on their axes so that the popliteal spaces face inward or anteriorly and the patellas outward or posteriorly, producing a single, fishlike structure. The bony pelvis is imperfectly developed, the anus imperforate, and the urogenital structures are malformed. Despite the association of this rare anomaly with the mermaids of fable, most recorded cases of sympodia are of the male sex.

The mermaid myths may have been inspired, as many believe, by the Sirenia, a vanishing order of mammals of the tropical waters of the Atlantic and Pacific Oceans: the Manatee, the Dugong, and the now extinct Steller's Sea Cow, endowed with small foreflippers, a wide flattened tail in lieu of hind limbs, and pectoral breasts. The last, it has been suggested, recalled to the suggestible minds of the seamen who saw them, thoughts of their ladies ashore. Fertile imagination and wishful thinking supplied the other attributes of the mermaids.

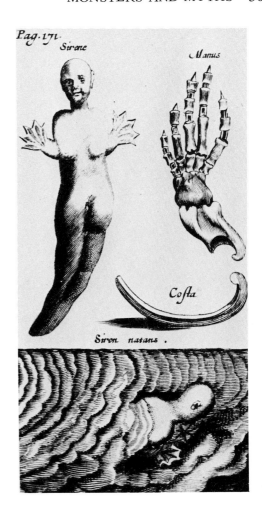

Fig. 14-9. A case of sympodia. Reported by Thomas Bartholin in 1654 in his *Historiarum anatomicarum rariorum*. The mermaid, endowed with webbed hands and full breasts, is shown floating on the waves.

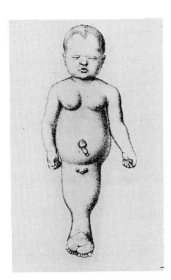

Fig. 14-10. Sympodia, with inversion of double foot. Illustration from Geoffroy Saint-Hilaire's atlas of congenital malformations, 1857.

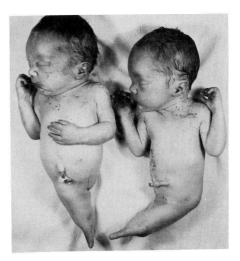

Fig. 14-11. Sireniform twins. Born in Long Beach, California, November 3, 1962.

JANICEPS

Janus, the god of good beginnings, like the month named for him, looked in two directions, fore and aft, at the old and to the new. His chief temple in Rome, running from east, where the day begins, to west, where the day ends, had two doors. Between them stood Janus' statue with two faces, one young, one old.

In the human janiceps, among the rarest forms of partial twinning, all of the facial features may be duplicated; or facial separation may be incomplete, a common median orbit being shared by the two sides.

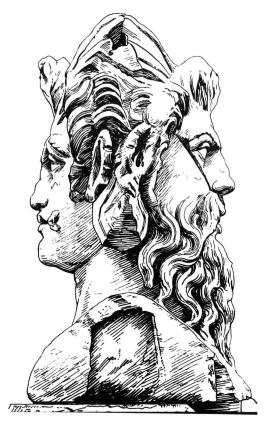

Fig. 14-12. Janiform bust. Musei Capitolini, Rome.

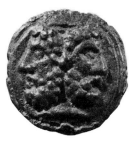

Fig. 14-13. Janus. As shown on a Roman coin, with one head and two bearded faces.

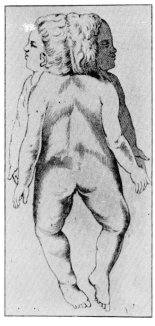

Fig. 14-14. Janiceps. A rare form of incomplete twinning.

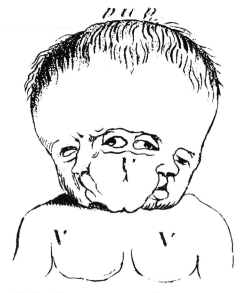

Fig. 14-15. Diprosopus or opodymus monster with two fused heads and two faces. Drawn from life by M. Meunier and illustrated in Geoffroy Saint-Hilaire's atlas of congenital malformations, 1857.

ACORMIA

King Polydectes, ruler of a small island, was in love with Danaë, the beautiful daughter of King Acrisius of Argos. But Danaë already had a grown son, Perseus, who had been sired by Zeus himself. Wishing to be rid of the young man, Polydectes told him of his longing to possess the head of one of the Gorgons, three monstrous sisters who lived on a remote island. All who gazed upon them, it was said, were instantly turned to stone.

And they are three, the Gorgons, each with wings
And snaky hair, most horrible to mortals.
Whom no man shall behold and draw again
The breath of life.

Lacking a gift for Polydectes at the betrothal celebration, Perseus promised to bring the head of Medusa, the only vulnerable Gorgon. Equipped with winged sandals, a magic cap to make him invisible, Hermes' sword which could be neither broken nor bent, and the polished bronze shield of Athene, Perseus flew across the sea to the island of the Gorgons. With never a direct glance at them, Perseus viewed the sleeping sisters in the mirror of his bright shield, as he cut through the neck of Medusa with one sweep of his sword. Heisod wrote,

The number of the Gorgons once were three,
Stheno, Medusa, and Euryale;
Of which two sisters draw immortal breath,
Free from the fears of age as free from death;
But thou, Medusa, felt a pow'rful foe,
A mortal thou, and born to mortal woe.

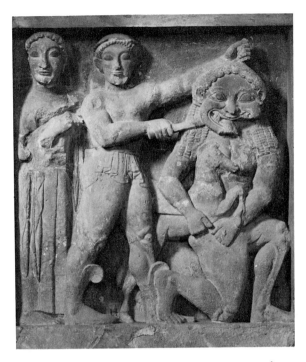

Fig. 14-16. Perseus beheading the Gorgon Medusa. Metope from Selinus, ancient city on the southern coast of Sicily (627–409 BC). Museo Civico, Palermo.

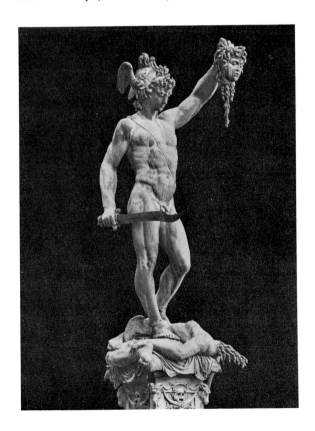

Fig. 14-17. Perseus holding Medusa's head. Bronze statue, 10½ feet tall, by Benvenuto Cellini (1500–1571), which took nine years to complete. Loggia dell' Orcagna, Piazza della Signoria, Florence.

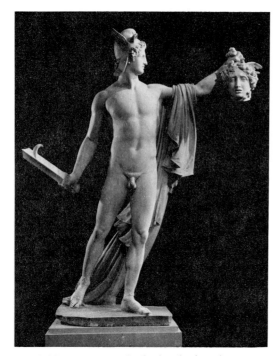

Fig. 14-18. Perseus with the head of Medusa. Carrara marble sculpture, 7 feet tall, by Antonio Canova (1757–1822). Carved between 1804 and 1808, it has been known as the Tarnowska Perseus after Valeria Tarnowska, the Polish noblewoman who commissioned it. An earlier version by Canova, completed in 1801, was purchased for the Vatican Museum by Pope Pius VII.

You by the conqu'ring hand of Perseus bled,
Perseus whose sword laid low in dust thy head;
Then started out, when you began to bleed,
The great Chrysaor, and the gallant steed. . . .
    [Thomas Cook's 1728 trans. of Hesiod:
        The Theogony. Eighth century BC.]

Thus,

. . . over the sea rich-haired Danaë's son,
Perseus, on his winged sandals sped,
Flying swift as thought.
In a wallet all of silver
A wonder to behold,
He bore the head of the monster,
While Hermes, the son of Maia,
The messenger of Zeus,
Kept ever at his side.

Fig. 14-19. Medusa beheaded. Vase painting, sixth century BC, depicting the three Gorgons after the flight of Perseus with Medusa's head. The two immortal sisters, with wings spread and knees bent, are about to start in pursuit of the slayer of Medusa, whose body is falling to the ground.

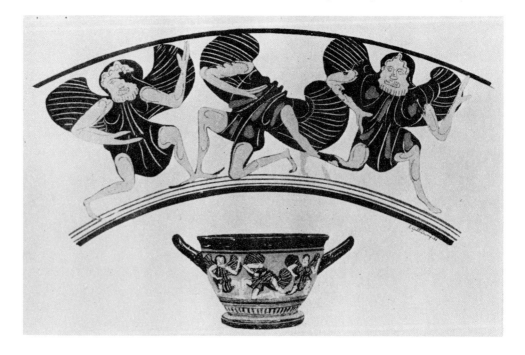

After rescuing the beautiful Andromeda from a sea serpent, Perseus returned to the island of Polydectes where his mother awaited him, and went directly to the palace. With Athene's shining buckler at his breast, Perseus stood at the entrance, drawing the attention of all the court. Before any could look away, he held up the Gorgon's head, at the sight of which the cruel Polydectes and his servile followers were turned into stone.

Medusa's head Perseus gave to Athene, who bore it upon the aegis, the shield she always carried for Zeus.

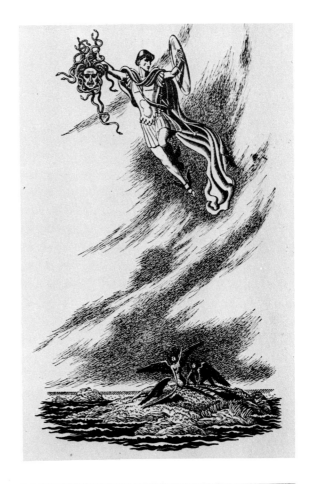

Fig. 14-20. Perseus in flight with Medusa's head, leaving behind on their little island the beheaded Medusa and her two sisters. Drawing by Steele Savage, 1942.

Fig. 14-21. The Head of Medusa. By Peter Paul Rubens (1577–1640).

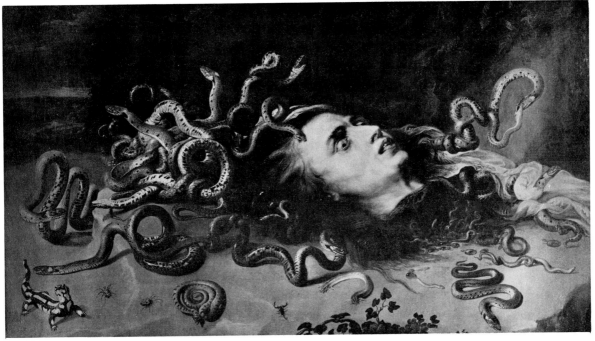

In multiple pregnancy, one fetus may be markedly stunted, developing into an acardiac monster. Covered with an exuberant growth of hair or with fronds of attached membranes, it may simulate a fetal head in some cases. In others, one of the blastocysts may be converted into a hydatidiform mole, while the second develops normally. Rarely, a parasitic fetus, consisting of only the upper part of the body, suggests a fetal head. It is doubtful, however, that a single human monster consisting of a head without a trunk has ever been observed.

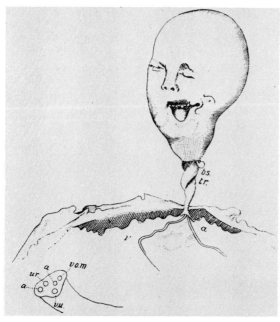

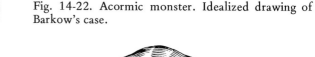

Fig. 14-22. Acormic monster. Idealized drawing of Barkow's case.

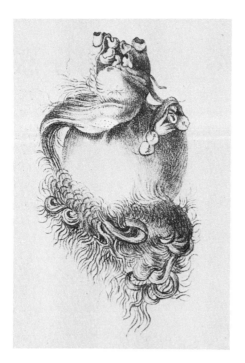

Fig. 14-23. Human *zoomyle,* a term coined by Geoffroy Saint-Hilaire for a variety of monsters, including uterine moles. Drawing from his atlas of congenital malformations, 1857, after a figure published by Sampson Birch in *Philosophical Transactions.* This type of malformation may have inspired the Medusa legend.

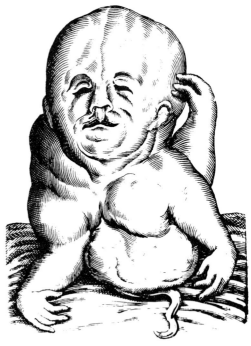

Fig. 14-24. Monster consisting of a head, three extremities, and a large omphalocele, born in Praust, Danzig, and reported by Joachim Olhaf in 1613. The product of a triplet pregnancy, the monster had two normally formed sisters. From C. Bauhin's *De hermaphroditorum,* Frankfort, 1613.

PHOCOMELIA

A hitherto rare type of human malformation, phocomelia, attracted wide attention in the fall of 1961, when a great increase in this anomaly was recorded and an association established between its development and the ingestion of a newly introduced sedative drug, thalidomide, by the mother during pregnancy. The distinctive feature of phocomelia is the absence of the proximal segment of one or more limbs. The malformation thereby simulates seals' flippers, from whence the name (*phoco,* seal; *melus,* limb).

Recent chromosomal studies have suggested that, in addition to the drug-induced anomalies, other cases of phocomelia may have a genetic basis. Phocomelia was probably recognized in the early years of Babylonian rule, for the teratologic records of Chaldea mention an infant with hands and feet like fish tails or fins. The 1675 French edition of the surgical text of Scultetus contains an illustration of a case of phocomelia with harelip, an association that has since been observed by others.

Wide renown was achieved by malformed Marc Cazotte, who went on public exhibition during the latter part of the eighteenth century, under the name *Pépin*. He lacked arms and legs; his hands were attached to his prominent shoulders, his feet to his hips. A clever man, with a mastery of four languages and with great manual dexterity, Pépin traveled over Europe on horseback, attracting large crowds. He died at age 62 in Paris, where his skeleton was preserved in the Musée Dupuytren.

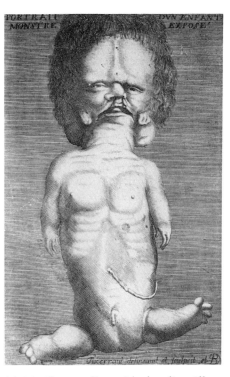

Fig. 14-25. Phocomelia, with harelip. Illustration from the 1675 French edition of Scultetus' textbook of surgery, *L'arcenal de chirurgie de Jean Scultet,* Lyon.

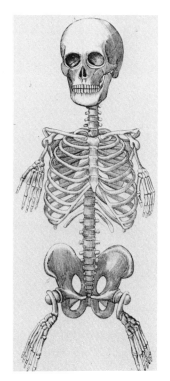

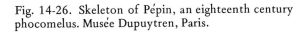

Fig. 14-26. Skeleton of Pépin, an eighteenth century phocomelus. Musée Dupuytren, Paris.

374 ICONOGRAPHIA GYNIATRICA

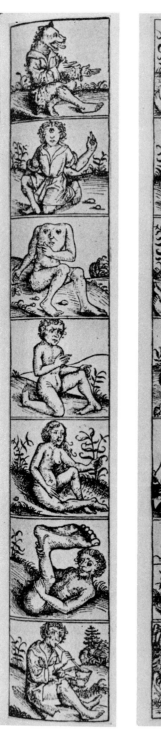
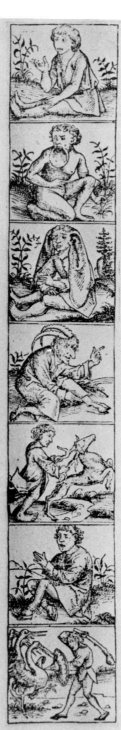

Fig. 14-27. Marvels of the East. Woodcuts from Hartmann Schedel's "Nuremberg Chronicle," 1493, illustrating the monstrous races of India.

FANTASTIC MALFORMATIONS

On the African coast of the Red Sea, Pliny tells us, near the country of the cave-dwelling Troglodytes, lived a race called Monocoli, men with but one median lower limb, who walked and jumped with great agility. Known also as Sciapodae, or shadow-feet, they shielded themselves from the sun while reclining, by using their foot as an umbrella. Other fantastic peoples were conjured up by Ktesias, a Greek physician, in a treatise on India published in the early part of the fourth century BC. This work perpetrated one of the greatest hoaxes of all time, the myth of these *monstrous races of India*, as they came to be known. The yarns of Ktesias, widely believed, were retold for hundreds of years. During the Middle Ages his fabulous creatures were described and pictured as *The Marvels of the East*. Woodcuts in Schedel's "Nuremberg Chronicle" (*Liber chronicarum*, 1493), based on those in the fourteenth century *Travels of Sir John Mandeville*, depict the Monocoli and others including,

The Cynocephali, dog-headed men, who barked instead of speaking;
Headless monsters with faces between their shoulders;
Men with tails, and men with horns;
And others with ears so large, they served their owners as blankets.

Widely known and often reproduced are some of the woodcuts from Paré's treatise on human monstrosities. The *bird-boy* pictured by him was said to have been born in 1512, shortly after a battle of France's Louis XII. Pictured as an hermaphrodite with the external genitalia of both sexes, the monster had a horned head, human trunk, wings, a fused lower extremity of a bird, and an extra eye in its knee. This creature was believed to portend the conquest of Italy by Louis XII.

Many are the references to monsters resulting from intercourse of humans with dogs, horses, and other species. A *dog-boy*, reputedly born in 1493 and illustrated by Paré, was said to be the product of sexual union of a woman and a dog. The offspring resembled, in its upper half, its human mother; in its lower, its canine father.

Paré further gave credence to, and published a woodcut illustrating, Lycosthenes' (Conrad Wolffhart's) account of an infant, stillborn in Cracow, Poland, in 1494, gnawed to death in utero by a serpent, which was still attached to its victim at birth. Credulity in other fantastic creatures, composites of human and bestial forms, persisted well into the nineteenth century.

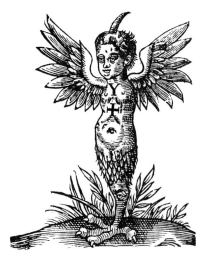

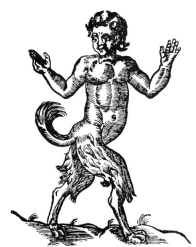

Fig. 14-28. Bird-boy. Illustrated by Paré, said to have been born in Ravenna, Italy, 1512. Figure reproduced from *The Works of that Famous Chirurgeon Ambrose Parey*, London, 1678. First appeared in P. Boaistuau's *Histoires prodigleusos les plus memorables*, Paris, 1560.

Fig. 14-29. Dog-boy. The alleged offspring of a woman and a dog, 1493, illustrated by Paré.

Fig. 14-30. Stillborn infant with live serpent attached. Said to have been born in Cracovia in 1494, reported by Conrad Wolffhart (Lycosthenes) in 1552, illustration reproduced by Paré.

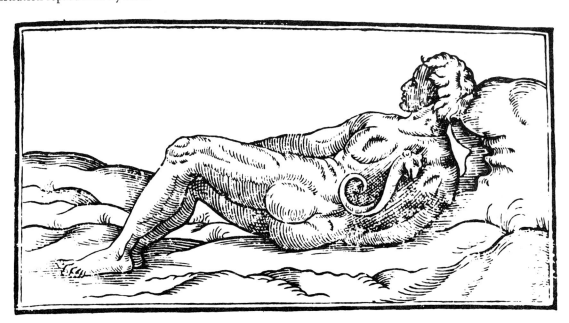

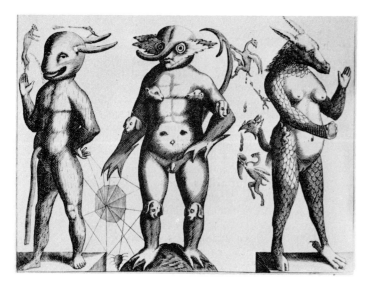

Fig. 14-31. Fantastic composites of human and animal forms. From the seventeenth century volume on monsters by Fortunio Liceti (1577–1657).

A FULL and PARTICULAR ACCOUNT of that most wonderful CHILD from Galloway; now exhibiting in this City, for the inspection of the curious; to which is added, a correct likeness, drawn from the life.

A YOUNG woman in Galloway having proved with child, laid the same to a respectable man of the name of John Woods, who denied being the father of the same, and persisted in his denial saying that he would never acknowledge the child, unless his name *was written at full length* on its face; and he accordingly gave his solemn oath before the Court to that effect. This made so much impression on the mind of the young woman, who was present, that his name and person remained constantly in her mind's eye, and when the child was born, the name of the father appeared in legible letters in the child's eyes, the name of "JOHN WOODS," on the right eye, and "BORN 1817," on the left eye. When John Woods, the alleged father, came to know this circumstance, he instantly absconded and has not since been heard of.

This wonderful child has now arrived in this city, and has been inspected by the Professors, and other learned Faculties of this city, and pronounced to be a most wonderful phenomenon of nature, and an astonishing dispensation of Providence in pointing out the truth against the wicked and perjured ways of men.

An inspection of this child will, it is hoped, be a salutary warning to all young persons of both sexes, first to beware of all such doings, and second to beware of perjury in their attempts to conceal their shame.

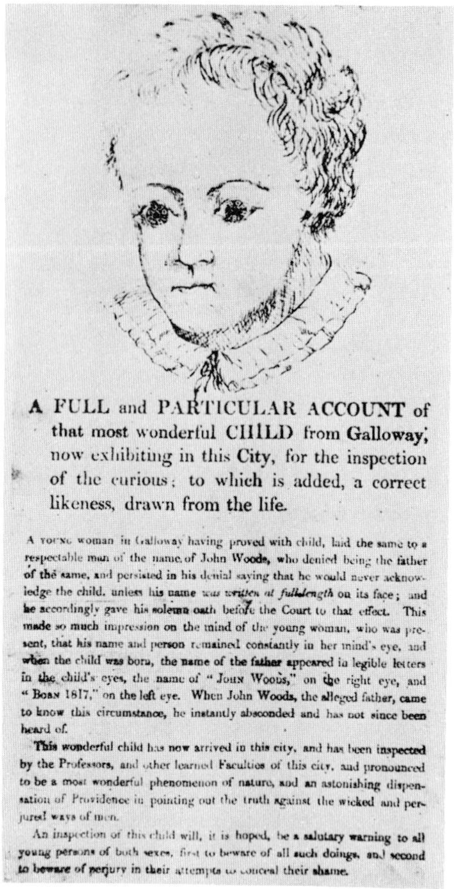

Fig. 14-32. Nineteenth century broadside advertising the public exhibition of a child allegedly marked by a maternal impression during pregnancy.

Until even more recently the gullible were duped by the belief that fetal malformations could be caused by maternal impressions. Remarkable for its audacity was the following advertisement of the public exhibition of a child from Galloway, Scotland:

"A young woman in Galloway having proved with child, laid the same to a respectable man of the name of John Woods, who denied being the father of the same, and persisted in his denial saying that he would never acknowledge the child, unless the name *was written at full length* on its face; and he accordingly gave his solemn oath before the Court to that effect. This made so much impression on the mind of the young woman, who was present, that his name and person remained constantly in her mind's eye, and when the child was born, the name of the father appeared in legible letters in the child's eyes, the name of JOHN WOODS, on the right eye, and BORN 1817, on the left eye. When John Woods, the alleged father, came to know this circumstance, he instantly absconded and has not since been heard of.

"This wonderful child has now arrived at this city, and has been inspected by the Professors and other learned Faculties of this city, and pronounced to be a most wonderful phenomenon of nature, and an astonishing dispensation of Providence in pointing out the truth against the wicked and perjured ways of men.

"An inspection of this child will, it is hoped, be a salutary warning to all young persons of both sexes, first to beware of all such doings, and second to beware of perjury in their attempts to conceal their shame."

Chapter 15

MULTIPLE PREGNANCY AND BIRTH

May any woman bear mo
Children in her at once but two?
A woman may bear kindly
Seven at once in her body,
For the matrice of woman,
If that thou understand can,
Hath seven chambers and no mo,
And each is departed other fro,
And she may have in each of tho
A child and with seven go,
If God's will be first thereto
And the kind of woman also.
If hot of kind be the woman
And great liking hath to man,
One chamber or two or three
Of thilke that in her matrice be
Of great will open there again
When that a man hath by her lain.

[*Sidrak and Bokkus,* medieval romance and book of knowledge, translated from French and put into verse by "Hugh of Campedone"; preserved in fifteenth century MS. Lansdowne 793, the British Museum, London.]

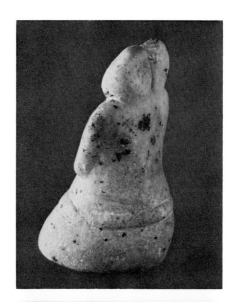

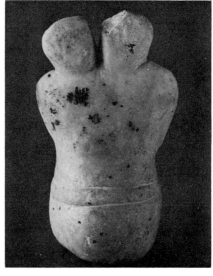

Fig. 15-1. Twin goddess. White marble figure, seventh millennium BC, recovered by James Mellaart from excavations in 1961, 1962, and 1963 in Çatal Hüyük, Shrine VI.A.10., on the Anatolian plateau, Turkey.

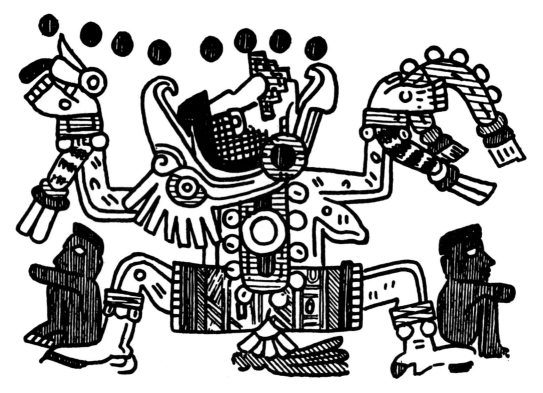

Fig. 15-2. Xochiquetzal, Mexican goddess of twins. According to Mexican legend, the first woman to give birth to twins was the goddess Xochiquetzal, who came, as told in song, "from the land of rain and mist... from Tamoanchan," the fabled home of mankind. She appears in birth posture, legs spread apart with a symbolic feather ornament protruding from her vulva. Strips of opossum hide, as were applied in labor to facilitate delivery, hang from her wrists. In one hand she holds a corn cob, in the other a jewelled ornament, and at her feet sit her twin children.

From the Biblical account of the birth of Jacob and Esau, our literary heritage, classical and contemporary, has portrayed twins in a variety of roles. A sampling of works of note in which twins figure prominently might include Shakespeare's *Twelfth Night* and his *The Comedy of Errors* (and the latter's modern musical adaptation *The Boys from Syracuse*), Poe's *Fall of the House of Usher*, Ariosto's *Orlando Furioso*, Calderón's *Devotion to the Cross*, Steinbeck's *East of Eden*, Iris Murdoch's *The Bell*, and Katherine Anne Porter's *Ship of Fools*.

Mythology likewise abounds with twins: Lugalgirra and Meslamtaea, the divinities in the Pantheon of ancient Mesopotamia; Ormazd and Ahrimen, the sons of the Persian Zervan; and in Greek and Latin legend: the Dioscuri, sons of Zeus; Apollo and Diana, offspring of Latona; and Romulus and Remus, twin sons of one of the Vestal Virgins. The offspring of multiple gestation never fail to arouse special interest, whether friendly or morbid.

The belief that twin birth results from a supernatural force has persisted through the centuries and still prevails in some cultures. It carried such force among certain tribes of American Indians, the Kiwai Papuans of British New Guinea, and several other primitive peoples that one of each twin pair was usually killed. In other civilizations, by contrast, twins have been held in high esteem, their mothers honored for their fertility. In the latter cultures twin amulets are found, and in some, twin goddesses.

Rare indeed are human multiple births of order higher than 3. If the frequency of twin birth is 1 in 80, a close approximation for the United States population, then the expectation of any higher birth multiple could be predicted, at least until recently,* by the ratio of $1 : 80^{x-1}$, where x presents the multiple of birth. This formulation, published in 1896 by the German physician Dionys Hellin, has since been known as Hellin's law.† Quadruplets, accordingly, might be expected once in about one-half million births, quintuplets, once in about 40 million.

The number of possible arrangements of the fetuses in utero increases in geometric ratio according to the number of fetuses. As with single gestations, the earliest representations of multiple pregnancies combined the crude drawings of the uterus with fanciful concepts of its occupants. Opportunities for liberty in illustration were compounded as the number of uterine occupants increased. Birth scenes of quadruplets, quintuplets, and multiples of even higher order have been depicted in woodcuts, paintings, and sculpture, and recorded in verse.

---

*Through the action of certain newly developed pharmacologic agents which often produce multiple ovulation in women, the frequency of multiple pregnancy appears to be increasing. On November 19, 1964 *The New York Times* reported the birth of two sets of quadruplets on the same day in Portland, Oregon and Baltimore, Maryland, respectively. On June 13, 1971 the first authenticated birth of nontuplets (nine babies) occurred, to an Australian woman who had been treated for infertility with a gonadotrophic hormone.

†Estimating the frequency of twin births at 1 in 90 rather than 1 in 80, Hellin predicted the frequency of other multiple births as $1 : 90^{x-1}$.

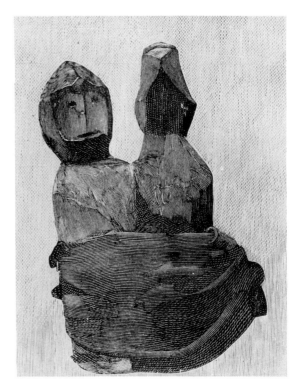

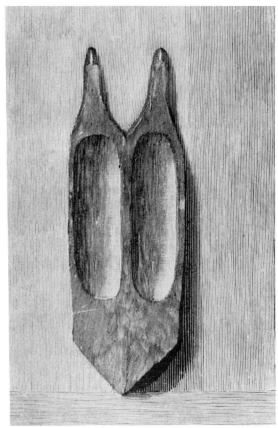

Fig. 15-3. Amulets used by the Goldi of Siberia at twin births. A carved wooden figure of a human and an animal wrapped together in cloth, and a carved wooden dish with two troughs.

380 ICONOGRAPHIA GYNIATRICA

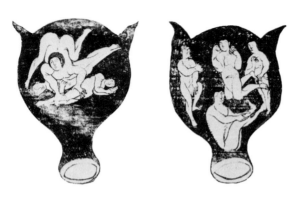

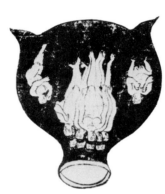

Fig. 15-4. Fetal positions in multiple pregnancies. Figures from a ninth century manuscript of Moschion, based on Soranus' *Gynecology*. The upper figures show a triplet and a quadruplet pregnancy, respectively, with the fetuses in various postures of repose and contortion. The lower figure, of a uterus containing 11 fetuses, suggests, if inverted, a fetal football team: a line of 5 flanked by 2 ends, and a backfield of 4. Bibliothèque de l'Academie Royale de Médecine de Belgique, Brussels.

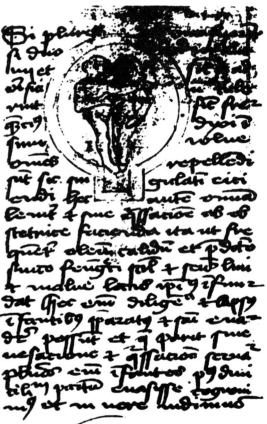

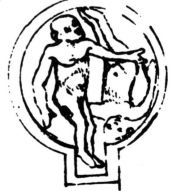

Fig. 15-5. Twins in utero. Page from the manuscript of Hermann Heyms, a fifteenth century Bavarian physician. Königliche öffentliche Bibliothek, Dresden.

Fig. 15-6. Twin pregnancy. As illustrated by Charles Estienne in his anatomy of 1545. Comfortably separated in the uterus and squatting side by side but facing in opposite directions, the twins are depicted like puppets, as though controlled by their umbilical cords suspended from their placentas, which the mother holds in her hand outside the uterus.

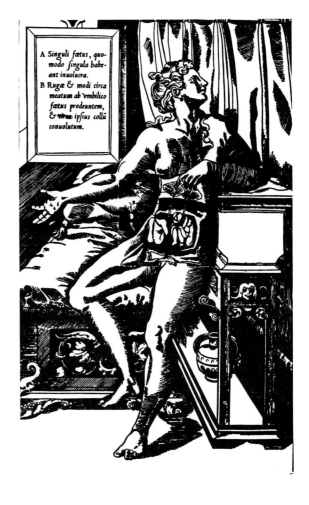

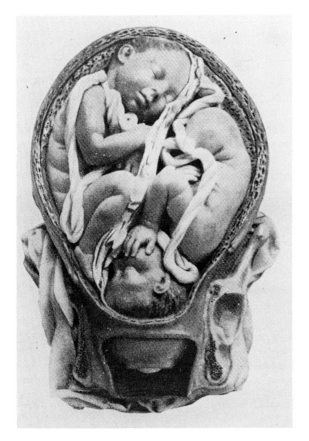

Fig. 15-7. Dichorial twins at term, uterus opened anteriorly in coronal plane. Wax figure by Gaetano Manfredini (d. 1870) based on an anatomic preparation by Carlo Mondino of Bologna. Museum of Medical Art, Hospital of Santo Spirito, Sassia, Rome. From L. Gedda: *Twins in History and Science,* 1961. Courtesy of Charles C Thomas, Publisher, Springfield, Ill.

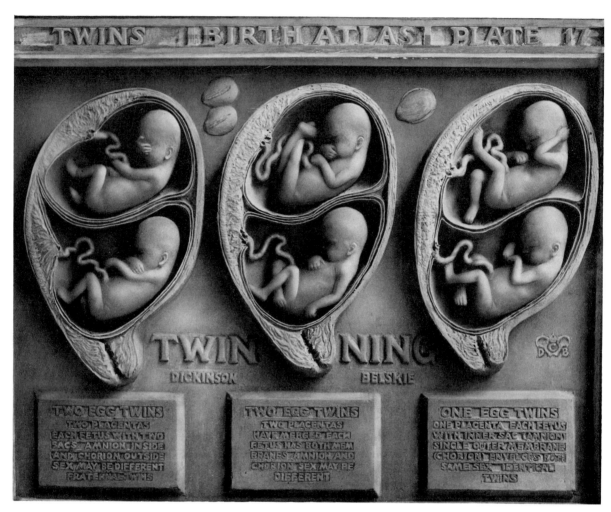

Fig. 15-8. Pregnant uteri in mid-trimester, showing the different relations of the placentas and membranes with fraternal and identical twins. Moulage by Robert L. Dickinson (1861–1950) and Abram Belskie (1907–   ). Fraternal or heterozygous twins, on the left and in the center, come from two eggs and two sperms, and may or may not be of the same sex. The placentas may be separate or fused, but each twin has its own sac of membranes (chorion and amnion). Identical or homozygous twins, on the right, come from one egg and one sperm and are always of the same sex. They usually share one large placenta and a common chorion, but almost always have separate amnions. Added here is Dickinson's personal touch, imparted to the fetal positions, to illustrate the old Japanese adage, "See no evil, hear no evil, speak no evil."

MULTIPLE PREGNANCY AND BIRTH 383

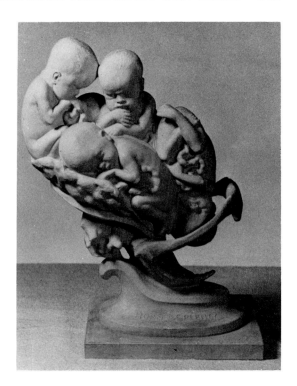

Fig. 15-9. The "Horn of Plenty." Reconstructed view of the Dionne quintuplets just before birth, moulage by Robert L. Dickinson and Abram Belskie. Born at Callander, Ontario, Canada, May 28, 1934, these quintuplets, all girls, were the first in history to survive to maturity. Cleveland Health Museum.

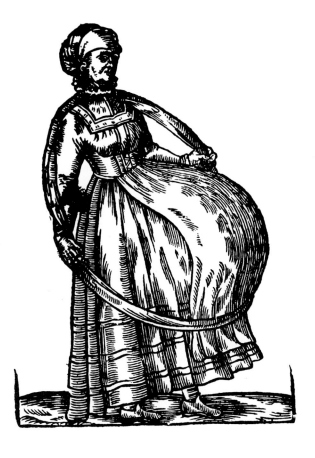

Fig. 15-10. Woodcut, from Paré's "Of Prodigies and Monsters," of Dorothea, an Italian woman of whom Franciscus Picus Mirandula wrote that she bore 20 children at two confinements, 9 at the first, 11 at the second. So big was she during the latter pregnancy "that she was forced to bear up her belly, which lay upon her knees, with a broad and large scarf tied about her neck." Mrs. Timothy Bradlee of Trumbull County, Ohio was said to have borne eight infants at one time, in 1872, all of whom survived; and the birth of nine infants to a woman in Dijon, France was reported in 1755, according to Gould and Pyle, in their *Anomalies and Curiosities of Medicine,* 1897. Earlier, Abulcasis mentioned a case in which 15 normally formed infants were delivered at one birth.

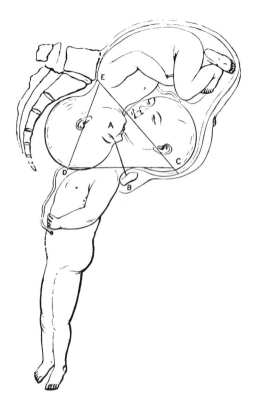
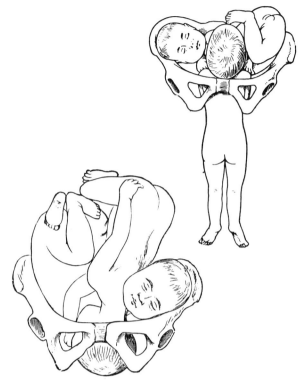

Fig. 15-11. Collision, compaction, interlocking. Rarely, perhaps once in one thousand cases of multiple pregnancy, is birth through the maternal pelvis impeded by collision, compaction, or interlocking of the infants. Countless types of entanglements are possible, of which three are shown here. The classic variety results when the chin of the partially born first fetus, delivering by the breech, impinges in utero against the chin of the second, presenting by the vertex.

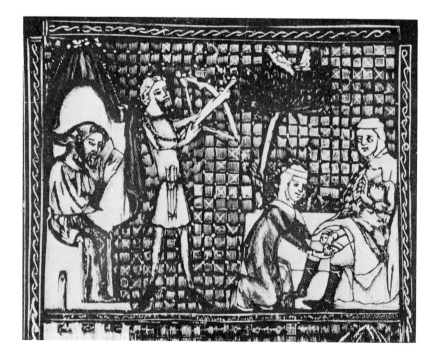

MULTIPLE PREGNANCY AND BIRTH 385

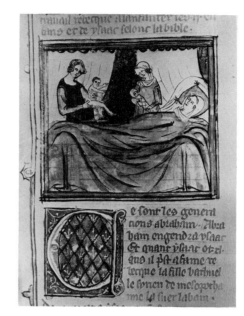

Fig. 15-13. The birth of Esau and Jacob. From a thirteenth century manuscript.

Fig. 15-14. The birth of Esau and Jacob. Engraving by Étienne Delaune (1518?–1583?). Jacob, partially born, is shown holding on to Esau's leg.

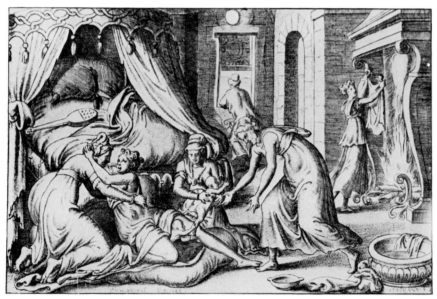

Fig. 15-12. The birth of Esau and Jacob.

"And Isaac intreated the Lord for his wife, because she was barren: and the Lord was intreated of him, and Rebekah his wife conceived. And the children struggled together within her; and she said, If it be so, why am I thus? And she went to enquire of the Lord. And the Lord said unto her, Two nations are in thy womb, and two manner of people shall be separated from thy bowels; and the one people shall be stronger than the other people; and the older shall serve the younger. And when her days to be delivered were fulfilled, behold, there were twins in her womb. And the first came out red, all over like an hairy garment; and they called his name Esau. And after that came his brother out, and his hand took hold on Esau's heel; and his name was called Jacob: and Isaac was threescore years old when she bore them." [Genesis 25:21-26]

Miniature from the Haggadah of Sarajevo, probably late thirteenth century. Read aloud at the Passover feast, the Haggadah tells of the deliverance of the Israelites from Egypt.

386 ICONOGRAPHIA GYNIATRICA

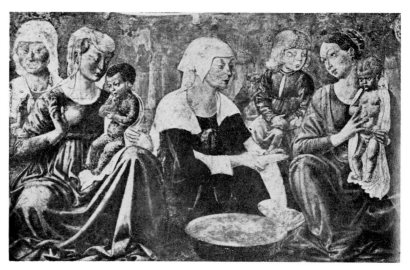

Fig. 15-15. Esau and Jacob at birth. From a fresco by the Tuscan artist Benozzo Gozzoli (1420–1497). Campo Santo, Pisa.

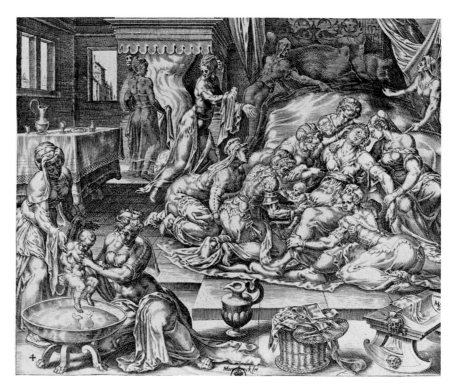

Fig. 15-16. The Birth of Pharez and Zarah.

"And it came to pass in the time of her [Tamar's] travail, that, behold, twins were in her womb. And it came to pass, when she travailed, that the one put out his hand: and the midwife took and bound upon his hand a scarlet thread, saying, This came out first. And it came to pass, as he drew back his hand, that, behold, his brother came out: and she said, How hast thou broken forth? this breach be upon thee: therefore his name was called Pharez. And afterward came out his brother, that had the scarlet thread upon his hand: and his name was called Zarah." [Genesis 38:27-30]

Engraving by Marten van Heemskerck (1498–1574). Bibliothèque Nationale, Paris.

MULTIPLE PREGNANCY AND BIRTH   387

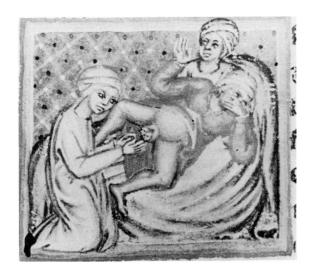

Fig. 15-17. Birth of twins, both heads emerging simultaneously. Miniature from a fourteenth century Latin manuscript of Abulcasis' "Surgery." Nationalbibliothek, Vienna.

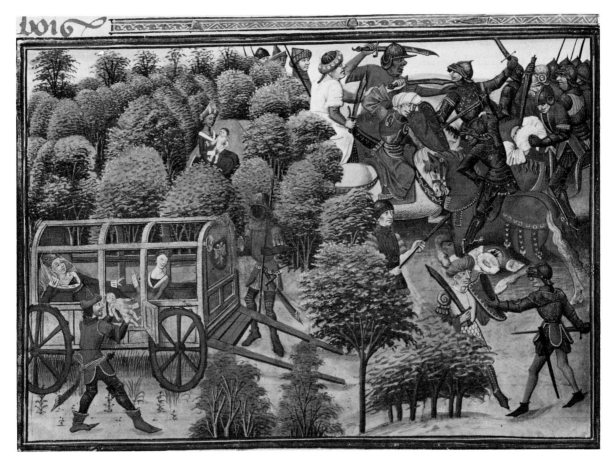

Fig. 15-18. The delivery of twin sons in the forest by the Duchess of Aigremont. Miniature from a narrative of the adventures of Renaud de Montauban (Rinaldo di Montalbano), famous seventeenth century figure of French and Italian romance. Reclining in an open wagon among the trees, the elegant parturient watches a soldier remove one of the infants. The other is held by a servant, in the background. On the right, a battle rages. Bibliothèque de l'Arsenal, Paris.

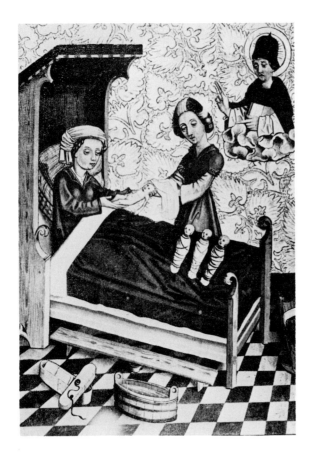

Fig. 15-19. The birth of quadruplets. By a German artist of the upper Rhein school, about 1450. The first three infants have already been swaddled. The parturient hands the fourth to the nurse. In the background, riding on a cloud, a saint blesses the scene. In the foreground, on the floor, are the bath for the newborn and a single cradle; quadruplets obviously were not expected.

Fig. 15-20. The birth of quintuplets. An illustrated broadside of 1566. Translated from the German by W. B. McDaniel, 2d, the woodcut's inscription reads,

"In a village situated halfway between Augsburg and Dillingen, about three miles from each, Emersacker by name, formerly subject and belonging to the posthumous sons of Master Ulrich von Knöringen, knight, it came about that on the 22d and 23d day of December of the 65th year just passed, Anna Rise, the wife of a poor peasant, Caspar Rise, dwelling in that place, a married housewife, gave birth to and was delivered of five living infants who were entirely complete and possessed of all the members. Namely, on the Sunday before Christmas, in the evening, she was delivered of a little boy, who lived about two hours. Subsequently, on the holy eve of Christ's birth, she gave birth to another son together with three little daughters, and thus, in two days, to five separate living children. But inasmuch as the aforesaid newborn children were very feeble, they were hastily baptized at home, following the Christian custom, and lived about two hours. After their death they were buried in the ground, as usual. The witnesses of the prodigious birth, who were themselves present and in attendance, were therefore examined by the chief magistrate. They are: first, the midwife, called and named, Hilaria Bützin; the godmother, Anna Gaugenriederin; also Anna Oertlein, magistrate's wife of that place; also Agatha Kratzeren and many more persons, all of whom gave competent information in connection with this case. It is also to be remarked that the above designated woman previously also had been delivered of three children at one birth.

"What now the Almighty God wishes to give us to understand through such and other wonderful dispensations, there is nothing final or conclusive thereon to write. For all that, it is well to wish—even diligently to implore and to pray—that, through His divine grace and omnipotence, He permit such wonder-works of His, in which we shall ever praise and commend Him, always to aid us to a just consideration of His divine majesty in true acknowledgement of our Christian faith and observance of His commands, through the merit of his only-begotten Son, our Redeemer and Savior, Jesus-Christ, who with Him and the Holy Spirit, reigns without end.

"Printed at Strassburg by Thiebold Berger at the Winemarket." [Library of the College of Physicians of Philadelphia.]

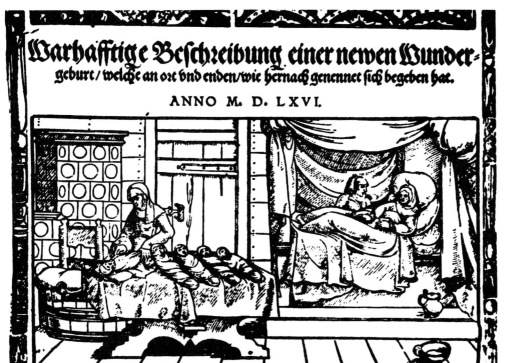

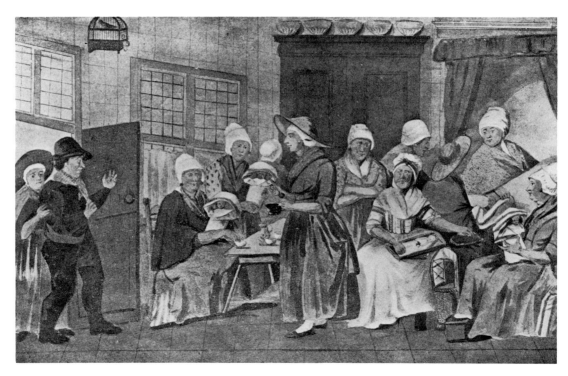

Fig. 15-21. The birth of quintuplets, four live, one stillborn, to Kniertje Roosendaal, in Scheveningen, Holland, January 5, 1719, Maria Semel, midwife. By an unknown Dutch artist. The parturient, her head concealed, lies in the canopy bed on the right, with the midwife at the foot of the bed. Shown are the surviving infants, three held by nurses, the fourth on the mother's bed. On the left, the excited father enters the birth chamber, accompanied perhaps by his mother-in-law.

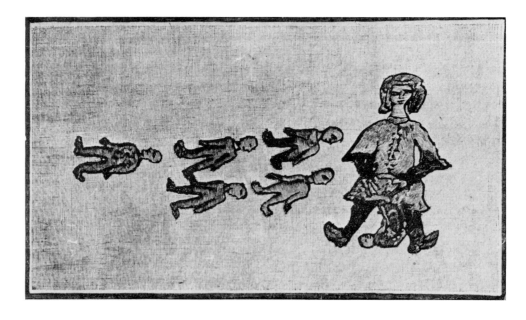

Fig. 15-22. The birth of sextuplets. Miniature from a thirteenth century Hebrew manuscript of the Passover Haggadah.

MULTIPLE PREGNANCY AND BIRTH 391

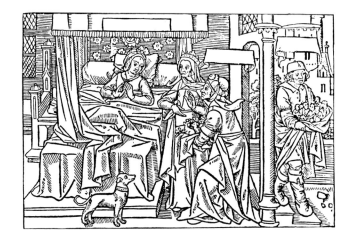

Fig. 15-23. The birth of septuplets. A satiric illustration from *Le vergier d'honneur* by André de la Vigne, about 1510. The completely credulous mother is shown a litter of seven puppies in place of her newly delivered septuplets which a servant is removing on the right. The tale of this canine birth was so widely believed that the Strasbourg medical faculty had to formally deny its possibility.

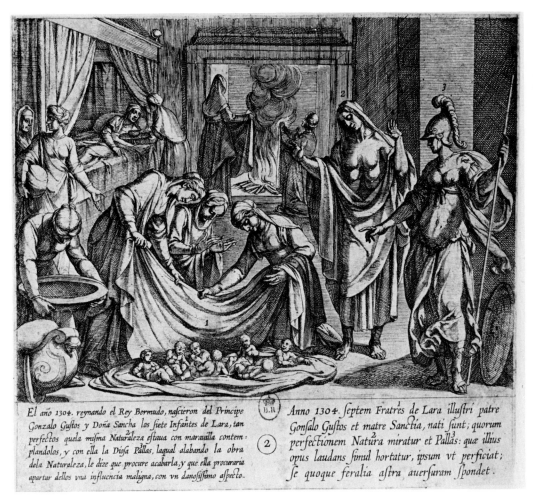

Fig. 15-24. The birth of the seven sons of Lara in the year 1304. One of a series of engravings made by Tempesta in 1612 to illustrate a Spanish legend. At the wedding of their uncle Rodriquez, so the legend goes, the children became embroiled in an argument with his new wife who thereupon reproached the boys' mother "for having borne seven sons, like a sow." When the boys then threatened to slash their new aunt's gown, Rodriquez avenged the insult by having the seven brothers put to death by the Moors.

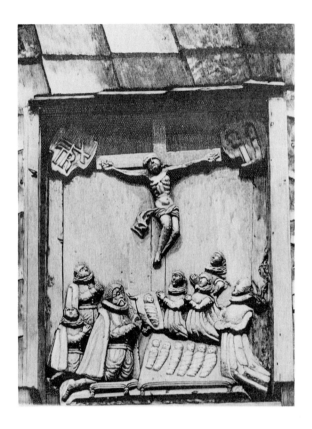

Fig. 15-25. Tombstone of the Roemer septuplets. The parents and friends are depicted kneeling around six of the swaddled infants; the father holds the seventh up toward the crucifix. The following inscription tells of their birth, in the Prussian city of Hameln, in the year 1600:

A citizen named Thiele Roemer in our town
His wife, too, Anna Breyers here well known,
As one counted 1600 years,
The ninth of January at 3 o'clock of the morn,*
Of her two baby boys, five little girls
At one time were born.
Have too received the Holy Baptism.
And then on the 20th at midday died happy.
May God give them the blessing
Vouchsafed to all believers.

[Ploss, Bartels, and Bartels, *Woman,* E. J. Dingwall, Ed., 1935.]

*The date of birth may have been January 19, according to Max Bartels, in which case the children would have lived but 33 hours, not 11 days.

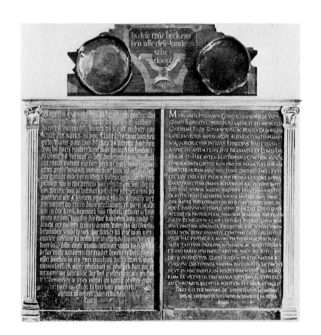

Fig. 15-26. The so-called multiple birth of the Countess of Henneberg, a case of hydatidiform mole. Dutch text on the left, Latin on the right, recounting the birth of 365 children to the 42 year old Countess Margaret on Good Friday of the year 1276. The "children" were baptized in two basins, all the boys being christened John, the girls Elizabeth. Their mother died too, probably of hemorrhage, on the day of their birth (molar expulsion),

"which has happened because of a poor woman who had carried 2 children of one gestation on her arms, of which the Countess, being amazed, declared that she could not have them by one man, and shook her off with contempt; whereupon this poor woman, being annoyed, cursed her with the wish that of one gestation as many children she might have as there were days in a whole year, which miraculously came to pass . . ."

MULTIPLE PREGNANCY AND BIRTH 393

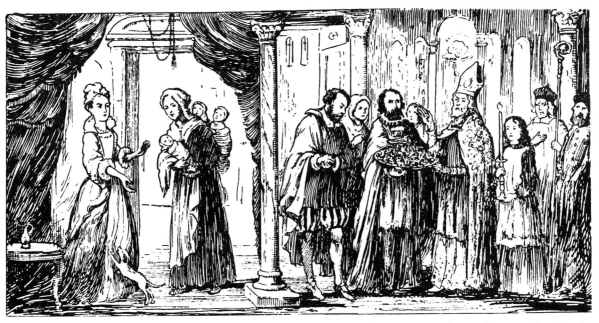

Fig. 15-27. Pen drawing. From a painting in the chapel of the Bavarian Castle of Thierberg illustrating the story of the Countess of Henneberg. The left panel shows the Countess wrangling with the poor woman who is carrying three infants and begging for alms. The right panel depicts the baptism of the countess' "365 children."

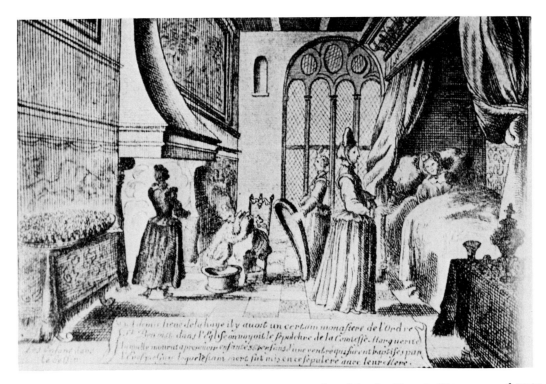

Fig. 15-28. The accouchement of the Countess of Henneberg. Anonymous sixteenth century engraving, reproduced in the *Magasin Pittoresque* of 1843. The 365 infants are shown in the large basin on the left.

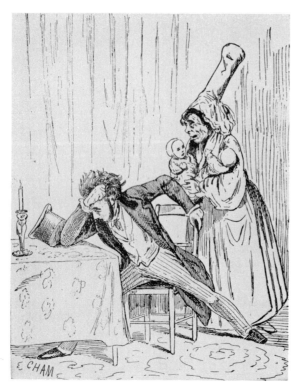

Fig. 15-29. A nineteenth century cartoon. By Cham (Amédée C. H. Moé, Compte de Cham, 1819–1879) depicting the despair of a father to whom the nurse has brought his newborn twins, saying, "Que bonheur, M'ssieu! Vous ne désirez qu'un garçon et Madame accouche de deux filles. (What luck, sir! You only wanted one boy and your wife delivers two girls.)"

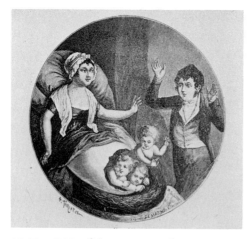

Fig. 15-30. "L'Oeuf de Paques" (The Easter Egg). A fantasy by the Belgian illustrator Jean Louis de Marne (1754–1829) showing the surprise of the father at the birth of triplets to his wife on Easter day.

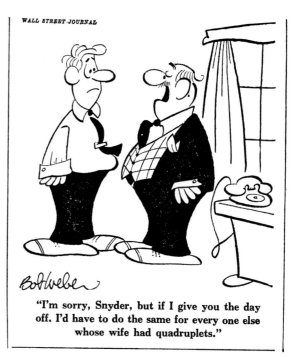

Fig. 15-31. *The Wall Street Journal* (Bob Weber), February 26, 1963.

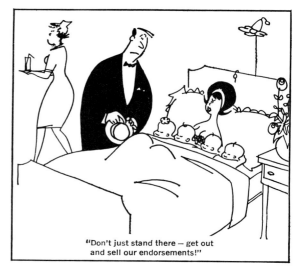

Fig. 15-32. *Modern Medicine* (Lawrence Katzman), October 11, 1965.

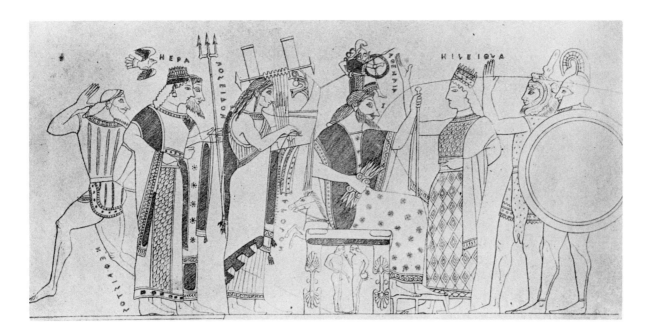

Fig. 15-33. The birth of Athene from the head of Zeus, in the presence of Hermes, Hephaistos, and two Eileithyia. Metis, a consort of Zeus, was pregnant with Pallas, Homer tells us. Zeus was warned by Ouranos and Gaia that this son-to-be would become the king of gods and men. The all-powerful Zeus thereupon persuaded the unsuspecting Metis to assume the form of a very small animal, then promptly swallowed her. In due time, full grown and in a panoply of gold,

Minerva [Athene], goddess of the martial train,
Whom wars delight, sprung from th'almighty's brain.

As told by Hesiod,

And now the king of gods, Jove [Zeus], Metis led,
The wisest fair one, to the genial bed;
Who with the blue-ey'd virgin fruitful proves,
Minerva [Athene], pledge of their celestial loves;
The sire, from what kind Earth and Heav'n reveal'd,
Artful the matron in himself conceal'd;
From her it was decreed a race should rise
That would usurp the kingdom of the skies;
And first the virgin with her azure eyes,
Equal in strength, and as her father wise,
Is born, th'offspring of th'almighty's brain:
And Metis by the god conceiv'd again,
A son decreed to reign o'er Heav'n and Earth,
Had not the sire destroy'd the mighty birth:
He made the goddess in himself reside,
To be in ev'ry act th'eternal guide.

[Hesiod's *The Theogony,* Thomas Cook, trans. (1728), eighth century BC.]

At Athene's birth, Homer relates,

All Olympus shooke
So terrible beneath her that it tooke
Up in amazes all the Deities there;
All Earth resounded with vociferous Feare;
The Sea was put up all in purple Waves,
And settld sodainly her rudest Raves;
Hyperion's radiant Sonne his swift-hov'd Steedes
A mighty Tyme staid, till her arming weedes,
As glorious as the Gods', the blew-eyd Maid
Tooke from her Deathlesse shoulders. But then staid
All these distempers, and heaven's counsailor, Jove,
Rejoic't that all things else his stay could move.

["Hymn to Pallas," *Chapman's Homer,* Allardyce Nicoll, ed. Pantheon Books, New York, 1956.]

Thus Pallas Athene whom no mother bore was the daughter of Zeus alone, and she became his favorite child. To her alone did he entrust his aegis and his devastating weapon, the thunderbolt. In poetry she became the embodiment of wisdom, reason, and purity. Known also as the Maiden Parthenos, chief of the three virgin goddesses, she was memorialized in her temple, the Parthenon.

396 ICONOGRAPHIA GYNIATRICA

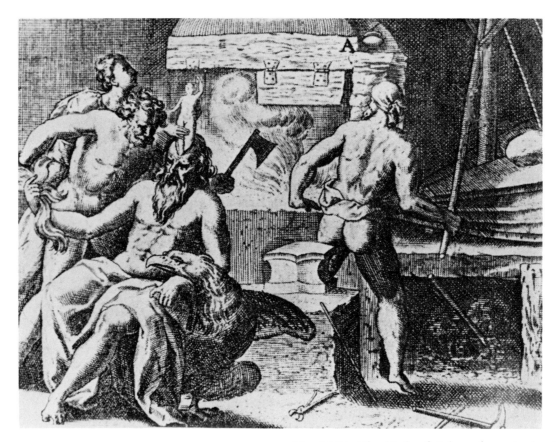

Fig. 15-34. The birth of Athene from the head of Zeus. Copper engraving, probably by Geerhardt de Jode, 1579.

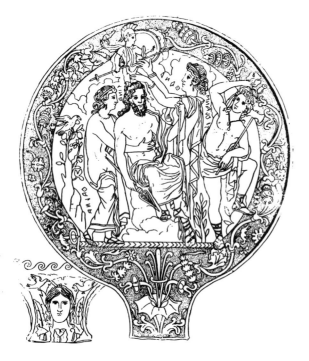

Fig. 15-35. The birth of Athene. Etruscan mirror.

INCOMPLETE TWINNING

Identical twins result from the splitting of the fertilized ovum early in its development, before the appearance of the primitive streak. If separation of the split halves is incomplete, a double monster results. Many varieties have been recorded, depending on the site of connection. Some incompletely separated twins are joined at the tops of their heads, others at the caudal region. Some have two heads and one trunk, sharing common inner organs, or are fused along the sides of their bodies; others are connected by only a slender stalk. Most double monsters are born dead or die in early infancy. Only a few have survived to adult life, and these have attracted wide interest. Like single monsters, incomplete twins have probably inspired some of the characters and legends of mythology such as the birth of Athene from the head of Zeus and the implantation of Dionysus into the latter's thigh.

Conjoined twins are classified according to their site of attachment. Most common is the pygopagus variety (from the Greek *pygē,* meaning rump), in which the twins are joined back to back, with parts of the buttocks, sacrum, and perineum in common; the thoracopagus, joined at the sternum; and the omphalopagus in which a part of the anterior abdominal wall is shared, the rest of the body being formed in duplicate. Unions of these and similar varieties have long been grouped under the generic term *Siamese twins,* so named after the celebrated Bunker brothers, Chang and Eng.

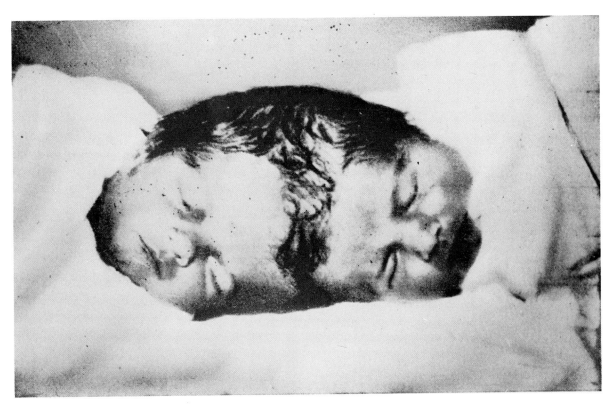

Fig. 15-36. Craniopagus twin sisters Kathleen and Lexie Smith, born in 1950 in Wynyard, Tasmania. From L. Gedda: *Twins in History and Science,* 1961. Courtesy of Charles C Thomas, Publisher, Springfield, Ill.

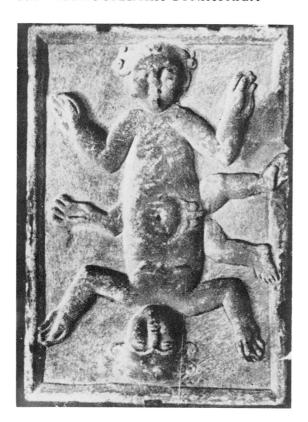

Fig. 15-37. Tablet of male ischiopagi, born in 1316 in Florence, Italy. Museum of San Marco, Italy. From L. Gedda: *Twins in History and Science,* 1961. Courtesy of Charles C Thomas, Publisher, Springfield, Ill.

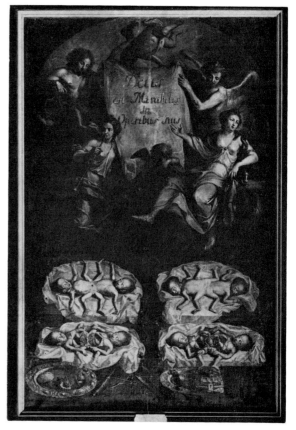

Fig. 15-38. Twins joined at the perineum. Painting by Nicolas Sauvage, 1704, commissioned by the city of Ghent, Belgium, after the dissection by Jean Palfyn. Museum of the History of Science, University of Ghent, Belgium.

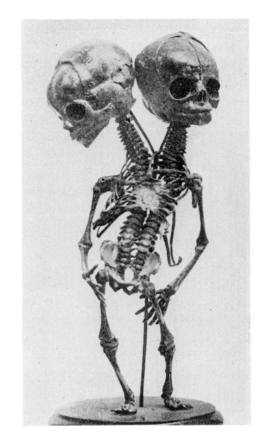

Fig. 15-39. Dicephalus dipus dibrachius. Skeleton of a monster with two heads, two arms, and two legs, Rome, 1802. Museum of the Hospital of Santo Spirito, Rome. From L. Gedda: *Twins in History and Science,* 1961. Courtesy of Charles C Thomas, Publisher, Springfield, Ill.

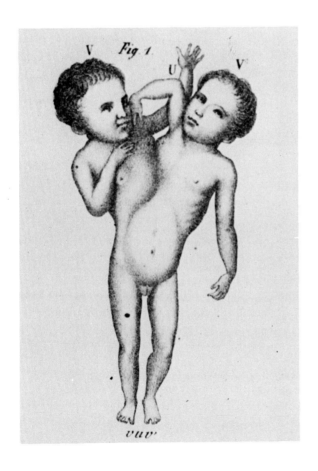

Fig. 15-40. Rita-Christina, perhaps the most widely known of the two-headed monsters: dicephalus dipus tetrabrachius (two heads, two legs, four arms). Born in Sassari, Sardinia, March 12, 1829, the incompletely separated twins were brought to Paris for public exhibition, survived eight and a half months, to November 23. Autopsy revealed two hearts within a single pericardium, fused livers, duplication of the digestive organs down to the distal ileum, and a double uterus.

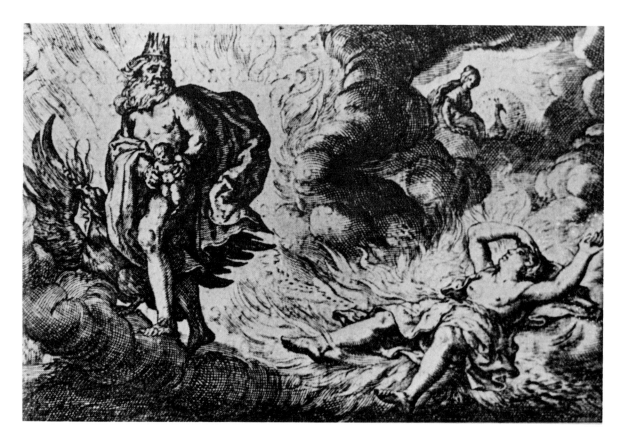

Fig. 15-41. The implantation of the fetus Dionysus into the thigh of Zeus. Copper engraving illustrating Heinsius' poem "Hymnus oft Lof-Sanck van Bacchus," 1614. In the foreground is the dying Semele; in the background Hera witnesses the result of her mischief. "Imperfectus adhuc infans genitricis ab alvo eriptur, patrioque tener (si credere dignum est) insuitur femori, maternaque tempora complet." (Ovid, book III, 310-312.)

Among the many consorts of the philandering Zeus, perhaps the most unfortunate was the princess Semele. In a moment of passion the king of the gods swore by the River Styx to fulfil her any wish, a vow that not even he could break. At the instigation of the immortal queen Hera, jealous wife of Zeus, Semele asked to see her lover in his full splendor, as Lord of the Thunderbolt. Although Zeus knew that no mortal could view him thus and survive, he was powerless to deny the wish of his beloved. In the fierce heat of his majestic rays Semele's abode was consumed and she too succumbed in the flames. With the help of Hermes, Zeus ripped from the belly of the dying Semele the fetus of six months that he had sired, and implanted the not yet viable infant into his own loin. There he hid his maturing son from Hera for three months, at the end of which time he bore the child Dionysus, god of the vine.

MULTIPLE PREGNANCY AND BIRTH   401

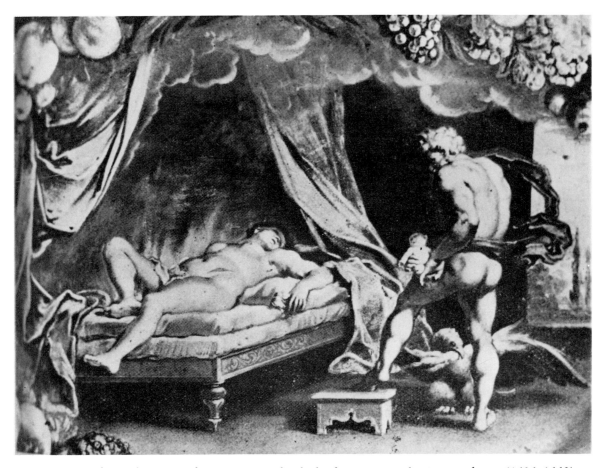

Fig. 15-42. The implantation of Dionysus into the thigh of Zeus. Fresco by Jean Boulanger (1606–1660).

Fig. 15-43. The birth of Dionysus. Antique bas-relief. Having reached full term, the infant is about to spring from the thigh of Zeus into the arms of Hermes. Vatican Museum.

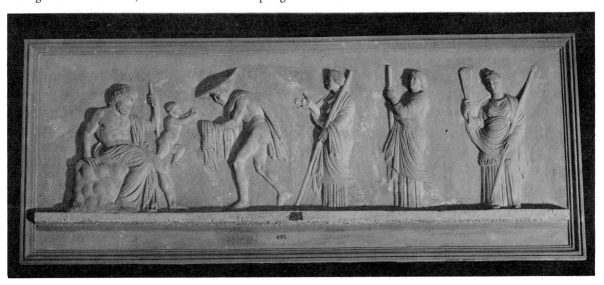

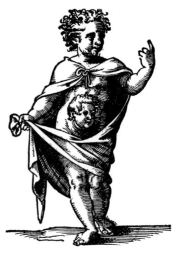

Fig. 15-44. Parasitic twin, its head attached at the umbilical region. Woodcut from Jacob Rueff's *De conceptu*, 1580.

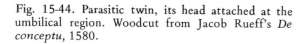

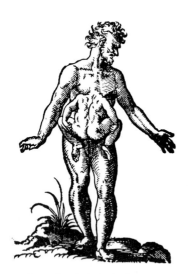

Fig. 15-45. Monster born in 1519. Woodcut from Jacob Rueff's *De conceptu*, 1580. Attached at the lower pectoral region was a parasitic twin, lacking only a head. Monsters of this general type may have inspired the myth of Dionysus' birth.

MULTIPLE PREGNANCY AND BIRTH 403

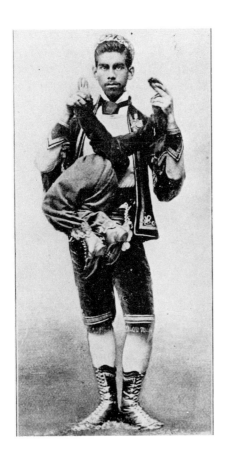

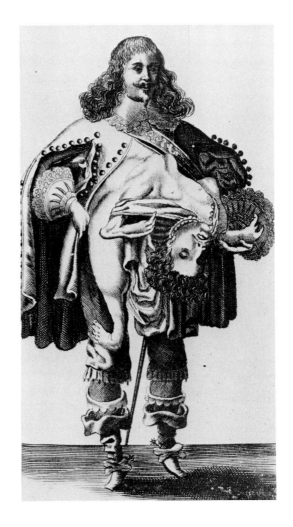

Fig. 15-46. "Laloo," a nineteenth century victim of incomplete twinning. Born in India, he went on public exhibition in the United States. The parasite was attached by bone to the lower sternum and by a fleshy pedicle to the upper abdomen. To enhance the morbid curiosity of the paying public, one of Laloo's exhibitors clad the parasite, although endowed with a penis, in female attire and advertised the monster as brother and sister.

Fig. 15-47. Lazarus-Joannes Baptista Colloredo, perhaps the most famous of the double monsters of the parasitic type, born in Genoa, Italy in 1617. Thomas Bartholin, the distinguished Dutch anatomist, examined Colloredo in life and described him thus, in his *Historiarum anatomicarum rariorum, Centuria I,* 1654:

"This Lazarus had a small brother with him, growing out of his breast and adhering to him . . . by a union of the xyphoid . . . with the sternum. The little brother had but one, and that the left leg and foot, which hung down; he had two arms, but only three fingers on each hand. When pressure was made against his chest, he moved his hands, ears, and lips. He received no food or nourishment except through the body of his larger brother Lazarus. . . . They had both been baptized, the larger one being named at the font Lazarus and the smaller Joannes Baptista. The head of the little brother was well formed and covered with hair but his eyes were closed, and his respiration weak, for when I held a feather to his mouth and nostrils, they gave it but little motion."

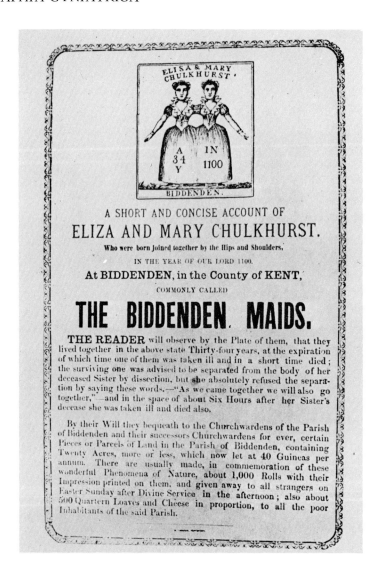

Fig. 15-48. Broadside describing the Biddenden Maids. Among the earliest recorded conjoined twins were Eliza and Mary Chulkhurst, said to have been born in the year 1100 in Biddenden, Kent, England, united at the hips and arms. When one of the twins died, at age 34, it was suggested that they be separated, but the surviving sister refused, so it is said, insisting, "As we came together, we will also go together"; and within six hours she too was dead. The Biddenden Maids bequeathed to the church wardens of their parish 20 acres of land, so the story goes, the proceeds from the rental of which were to be used for the purchase of bread, cheese, and cakes, to be distributed every Easter to the poor. For many years, cakes bearing the girls' images and names, the date 1100, and their age at death, were provided in the church, immediately after the Easter service; but the custom was ultimately discontinued because of the disturbance it caused.

Doubt has been cast upon the authenticity of the Biddenden Maids, for three principal reasons: first, because of the remoteness of the year 1100 and the unreliability of tales dating from that era; second, because of the possibility of a retrospective fabrication, for William Rufus, King of England, was killed in the same year and according to the Anglo-Saxon Chronicle his death was preceded by several prodigies; and third, because of the unique union of the twins by the arms. J. W. Ballantyne, the renowned pediatric pathologist, suggested, on the other hand, that the girls were united only at the hips, but were depicted as joined by the arms because of their custom of walking with their arms about each other's shoulders.

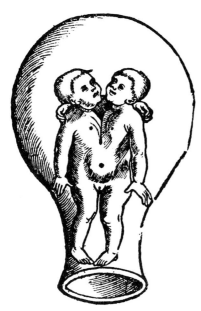

Fig. 15-49. Omphalopagus conjoined twins, each with two arms and one leg. Woodcut from Eucharius Rösslin's *Rosengarten*, 1513.

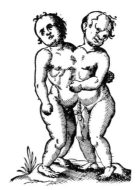

Fig. 15-50. Omphalo-thoracopagus twins, joined at chest and abdomen, each infant having two legs as well as two arms. Woodcut from Jacob Rueff's *De conceptu*, 1580.

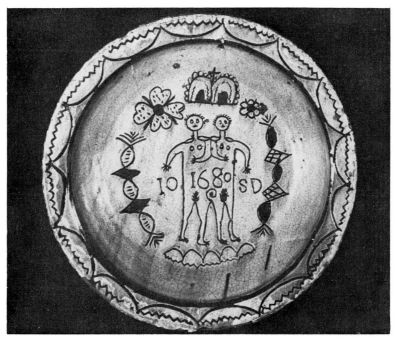

Fig. 15-51. Sgraffito plate of red clay covered with yellow glaze, 13½ inches in diameter, to commemorate the birth of Aquila-Priscilla. On May 19, 1680 at Ile Brewers near Langport, England, were born twin sisters named Aquila and Priscilla joined side to side from the chest to the upper level of the sacrum. When seen by the Reverend Andrew Paschall, vicar of Chedzoy, 10 days after their birth, the twins were adjudged "well and likely to live"; but soon they were taken away from their mother by one Henry Walrond and a Sir Edward Phelips and placed on public exhibition, and after several months they died. Somerset County Museum, Taunton, England.

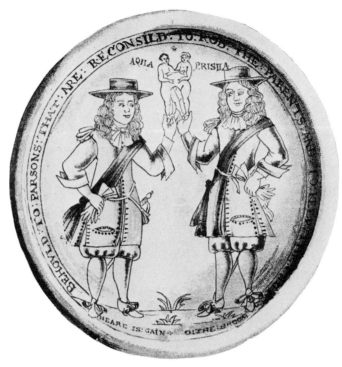

Fig. 15-52. Delft plate with figure of the conjoined twins Aquila and Priscilla being held by two men in military uniform, alleged abductors of the infants. An inscription around the figure reads, "Behould: To Parsons That Are Reconsild To Rob The Parents And To Keep The Child." The Wellcome Historical Medical Museum, London.

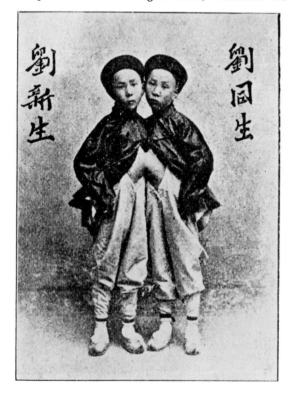

Fig. 15-53. Liu Soo San and Liu Tang San, thoracopagus twins, widely shown for 13 years in the Barnum and Bailey Circus. Joined at the sternum, they were regarded in their birthplace, Kiangsi Province, China, as the product of the god Khango's intervention.

MULTIPLE PREGNANCY AND BIRTH 407

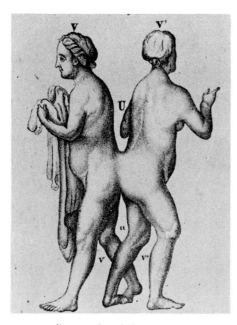

Fig. 15-54. Hélene and Judith, **pygopagus** twins born in Szony, Hungary in 1701. Exhibited from age seven in Germany, Italy, France, Holland, and England, they died in a convent in Pressburg, Hungary in their 22nd year. From an engraving by B. Cole, about 1715.

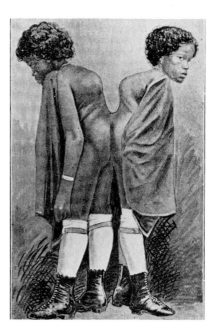

Fig. 15-55. Millie and Christine, pygopagus twins born of slave parents July 11, 1851 in Columbus County, North Carolina. Exhibited in Paris in 1873, they danced, sang, and accompanied themselves on the guitar.

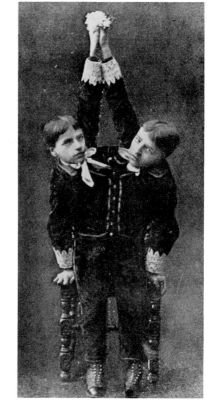

Fig. 15-56. The Tocci brothers, Giovanni-Battista and Giacoma, omphalo-pygopagus twins born in 1877 in Turin, Italy. Joined at the abdomen and pelvis, they had three buttocks, a single anus, one penis, and two legs. They could not walk, however, for each of the twins could control but one leg.

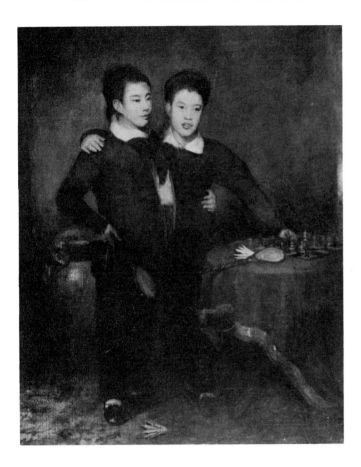

Fig. 15-57. Chang and Eng. Oil painting by Irvine. Most famous of all conjoined twins were Chang and Eng. Born near Bangkok in 1811 to a Chino-Siamese mother and a Chinese father, they were subsequently known as the Siamese Twins. Attached to each other at the lower chest and upper abdomen, the brothers gained increasing freedom of movement as the short, rigid ligament that joined them softened and stretched, permitting them eventually to stand side by side, back to back, and even to run, jump, and swim. In 1829 at age 18, the twins were exhibited in England and the United States where they aroused great interest among the medical profession as well as the general public. They soon came under the artful management of the master showman P. T. Barnum who advertised them with the verse,

The Twins of Siam —
Rarest of Dualities,
Two ever Separate
Ne'er apart Realities.

Surgical separation of the twins, carefully considered but adjudged too hazardous by most authorities, was never attempted.

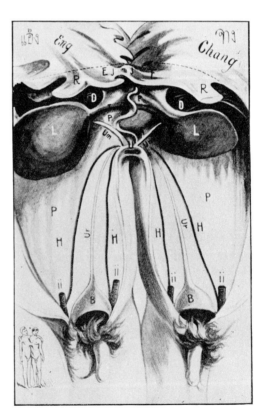

Fig. 15-58. The internal anatomy of Chang and Eng (after Pancoast). (U) umbilicus, (Ur) urachus, (H) hypogastric artery, (Um) umbilical vein, (L) liver, (B) bladder, (ii) internal iliac artery, (P) peritoneal pouch, (D) diaphragm.

Chapter 16

FERTILITY AND ITS CONTROL

"Men and women have always longed for both fertility and sterility, each at its appointed time and in its chosen circumstances.... While women have always wanted babies, they have wanted them when they wanted them. And they have wanted neither too few nor too many." [Norman E. Himes: *Medical History of Contraception*. Gamut Press, New York, 1936.]

FERTILITY DEITIES

Fertility of family as well as soil became important to man when he adopted an agrarian life, perhaps 6000 or 7000 years ago. In an economy based on hunting alone, fellow man had been a competitor, for food was dearly won, but in cultivating his fields and tending his flocks, man now needed help. Specific deities were invoked to augment the family and for other favors. To please his gods man offered gifts, wore amulets, and performed rituals. Religious cults, ceremonies, and deities were passed on from generation to generation. The deities often underwent change of name with the conquest of nation over nation and the assimilation of one culture by another. The Egyptians, for example, who acquired much of their mythology from the Sumerians and Chaldeans provided the Greeks with many of their gods and much of their religious heritage.

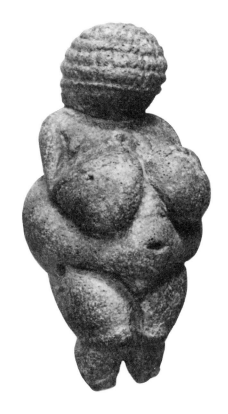

Fig. 16-1. "Venus of Willendorf," a fertility goddess. Limestone statuette of a nude woman, about 4½ inches tall, emphasizing the breasts, abdomen, buttocks, and thighs. The almost faceless head is wound with plaited hair. This figure from the Middle Aurignacian period of the Old Stone Age (40,000–16,000 BC) is believed to be one of the earliest known representations of the human form. It was unearthed in 1908 in Willendorf, Austria, a village on the Danube. Naturhistorisches Museum, Vienna.

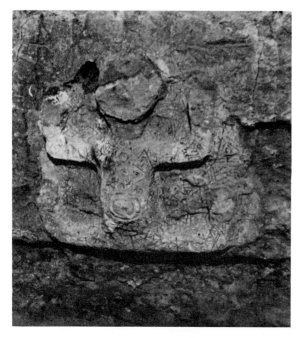

The primitive deities were usually represented in human form, not much different from that of the worshipper, the fertility goddesses most often in frontal view, emphasizing the breasts and pudenda.

The goddess of love, beauty, and fertility was known to the Semitic peoples of Mesopotamia as Ishtar. To the Phoenecians she was Astarte. In other cultures she was called by still other names, for instance, Venus, by the Romans and Aphrodite, by the Greeks who regarded her initially as a sea-divinity. She is often portrayed with the water of life, a symbol of fertility.

Isis, daughter of Qêb and Nut, sister of

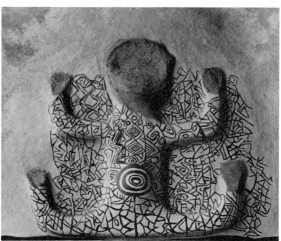

Fig. 16-2. Painted plaster reliefs of pregnant goddess. Seventh millennium BC, unearthed by James Mellaart in excavations in 1961, 1962, and 1963 at Çatal Hüyük, a neolithic city in Anatolia.

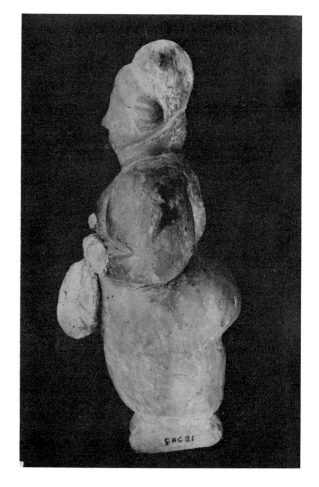

Fig. 16-3. Pregnant goddess. Alabaster figure, seventh millennium BC, recovered by James Mellaart in Çatal Hüyük (Shrine E.IV.4).

Osiris, and mother of Horus, was the Egyptian goddess of fertility and love and protectress of women in the vicissitudes of life. She is usually depicted wearing a crown of two horns embracing a solar disc and often holding a papyrus scepter. After the twenty-fifth Dynasty (663 BC), Isis was commonly shown as a nursing mother with Horus.

With the introduction of Christianity into Egypt, many saw marked similarities between the new religion and the moral system of the old cult. Transferring their allegiance from Osiris to Jesus, they identified Isis and her son Horus with the Virgin Mary and her Child.

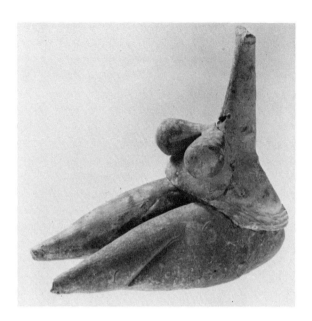

Fig. 16-4. A neolithic fertility goddess. Clay figurine, about 6,000 BC, found by Robert J. Braidwood in diggings at Sarab, an early village site near modern Kermanshah in Iran. Missing are the head and feet; disporportionately large, the breasts and thighs. Oriental Institute, University of Chicago.

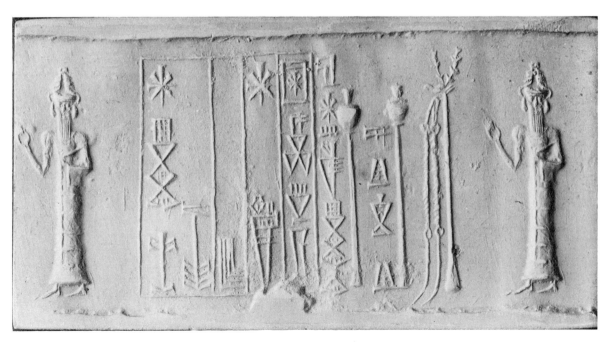

Fig. 16-5. Invocation to the god of childbirth. On the seal of Urlugaledinna, a physician or male midwife, in Lagash (or Shipurla), Sumerian city in southern Babylonia about 3,000 BC. Musée du Louvre, Paris.

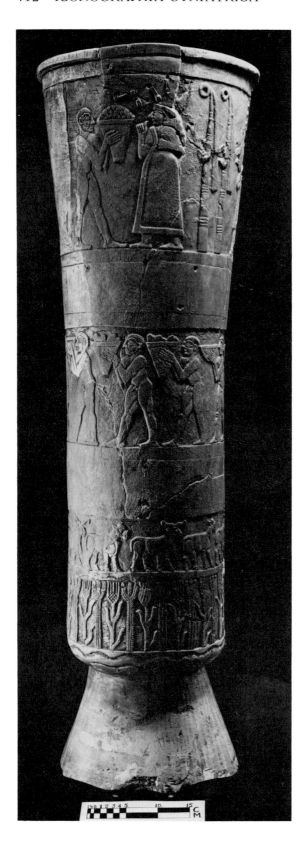

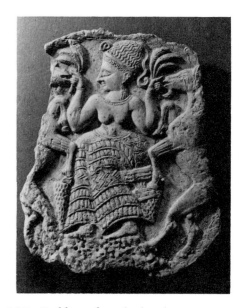

Fig. 16-6. An offering to Inanna, Sumerian goddess of fertility. Alabaster vase about 2300 BC found at Uruk (Erech), ancient Sumerian city in southern Babylonia on the Euphrates. The upper and middle panels show gifts being brought to the goddess; the lowermost symbolizes nature's bounty. Iraq Museum, Baghdad.

Fig. 16-7. Goddess of motherhood. Mycenaean ivory about 1400 BC found at Ras Shamra, site of ancient city near Syrian coast. Musée du Louvre, Paris.

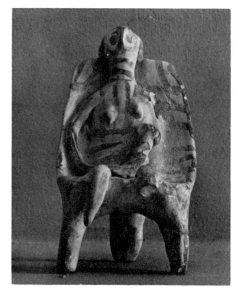

Fig. 16-8. Goddess of motherhood. Mycenaean terra cotta figure. Musée du Louvre, Paris.

FERTILITY AND ITS CONTROL 413

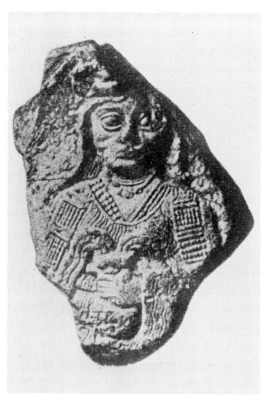

Fig. 16-9. Ishtar. Clay bas-relief found at Telloh, a village in southern Mesopotamia, now Iraq. The goddess holds a vase from which flows the water of life. Musée du Louvre, Paris.

Fig. 16-10. Ishtar as a winged goddess. Babylonian terra cotta bas-relief. Musée du Louvre, Paris.

Fig. 16-11. Ishtar depicted in Oriental motif. Musée du Louvre, Paris.

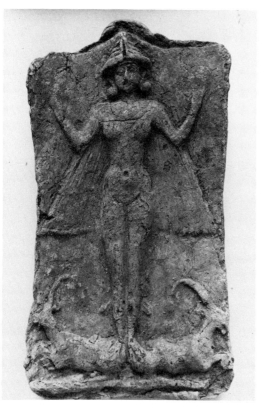

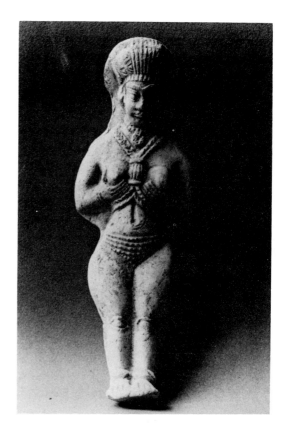

414 ICONOGRAPHIA GYNIATRICA

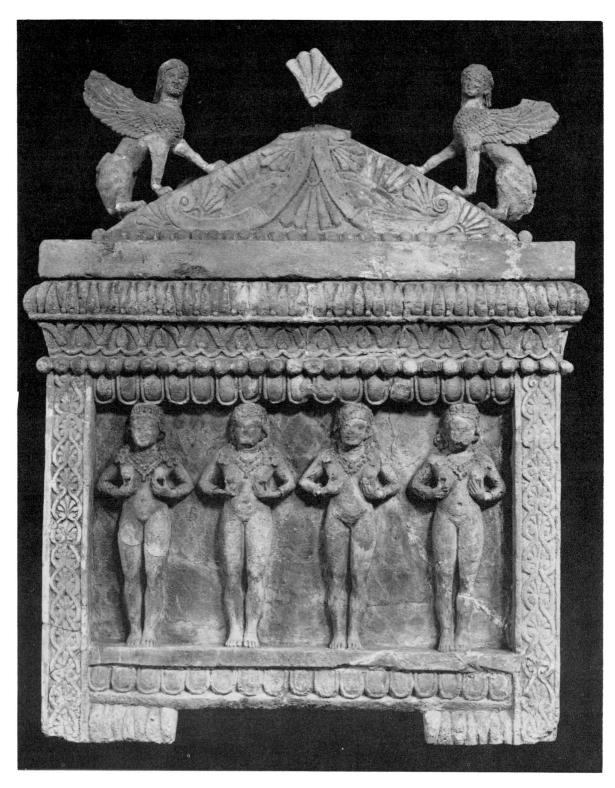

Fig. 16-12. Astarte. Limestone sarcophagus from Cyprus 600–550 BC portraying the goddess in a blend of Greek and Oriental styles. The Metropolitan Museum of Art, New York.

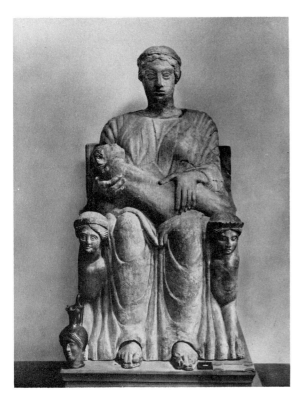

Fig. 16-13. Mater Matuta, goddess of motherhood. Etruscan stone figure, fifth century BC. Museo Archeologico, Florence.

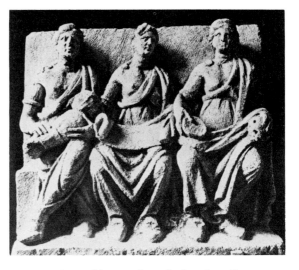

Fig. 16-14. Goddesses of motherhood. Gallo-Roman column. The goddess on the left supports an infant on her lap; the center goddess unrolls a swaddling band; the goddess on the right holds a sponge. Musée de Chatillon-sur-Seine, France.

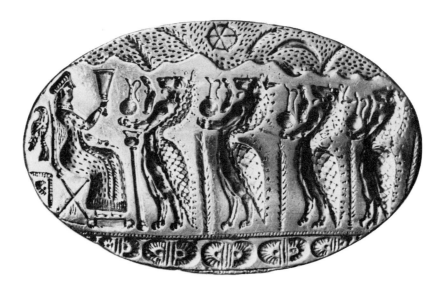

Fig. 16-15. Minoan goddess of fertility. The face of a gold signet ring from Tiryns, a prehistoric citadel in southern Greece, destroyed about 469 BC. The goddess is seated on a chair, a bird perched behind her. Before the goddess stand stalks of wheat and a procession of demons bearing water, symbols of fertility. National Archaeological Museum, Athens.

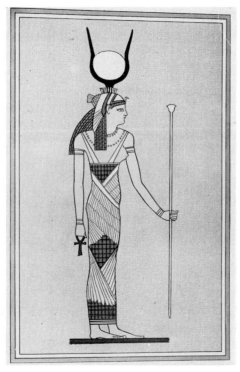

Fig. 16-16. The goddess Isis.

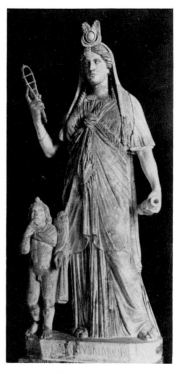

Fig. 16-18. Isis with Horus. Ancient marble statue.

Fig. 16-17. Isis nursing Horus in the papyrus swamp.

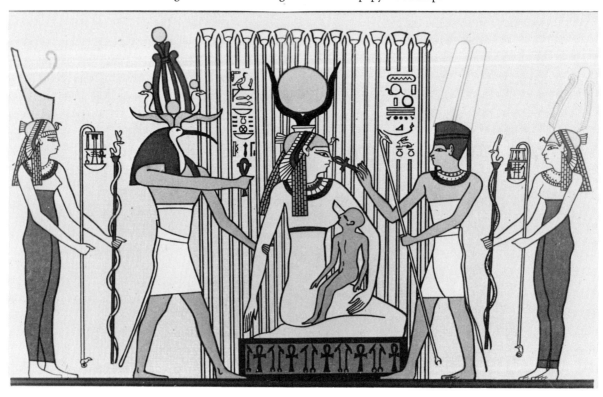

FERTILITY AND ITS CONTROL 417

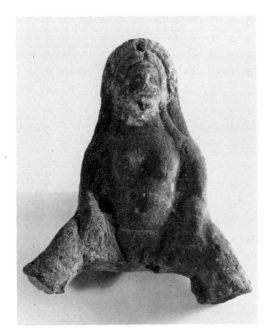

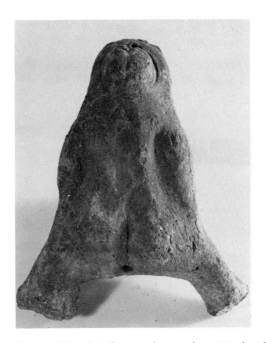

Fig. 16-19. Baubo, Greek female fertility goddess. Terra cotta. Baubo was usually represented in a sitting posture, her thighs spread to emphasize the pudenda. According to legend, when Isis was mourning for Osiris, Baubo assumed the attitude depicted in this figure, thus making Isis laugh and thereby ending her lamentation. In addition, Baubo was often shown with an elaborate headdress. University College, London.

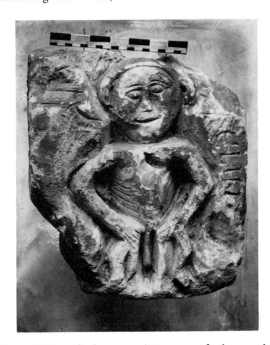

Fig. 16-20. *Sheila-na-gig* (Woman of the castle), female fertility idol. Clunch stone figure found embedded in the wall of Easthorpe Church, Essex, England. Colchester and Essex Museum, Colchester, England.

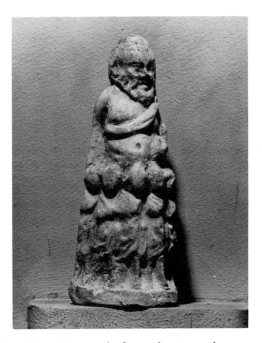

Fig. 16-21. Gigon, god of reproduction and protector of male infants. Terra cotta figure from Cyrenaica, ancient country of North Africa, now Libya. Musée du Louvre, Paris.

418   ICONOGRAPHIA GYNIATRICA

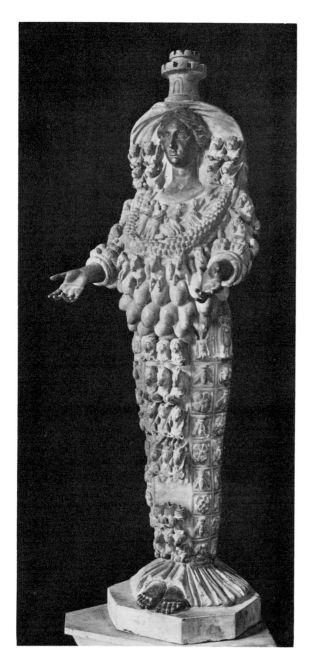

Fig. 16-22. Artemis of Ephesus, Greek goddess of fertility (called Diana by the Romans). Marble statue with head and hands of bronze. Her multiple breasts symbolized the goddess' reproductive prowess. Musei Capitolini, Rome.

Fig. 16-23. Entrance to the Temple of Amenerdais, ecclesiastic ruler of Thebes, ruined city of Upper Egypt under the last Ethiopian monarch. In ancient Egypt, Greece and Rome women sought relief from infertility by visits to the temples. If conception ensued, impregnation was attributed to a god often in the form of a serpent. The Temple of Amenerdais was built as his funerary edifice by Queen Shepenupt II, his adopted daughter. The relief above the entrance states that the chapel was for the benefit of childless women and expectant mothers. The Wellcome Historical Medical Museum, London.

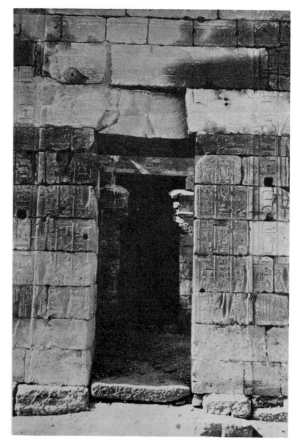

Fig. 16-24. Toueris, Egyptian symbol of fecundity and protectress of the pregnant and parturient. Not until relatively late in Egyptian history were animals worshipped, but they were always accorded a special status close to that of the gods because of their intimate knowledge of nature's laws. In the guise of a pregnant hippopotamus, Toueris is usually shown standing on her hind legs and holding the hieroglyph meaning protection in one paw, the sign for life in the other. Small figures of Toueris were popular as amulets. Egyptian Museum, Cairo.

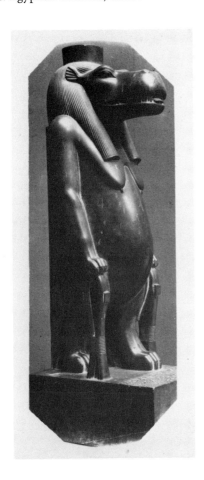

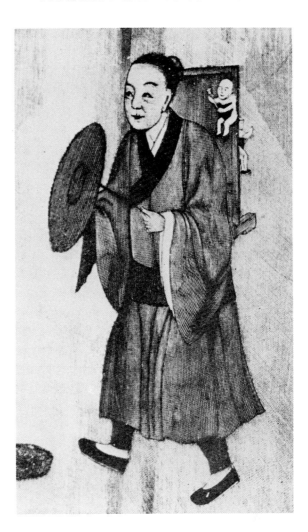

Fig. 16-25. Woodcut of a Chinese priestess who brought fecundity to barren women. Courtesy of Ciba Symposia, formerly published by CIBA Pharmaceutical Company, Summit, New Jersey.

420 ICONOGRAPHIA GYNIATRICA

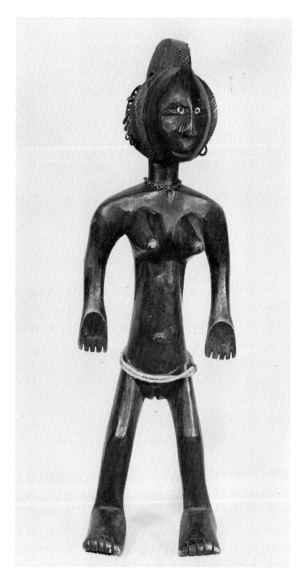

Fig. 16-26. Bambara goddess of fertility. Twentieth century woodcarving from French Sudan (since 1960, Republic of Mali), Africa. The Brooklyn Museum, New York.

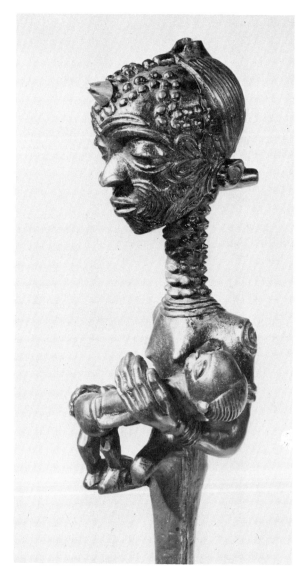

Fig. 16-27. Bena Lulua fertility goddess. Twentieth century woodcarving from Republic of the Congo, Africa. The Brooklyn Museum, New York.

FERTILITY AMULETS, DOLLS, FETISHES, AND VOTIVES

So long as man conceived of his dieties in human form not unlike his own, it seemed but natural to endow them with human emotions. Gods and goddesses, like men and women, would surely be flattered by images created in their honor and would be influenced, it was hoped, by gifts. Figures and ornaments to curry favor of the gods date back to prehistoric time; members of primitive cultures still resort to them to enhance fertility.

Votive tablets and free will offerings, usually in the form of the genital organs, together with torches and wreaths were carried by the women of ancient Rome and Greece to their temples, beseeching fecundity and easy delivery. Worshipped in many primitive communities, particularly in Africa, fetishes, usually woodcarvings in human form, were considered to be the seat of magic power or the abode of a spirit. The fetish was almost always endowed with an orifice into which the owner could place his prayerful offerings. Amulets worn as jewelry were likewise endowed with magic properties and were restricted to a single function, to ward off evil such as infertility. Masks of clay, wood, and animal horns have been worn among primitive tribes of Africa, New Guinea, and South and Central America for the past 4,000 years, to dispel the spirits of sickness and death and bring the blessings of fertility. Fertility dolls of clay and of beads still play an important role in the culture of certain tribes of South Africa.

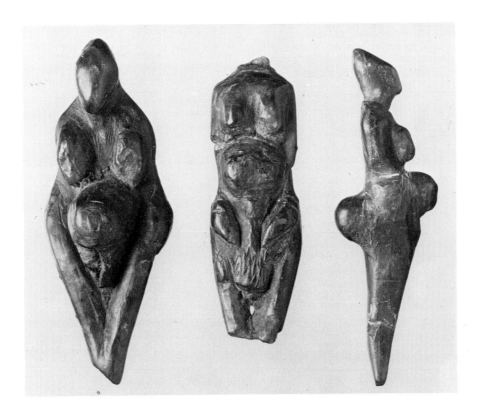

Fig. 16-28. Venus. Three prehistoric statuettes depicting the fertility goddess in advanced stages of pregnancy. Probably used as amulets, these figures were discovered in the caves of Grimaldi in Ventimiglia, Northwest Italy, the home of a Negroid race of the late paleolithic period (before 2500 BC) whose anthropologic features are reflected in Venus' ovoid head and protuberant buttocks.

422 ICONOGRAPHIA GYNIATRICA

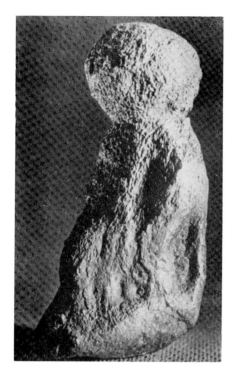

Fig. 16-29. Sitting pregnant woman. A fertility figure, 21 cm high, carved from a mammoth's tusk. Found in Czechoslovakia, it dates back to the early Aurignacian period, ice age.

Fig. 16-30. Pair of modeled breasts, right, and bull's head with horns alongside. Female and male fertility symbols, seventh millennium BC, uncovered by James Mellaart 1961, 1962, and 1963 at Çatal Hüyük, a neolithic city in Anatolia (Shrine VI.10.).

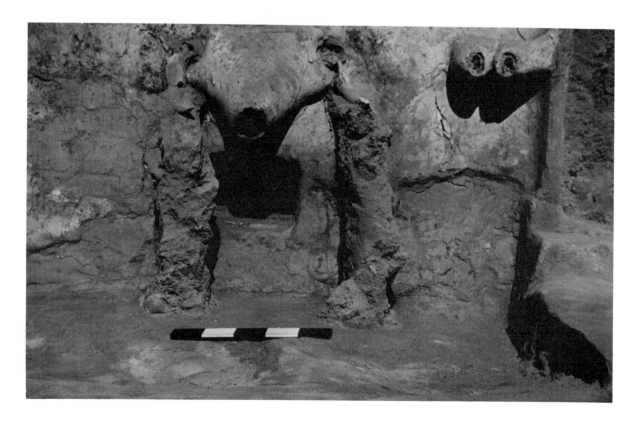

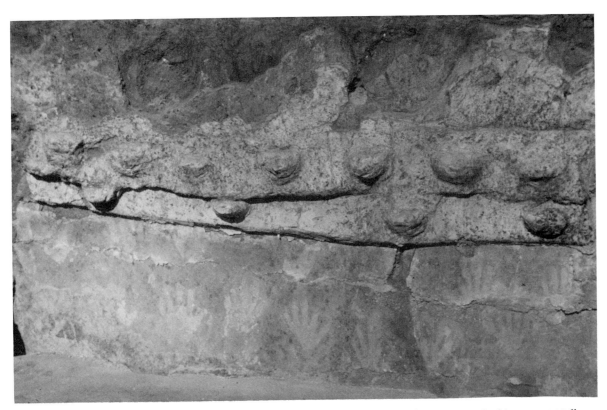

Fig. 16-31. Rows of modeled breasts, female fertility symbols, over jaws of wild boars and broken bulls' heads, male fertility symbols, and paintings of hands. Seventh millennium BC, unearthed by James Mellaart at Çatal Hüyük (Shrine VI. 8.).

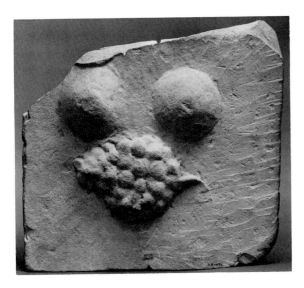

Fig. 16-32. Female torso. Marble fragment from Cyprus, after 300 BC. The bunch of grapes below the breasts identifies the tablet as a fertility symbol. The Metropolitan Museum of Art, New York.

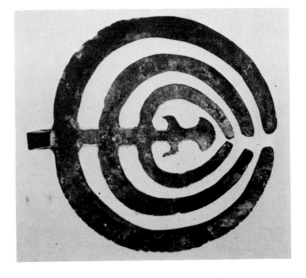

Fig. 16-33. Bronze fertility amulet representing a fetus in utero. Umbrian, eighth to seventh century BC.

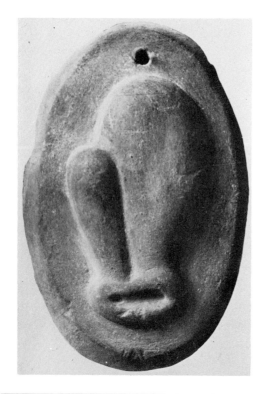

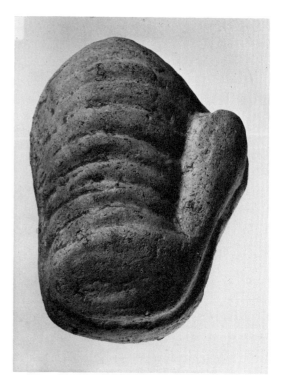

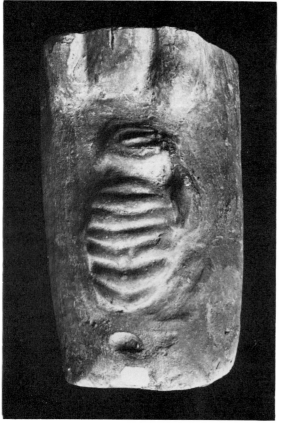

Fig. 16-34. Ex-voto of uterus with urinary bladder attached. From the Island of Kos off the Bodrum Peninsula, southwest Turkey, birthplace of Hippocrates.

Fig. 16-35. Etruscan pottery ex-voto of a uterus. Third century BC. The structure on the right may represent an adnexal inflammatory mass, ovarian tumor, or uterine fibromyoma. The British Museum, London.

Fig. 16-36. Terra cotta ex-voto of female trunk emphasizing the genitalia. The transverse folds probably represent the vaginal rugae covering a prolapsed uterus or cystocele. Museo Archeologico, Florence.

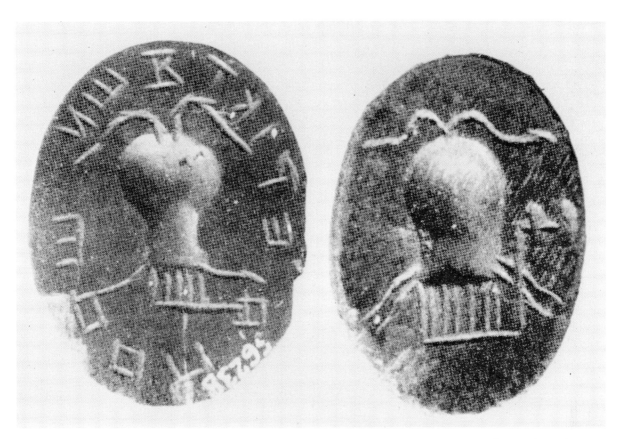

Fig. 16-37. Gnostic gems, the center of each occupied by a uterus. The parallel lines under the cervix have been interpreted as the bit of a key either to unlock the uterus to alleviate sterility or to lock the organ to prevent conception. When worn by a man such gems were supposed to render his wife invulnerable to approach by any other man. Gnosticism, a mystic religion of the early centuries of the Common Era based on oriental mythology and embracing countless spirits and demons, focussed much attention on the uterus, called *metra* or *matrix*. Assimilated into Gnosticism was Isis, the Egyptian goddess of fertility. The union of Darkness and Spirit, according to Gnostic belief, resulted in Metra who gave to heaven and earth their womblike shape. Amulets, mostly in the form of intaglios, figures engraved in stone or hard metal, were passed on from one generation to the next.

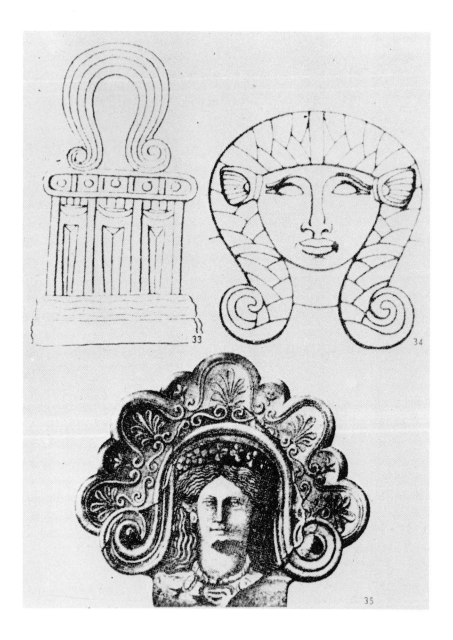

Fig. 16-38. Outlines of the uterus as a fertility symbol (upper left) were included among the altar decorations of the temple of Babylon in addition to forms of the deities. The Egyptians later placed the face of Hathor, their mother goddess, within this uterine form which thus came to be known as Hathor's hairdress (upper right). In an Etruscan terra cotta figure (below) the head of the fertility goddess is surmounted by a crown of embellished uteri.

FERTILITY AND ITS CONTROL 427

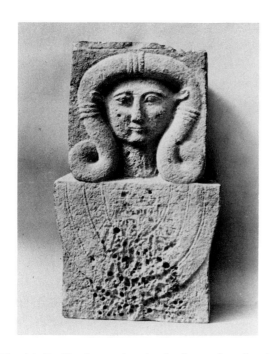

Fig. 16-39. Limestone stele with Hathor head. Cypriote, c. 600–550 BC. Metropolitan Museum of Art, New York.

Fig. 16-40. Uterine votives in the form of toads. The figures are provided with a base, permitting them to stand as shown, and with a constriction at the neck to accommodate a string for hanging. In folklore as late as the nineteenth century, the human uterus was commonly represented by the toad, but no satisfactory explanation has been proposed for this identification.

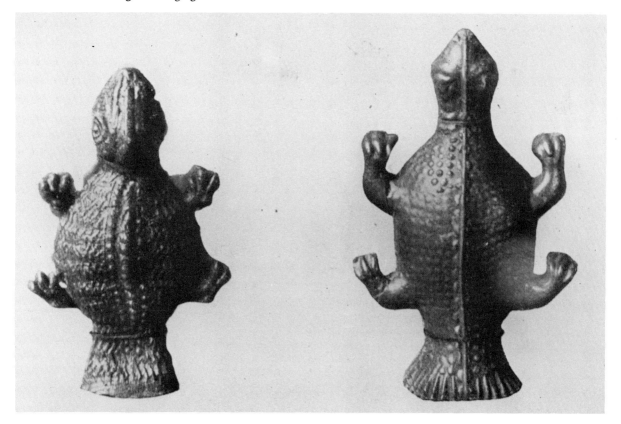

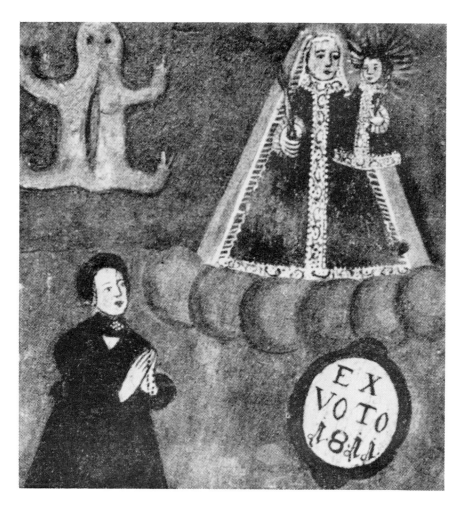

Fig. 16-41. Votive picture denoting prayer for fertility. Austria, 1811. Shown in the upper left is the form of a toad, symbolizing the uterus.

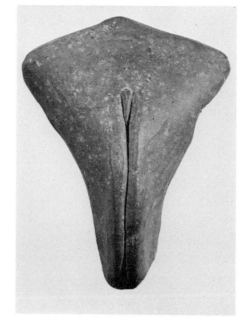

Fig. 16-42. Terra cotta ex-voto representing the vulva. Museo Nazionale di Villa Giulia, Rome.

FERTILITY AND ITS CONTROL 429

Fig. 16-43. Pregnant woman with exaggerated navel, presumably a fertility figure. Statuette unearthed by an archeological expedition during the mid 1960s from a cave at Safadi in the Israeli Negev. This figure has been attributed to a troglodyte culture dating back to 3500 BC, 15 centuries before Abraham settled in Beersheba.

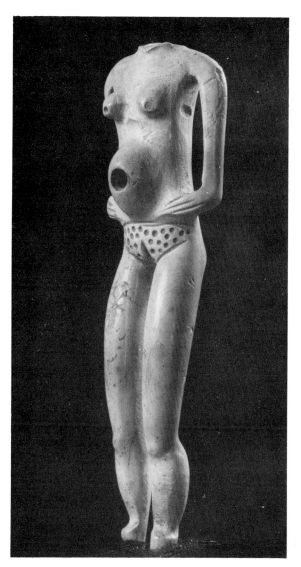

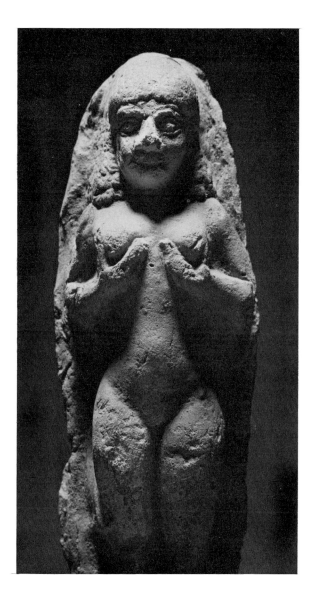

Fig. 16-44. Fertility idol from Ur. About 2000 BC.

430 ICONOGRAPHIA GYNIATRICA

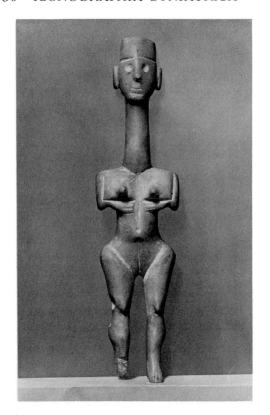

Fig. 16-45. Marble fertility figure emphasizing the breasts. From the Cyclades (South Aegean Sea), third millennium BC. The Metropolitan Museum of Art, New York.

Fig. 16-46. Terra cotta fertility figures from Cyprus, 2000–1200 BC. The Metropolitan Museum of Art, New York.

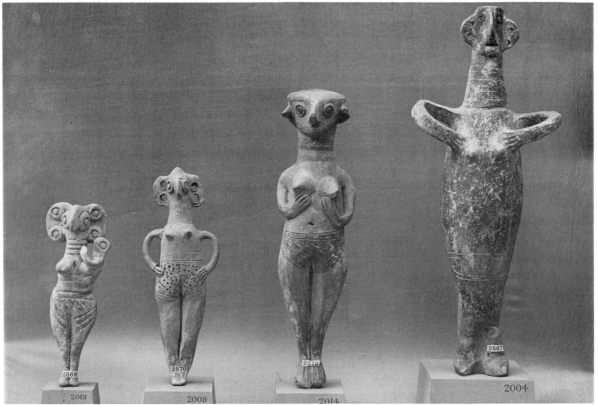

FERTILITY AND ITS CONTROL 431

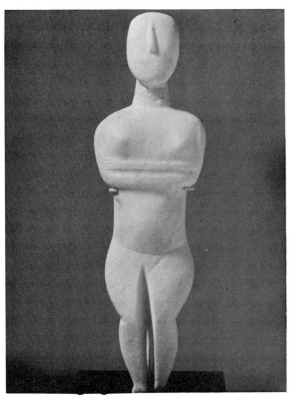

Fig. 16-47. Marble fertility figure. Cycladic sculpture, second or third millennium BC. The Brooklyn Museum, New York.

Fig. 16-48. Mexican clay fertility figure. From the Tlatilco Valley, first or second millennium BC. The Brooklyn Museum, New York.

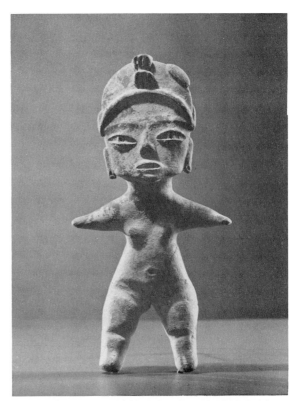

Fig. 16-49. Mexican fertility symbol. From the Tlatilco Valley, first or second millennium BC. Clay figurine of mother and child found in a grave almost 4,000 years old, probably having been placed there as an offering to the dead to assure fertility for the living. The Brooklyn Museum, New York.

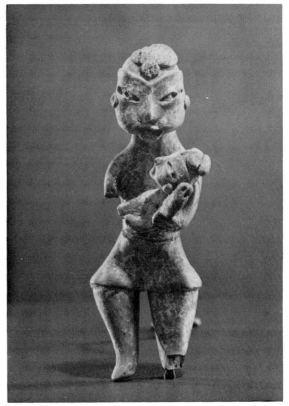

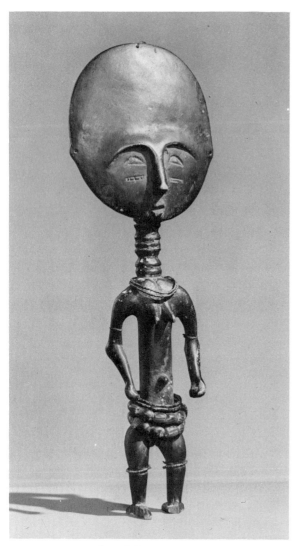

Fig. 16-50. Fertility doll. From Ashanti, the wooded interior of what is now Ghana, West Africa. Among some African tribes in which a woman's ability to bear children takes precedence over all other wifely functions, a doll is given her when she is about to marry. Believed endowed with magic powers of fertility, the doll is sometimes worn as a necklace or bound to the woman's body, under her clothes, to help her to become pregnant. Museum of Primitive Art, New York.

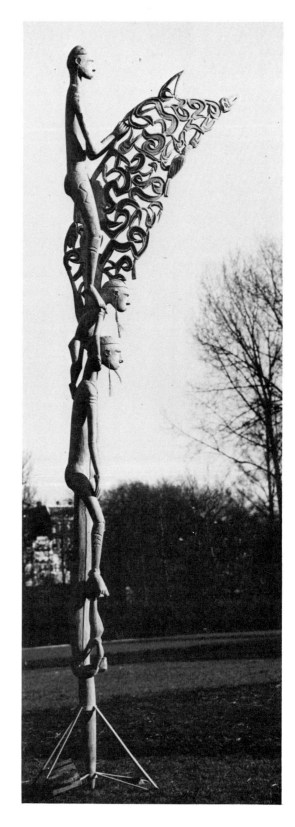

Fig. 16-51. The Bisj-pole. A fertility symbol from the Asmat district of Southwest New Guinea. Elaborate woodcarving displayed during the ritual to enhance the fertility of man, his animals, and his crops. Tropenmuseum, Amsterdam.

FERTILITY AND ITS CONTROL   433

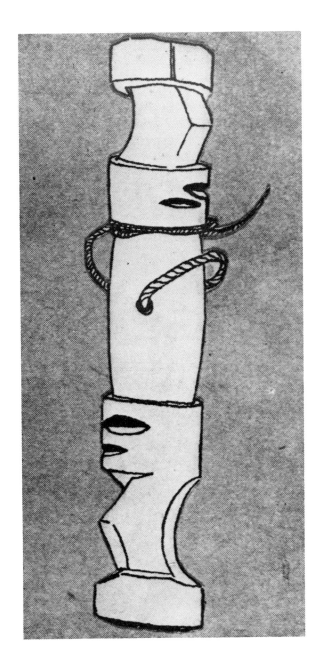

Fig. 16-53. Maori fertility symbol. Carving of a male and female figure on a house post, New Zealand.

Fig. 16-52. *Katwame*. A twin figure used as a fertility amulet by the Chokve tribe of Angola, Southwest Africa. Courtesy of Ciba Symposia, formerly published by CIBA Pharmaceutical Company, Summit, New Jersey.

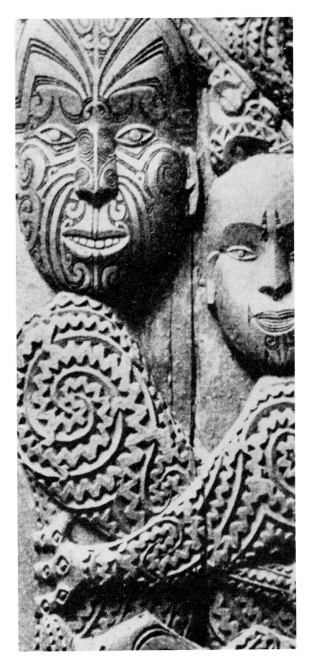

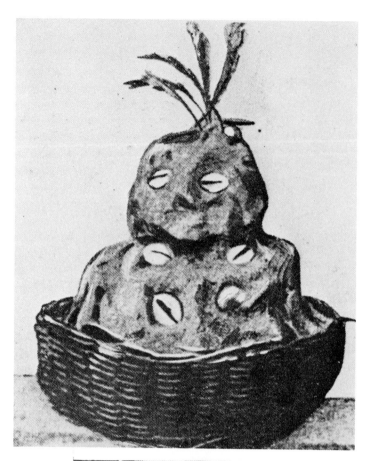

Fig. 16-54. *Se.* A clay fertility figure containing cowrie shells and chicken feathers, used in the rites of the Ewe tribe, African West Coast.

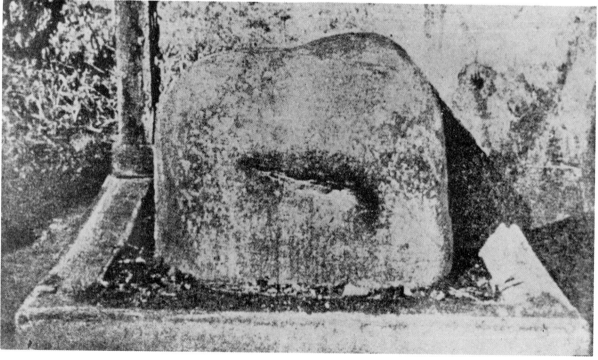

Fig. 16-55. *Onna-ishi.* A stone shrine in Kamakura, Southeast Honshu, Japan, visited by women in quest of fertility.

FERTILITY AND ITS CONTROL 435

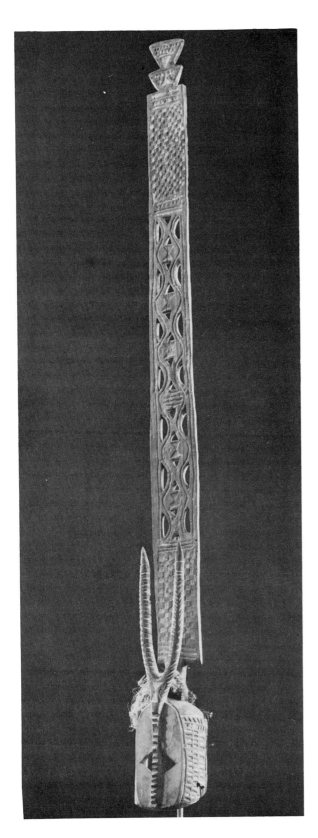

Fig. 16-56. Wango Society mask. Mossi Tribe, Upper Volta, West Africa, twentieth century. Bearing a crown of antelope horns, this mask was worn by the men during their ritual dances to ensure to the tribe energy, health, and fecundity. The Brooklyn Museum, New York.

Fig. 16-57. *Debata idup*. Carved wooden male and female figures of the deities of life carried on the backs of the Battak women, an agricultural group of Indonesians of the highlands of Sumatra, to bring them fertility. Museum für Völkerkunde, West Berlin.

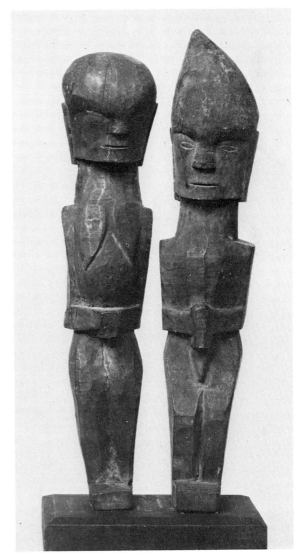

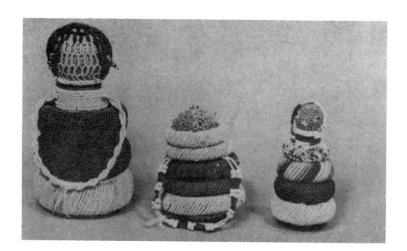

Fig. 16-58. Beaded fertility dolls from South Africa, obtained by Karl Hechter-Schulz. Brides often received such dolls on their wedding day and wore them hanging from a bead necklace or inside their clothing. Copies are now mass-produced for sale to tourists. Left: Blue, red, and white doll, old, 6¼ inches tall from north of Pretoria. Made by the grandmother of a childless Ndebele wife, it was kept in a niche in the wall of the young woman's hut and secretly fondled. Obtained in 1957.

Fig. 16-59. Beaded fertility dolls from South Africa, obtained by Karl Hechter-Schulz. Left: Multicolored old doll, 6¾ inches tall, obtained in 1960 from a Xosa (Tembu) woman near Pedie in the Transkei. Right: Multicolored doll, 11 inches tall, made for Hechter-Schulz in 1965 by a woman of the Makatees clan of the Pedi near Denilton in the Eastern Transvaal.

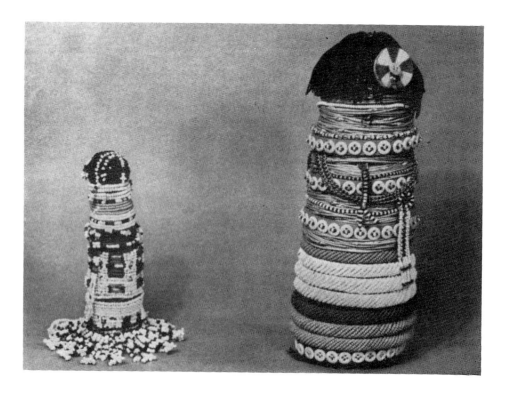

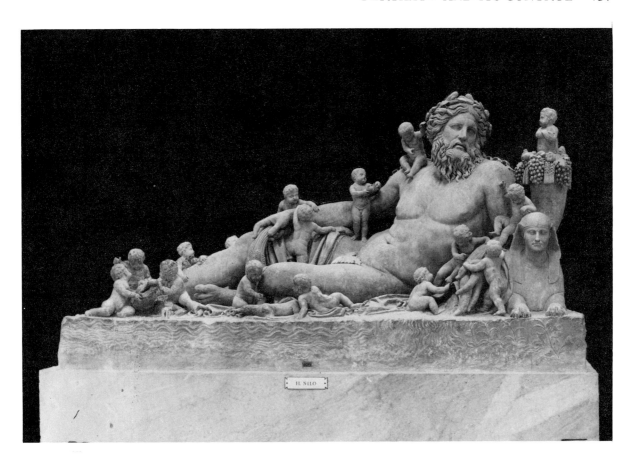

Fig. 16-60. Sculpture of Father Nile, symbol of fertility. The Vatican.

INFERTILITY

"Be fruitful, and multiply, and replenish the earth." [Genesis 1:28]

Guided by a literal interpretation of this Biblical injunction and placing a high premium on his reproductive prowess, man has ever regarded infertility as the curse supreme, exemplified by Jeremiah's quotation of the Lord, "Write ye this man childless" (Jeremiah 22:30) and Rachel's entreaty to Jacob, "Give me children, or else I die" (Genesis 30:1). God was the source of sterility as well as fertility, closing the wombs of Sarah (Genesis 16:2), Hannah (1 Samuel 1:6), Michal (2 Samuel 6:23), and the women in Abimelech's household (Genesis 20:18), while opening up the wombs of Leah (Genesis 24:31) and Rachel (Genesis 30:22); and prayer remained man's principal resort for relief from infertility until he began to understand the physiologic factors in reproduction.

There were many gods and goddesses to which the early Greeks and Romans, men and women alike, appealed for help in performing their respective parts in the reproductive process. Not content with the aid of their divinities alone, however, they resorted to theurgic devices as well including magic formulas, songs and incantations, and the laying-on of hands.

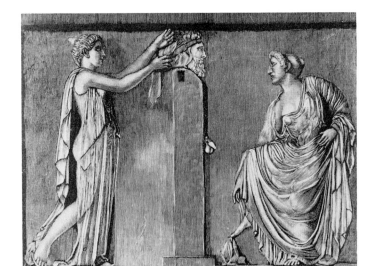

Fig. 16-61. Women honoring Hermes. Relief of a fertility rite. The scantily clad maiden on the left is about to place a wreath on the Hermes column while the woman on the right raises her dress to present herself to the god of fertility whose genitals are prominently exposed. Glyptothek, Munich.

Fig. 16-62. The Trinity presents a man and wife with a child. Miniature from a fifteenth century manuscript bearing the inscription "*Faciamus hominem ad ymaginem et simultudinem nostram* (We make man in our own image)." Bibliothèque de l'Arsenal, Paris.

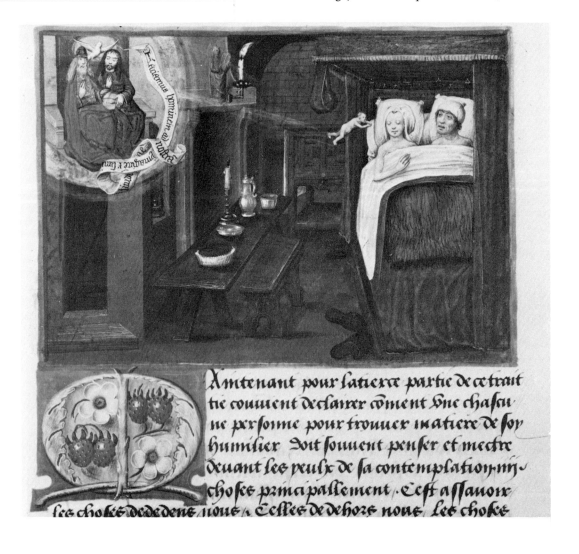

FERTILITY AND ITS CONTROL   439

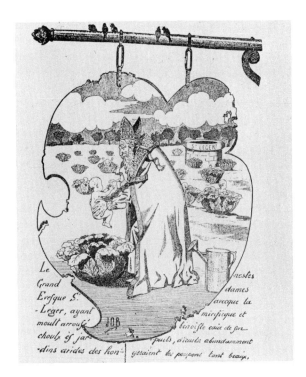

Fig. 16-63. The Bishop St. Léger finding chubby babies among the cabbages at Pougues, France. The scene a testimonial to the region's waters, renowned as a cure for sterility.

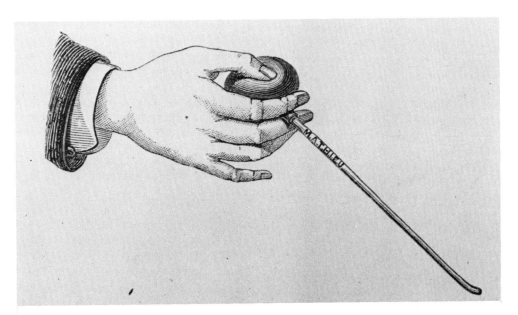

Fig. 16-64. *Fécondateur* of French obstetrician Charles Pajot (1816–1896). Syringe for artificial insemination. So long as the husband could perform the conjugal act, infertility in a marriage was ascribed to the wife. Male potency implied virility. Only when coitus could not be consummated because of impotence or anatomic aberration was the husband's role in the reproductive process impugned. The obvious resort was artificial insemination. This was first attempted in 1680 without success by the Dutch anatomist Jan Swammerdam, with the eggs and sperm of fish. Ludwig Jacobi was successful in 1742. Not until 1780 was artificial insemination fruitful in mammals. In that year the Italian anatomist Lazaro Spallanzani impregnated a bitch with the semen of a dog. At about the same time, the illustrious John Hunter impregnated the wife of a man with hypospadias by vaginal injection of her husband's semen.

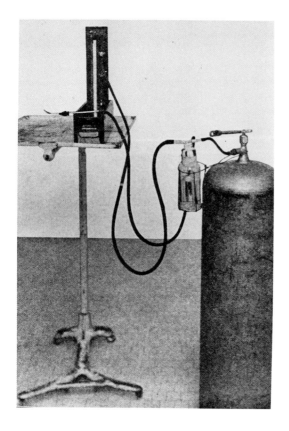

Fig. 16-65. The original apparatus, 1919, used by Isidor Clinton Rubin (1883–1958) in his tests of tubal patency. Before Rubin's experiments, the office diagnosis of tubal patency or obstruction depended upon the clinical acumen of the examiner and was subject to frequent error. Rubin initially used oxygen for tubal insufflation but switched later to the more rapidly absorbed carbon dioxide.

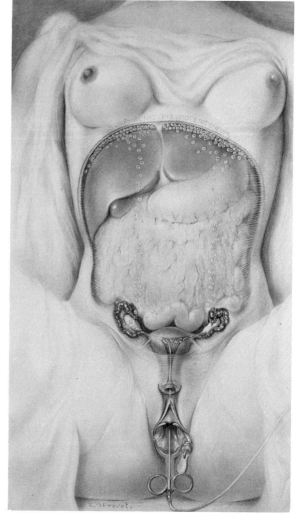

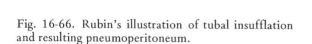

Fig. 16-66. Rubin's illustration of tubal insufflation and resulting pneumoperitoneum.

CONTRACEPTION

"The desire for [conception] control is neither time nor space bound. It is a universal characteristic of social life." (N.E. Himes: *Medical History of Contraception*. Gamut Press, New York, 1963, p. 55.)

Man's unbridled fertility has produced perhaps his most urgent problem. Of the earth's three billion inhabitants, more than one third are sorely malnourished for lack of food. Starvation takes its relentless toll of countless numbers. These underfed masses of the underprivileged and overpopulated areas refute the oft-repeated assurance, "if God sends another mouth to fill, He will find means to fill it." Since 1954 in the United States alone, more than 4.2 million live births have occurred each year, 11,520 each day, 480 each hour, 8 each minute. Almost 98 per cent of all liveborn infants now survive. At the current rate of increase of 1.3 per cent annually, the world's population will double in less than 35 years. Demographers, statesmen, theologians, physiologists, chemists, and physicians have joined hands at long last in a hopeful effort to stem this tide, which threatens to engulf mankind.

Thomas Robert Malthus (1766–1834),

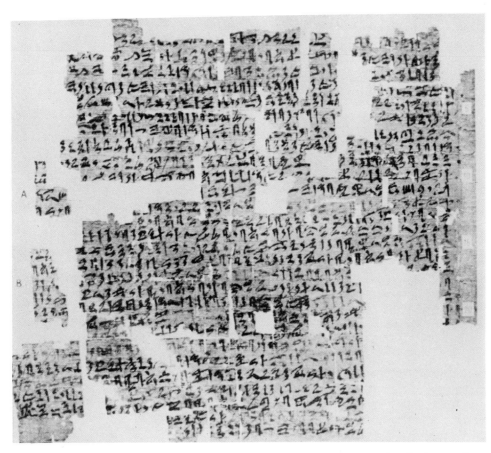

Fig. 16-67. The earliest known contraceptive prescriptions. From the Petrie Medical Papyrus, an ancient Egyptian manuscript of three large pages, 39½ inches by 12¾ inches, from 1950 BC or earlier. Found at Kahoun in 1889, it is known also as the Kahoun Papyrus. The third page, shown here, was reconstituted from 46 separate pieces. It contains 17 recipes for various gynecologic problems plus the single incantation in the papyrus. See also Fig. 19-1.

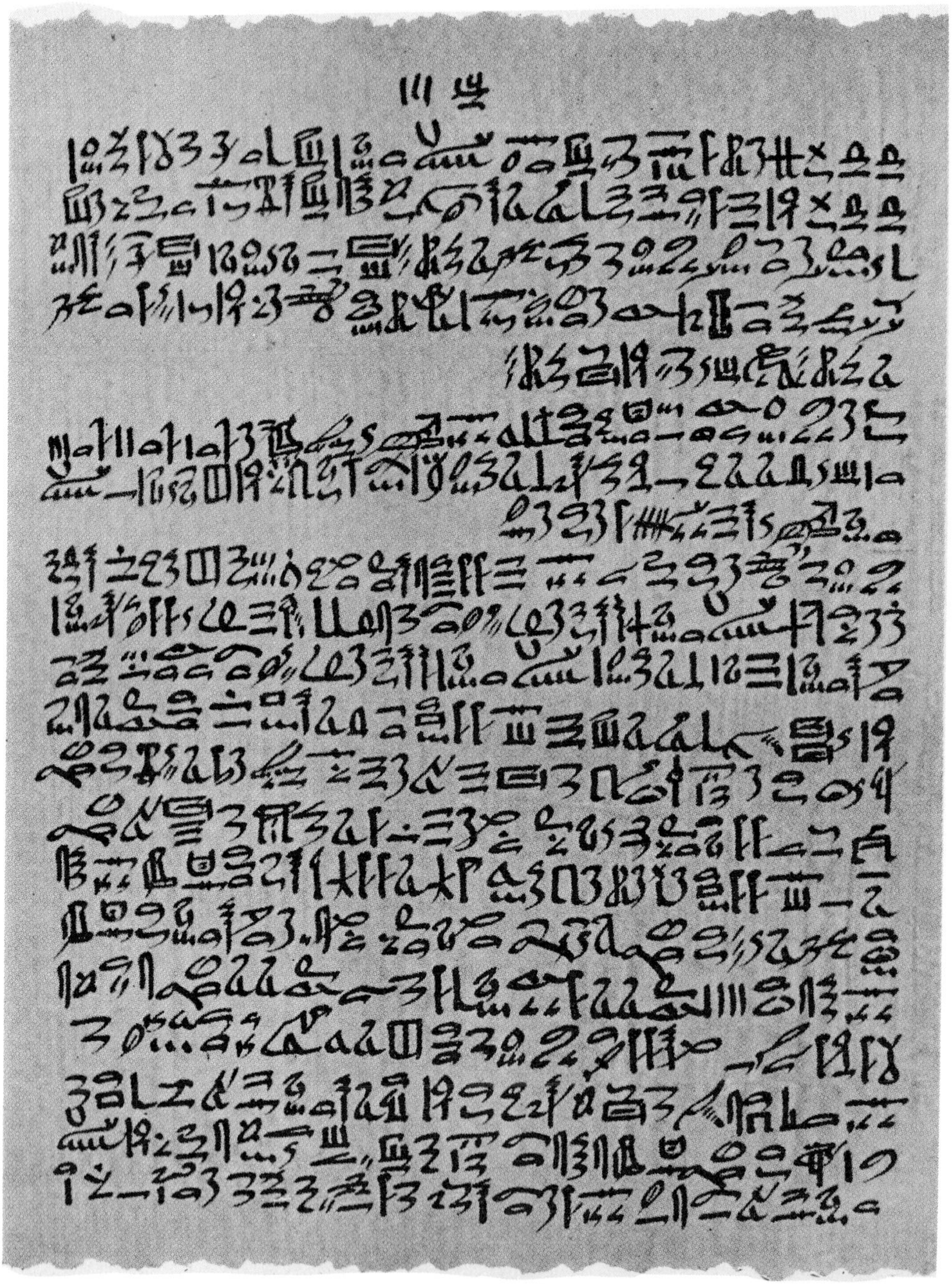

Fig. 16-68. Prescription for a medicated tampon to prevent conception. From the Ebers Papyrus, 1550 BC, a mixture of honey and the tips of the acacia shrub made into a vaginal suppository. A product of acacia's fermentation, lactic acid is an important spermicidal ingredient of several contraceptive jellies of the mid twentieth century.

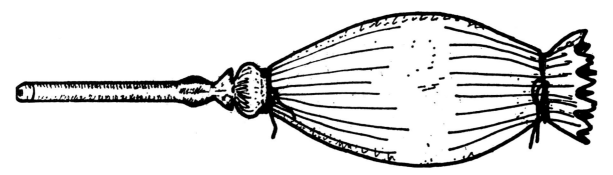

Fig. 16-69. A thirteenth century douche bag made of a sow's bladder with wooden nozzle attached. A popular but inefficient contraceptive device. From L. Heister's *A General System of Surgery*, London, 1743.

English clergyman turned economist, in his *Essay on the Principles of Population* published in 1798, called attention to the disparity between the geometric rate of population increase and the slower increase of the food supply. War and disease, he pointed out, were the only alternatives to voluntary limitation of family size. Extending the teachings of Malthus, the English sociologist Francis Place beginning in the 1820s advocated contraceptive measures for the restriction of population increase. His writing and lecturing, the beginning of the birth control movement, drew attention to contraception as a social issue. Place wrote,

"Many young men who fear the consequences which a large family produces, turn to debauchery, and destroy their own happiness as well as the happiness of the unfortunate girls with whom they connect themselves.

"Other young men, whose moral and religious feelings deter them from this vicious course, marry early and produce large families, which they are utterly unable to maintain.... But when it has become the custom ... to limit the number of children, so that none need have more than they wish to have, no man will fear to take a wife, all will be married while young—debauchery will diminish—while good morals, and religious duties will be promoted."

John Stuart Mill wrote a half-century later in his *Principles of Political Economy* (1848),

"There is room in the world, no doubt, and even in old countries, for a great increase of population, supposing the arts of life to go on improving, and capital to increase. But even if innocuous, I confess I see very little reason for desiring it. The density of population necessary to enable mankind to obtain, in the greatest degree, all the advantages both of co-operation and of social intercourse, has, in all the most populous countries, been attained. A population may be too crowded, though all be amply supplied with food and raiment. It is not good for man to be kept perforce at all times in the presence of his species. A world from which solitude is extirpated, is a very poor ideal. Solitude, in the sense of being often alone, is essential to any depth of meditation or of character; and solitude in the presence of natural beauty and grandeur, is the cradle of thoughts and aspirations which are not only good for the individual, but which society could ill do without. Nor is there much satisfaction in contemplating the world with nothing left to the spontaneous activity of nature; with every rood of land brought into cultivation, which is capable of growing food for human beings; every flowery waste or natural pasture ploughed up, all quadrupeds or birds which

De Morbo Gallico. 52

uerucam, & mediam partem glandis excessit: sed quia ego dixi quòd caries oritur per contagium. sciatis quòd etiam oriri solet ratione hæpatis transmittentis: dimittamus hanc secundam speciem loquamur de prima, atque quo iuuenis coiens cum infecta ab hac præseruetur, & cariem non sentiat.

De præseruatione à carie Gallica. CAP. LXXXVIIII.

Ego nihil fecisse uideor nisi doceam uos, quomodo quis uidens pulcherrimam sirenam, & coiens cum ea, etiam infecta, à carie, & lue Gallica præseruetur. Ego semper fui huius sententiæ, quòd adsit ratio præcauendi, ne per contagium, huiusmodi ulcera oriantur: sed quæ est ista ratio? Ego dixi quòd nascitur caries hæc per communicata corpuscula saniosa, quæ imbibita poris glandis faciunt cariem, ideò opus est, ut statim saniem a glãde expurgemus, sed si imbibita sit in poris licet uino, lotio, uel aqua detergamus priapum, tamen eam detergere non possumus. & hoc sæpe accidit in tectis, & mollibus glandibus. Quomodo ergo agendum? semper fui istius sententiæ, quòd ponamus aliquod habens uim penetrandi corium, & dissipande materiæ, uel extrahendæ, uel siccandæ & uincendæ natura sua. ideò inuestigaui hoc medicamentum. Sed quia oportet etiam Meretricum animos disponere, non licet nobiscum unguenta domo afferre. propterea ego inueni linteolum imbutum medicamento, quod potest commodè asportari, cum femoralia iam ita uasta feratis, ut totam apotecam uobiscum habere possitis: Quoties ergo quis coiuerit abluat (si potest) pudendum, uel panno detergat: postea habeat linteolum ad mensuram glandis præparatum; demum cum coiuerit ponat supra glandem, & recurrat præputium: si potest madere sputo, uel lotio bonum est, tamen non refert: si timetis, ne caries oriatur in medio canali, habeatis huius lintei inuolucrum, & in canali ponatis, ego feci experimentum in centum, & mille hominibus, & Deum testor immortalem nullum eorum infectum. Notate autem obiter, quòd quælibet species lienteoli mundi tantam habet uim in præseruatione, ut nihil magis [addite quòd gossipium nouum, molle, fidibus bene concussum glandi optimè lotæ detergentibus, obuolutum mirum in modũ præseruat. & quum quis Gallicis scopulis lignum percussit post ablationem inspiciat: uidebit enim inuolucrum illud saniosum, aut citrino, aut pallido, uel subnigro colore infectum] ideò semper quis paruo linteolo obuoluat glandem per spatium quatuor, aut quinque horarum, & hoc non est molestum mulieribus: sed tamen præparati lintei ratio est præstantissima. Præparatur autem hoc modo.

Nota de præseruatione.

Linteoli mundum. Gossipiũ.

Præparatio lintei.

Fig. 16-70. First published description of the linen sheath, forerunner of the condom. From *De morbo gallico* of Gabriele Falloppio, 1564. Penile sheaths were used initially for protection against venereal disease. Not until the eighteenth century did the membranous condom, usually fashioned from an animal's cecum, become popular for contraception.

With the vulcanization of rubber in 1884 contraception achieved an explosive popularity because of the sudden cheapness of the new product which virtually replaced its membranous antecedent. At mid-twentieth century the condom was the most widely used of all artificial contraceptives.

are not domesticated for man's use exterminated as his rivals for food, every hedgerow or superfluous tree rooted out, and scarcely a place left where a wild shrub or flower could grow without being eradicated as a weed in the name of improved agriculture. If the earth must lose that great portion of its pleasantness which it owes to things that the unlimited increase of wealth and population would extirpate from it, for the mere purpose of enabling it to support a larger, but not a better or a happier population, I sincerely hope, for the sake of posterity, that they will be content to be stationary, long before necessity compels them to it."

In primitive societies contraception was probably of little importance. Pregnancy was prevented by sexual taboos, and unwanted issue were eliminated by abortion or infanticide, accepted by most of the early Greek philosophers as essential to the ideal state. The earliest known formulas for the prevention of conception are found in the Petri Papyrus, written in ancient Egypt nearly 4000 years ago, about 1950 BC. Recommended among other prescriptions were contraceptive pessaries of crocodile dung and honey and vaginal fumigations with minnis, an ancient drug. Two thousand years later Soranus of Ephesus advocated, as a barrier to conception, mixtures of honey or cedar wood oil with figs or pomegranate pulp. Blossoms of the palash flower, mentioned as an orally effective contraceptive in the *Kama-Sutra*, a fourth century Hindu love manual, were tested on rats by the Indian Council for Medical Research in the 1960s and found to prevent conception in 80 per cent of the animals.

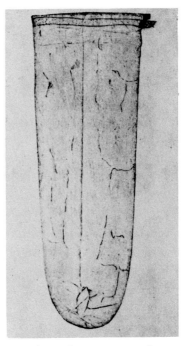

Fig. 16-71. Eighteenth century condom, 9½ x 3 in, made from the cecum of a sheep.

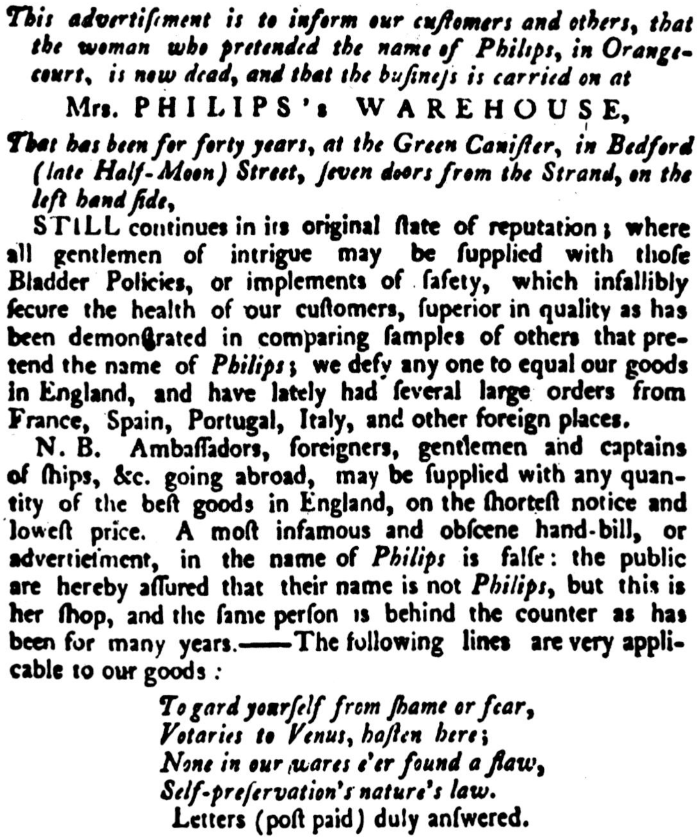

This advertisement is to inform our customers and others, that the woman who pretended the name of Philips, in Orange-court, is now dead, and that the business is carried on at

Mrs. PHILIPS's WAREHOUSE,

That has been for forty years, at the Green Canister, in Bedford (late Half-Moon) Street, seven doors from the Strand, on the left hand side,

STILL continues in its original state of reputation; where all gentlemen of intrigue may be supplied with those Bladder Policies, or implements of safety, which infallibly secure the health of our customers, superior in quality as has been demonstrated in comparing samples of others that pretend the name of *Philips*; we defy any one to equal our goods in England, and have lately had several large orders from France, Spain, Portugal, Italy, and other foreign places.

N. B. Ambassadors, foreigners, gentlemen and captains of ships, &c. going abroad, may be supplied with any quantity of the best goods in England, on the shortest notice and lowest price. A most infamous and obscene hand-bill, or advertisement, in the name of *Philips* is false: the public are hereby assured that their name is not *Philips*, but this is her shop, and the same person is behind the counter as has been for many years.——The following lines are very applicable to our goods:

To gard yourself from shame or fear,
Votaries to Venus, hasten here;
None in our wares e'er found a flaw,
Self-preservation's nature's law.
Letters (post paid) duly answered.

Fig. 16-72. An eighteenth century advertisement of condoms.

TO
THE MARRIED OF BOTH SEXES
IN
Genteel Life.

Among the many sufferings of married women, as mothers, there are two cases which command the utmost sympathy and commiseration.

The first arises from constitutional peculiarities, or weaknesses.

The second from mal-conformation of the bones of the Pelvis.

Besides these two cases, there is a third case applicable to both sexes: namely, the consequences of having more children than the income of the parents enables them to maintain and educate in a desirable manner.

The first named case produces miscarriages, and brings on a state of existence scarcely endurable. It has caused thousands of respectable women to linger on in pain and apprehension, till at length, death has put an end to their almost inconceivable sufferings.

The second case is always attended with immediate risk of life. Pregnancy never terminates without intense suffering, seldom without the death of the child, frequently with the death of the mother, and sometimes with the death of both mother and child.

The third case is by far the most common, and the most open to general observation. In the middle ranks, the most virtuous and praiseworthy efforts are perpetually made to keep up the respectability of the family; but a continual increase of children gradually yet certainly renders every effort to prevent degradation unavailing, it paralizes by rendering hopeless all exertion, and the family sinks into poverty and despair. Thus is engendered and perpetuated a hideous mass of misery.

The knowledge of what awaits them deters vast numbers of young men from marrying and causes them to spend the best portion of their lives in a state of debauchery, utterly incompatible with the honourable and honest feelings which should be the characteristic of young men. The treachery, duplicity, and hypocrisy, they use towards their friends and the unfortunate victims of their seductions, while they devote a large number of females to the most dreadful of all states which human beings can endure extinguishes in them to a very great extent, all manly, upright notions; and qualifies them to as great an extent, for the commission of acts which but for these vile practices they would abhor, and thus to an enormous extent is the whole community injured.

Marriage in early life, is the only truly happy state, and if the evil consequences of too large a family did not deter them, all men would marry while young, and thus would many lamentable evils be removed from society.

A simple, effectual, and safe means of accomplishing these desirable results has long been known, and to a considerable extent practised in some places. But until lately has been but little known in this country. Accoucheurs of the first respectability and surgeons of great eminence have in some peculiar cases recommended it. Within the last two years, a more extensive knowledge of the process has prevailed and its practice has been more extensively adopted. It is now made public for the benefit of every body. A piece of soft sponge about the size of a small ball attached to a very narrow ribbon, and slightly moistened (when convenient) is introduced previous to sexual intercourse, and is afterwards withdrawn, and thus by an easy, simple, cleanly and not indelicate method, no ways injurious to health, not only may much unhappiness and many miseries be prevented, but benefits to an incalculable amount be conferred on society.

Fig. 16-73. A handbill distributed by Francis Place, 1823, advocating contraception as a safeguard to family life. "A piece of soft sponge ... slightly moistened ... is introduced previous to sexual intercourse, and is afterwards withdrawn ..."

Advocates of artificial control of conception, traditionally opposed by the Catholic Church, received hearty encouragement in 1958 by the Lambeth Conference of Bishops of the Anglican Communion. These churchmen resolved,

"The responsibility for deciding upon the number and frequency of children has been laid by God upon the consciences of parents everywhere ... the means of family planning are in large measure matters of clinical and aesthetic choice ... scientific studies can rightly help, and do, in assessing the effects and usefulness of any particular means; and Christians have every right to use the gifts of science for proper ends."

By the end of 1971 contraceptive advice was being offered by the International Planned Parenthood Federation in 109 countries, on every continent. In the United States during the year 1970, 620 Planned Parenthood-World Population clinics provided contraceptive service for 407,000 women. At the same time, however, about three-fourths of the medically indigent women of this favored land still lacked counsel in the principles and techniques of family planning.

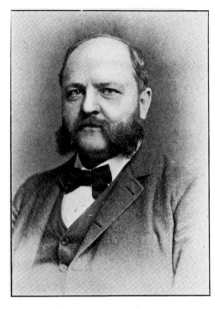

Fig. 16-74. Anthony Comstock (1844–1915). Anti-sin crusader for whom the federal postal law of 1873 prohibiting the dissemination of birth control information and contraceptive materials through the United States mail was named. Later, as a special agent of the Post Office he ordered the destruction of 160 tons of contraceptive literature, which he branded as "lewd, lascivious, and obscene."

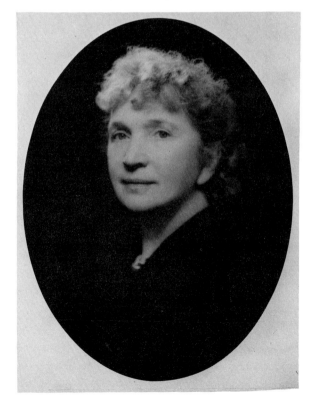

Fig. 16-75. Margaret Higgins Sanger (1883–1966). Leading lay advocate of contraception in America, she founded its first birth control clinic in the Brownsville section of Brooklyn, New York in 1916. Later she helped organize birth control organizations throughout the world. At her death in 1966 the Planned Parenthood Federation, sparked by her, had spread to 88 countries. Named for her, the Planned Parenthood Federation's Margaret Sanger Research Bureau in New York City by 1966 was giving contraceptive advice to more than 2,000 new applicants each year, providing counsel to over 500 infertile couples and premarital guidance to nearly 1,000, and operating a laboratory for evaluation of new contraceptives.

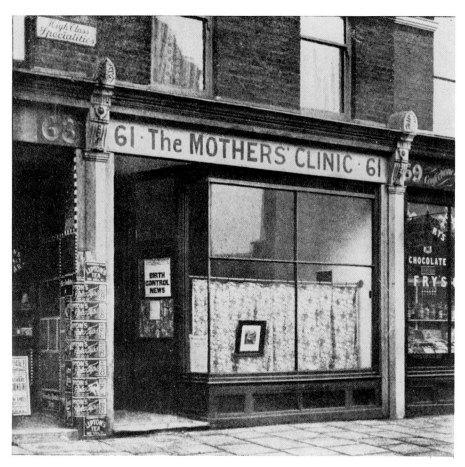

Fig. 16-76. The first British birth control clinic, established in 1921 by Marie Carmichael Stopes and her husband H. V. Roe at 61 Marlborough Road, Holloway, London, where counsel in contraception was offered to,

"(a) All women who have experienced serious shock or danger in childbirth,
(b) All parents who are obviously suffering from hereditary disease or defect or too debilitated,
(c) All married people whose economic conditions obviously preclude their doing justice to more children,
(d) All married men and women who ask for it."

Not until 44 years later in 1965 did the Supreme Court of the United States make such clinics possible everywhere in this country when it declared unconstitutional Connecticut's law banning the dissemination of contraceptive advice.

Fig. 16-77. Vaginal contraceptive devices. Early twentieth century. (1) Cervical occlusive cap with inflated rim. (2–3) Cervical occlusive caps with solid rim. (4) Dutch cap with metal spring. (5) Mizpah cap. (6) "Pro Race" cervical cap. (7) Dumas cap. (8) Sponge-covered cap. (9) Matrisalus cap. (10) Female sheath or *Capote anglaise*.

FERTILITY AND ITS CONTROL 449

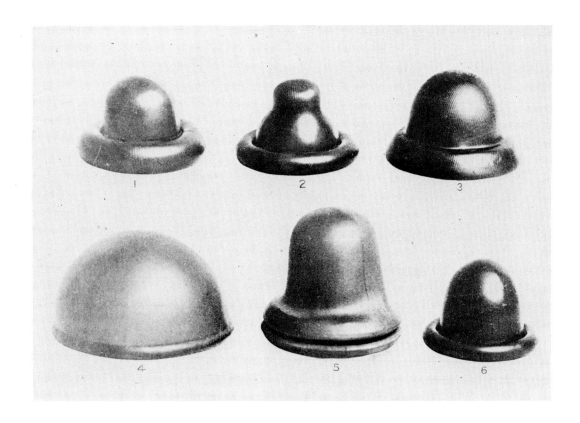

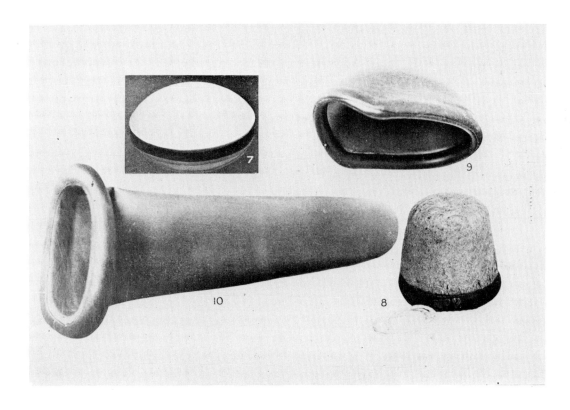

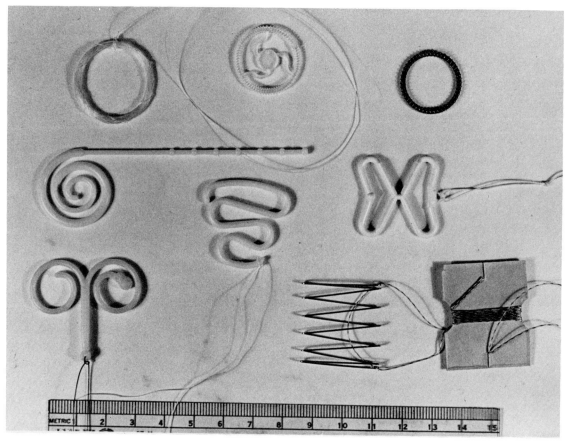

Fig. 16-78. Intrauterine contraceptive devices. In 1930 Ernst Gräfenberg, a German gynecologist, devised a flexible silver ring for insertion into the uterus to prevent conception. The Gräfenberg ring found little favor and was greeted with scorn in most medical circles. Three of Gräfenberg's associates, Herbert H. Hall, later of New York, W. Oppenheimer of Israel, and Atsumi Ishihama of Japan, experimented further with intrauterine contraceptives. From their efforts evolved a variety of devices, rings, loops, and bows of stainless steel or plastic, which can be retained within the uterus for indefinite periods by most women. Complications are occasional, failures, few, and mode of action, mysterious. Top from left, Zipper ring (Jaime Zipper), Ota ring (Tenrei Takeo Ota), Hall-Stone ring (Herbert H. Hall and Martin L. Stone); middle from left, Margulies spiral (Lazar C. Margulies), Lippes loop (Jack Lippes), Birnberg bow (Charles H. Birnberg); bottom from left, *Saf-T Coil* (invented by Ralph Robinson, manufactured by Deseret Pharmaceuticals, distributed by Julius Schmid Pharmaceuticals), Majzlin spring (Gregory Majzlin).

Fig. 16-79. Tubal sterilization. Illustrations of some common methods from R. L. Dickinson and L. S. Bryant: *Control of Conception*, 1932. Dickinson and C. J. Gamble in 1950 wrote in their monograph *Human Sterilization* that the field for sterilization includes,

"all those who because of heredity and physical condition are totally unfit to have children, as well as those parents for whom another child would be very unwise, or an actual danger, and who lack intelligence or persistence to use other means of control."

In women, termination of the reproductive capacity is accomplished most simply and with least disturbance of other functions by bilateral division of the fallopian tubes. James Blundell first recommended this procedure in the early nineteenth century as a means of preventing the hazards of dystocia in women with contracted pelvis. Cesarean section, because of its high mortality, had not yet been embraced by the obstetrician. Blundell wrote,

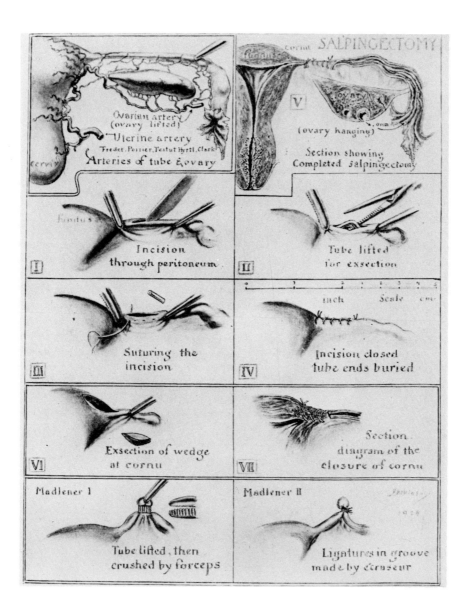

"If the pelvis be contracted in so high a degree that parturition, by the natural passages, is impossible ... the shortest way to avoid the necessity of the operation [cesarean section], would be by abstinence altogether from intercourse with the other sex. The most solid resolution, however, may sometimes thaw; and when a woman is married, she may be placed under those circumstances in which it is not very easy to adhere to this advice, her life perhaps falling a sacrifice to her neglect.... If a woman were in that condition, in which delivery could not take place by the natural passage ... I would advise an incision of an inch in length in the linea alba above the symphysis pubis ... that the fallopian tube on either side should be drawn up to this aperture ... that a portion of the tube should be removed, an operation easily performed, when the woman would for ever after, be sterile." [J. Blundell: *The Principles and Practice of Obstetricy,* T. Castle, ed. E. Cox, London, 1834, 579–80.]

CHASTITY BELTS

In the years of the Crusades when women were viewed as private property, men designed belts and girdles for their wives, mistresses, and unmarried daughters to be worn during their master's absence to frustrate the advances of other men. Known as chastity belts or girdles of chastity, they were made of metal, covered in part by leather, and worn in such a manner as to guard the entrances to the vagina and rectum. A probable forerunner of these devices in the form of a pudendal shield called *kumaz* is mentioned in the Bible (Exodus 35:22 and Numbers 31:50) and in the tractate Sabbath of the Talmud and is described by Rashi in his commentary as an "ornament in the form of the womb, worn by the women upon their flesh." European models of these shields, fashioned after their oriental counterparts, were designed as guards rather than ornaments.

The chastity belt consisted of a waistband from which was suspended a metal plate, more often two, fore and aft, connected at a joint between the wearer's legs. In each plate was a small serrated opening which provided a portal of egress for the bladder, bowel, and uterus but prevented the approach of a man. Secured with a lock, the plates could be removed only at the pleasure of the keyholder. In this way some Medieval men guarded the chastity of their women. As recently as December 1933 the League of Awakened Magyars advocated, as Point 19 of their National Program, that all unmarried Hungarian girls of age 12 or older be required to wear a chastity girdle, the father or other competent authority maintaining custody of the key.

Fig. 16-80. Chastity belts. The lower one consists of a serrated ivory plate fastened to a leather-covered steel belt closed by a lock.

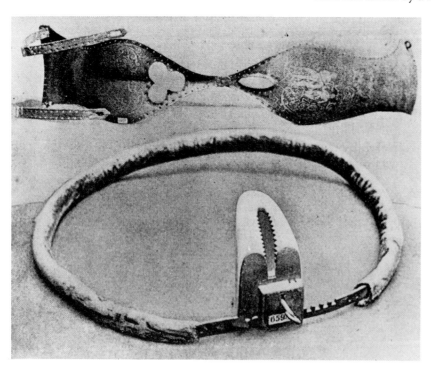

FERTILITY AND ITS CONTROL 453

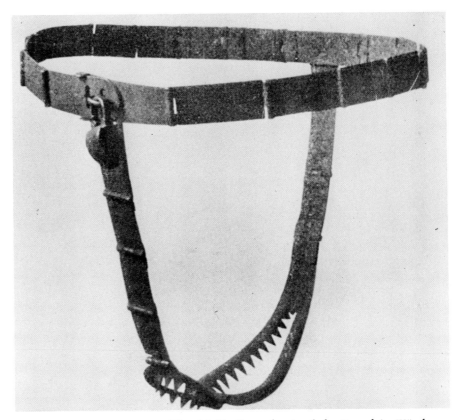

Fig. 16-81. Iron chastity belt. Found in Würzburg, Germany, 1885.

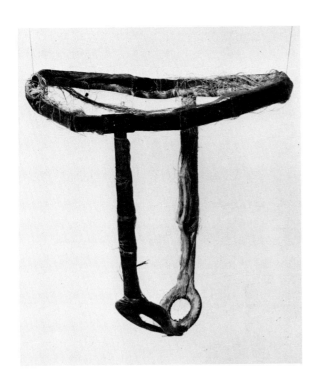

Fig. 16-82. Leather-covered chastity belt.

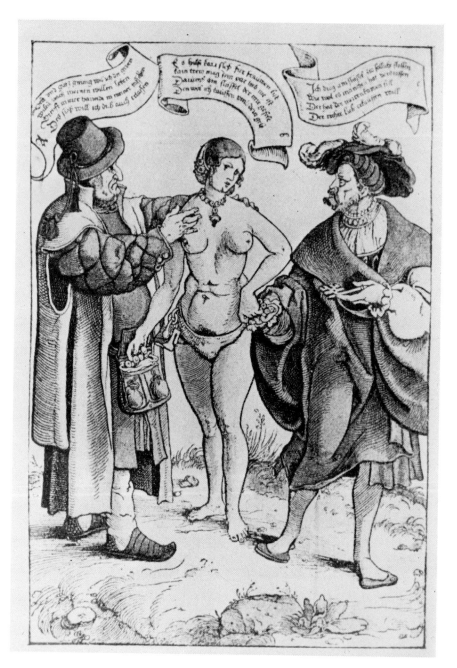

Fig. 16-83. The girdle of chastity. Sixteenth century woodcut attributed to Heinrich Vogtherr (1490–1556). With one hand the woman, wearing a chastity belt, is taking money from the purse of the man on her right, who fondles her, while with the other hand she gives the coins to the man on her left who holds the girdle's key. To the latter she says,

It boots no key 'against wifely art,
No faith can be where love's apart,
And the key which now you hold,
That I will buy and with thy gold.

Chapter 17

GYNECOLOGY

An essential part of modern gynecology is its surgery. Surgical operations may be grouped into three general categories—diagnostic, extirpative, and reparative. The principal distinctive operations of gynecology thus comprise (1) uterine curettage, (2) the excision of genital neoplasms and the aftermath of pelvic inflammations, and (3) the repair of genital relaxations, hernias, and childbirth injuries, including fistulas.

Although minor operations on the female genitalia date back to antiquity, gynecology remained an essentially nonsurgical discipline until the nineteenth century and gynecologic operations were rare until its latter decades. From 1848 to 1851, for example, not a single gynecologic surgical procedure was performed at the New York Hospital. Even a quarter century later, in the year 1874, New York's Presbyterian Hospital reported all its gynecologic cases from its medical division, none from its surgical.

The earliest gynecologic instruments from the Hippocratic era and before consisted of dilators and speculums for intravaginal fumigation and medication and pessaries for the correction of uterine prolapse. Galen, in the second century AD, attributed virtually every type of female complaint to uterine displacement. Amputation of the completely prolapsed cervix was undertaken occasionally in the seventeenth and eighteenth centuries, but abdominal surgery was out of the question. Indeed, hysterectomy was believed incompatible with survival until 1768 when Joseph Cavallini, having successfully excised the uteri of pregnant dogs and sheep, speculated that future generations would demonstrate that the womb "may be plucked out with impunity from the human body."

Physicians seldom discovered organic gynecologic disease early until the mid nineteenth century, for they subjected women to the embarrassment of an internal examination only when urgently indicated, and even then under drapes that concealed the patient's genitalia from the examiner's eyes. Inflammations of the genital organs were commonly treated by the application of leeches to the cervix.

The modern era of gynecologic surgery began a few days before Christmas, 1809, when Mrs. Jane Crawford set out on her fateful ride some 60 miles on horseback to her rendezvous with Dr. Ephraim McDowell. Throughout the preceding century, wrote Sir Thomas Spencer Wells, "surgeons stood and trembled on the brink of ovarian waters." Ovarian cysts had been regarded as incurable. Uniform fatality had been the result in the few cases in which excision was attempted. To withdraw, by tapping, the rapidly reaccumulating fluid could offer the hapless sufferer only temporary palliation. One case report tells of a patient whose cyst was tapped 299 times for the removal of 9867 pounds of fluid. An attitude of fatalism toward ovarian cysts prevailed until McDowell's successful operation on Mrs. Crawford. This marked the birth of abdominal surgery. Encouraged by McDowell's triumph, others cautiously attempted ovarian excision, especially in England, and by the middle of the nineteenth century the operation was an established procedure. Known initially as *ovariotomy*, it has since been superseded by the etymologically and surgically correct term, *oophorectomy*.

Just as Ephraim McDowell was to be named the founder of abdominal surgery, James Marion Sims came to be known as the father of American gynecology. For centuries physicians had struggled with vesicovaginal fistulas, exhausting their ingenuity on countless mechanical devices and surgical procedures in efforts, usually vain, to reclaim those social outcasts, victims of childbirth injuries, who soon became a source of disgust even to themselves, unable to escape from the uriniferous odor in which they were constantly steeped.

Hendrik van Roonhuyze in one of the earliest texts on operative gynecology published in 1663 and translated into English in 1676 under the title *Medico-Chirurgical Observations,* suggested a method for the cure of vesicovaginal fistula, by exposure of the fistula with a speculum, denudation of the fistula's margins, and approximation of the denuded edges with stiff swan's quills. Although van Roonhuyze may never have performed the operation himself, cures by this technique were probably achieved by Johann Fatio in 1675 and 1684, as evidenced by a posthumous report in 1752. Ignorant of asepsis, without benefit of anesthesia, and with poor exposure, inadequate instruments, and faulty suture material, however, only rarely were surgeons successful in their attempts at fistula repair. Velpeau in his *Operative Surgery* lamented,

"To abrade the borders of an opening when we do not know where to grasp them, to shut it up by means of needles or threads when we have no point apparently to sustain them, to act upon a movable partition placed between two cavities hidden from our sight, and upon which we can scarcely find any purchase, has appeared to be calculated to have no other result than to cause unnecessary suffering to the patient." [*New Elements of Operative Surgery,* first American from last Paris edition, P. S. Townsend, trans., Samuel S. & William Wood, New York, 1847.]

Attacking the problem freshly in 1845 Sims, a young physician in Montgomery, Alabama, began a series of surgical experiments on the now legendary slaves Anarcha, Betsy, and Lucy. After repeated failures, about 40 in number, the persistent Sims with the aid of silver sutures, the rediscovered knee-chest position, and a vaginal speculum subsequently named for him, developed a successful technique for vesicovaginal fistula repair. Sims reported his historic achievement in 1852, moved to New York the following year, and in 1855 founded a hospital for women, the forerunner of the Woman's Hospital of the State of New York. Here Sims and his colleagues Thomas Addis Emmet, E. R. Peaslee, and T. Gaillard Thomas achieved a brilliant record for their fistula repairs and vaginal plastic operations. Gynecology had become a surgical specialty.

THE VAGINAL SPECULUM

This device, in many forms, has been used for both inspecting and dilating the vagina. The Talmud instructs women in the use of a tube through which a cotton-tipped rod can be passed into the vagina to ascertain the presence of blood. Earliest of the known speculums are the bronze instruments among the surgical paraphernalia recovered from the ruins of Pompeii which was destroyed in AD 79.

GYNECOLOGY 457

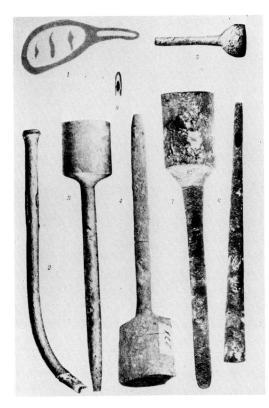

Fig. 17-1. Uterine drainage tubes and vaginal irrigators. From the Hippocratic period.

Fig. 17-2. Surgical and gynecological instruments found at Pompeii. At right, a four-bladed vaginal speculum operated by a central screw. Alongside it, a speculum with three blunt blades and a central screw mechanism, the prototype of many later models. Museo Nazionale, Naples.

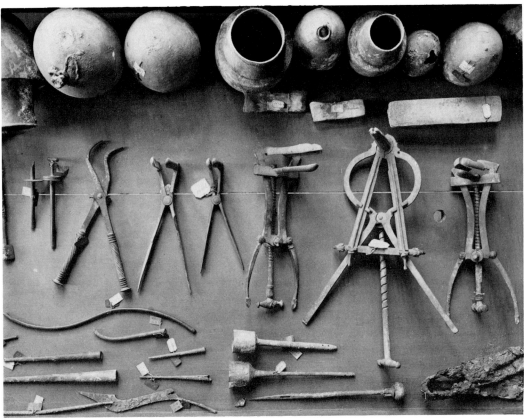

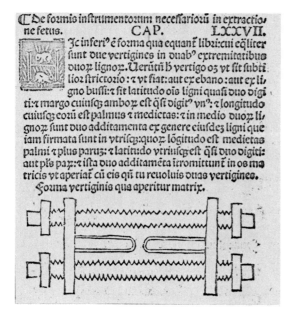

Fig. 17-3. Wooden dilator of Abulcasis (936–1013). Pictured in a manuscript of Guy de Chauliac, 1500. This figure appeared in chapter 77 of Abulcasis' manuscript ("Instrument for extracting the fetus") and bore the caption, "A type of screw for opening the uterus."

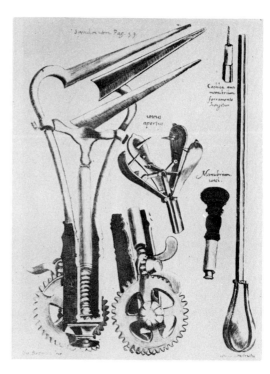

Fig. 17-4. Vaginal speculum and tenaculum. Illustrated by Fabricius ab Aquapendente (1537–1619).

Fig. 17-5. Vaginal speculum, nineteenth century. Used for the application of leeches to the cervix in the treatment of pelvic inflammation.

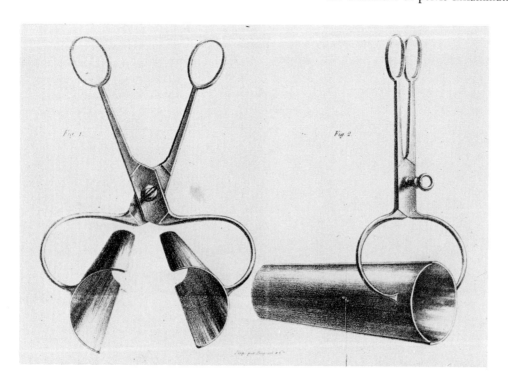

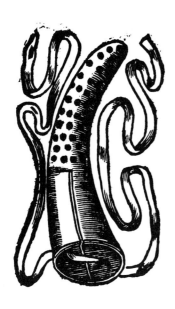 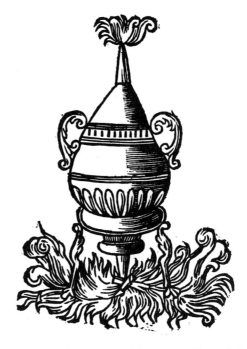

Fig. 17-6. Perforated canister for the intravaginal application of perfumes, left, and kettle for fumigating the uterus, right. From Mercurio's *La Comare,* 1596.

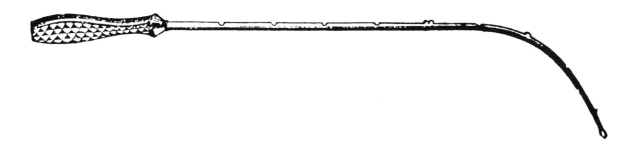

Fig. 17-7. The uterine sound of James Young Simpson (1811–1870). Its uses:

"I. The Sound increases to a great degree our power of making a perfect and precise tactile examination of the Fundus, Body, and Cervix of the Uterus . . . [by] giving sufficient *resistance* to the organ for its exploration by the fingers; and . . . of altering the *position* of its parts, so as to bring them each successively within the reach of tactile examination. . . . II. The previous introduction of the Sound facilitates and simplifies the subsequent visual examination of the Cervix Uteri with the Speculum. . . . After making such tactile examination as may be required with the sound, leave it in the uterine cavity, and using it as a general guide, slip the uterine extremity of the speculum, whether tubular or bladed, over its handle and along its stem, till the instrument be fully introduced. . . . III. By the use of the Uterine Sound we may, in many instances of Pelvic and Hypogastric or Abdominal Tumors, ascertain the connection or nonconnection of these Tumors with the Uterus." [*The Obstetric Memoirs and Contributions of James Y. Simpson, M.D., F.R.S.E.,* W. O. Priestly and H. R. Storer, eds., J. B. Lippincott, Philadelphia, 1855, 60–69.]

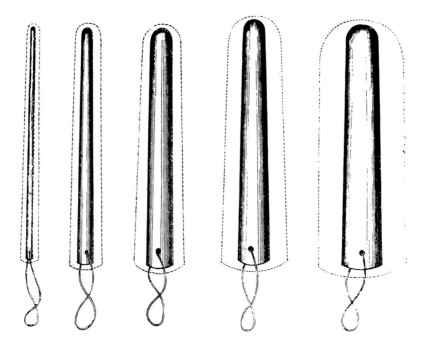

Fig. 17-8. Tupelo tents made from the spongy wood of the roots of the tree *Nyssa uniflora* or related species. The dotted lines indicate the tent's size after expansion which resulted from fluid absorption while in the cervix.

CERVICAL DILATORS

Graduated dilators for introducing medicaments into the uterus were described in the writings of Hippocrates. Made of tin or lead, they were hollow at one end and mounted on long wooden handles. Sponges, laminaria, and tupelo tents were subsequently used as cervical dilators to alleviate dysmenorrhea or produce abortion, as well as to permit access to the uterine cavity. Advocated T. Gaillard Thomas, Professor of Gynecology in New York's College of Physicians and Surgeons, in one of his popular clinics in 1873, for a girl of 17 years suffering from dysmenorrhea,

"She should be put under an anesthetic and a delicate sponge tent introduced into the uterus, and left there for 4 days. It should then be replaced by another a little larger and this should be left in position for 4 days. This should be followed by a still larger one and so on until the uterus is dilated. The irritation brought on by this will cause congestion of the uterus and increased nutrition."

From this type of treatment severe parametritis often resulted. The sponges and laminary tents of yesteryear have been superseded by steel dilators of two principal types, named for Alfred Hegar (1830–1914) and William Goodell (1829–1894).

GYNECOLOGY 461

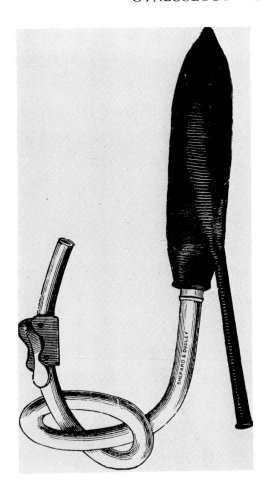

Fig. 17-9. Emmet's water dilator. A distensible rubber bag designed by Thomas Addis Emmet (1820–1919) for dilating the cervix.

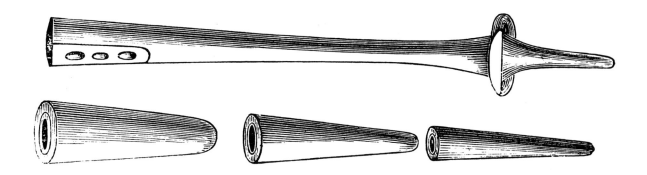

Fig. 17-10. Tait's dilators. Graduated vulcanite cones attached to a perforated handle, designed by Robert Lawson Tait (1845–1899). Elastic bands which passed through the perforations in the handle and attached to a belt around the patient's waist caused the cone to advance gradually into the cervix.

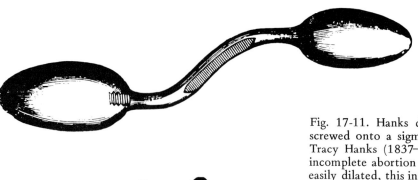

Fig. 17-11. Hanks dilator. Graduated metal ovoids screwed onto a sigmoid handle, designed by Horace Tracy Hanks (1837–1900). Used chiefly in cases of incomplete abortion in which the cervix was soft and easily dilated, this instrument permitted digital access to the uterine cavity.

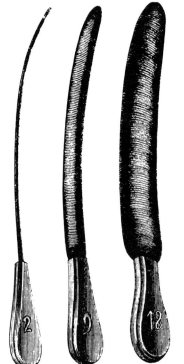

Fig. 17-12. Hegar dilators. Named for Alfred Hegar (1830–1914), German gynecologist.

Fig. 17-13. Goodell dilator. Named for William Goodell (1829–1894), modification of an earlier model by Leopold Ellinger, nineteenth century German gynecologist.

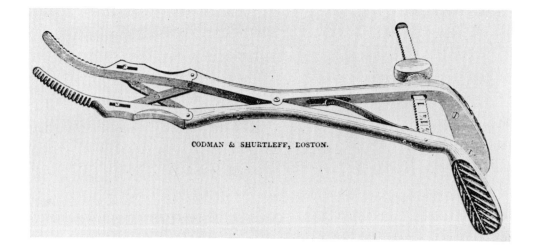

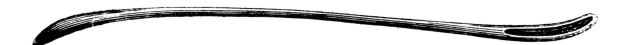

Fig. 17-14. The original uterine curette introduced in 1843 by Joseph Claude Anthelme Récamier (1774–1852). He used the instrument, a small scoop attached to a long handle, to scrape *fungous growths* from the endometrial cavity in cases of metrorrhagia. The operation he called *curettage*.

UTERINE DISPLACEMENTS

Prolapse. Many treatments have been used for uterine prolapse: manual reposition, vaginal tamponade, the wearing of utero-abdominal supporters, the insertion of pessaries of countless shapes, the application of astringents, cold sitz baths, sea water douches, postural exercises, and leeching. The Ebers Papyrus (about 1550 BC) prescribed a paste of honey and other ingredients to be smeared on the fallen womb before its replacement within the vagina. Recommended also to facilitate reposition was that an ibis of wax be heated on coals, and that the fumes thereof be permitted to penetrate into the woman's sex organs. Aretaeus the Cappadocian (AD 81-138), discussed prolapse of the womb in his book *Chronic Diseases*.

"The whole uterus is protruded from its seat and lodged between the woman's thighs—an incredible affliction.... It takes place from abortion, great concussions, and laborious parturition.... If it does not prove fatal, the woman lives for a long time, seeing parts that ought not to be seen, and nursing externally and fondling the womb.... Sometimes the mouth of the womb only, as far as its neck, protrudes, and retreats inwardly if the uterus be made to smell a fetid fumigation, and the woman also attracts it in if she herself smells fragrant odors. But by the hands of the midwife it readily returns inward when gently pressed, if anointed beforehand with the emollient plaster...."

Similarly varied in the treatment of prolapse were the surgical measures of the nineteenth and early twentieth centuries which included shortening of the round ligaments, scarification of the vagina, partial colpocleisis, suturing together of the labia majora, cervical amputation, several types of colporrhaphy, uterine ventro-fixation, interposition operations, and hysterectomy, both vaginal and abdominal. Alwin Mackenrodt (1859–1925) made a major contribution toward an understanding of uterine prolapse with his anatomic studies of the pelvic fascia, published in 1895. His recognition of the importance of the cardinal ligaments led to the utilization of these structures by William Edward Fothergill (1865–1926) in the procedure that came to be known as the Manchester operation. It shares with vaginal hysterectomy, in the late twentieth century, the foremost position in the surgical treatment of uterine descensus.

Inversion. Rarer than prolapse and occasionally fatal is uterine inversion, usually an accident of parturition. Repositors of various design were used during the nineteenth century to replace the inverted womb when manual efforts failed.

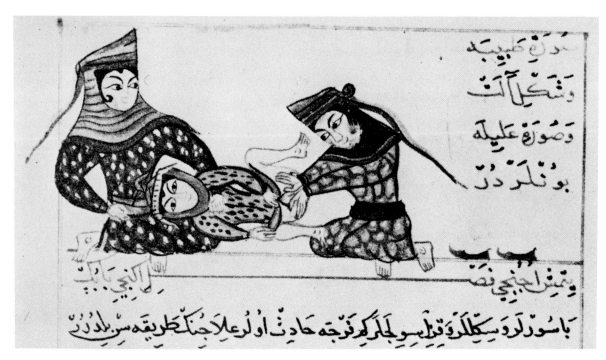

Fig. 17-15. Reduction of a prolapsed uterus by an Arabian midwife. Illustration from the 1465 Turkish surgical manuscript of Charaf Ed-Din.

Fig. 17-16. The treatment of uterine prolapse as illustrated in the sixteenth century German manuscript of Caspar Stromayr. The examination.

Fig. 17-17. The reposition of uterine prolapse, from Stromayr's manuscript.

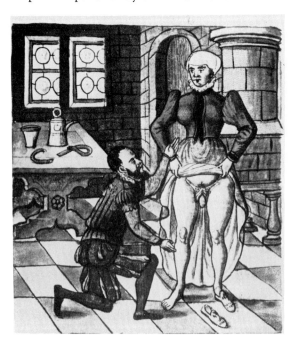

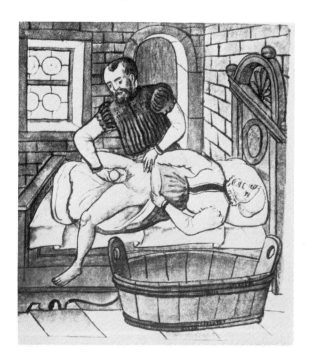

GYNECOLOGY 465

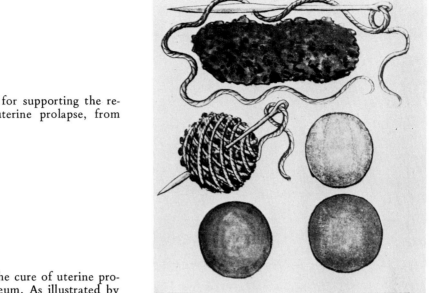

Fig. 17-18. Vaginal tampons for supporting the replaced uterus in cases of uterine prolapse, from Stromayr's manuscript.

Fig. 17-19. Instruments for the cure of uterine prolapse and repair of the perineum. As illustrated by Pierre Dionis, 1708.

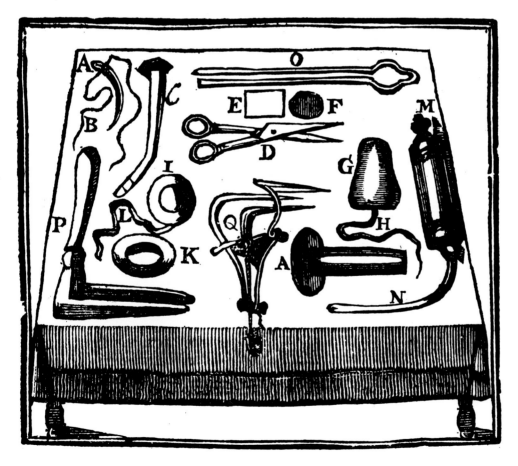

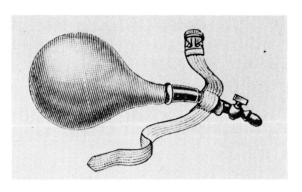

Fig. 17-21. Colpeurynter of Carl Braun (1822–1891). The bag, well greased and containing about an ounce of water, was introduced into the vagina, then distended with air. Thus inflated, it supported the uterus within the vagina and was less likely to produce vaginal ulceration than were various other pessaries.

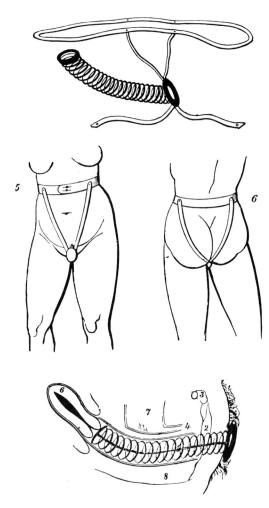

Fig. 17-20. Pessary designed by Charles Clay in 1842 for the alleviation of uterine prolapse. A silver wire coil covered with oiled silk held the uterus in proper position and was itself secured by four straps attached to a waist belt

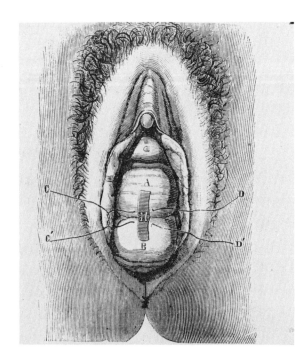

Fig. 17-22. Illustration of partial colpocleisis for uterine prolapse by Léon Le Fort (1829–1893). From his paper of 1877 showing a stage in the operation that bears his name.

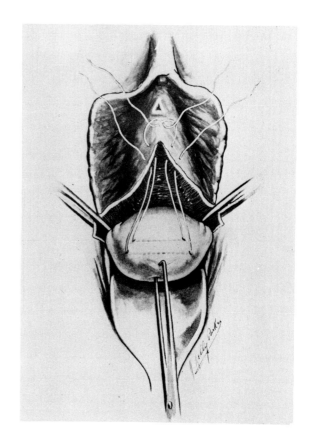

Fig. 17-23. Illustration from the 1906 paper of Thomas James Watkins (1863–1925) showing a step in his interposition operation.

Fig. 17-24. Inversion of the uterus in coronal section. Illustration from an essay by John Green Crosse, 1845–1847.

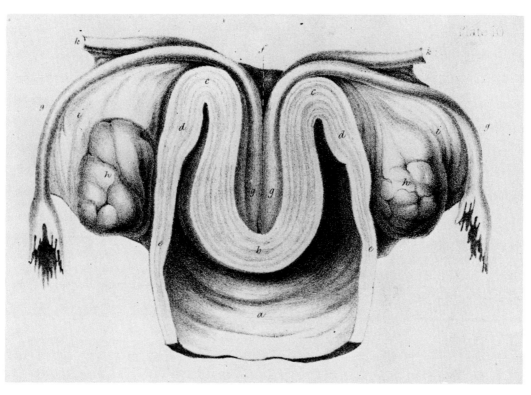

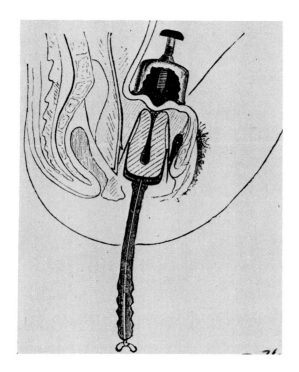

Fig. 17-25. Byrne's repositor. A piston in the lower cup pushed the uterine fundus up while a bell-shaped instrument with screw adjustment, applied against the abdominal wall, made counterpressure and dilated the cervix from above.

Fig. 17-26. White's repositor. This nineteenth century instrument for the correction of uterine inversion consisted of a rubber cap attached by a stiff metal rod to a spiral spring. The cup was placed against the fundus of the inverted uterus, the spring, against the chest of the operator who was thus able to apply continuous pressure while manipulating the uterus back into place.

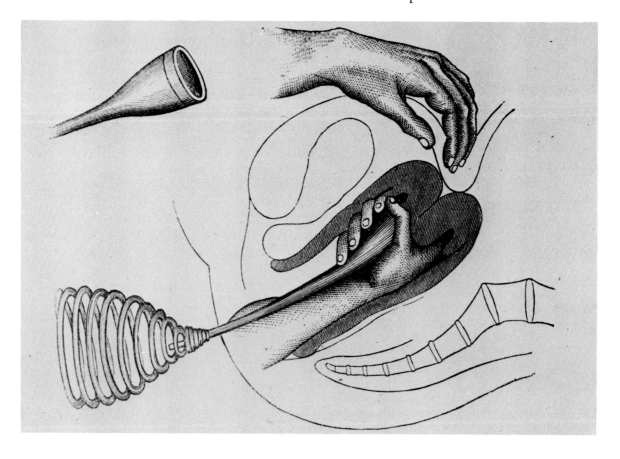

Retroversion. Long forgotten or ignored, Galen's belief that displacements of the uterus are the principal cause of women's complaints was revived toward the middle of the nineteenth century when female ills of all sorts were interpreted as *uterine sympathies.* Much of gynecologic practice then focussed on the correction of uterine retroversion by the insertion of various vaginal and uterine devices.

The vaginal pessary is among the oldest of all medical instruments; no one knows when the first was invented. Pessaries have been fashioned of wood, leather, glass, metal, rubber, and plastics, in many shapes and sizes. Hugh Lenox Hodge (1796–1873), who designed one of the most popular models, spoke for a large segment of the medical profession when he stated in 1860,

"The mechanical treatment of uterine displacements by intra-vaginal supports is essential, a 'sine qua non,' for their perfect relief; that by pessaries, of suitable material, size, and form, the uterus may very generally be replaced and be maintained in situ; that the local symptoms of weight, pain, etc., the leucorrhoea, the menorrhagia, the dysmenorrhoea, and all the innumerable direct and indirect symptoms of spinal and cerebral irritation, including neuralgia, nervous headache, nervous affections of the larynx, lungs, heart, stomach, bowels, etc., as also spasms, cramps, and convulsions, may often thus be dissipated; that the intellectual and spiritual being may be elevated from the lowest states of depression, bordering on melancholy, or be delivered from the highest degree of maniacal excitement; and that the whole economy may thus be revolutionized."

Later in the nineteenth century and in the early years of the twentieth century, during a period that some derisively referred to in retrospect as "the dark ages of operative furor," leading gynecologists devised a variety of surgical procedures for the cure of uterine

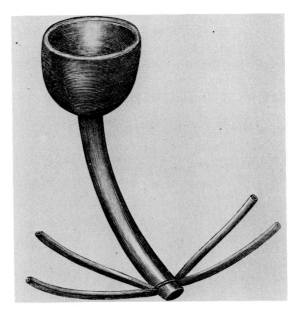

Fig. 17-27. Cup-and-stem pessary. Held in place by elastic bands and a belt for the reduction of uterine inversion by continuous gentle pressure.

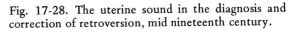

Fig. 17-28. The uterine sound in the diagnosis and correction of retroversion, mid nineteenth century.

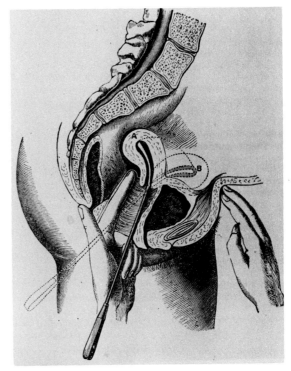

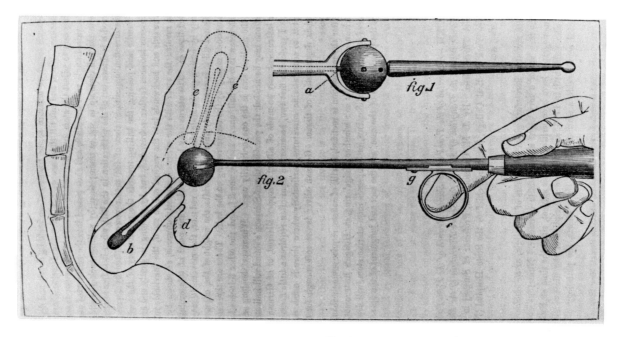

Fig. 17-29. Repositor of James Marion Sims, 1858, for the correction of uterine retroversion.

Fig. 17-30. Intrauterine stem pessary of Robert Greenhalgh (1819–1887) for the treatment of *acute anteflexion*.

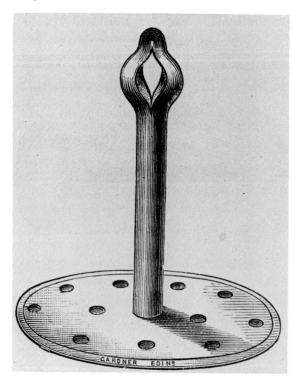

retroversion. In the words of C. Frederic Fluhmann, "the round ligaments were folded, ligated, plicated, shirred, plaited, planted, transplanted, replanted, drawn over, above, and through the broad ligaments and fastened to the back of the uterus." So popular had suspension operations become, according to Mr. William Alexander of Liverpool, inventor of one of the best known procedures, that when a visiting surgeon asked him to demonstrate it in 1911, each of Alexander's four assistants whom he sent into the north, east, south, and west sectors of the city to find a suitable subject returned after an unsuccessful search stating that in all of Liverpool no woman could be found who had not already had her uterus suspended by the Alexander operation! During the second quarter of the twentieth century suspension operations for uterine retroversion fell rapidly in favor and by mid-century had been virtually abandoned.

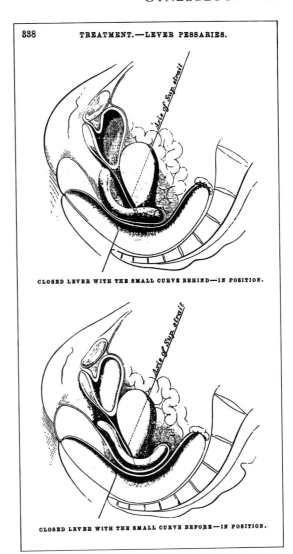

Fig. 17-31. The Hodge pessary for uterine retroversion. Hodge's illustrations from his textbook of 1860.

Fig. 17-32. The Alexander operation. Steps in the uterine suspension procedure of William Alexander (1844–1919) showing the plication of the round ligament in the inguinal canal.

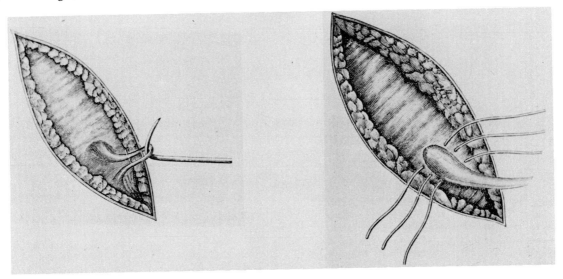

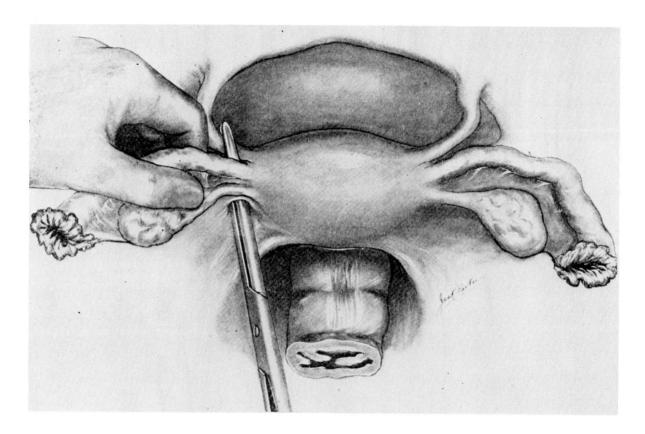

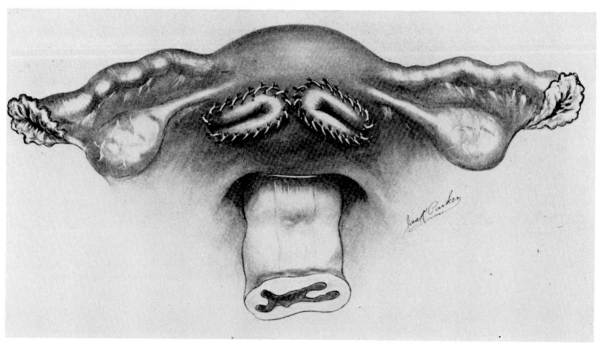

Fig. 17-33. The uterine suspension of John Clarence Webster (1863–1950). The round ligaments were drawn through a perforation in the broad ligament and sutured to the posterior surface of the uterus.

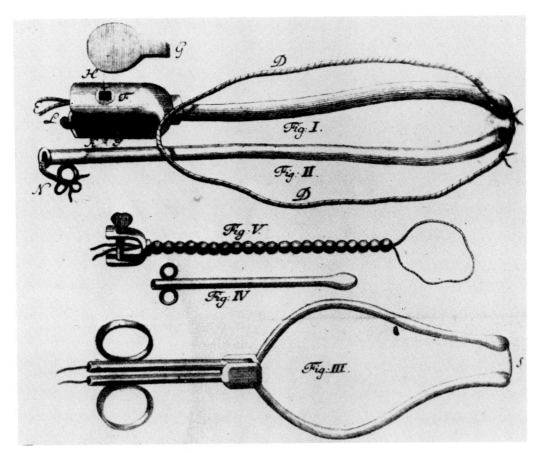

Fig. 17-34. Instruments designed by Georges Herbiniaux, a Belgian surgeon of the late eighteenth century, for avulsing uterine polyps. From *Chirurgische Bibliothek,* Göttingen, 1789.

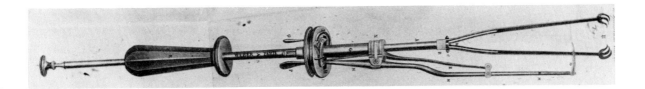

Fig. 17-35. Instrument devised in 1828 by Marc Colombat (1797–1851), known also as Colombat-de-L'Isere, for amputating a cancerous cervix.

474 ICONOGRAPHIA GYNIATRICA

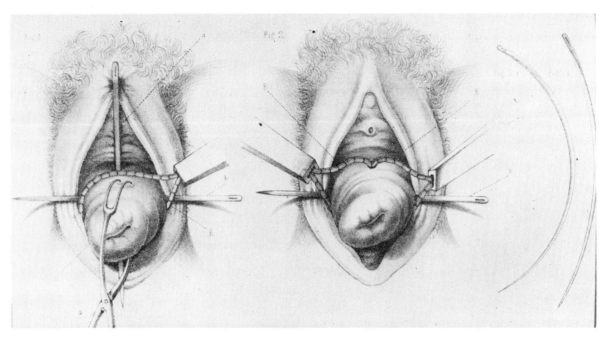

Fig. 17-36. Amputation of a prolapsed cervix. Technique of Gustav Simon, 1859. The cervix, transfixed with pins, was encircled with a crushing chain.

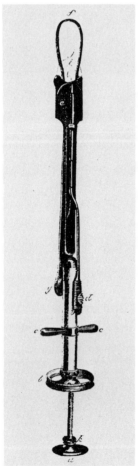

Fig. 17-37. The uterine guillotine of James Marion Sims for cervical amputation. From an 1867 catalogue of surgical instruments.

Fig. 17-38. Metrotome of James Young Simpson (1811–1870). A scissors-like instrument for dividing the cervix in cases of uterine anteflexion and cervical stenosis to which were attributed dysmenorrhea and infertility.

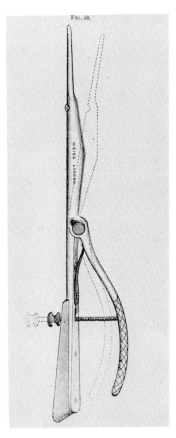

Fig. 17-39. Ovarian cyst containing 78 liters of fluid in a girl aged 17. Patient of Dr. H. Dayot successfully treated by *ovariotomy* in 1893.

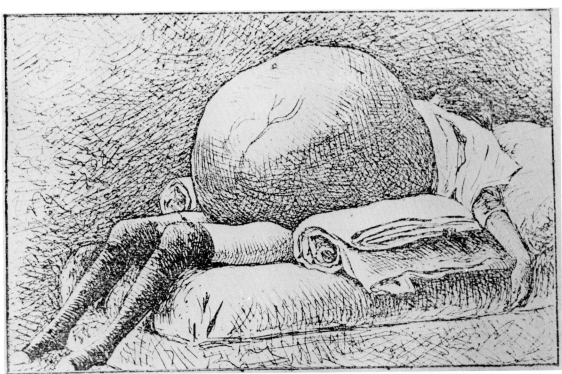

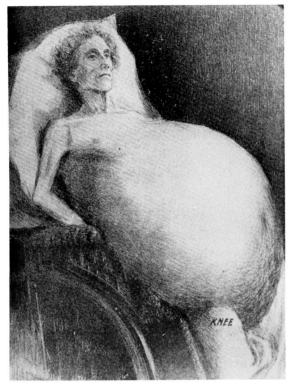

Fig. 17-40. Ovarian cyst weighing 176 pounds. Patient of Dr. D. Tod Gilliam pictured in his early twentieth century textbook.

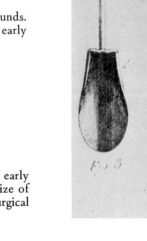

Fig. 17-41. Trocars for tapping ovarian cysts, early nineteenth century. Because of the enormous size of some cysts, tapping was necessary before surgical removal was feasible.

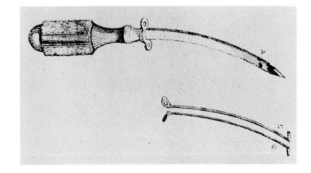

Fig. 17-42. Ovarian trocar and retention catheter of Jacques-Gilles-Thomas Maisonneuve (1809–1897), about 1860. Catheters were often inserted into ovarian cysts to provide continuous drainage for the rapidly accumulating fluid.

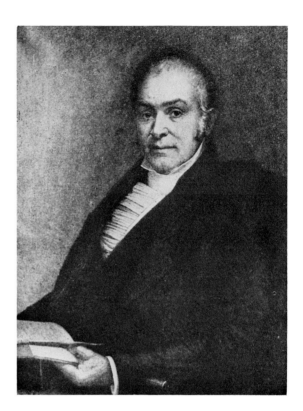

Fig. 17-43. Ephraim McDowell (1771–1830). Born in Augusta County, later named Rockbridge County, Virginia, he studied medicine under Dr. Alexander Humphreys of Staunton, later with the illustrious John Bell at Edinburgh, Scotland. He then entered practice in Danville, Kentucky, 1,000 miles from the nearest hospital, covering several hundred square miles by horseback. He removed a urinary bladder stone from James K. Polk who later became President of the United States. McDowell also helped found and served on the first board of trustees of Center College. His most memorable achievement, however, was his operation on Mrs. Jane Todd Crawford in 1809, the first successful removal of an ovarian cyst.

Robert Houstoun, of Scotland, (Philosophical Transactions 7:541, 1734) successfully evacuated a large ovarian cyst, probably a mucinous cystadenoma, by laparotomy in August, 1701 but without removal of the ovary. The patient, aged 58, lived in good health until October, 1714 when she died of an unknown cause.

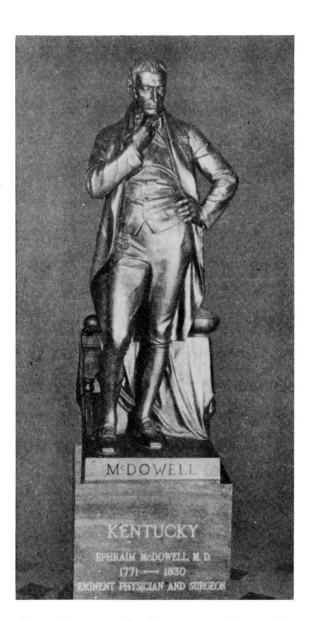

Fig. 17-44. Statue of Ephraim McDowell erected in McDowell Park, Danville, Kentucky in 1879.

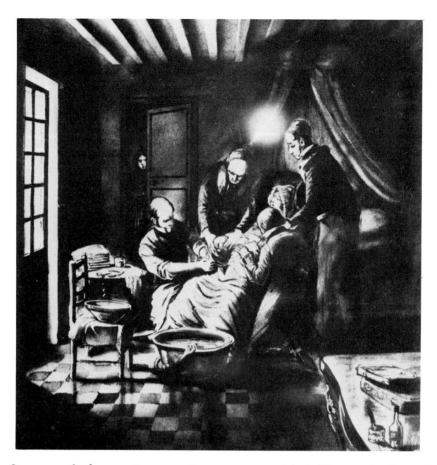

Fig. 17-45. The first removal of an ovarian tumor in France, May 1, 1844 by Dr. Roch Woyerkowski at Quingey, Doubs. Watercolor by Dr. H. K. Wagner based on the recollection of Dr. F. Jayle. The ovarian tumor weighed 8½ pounds, the patient's abdomen contained 30 liters of ascitic fluid, the operation took eight minutes. The patient made a complete recovery and subsequently bore two children.

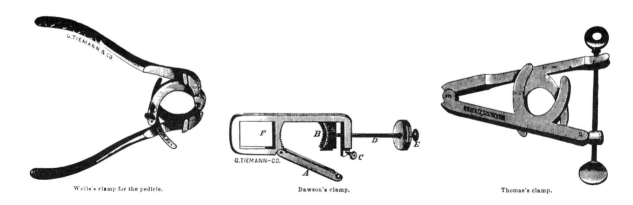

Fig. 17-46. Types of *ovariotomy clamps* which were applied to the ovarian pedicle.

GYNECOLOGY 479

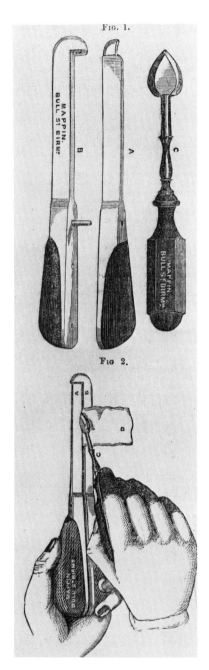

Fig. 17-47. Ovarian pedicle clamp and cautery knife of John Clay (1821–1894).

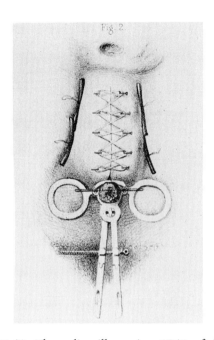

Fig. 17-48. The earliest illustration, 1865, of abdominal closure after oophorectomy. The ovarian pedicle is held up through the lower end of the wound by the ovariotomy clamp. The incision is closed by linen thread entwined about stay pins inserted through the wound edges.

Fig. 17-49. An operation for ovarian cyst, about 1890.

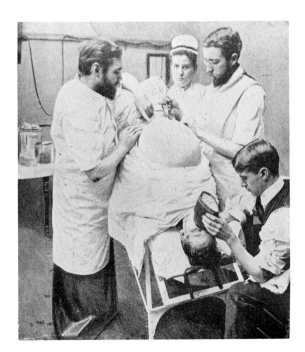

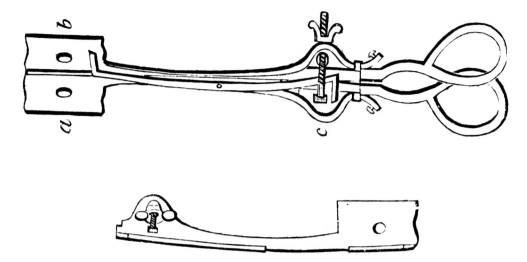

Fig. 17-50. A clamp used in the early nineteenth century for closing vesicovaginal fistulas. The edges of the fistula were brought together between the jaws of the clamp which was left within the vagina for days or weeks with the detachable handle removed. Healing of the fistula occasionally occurred.

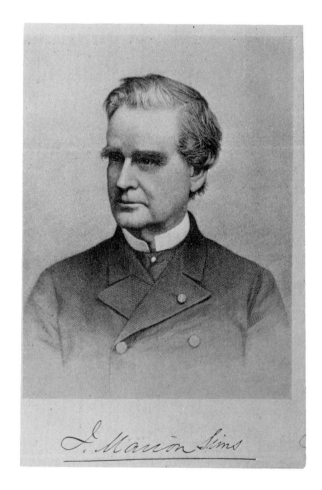

Fig. 17-51. James Marion Sims (1813–1883). Born in Hanging Rock, Lancaster County, South Carolina, Sims studied briefly with Dr. Churchill Jones, a local surgeon, took a 14 week course in the Medical College of Charleston, then transferred to Jefferson Medical College in Philadelphia from which he graduated in 1835. He achieved a large surgical practice in Montgomery, Alabama where he began his experiments on, and ultimate success in the cure of, vesicovaginal fistulas. In 1853 he moved to New York, founded the Woman's Hospital, popularized silver sutures, and attained international renown as America's foremost gynecologist. Proud, sensitive, and rigid, Sims resigned from the Woman's Hospital in 1874 after becoming embroiled in controversy with the hospital's board of lady managers over their policy of refusing admission to cancer patients and over their attempts to limit the number of visitors in his operative clinics. He served as president of the American Medical Association in 1875–1876. Sims made a number of trips abroad, received decorations from several European governments and honorary citations from many learned societies.

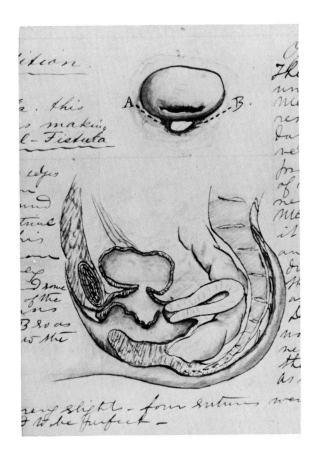
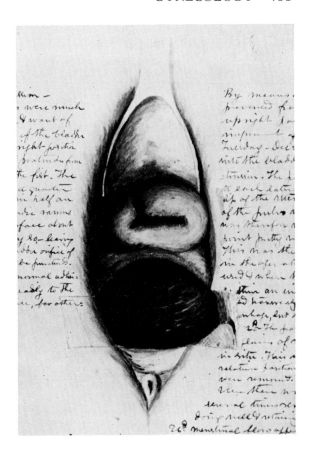

Fig. 17-52. Drawings of vesicovaginal fistulas by Thomas Addis Emmet. From the notes of operations at which he assisted J. Marion Sims, 1855–1857.

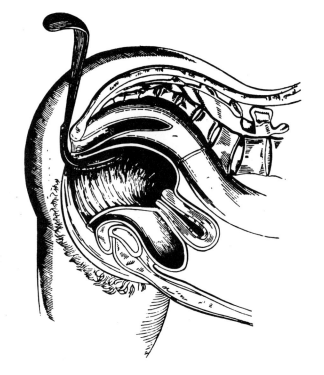

Fig. 17-53. Illustration from Sims's historic paper of 1852 on the treatment of vesicovaginal fistula, showing the patient in the knee-chest position and the use of the Sims speculum.

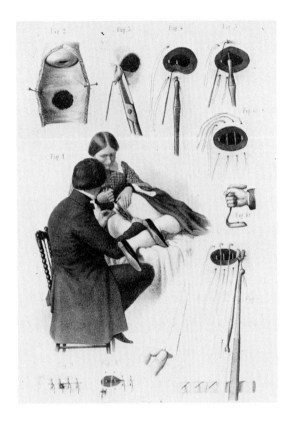

Fig. 17-54. James Marion Sims repairing a vesicovaginal fistula. Illustration by J. B. Léveillé made under Sims's supervision.

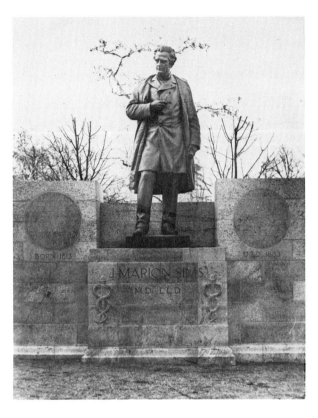

Fig. 17-55. Statue of James Marion Sims in New York's Central Park at Fifth Avenue and 103rd Street.

UTERINE MYOMAS, MYOMECTOMY, AND HYSTERECTOMY

Abdominal hysterectomy was successfully accomplished for the first time in June, 1853, by Walter Burnham of Lowell, Massachusetts. All previous attempts in the era before anesthesia and asepsis, when speed took precedence over hemostasis, ended in failure. The illustrious Sir James Young Simpson referred to abdominal hysterectomy as late as 1863 "as an utterly unjustifiable operation in surgery." Loathe to undertake an abdominal approach to uterine tumors, many gynecologists of the early and mid nineteenth century attained proficiency at vaginal myomectomy, removing tumors of any size, provided that they could be approached through the uterine cavity. In preparation for the operation they would dilate the cervix with metal dilators, metreurynters, or laminary tents, for several days in the case of large tumors. The operation itself entailed incision of the tumor capsule from below, application of traction with a tenaculum, and excision of the mass in stages, contractions of the uterus being depended upon for help in delivering the tumor into the vagina.

GYNECOLOGY 483

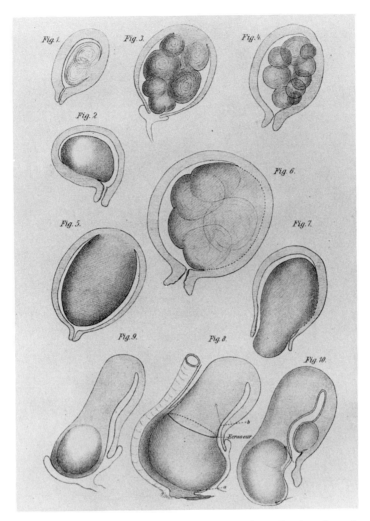

Fig. 17-56. Uterine myomas considered amenable to vaginal enucleation, late nineteenth century.

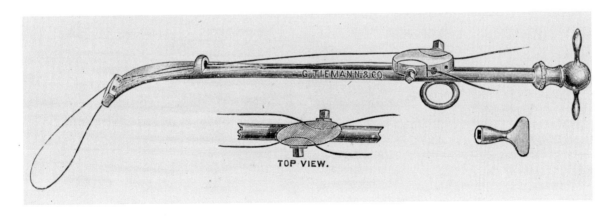

Fig. 17-57. An *écraseur* or snare for removing uterine tumors through the vagina. The steel wire was looped around the pedicle and tightened until the tumor was avulsed.

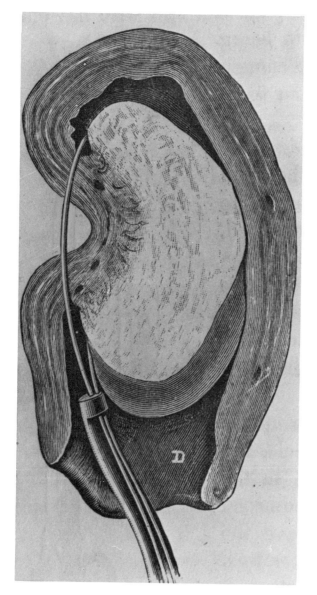

Fig. 17-58. A complication from the use of the *écraseur*, the inadvertent excision of the myometrium and perforation of the uterus. This type of accident was not rare. Using a similar instrument for the amputation of a cancerous cervix in 1860, James Marion Sims noticed, after removing the *écraseur*, that air was rushing in and out of the vagina "with all the regularity of, and synchronously with, inspiration and expiration." On further inspection he found, greatly to his horror, an "immense hole of a semi-lunar form" in the cul-de-sac through which the abdominal viscera were clearly visible.

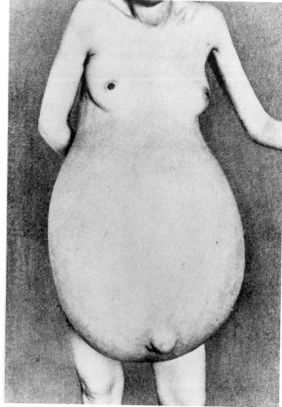

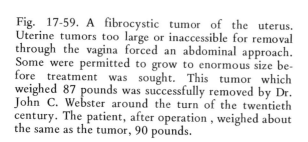

Fig. 17-59. A fibrocystic tumor of the uterus. Uterine tumors too large or inaccessible for removal through the vagina forced an abdominal approach. Some were permitted to grow to enormous size before treatment was sought. This tumor which weighed 87 pounds was successfully removed by Dr. John C. Webster around the turn of the twentieth century. The patient, after operation, weighed about the same as the tumor, 90 pounds.

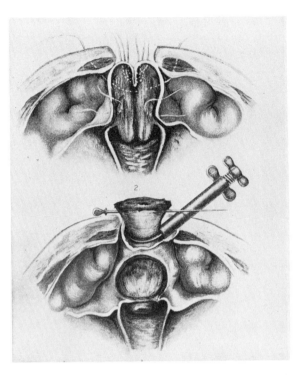

Fig. 17-60. The cervical stump in abdominal hysterectomy, two methods of management in the late nineteenth century. The lower figure shows the stump transfixed by a pin with the snare applied. In the upper figure the cervical stump is sutured to the abdominal wall, the uterine vessels having been ligated.

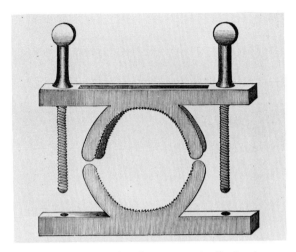

Fig. 17-61. Thomas' clamp (T. Gaillard Thomas, 1831–1903) for securing the cervical stump in hysterectomy for myomata uteri. The clamp provided hemostasis and held the pedicle up through the abdominal incision.

Fig. 17-62. Wilhelm Alexander Freund (1833–1918). He performed the first complete abdominal hysterectomy for uterine cancer on January 30, 1878.

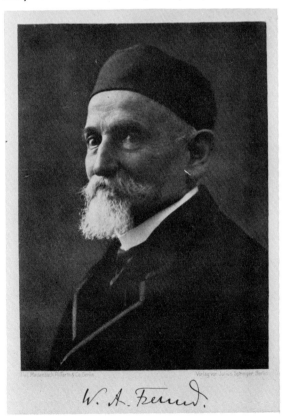

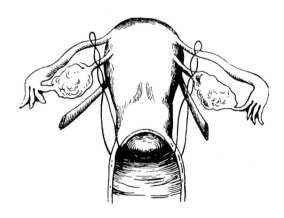

Fig. 17-63. Freund's method of suturing the broad ligament and uterine adnexa in complete abdominal hysterectomy.

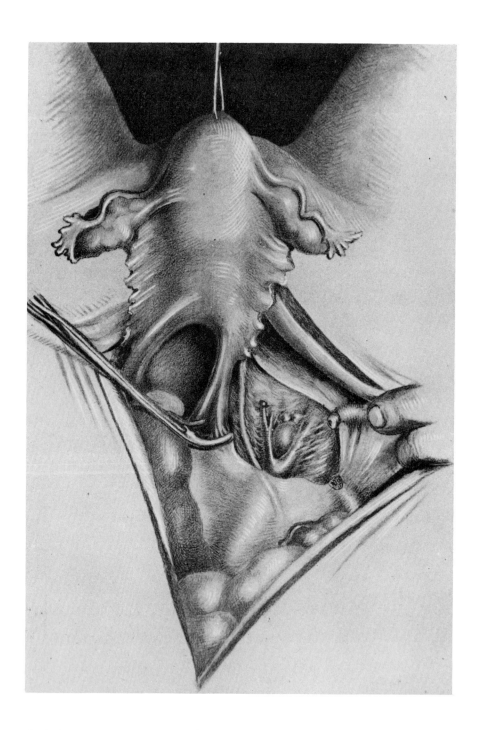

Fig. 17-64. Radical hysterectomy. A stage of the operation popularized by Ernst Wertheim (1864–1920), Viennese gynecologist. Extension of Freund's hysterectomy technique with dissection of the pelvic lymph nodes was suggested for the treatment of uterine (cervical) cancer by Emil Reis, one of Freund's students, in 1895. This extended operation, radical hysterectomy, was first performed that year by John G. Clark at The Johns Hopkins Hospital in Baltimore.

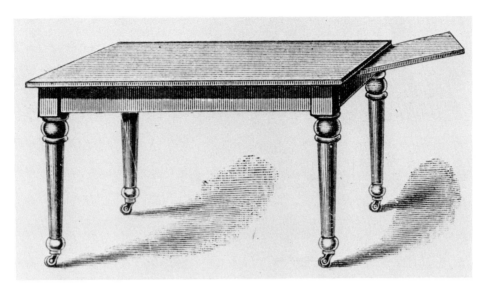

Fig. 17-65. Gynecologic examining table designed by Dr. F. H. Davenport, Boston, late nineteenth century. The head end of the table was slightly lower than the foot to permit the patient's abdominal viscera to recede from the pelvis. A wooden board which protruded at an angle of 45 degrees supported the feet while the patient assumed the lateral Sims position.

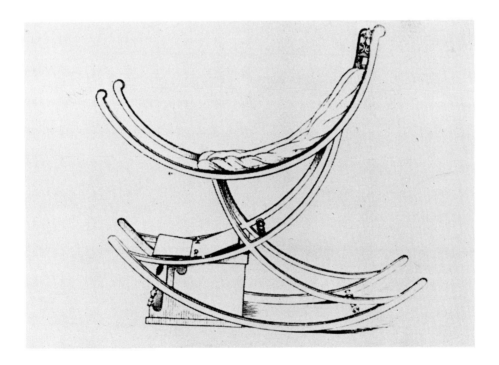

Fig. 17-66. A gynecologic examining chair on a rocker base, in use about 1860.

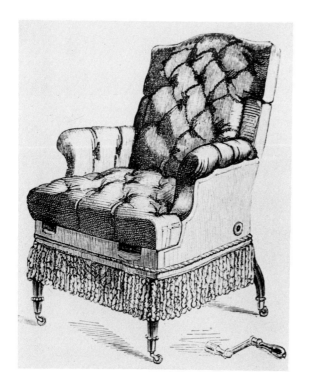 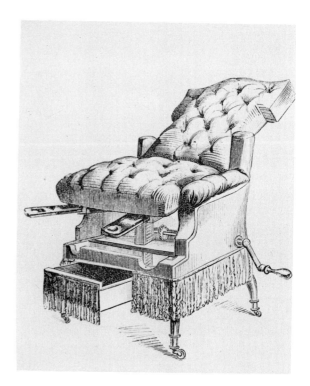

Fig. 17-67. An upholstered adjustable examining chair of the late nineteenth century.

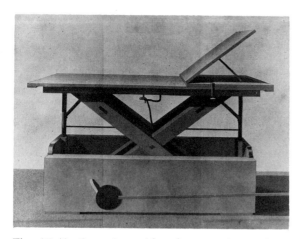

Fig. 17-68. Operating table of Herman von Alten, 1820.

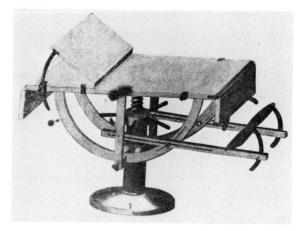

Fig. 17-69. Operating table, mid nineteenth century.

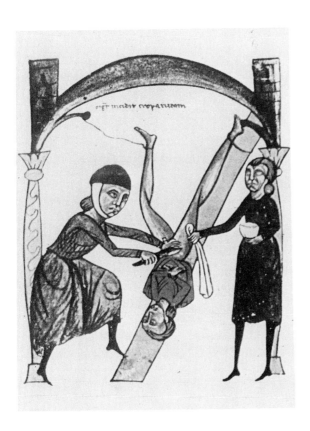

Fig. 17-70. The inclined position. As illustrated in a manuscript, about 1300, of *Practica chirurgiae* (or *Post mundi fabricam*) of Roger of Salerno and Roland of Parma, showing the repair of an inguinal hernia. Most gynecologic laparotomies are performed with the patient in an inclined or Trendelenburg position which lowers the head and chest and elevates the hips, allowing the intestines to gravitate toward the diaphragm, thereby facilitating access to the pelvic viscera. This position was used as early as 40 BC in the treatment of abdominal injuries, for replacing eviscerated intestines. Casanatense Library, Rome.

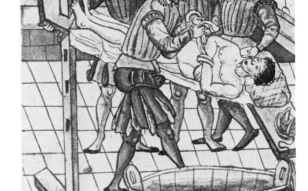

Fig. 17-71. The inclined position. As illustrated in Caspar Stromayr's manuscript of 1559.

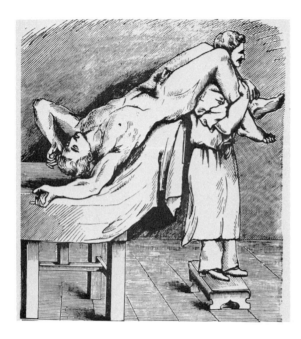 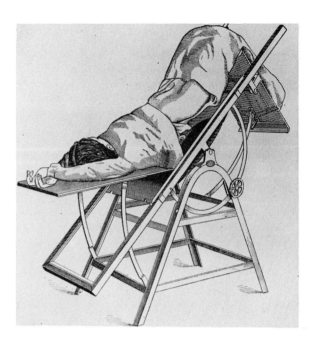

Fig. 17-72. The Trendelenburg position. Woodcut from Willy Meyer's paper of 1884 which first described Friedrich Trendelenburg's use of the inclined position. An assistant supported the patient's legs to elevate the pelvis.

Fig. 17-73. The Trendelenburg position produced by an adjustable operating table, late nineteenth century.

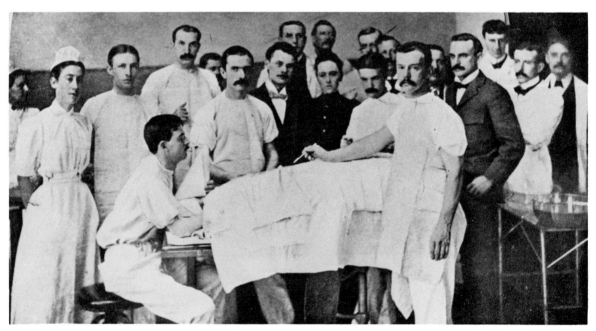

Fig. 17-74. Howard Atwood Kelly (1858–1943), Gynecologist in Chief, The Johns Hopkins Hospital, Baltimore about to operate in 1897. At the foot of the table in street clothes stands John G. Clark who performed the first radical hysterectomy. In the center, also in street clothes, Max Brödel, distinguished medical artist; at his right Thomas S. Cullen, Kelly's successor at the Hopkins. Caps, masks, and gloves were yet to come.

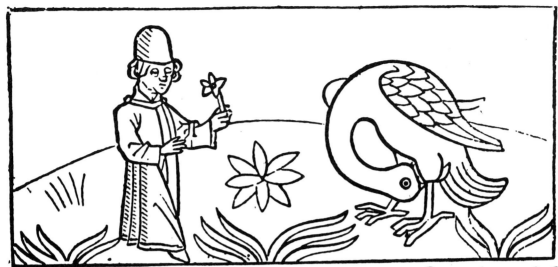

Fig. 17-75. The ibis purging itself. Fifteenth century woodcut. The ancient Egyptians are said to have conceived of the enema from their observations of the ibis, a type of stork. When the ibis is disturbed by abdominal distress, the Egyptians believed, it proceeds to the edge of the sea and fills its long neck with water which it then injects through its beak into the anus, thus relieving its constipated bowel. Ornithologists have since reinterpreted these actions of the bird as an aid in dressing its feathers: it wets its bill in the water, then presses it against the oil glands alongside the anus to obtain their secretion.

THE DOUCHE AND ENEMA

Indispensable to countless generations of women in the maintenance of their hygiene and to their physicians in the management of myriad maladies, were the douche and enema. Passed, happily, is the day of promiscuous purging.

Especially in France, the enema achieved popularity in medical treatment. The vaginal douche similarly enjoyed great favor in the daily routine of the women of that country. The bidet lingers there yet. The toilet accessories of sixteenth century France commonly included syringes of porcelain, mother-of-pearl, and gilded silver. Madame de Pompadour is said to have kept an assortment of ornate syringes on display in her perfumed boudoir, as part of its decor. An apparatus with a long hose and interchangeable cannulas for self-administration of either rectal or vaginal irrigations, invented by the illustrious Dutch anatomist and physiologist Reinier de Graaf (1641–1673), was highly publicized by the satirical plays of Molière during the reign of Louis XIV when women of the aristocracy resorted to enemas as often as three or four times daily to improve their complexion and retain their youthful appearance. The clyster had become the fountain of youth. Apothecaries vied with one another in the formulation of colorful and fragrant enema solutions made from orange blossoms, roses, bergamot, and lilies. Female attendants in the court of Louis XVI, so it is said, were required to submit to multiple enemas before undertaking their daily duties, to avoid any interference with their service.

The use of the enema in obstetrics is at least two centuries old. Thomas Denman (1733–1815) in his *An Introduction to the Practice of Midwifery* (1795) advocated "repeated exhibition of emollient clysters" in the treatment of prolonged labor associated with excessive uterine distention and the addition of salts in other cases of uterine inertia to "rouse the dormant powers into action." Enemas of linseed or of flour and water were used during pregnancy; clysters of opium were given to soothe the irritated rectum.

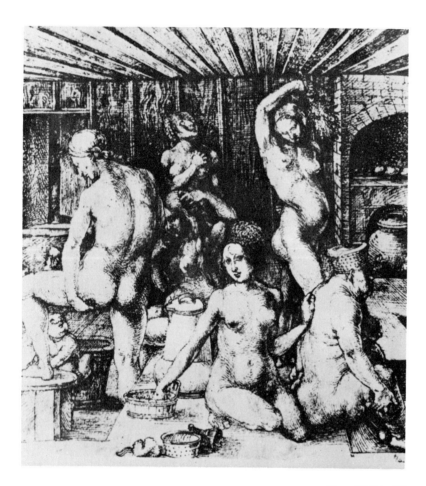

Fig. 17-76. The Steam Baths. Painting (1496) by Albrecht Dürer (1471–1528). The woman on the left is fumigating her genitalia.

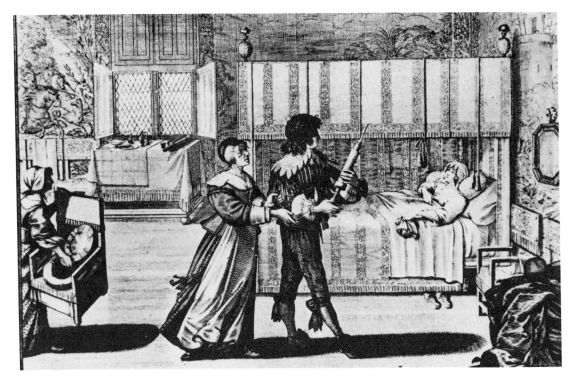

Fig. 17-77. The Enema. Engraving by Abraham Bosse (1602–1676).

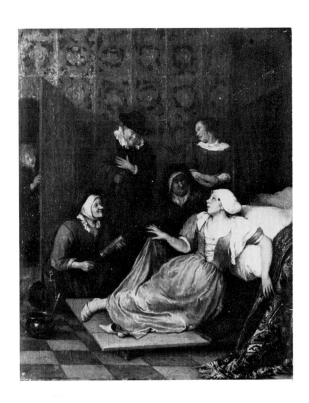

Fig. 17-78. The patient receives an enema. Painting by Jan Steen (1626–1679). Formerly in Museum der Bildenden Künste, Leipzig, missing since 1965.

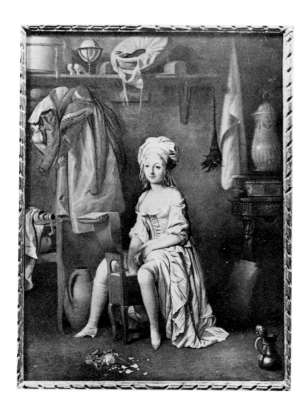

Fig. 17-79. *Femme à sa Toilette.* Painting by Louis Leopold Boilly (1761–1845). The woman is taking a douche. The back of the bidet stool holds her toilet accessories.

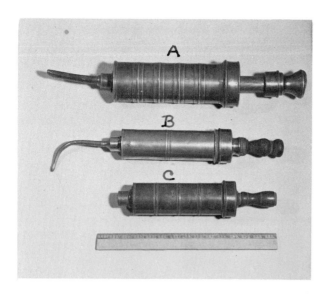

Fig. 17-80. Pewter enema syringes, about 1800. The uppermost (A) weighs 6 pounds, measures 2½ feet with its plunger extended. Before the syringe was invented, enema solutions were blown into the rectum by mouth, through a tube.

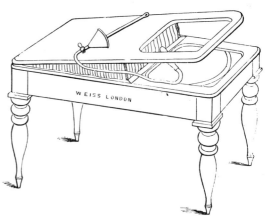

Fig. 17-81. Douching apparatus, advertised in 1867 by a London instrument manufacturer as "easy of application and self acting." The woman, with the douche nozzle in her vagina, sat on a water-filled rubber bag covered by a wooden lid, her weight forcing the water from the bag into her vagina.

Chapter 18

HOSPITALS FOR WOMEN

Within these gray walls Life begins and ends,
Here, in this harbor, worn, sea-weary ships
Drop anchor, as the fading sun descends,
And new-launched vessels start their outbound
  trips.

  [E. O. Laughlin: "Inscription
     for a Hospital"]

Hospitals have served the feeble and the fallen, the senile and the sick, for 2400 years. They offered shelter, sustenance, and solace in Ceylon during the fifth century BC, in India as early as 260 BC. Not until the Middle Ages did Christian endeavor produce hospitals for the Western World. During the early years of that era (AD 500–1500), charitable institutions, staffed almost exclusively by monks and nuns, housed the indigent and aged, providing hospitality, rather than healing, for "God's poor." Earliest among the hospitals of Europe were the Hôtel-Dieu of Lyon created about 542 by Childebert I, King of the Franks, the Hôtel-Dieu of Paris founded about 652 by St. Landry, the twenty-eighth Bishop of Paris, which welcomed "soldiers and citizens, religious and laymen, Jews and Mohammedans, and all who bore marks of poverty and wretchedness," the hospital of Santa Maria della Scala established in Siena, Italy in 898, the Ospedale di Santo Spirito of Rome consecrated in 1198 by Pope Innocent III, and St. Bartholomew's Hospital organized in London in 1123.

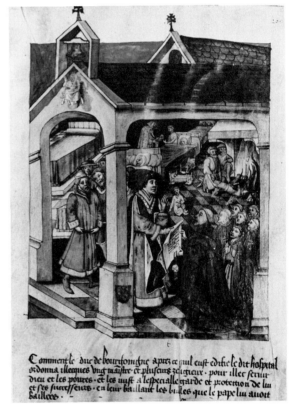

Fig. 18-1. Obstetric ward, Hôpital de Dijon, France. From a fifteenth century manuscript of Saint-Esprit.

495

Separate hospitals were designated during the eighteenth century, and in increasing number during the nineteenth, for the sick with diseases too troublesome or hazardous for general hospitals such as lunacy and smallpox and for groups that were beginning to stimulate specialized medical interest, such as children and the parturient. Lying-in hospitals served the double function of providing a haven for the poor and subjects for the clinical teaching of medical students and midwives.

The first obstetric hospital was established in 1728 in Strasbourg with Johann Jacob Fried as director and lecturer. Soon thereafter, Britain's Sir Richard Manningham proposed

"that proper measures be taken by the Legislature for establishing a national public hospital for all sorts of women promiscuously; for amongst the unhappy wretches of ill-fame there are doubtless many objects of compassion who, I think, are as properly the concern and care of the Legislature as a profligate child is that of its parents."

Manningham failed to achieve immediate implementation of his plan, but in 1739 he did succeed in establishing a small lying-in ward, among the first in the British Isles, where midwives were given practical instruction, in the parochial Infirmary of St. James, Westminster.

Most American hospitals devoted to obstetrics and gynecology, such as the Woman's Hospital of the State of New York and the Sloane Hospital for Women which gained renown during the late nineteenth and early twentieth centuries, have since been incorporated into general medical centers.

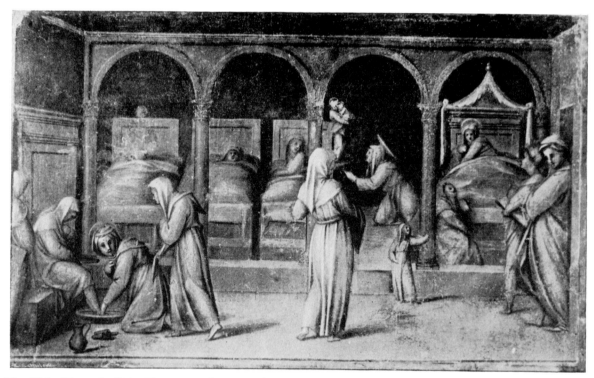

Fig. 18-2. Women's clinic, Florence, Italy. By Andrea del Sarto (Andrea d'Agnolo), 1486–1531. Although the first true lying-in hospital was not established until 1728 in Strasbourg, this and the preceding figure show that isolated facilities for the care of women existed earlier, in France and Italy, for example. The Hôtel-Dieu in Paris and Germany's Nürnberg Krankenhaus were among the first institutions to create separate obstetric divisions.

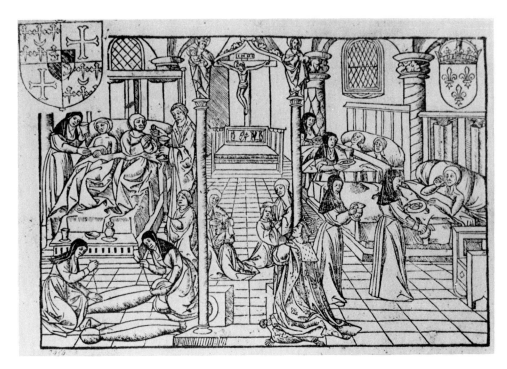

Fig. 18-3. The interior of the Hôtel-Dieu of Paris, about 1500. Woodcut from a letter from the Archbishop of Bourges to the hospital's benefactors.

THE HÔTEL-DIEU OF PARIS

Founded at the beginning of the seventh century, this famous Parisian hospice acquired the character of a general hospital by the middle of the twelfth century, subsequently grew to one of the largest in Europe. In the eighth century the Hôtel-Dieu established a special section for parturients, the only facility of its kind in Paris, a small ward staffed by one midwife and a few pupils. This later became the great Parisian center for the training of midwives and a few male accoucheurs, most famous of whom were François Mauriceau (1637–1709), Pierre Dionis (died 1718), and Paul Portal (died 1703).

During the reign of Louis XI in the 15th century, the Hôtel-Dieu contained 5 large wards and was staffed by 12 priests, 6 clerks, 2 chaplains, 14 nuns and an equal number of novitiates, and several physicians, barber-surgeons, and midwives. In the basement was the 24 bed obstetric ward. As always with hospitals, these facilities eventually proved inadequate. Incredibly poor were the hygienic conditions. A record of February 6, 1660 stated that pregnant and puerperal women were lying four and five in a bed. In addition to its overcrowding, the obstetric ward suffered from the periodic overflow and stench of the Seine on the banks of which the Hôtel-Dieu was situated and into which it discharged its sewage. Puerperal fever was common; only one woman in 20 survived an epidemic in 1746. Major fires occurred in 1737, 1742, and 1772, the hospital being largely destroyed, providentially, by the last. When rebuilt, the Hôtel-Dieu incorporated the changes recommended by a commission of 1788, headed by Lavoisier, to rectify the previously intolerable conditions.

498 ICONOGRAPHIA GYNIATRICA

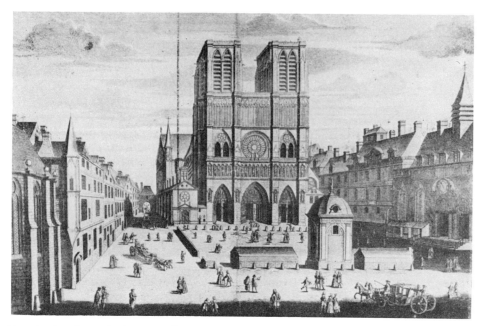

Fig. 18-4. The Hôtel-Dieu of Paris, seventeenth century.

Fig. 18-5. The burning of the Hôtel-Dieu, Paris, 1772. Painting by Nicolas and Jean-Baptiste Raguenot, father and son, eighteenth century artists.

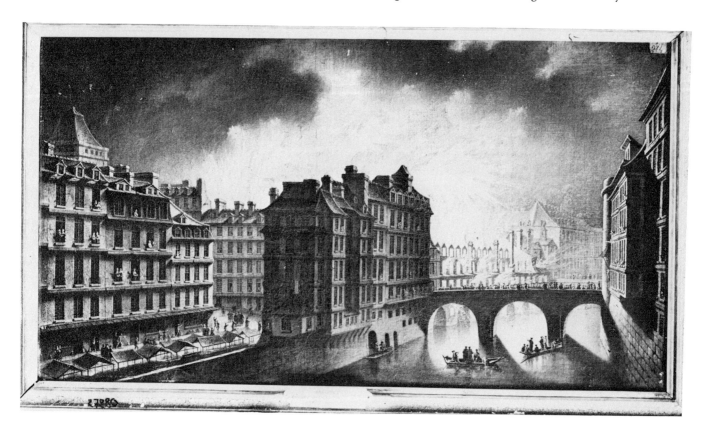

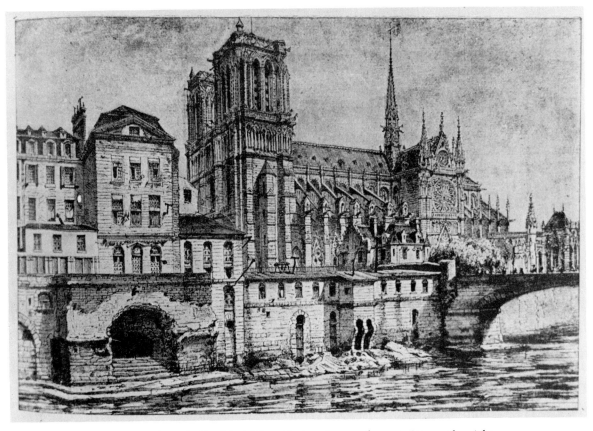

Fig. 18-6. The rebuilt Hôtel-Dieu, Paris, nineteenth century, on the right bank of the Seine. Etching by Alfred-Louis Brunet-Debaines (born 1845).

THE DUBLIN ROTUNDA

Oldest of Great Britain's hospitals with maternity services is the Edinburgh Royal Infirmary in Scotland dating back to 1736. But the first institution in the British dominion devoted exclusively to the care of obstetric patients was a small hospital of 10 beds in George's Lane, Dublin, Ireland which opened on March 15, 1745 as the Hospital for Poor Lying-in Women in a three storied house of 15 rooms previously used as a theatrical school.

Bartholomew Mosse, the son of a rector in Maryborough, Queen's County, Ireland, having completed his studies as a surgeon's apprentice in 1733, then satisfied his military obligation and traveled through Europe to perfect himself in surgery and midwifery before beginning practice in Dublin. A man-midwife, Mosse was appalled by the city's lack of obstetric facilities for the indigent, noting that

"the misery of the poor women of the city of Dublin, at the time of their lying-in, would scarcely be conceived by any who had not been an eye witness of their wretched circumstances; that their lodgings were generally in cold garrets, open to every wind, or in damp

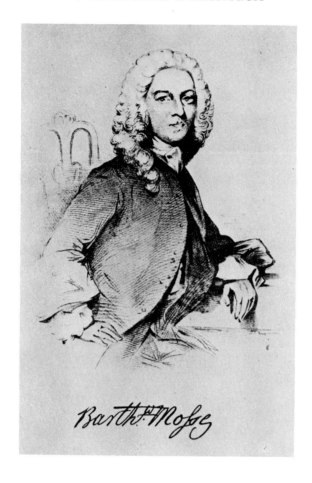

cellars, subject to floods from excessive rains; destitute of attendance, medicines, and often of proper food, by which hundreds perished with their little infants."

Mosse envisioned a maternity hospital for Dublin's poor; his determination culminated in the creation of the Dublin Lying-in Hospital, forerunner of the Rotunda. By the end of its first year the hospital had grown to 28 beds, admitted 209 women, 208 of whom delivered infants, and had established a record admirable for its time: the loss of only one mother from puerperal fever and the discharge of 190 live infants. The little hospital prospered, its fame spread, and during the next few years several similar institutions were established in London, patterned after Mosse's model: the Brownlow Street Hospital, 1749 (from 1756 known as the British Lying-in Hospital); the City of London Lying-in Hospital, 1750; the General Lying-in Hospital, 1752 (later renamed Queen Charlotte's Lying-in Hospital); the Westminster Lying-in Hospital, 1765 (subsequently designated the General Lying-in Hospital); and a number of other maternities that closed their doors after varying periods and no longer exist.

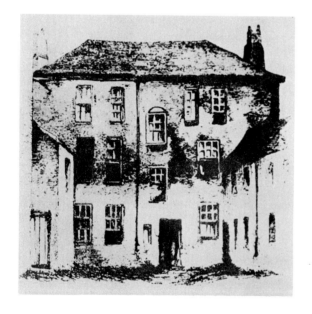

Fig. 18-7. Bartholomew Mosse (1712–1759) founder and first Master of Dublin's Hospital for Poor Lying-in Women. Among the subsequent Masters were Fielding Ould (c. 1710–1789), Robert Collins (died 1868), Evory Kennedy (1807?–1886), Alfred McClintock (1822–1881), George Johnston (1815–1889), William Smyly (1850–1929), Ernest Hastings Tweedy (1862–1945), and Bethel Solomons (1885–1965).

Fig. 18-8. Original home of the Hospital for Poor Lying-in Women, George's Lane, Dublin which opened on March 15, 1745. From a sketch made in 1846.

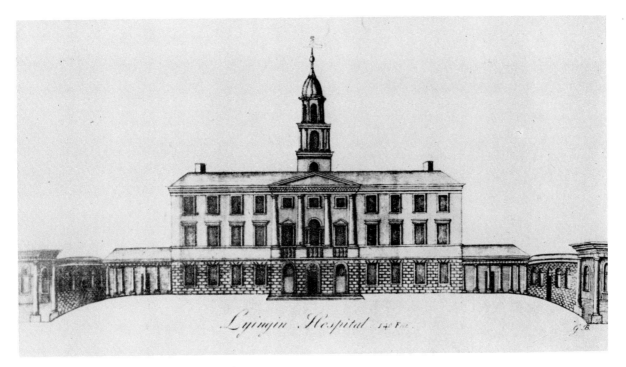

Fig. 18-9. The Dublin Lying-in Hospital, new quarters, occupied December 8, 1757.

Fig. 18-10. The enlarged Dublin Lying-in Hospital, about 1785, later known as The Rotunda Hospital.

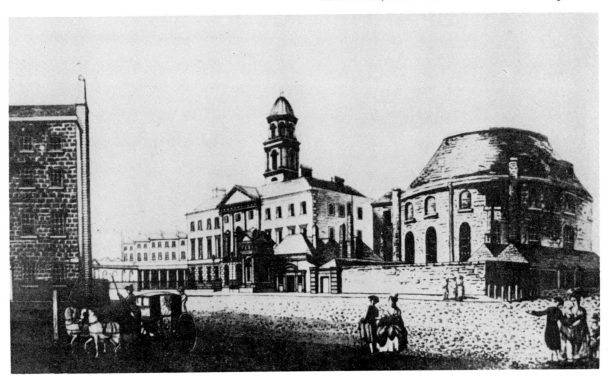

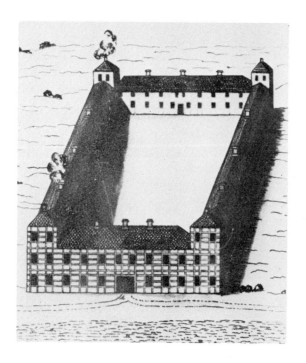

Fig. 18-11. The original Charité on the Spree River in Berlin in 1730, 20 years after its founding. Medical center of the Humboldt-Universität, it became the most famous hospital in Germany.

Fig. 18-12. The rebuilt Charité, its construction begun in 1785 by Friedrich the Great, completed in 1800 under Friedrich Wilhelm III. A department of obstetrics was created in the medical faculty of the Berlin University in 1812 with Adam Elias von Siebold as Professor, a lying-in hospital erected in 1817, and a gynecologic division established by Eduard Martin who assumed direction of the department in 1858. Among the physicians and scientists who subsequently added luster to the institution were Carl Credé, Carl Schröder Adolf Gusserow, Robert von Olshausen, Ernst Bumm, and Walter Stoeckel in clinical obstetrics and gynecology; Robert Meyer in gynecologic pathology; and Selmar Aschheim and Bernhard Zondek in experimental endocrinology.

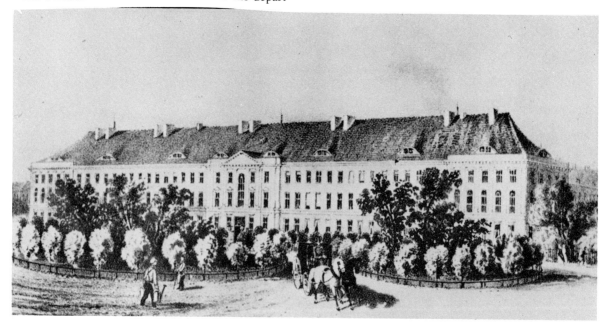

HOSPITALS FOR WOMEN 503

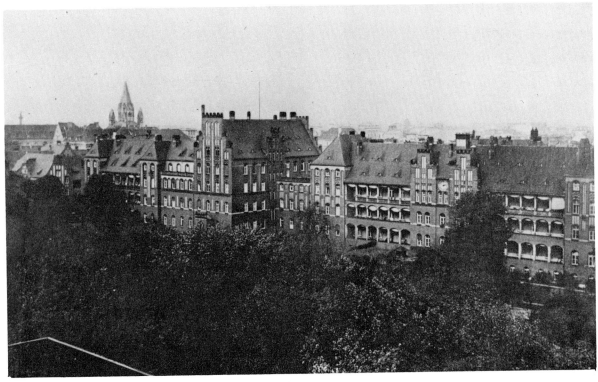

Fig. 18-13. The Charité, Berlin, during the first half of the twentieth century.

Fig. 18-14. The Universitätsfrauenklinik (Women's clinic) of the Charité, 1960. (Brochure commemorating 250th anniversary.)

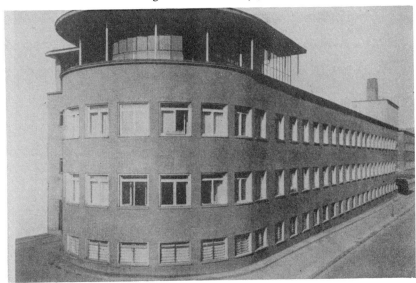

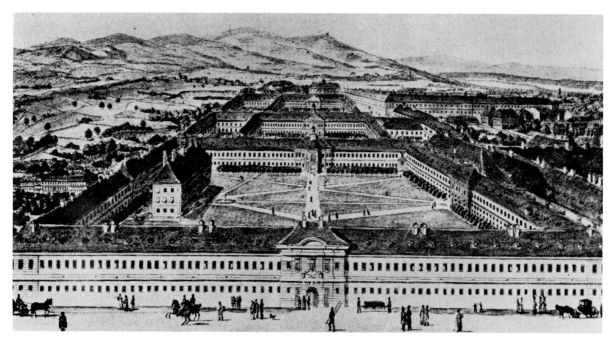

Fig. 18-15. The Allgemeines Krankenhaus (General Hospital) in Vienna, about 1800. Founded in 1784 by the Austrian Emperor Joseph II, son of Maria Theresa, it became the home of Europe's largest obstetric service.

Fig. 18-16. The Viennese Allgemeines Krankenhaus, entrance on the Alserstrasse. Here Ignaz Philipp Semmelweis (1818–1865) helped combat puerperal fever; later, in the Universitäts-Frauenklinik, major advances were made in gynecologic surgery.

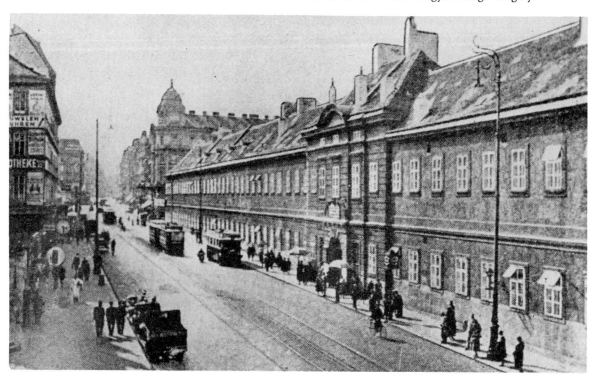

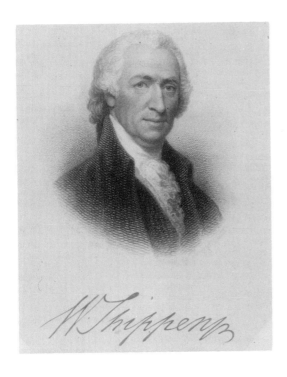

Fig. 18-17. William Shippen, Jr. (1736–1808). After studying anatomy in London under William and John Hunter and obstetrics under Colin MacKenzie, he returned to his native Philadelphia where he gave courses in these subjects, helped organize Colonial America's first medical school, and established its first lying-in hospital.

AMERICAN HOSPITALS

Institutional obstetrics in America originated in the junior William Shippen's pioneer medical school, established in Philadelphia in 1762. After teaching anatomy for three years, Shippen proclaimed himself a man-midwife, offered a course in midwifery, and provided accommodations for the housing and delivery of a few poor women. During the next 100 years several small lying-in hospitals were created and separate wards designated for maternity patients in a few general hospitals, intended primarily as asylums for the poor but not for the training of medical students or physicians. Among the earliest of America's obstetric facilities were the lying-in wards of the New York Almshouse, established in 1799, of the Philadelphia Almshouse, opened in 1802, and of the Pennsylvania Hospital, in 1803; the New York Lying-in Hospital, founded in 1798; the New York Asylum for Lying-in Women, known also as the Marion Street Maternity, 1822; and the Boston Lying-in Hospital, 1832. The first obstetric hospital in the United States to offer student training was opened at Baltimore's College of Physicians and Surgeons in 1822. Small and poorly equipped, it survived but briefly.

Although every general physician was required to be an obstetrician as well, almost none acquired any practical experience before receiving his medical diploma. Special training in obstetrics required a trip to Europe after graduation. Sensitive to this lack in American medical education, James W. McLane, Professor of Obstetrics and the Diseases of Women in New York's College of Physicians and Surgeons and physician to the affluent Vanderbilt and Sloane families, obtained in 1886 the endowment for the Sloane Maternity Hospital (known later as The Sloane Hospital for Women), to provide for medical students practical training in obstetrics; for the medically indigent, a modern maternity hospital; and for American medicine, an institution for the special training of advanced students and physicians in the art and science of obstetrics.

Doctor SHIPPEN, junior,

HAVING been lately called to the Aſſiſtance of a Number of Women in the Country, in difficult Labours, moſt of which were made ſo by the unſkilful old Women about them; the poor Women have ſuffered extremely, and their innocent little Ones were entirely deſtroyed, whoſe Lives might have been eaſily ſaved by proper Management: And being informed of ſeveral deſperate Caſes in the different Neighbourhoods, which had proved fatal to the Mothers as well as their Infants, and were attended with the moſt painful Circumſtances, too diſmal to be related! he thought it his Duty immediately to begin his intended Courſe of Lectures on Midwifery, and has prepared a proper Apparatus for that Purpoſe, in order to inſtruct thoſe Women who have had Virtue enough to own their Ignorance, and apply for Inſtruction, as well as all thoſe young Gentlemen now engaged in the Study of that uſeful and neceſſary Branch of Surgery, who are taking Pains to qualify themſelves to practiſe in different Parts of the Country, with Safety and Advantage to their Fellow Creatures.

The Doctor propoſes to begin his firſt Courſe as ſoon as a Number of Pupils ſufficient to defray the neceſſary Expence ſhall apply. A Courſe will conſiſt of about 20 Lectures, in which he will treat of that Part of Anatomy which is neceſſary to underſtand that Branch, explain all Caſes in Midwifery, natural, difficult, and preternatural, and give Directions how to treat them with Safety to Mother and Child; deſcribe the Diſeaſes incident to Women and Children in the Month, and direct to proper Remedies; will take Occaſion, during the Courſe, to explain and apply thoſe curious anatomical Plates and Caſts of the gravid Uterus at the Hoſpital, and conclude the whole with neceſſary Cautions againſt the dangerous and cruel Uſe of Inſtruments.

In order to make the Courſe more perfect, a convenient Lodging is provided for the Accommodation of a few poor Women, who otherwiſe might ſuffer for Want of the common Neceſſaries on thoſe Occaſions, to be under the Care of a ſober honeſt Matron, well acquainted with lying-in Women, employed by the Doctor for that Purpoſe.

Each Pupil to attend two Courſes at leaſt, for which he is to pay Five Guineas. Perpetual Pupils to pay Ten Guineas.

The female Pupils to be taught privately, and aſſiſted at any of their private Labours when neceſſary.

The Doctor may be ſpoke with at his Houſe, in Front-ſtreet, every Morning, between the Hours of Six and Nine, or at his Office, in Letitia-Court, every Evening.

Fig. 18-18. Shippen's advertisement in the *Pennsylvania Gazette* of January 31, 1765 announcing his course in midwifery and the establishment of his lying-in hospital, offering

"a convenient Lodging . . . for the Accommodation of a few poor Women, who might otherwise suffer for Want of the common Necessaries on those Occasions, to be under the Care of a sober honest Matron, well acquainted with lying-in Women. . . . "

Fig. 18-19. Bellevue Hospital, New York, established in 1826 as an outgrowth of the New York Almshouse which provided the city's first obstetric service, a lying-in ward, in 1799.

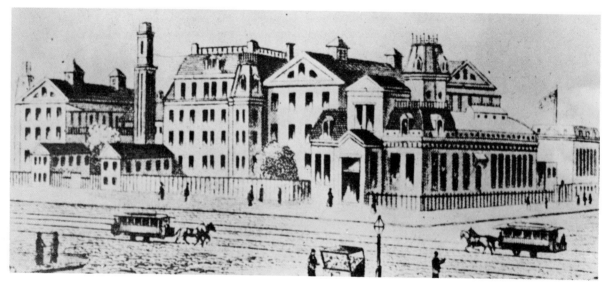

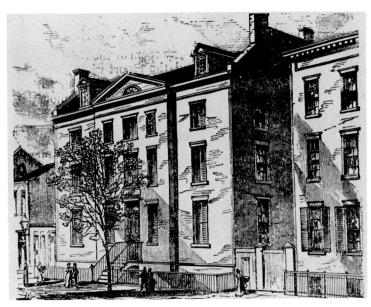

Fig. 18-20. The New York Asylum for Lying-in Women, known also as the Marion Street Maternity. Established in 1822, it provided a home delivery service in addition to its indoor ward facilities.

The first American institution devoted exclusively to the treatment of gynecologic disorders was the Woman's Hospital in New York City, founded by James Marion Sims in 1855. Similar hospitals opened during the next quarter century: in Chicago, the Chicago Hospital for Women and Children and the Women's Hospital of the State of Illinois (1870); in Boston, the Northeastern Hospital for Women and Children (1863) and the Free Hospital for Women (1875); in Philadelphia, Howard A. Kelly's Kensington Hospital (1883). Of these, only New York's Woman's Hospital (now a division of St. Luke's Hospital) and Boston's Free Hospital (now combined with the Boston Lying-in Hospital as the Boston Hospital for Women) remain.

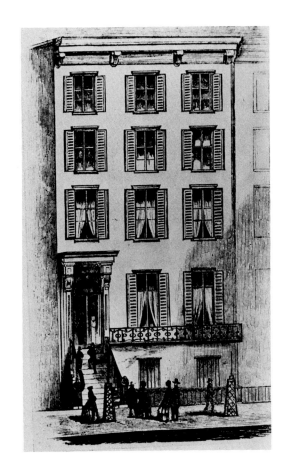

Fig. 18-21. New York's Woman's Hospital, 1855, at 83 Madison Avenue, founded by James Marion Sims. Here Sims achieved renown for his vaginal fistula repairs, and with his associates Thomas Addis Emmet, T. Gaillard Thomas, and Edmund Randolph Peaslee, brought fame to the institution for its gynecologic surgery.

508 ICONOGRAPHIA GYNIATRICA

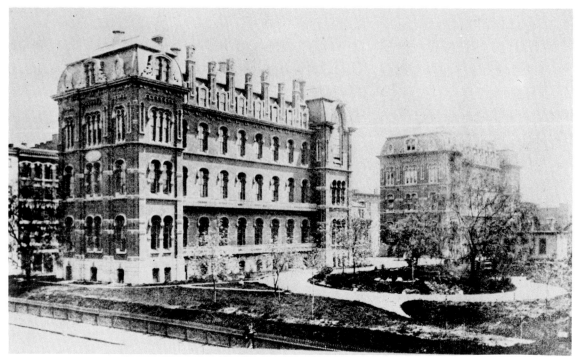

Fig. 18-22. The Woman's Hospital of the State of New York, 1867, ten years after being so chartered, at Park Avenue and 50th Street, New York City, now the site of the Waldorf-Astoria Hotel.

Fig. 18-23. The Woman's Hospital of the State of New York, 1949, at West 110th Street, New York City.

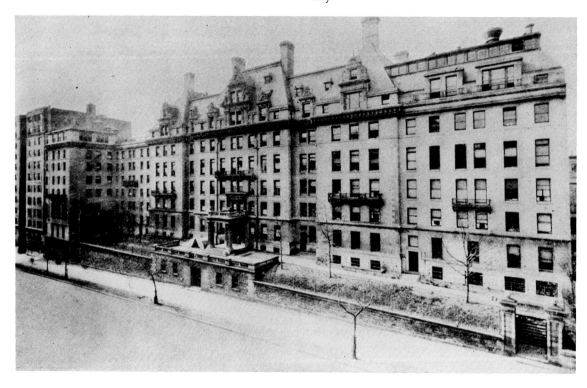

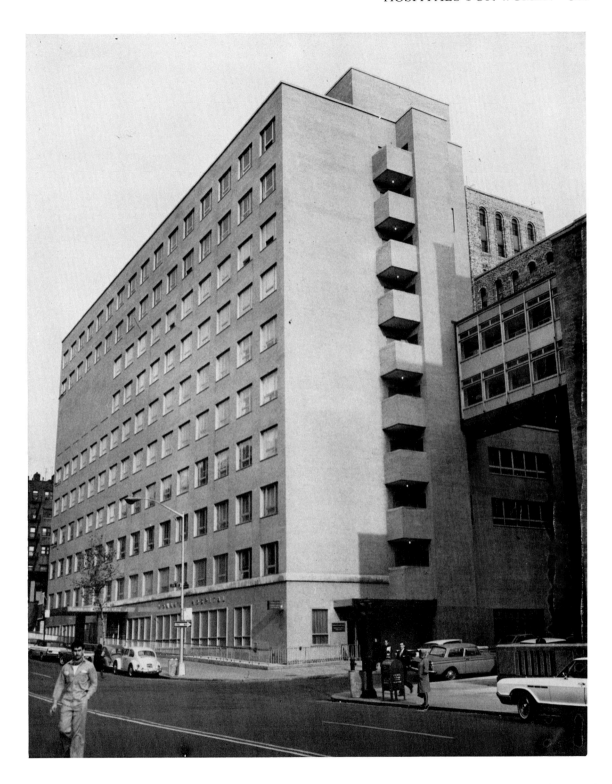

Fig. 18-24. The Woman's Hospital Division of St. Luke's Hospital, New York. New quarters of the Woman's Hospital at 114th Street and Amsterdam Avenue, occupied in August 1965, after the consolidation of the two institutions.

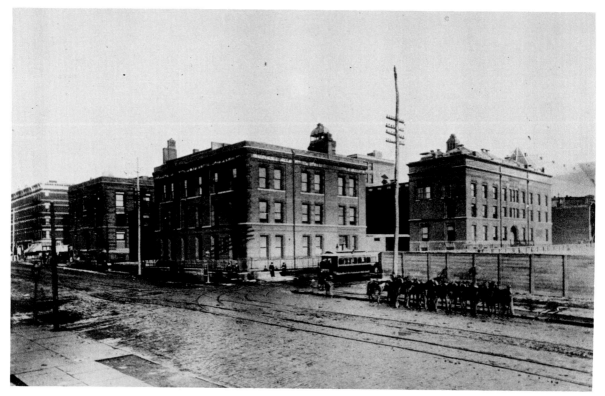

Fig. 18-25. The Sloane Maternity Hospital (later the Sloane Hospital for Women), established in 1887 at the southeast corner of Fifty-ninth Street and Tenth Avenue, New York City, through the efforts of James Woods McLane (1839–1912) and the benefaction of William Douglas Sloane (1844–1915) and his wife Emily Thorn Vanderbilt Sloane (1852–1946). At right, College of Physicians and Surgeons; at left, Vanderbilt Clinic. The Sloane Hospital for Women merged with New York's Presbyterian Hospital in 1925, moved into its present home on West 168th Street in 1928, as part of the Columbia-Presbyterian Medical Center. McLane served as the Sloane Hospital's first Director, his successors: Edwin Bradford Cragin (1859–1918), William Emery Studdiford (1867–1925), Benjamin Philp Watson (1880–   ), Howard Canning Taylor, Jr. (1900–   ), John George Moore, Jr. (1917–   ), and Raymond L. Vande Wiele (1922–   ).

Chapter 19

OBSTETRIC AND GYNECOLOGIC TEXTS

"The progress of science has rendered obsolete even those books that most helped that progress. As they are no longer of any utility, youth believes in good faith that they have never been of any use; it despises them... it laughs at them." [Anatole France: *The Crime of Sylvestre Bonnard.*]

Recorded obstetric and gynecologic knowledge dates back to ancient Egyptian papyri, the earliest known of which is the Petrie or Kahoun Papyrus, 4000 years old. Scientific periodicals, the principal medium for modern medical communication, did not originate until the mid seventeenth century; journals devoted exclusively to obstetrics and gynecology did not appear until 100 years later.

Foremost among the early efforts at obstetric and gynecologic teaching was the work of Soranus, regarded as authoritative for 1500 years. Educated in Alexandria, Soranus practiced in Rome in the early part of the second century AD. His treatise, written in Greek, included chapters on the female anatomy, menstruation, fertility, signs of pregnancy, antepartum care, labor, the obstetric chair, the newborn, amenorrhea, dysmenorrhea, uterine hemorrhage, and the vaginal speculum. This work served as the basis for Moschion's sixth century Latin manuscript, essentially a translation from Soranus' Greek, illustrated similarly with drawings of the female genitalia and of the fetal positions in utero. Nothing significant was added to obstetric teaching until the invention of printing from moveable type in the mid fifteenth century. Thereafter as never before, multiple copies could be produced easily. During the sixteenth century, the textbook rapidly replaced the manuscript as an instrument of record and teaching.

Eucharius Rösslin, whose name appears in various spellings—Röslin, Roeslin, Roesslin, and the Latin version, Rhodion—had worked as an apothecary in Freiburg im Breisgau during the years 1493–1498, then became a physician in Worms, later in Frankfurt-am-Main. Whether he ever practiced obstetrics is not known, but he assiduously studied the writings of the ancients, restated much of the obstetric teaching of Soranus, and employed an artist, Erhard Schön, to redraw many of the figures from the manuscripts of Soranus and Moschion. From these efforts came the first printed obstetric textbook, published in German in 1513 under the title *Der Swangern Frauen und Hebamen Rosegarten,* which Rösslin dedicated to the Duchess of Brunswick and Lüneberg whose service he had entered five years before. Three editions appeared in the same year, each with distinctive frontispiece. Which was published first cannot be determined. Popularly known as

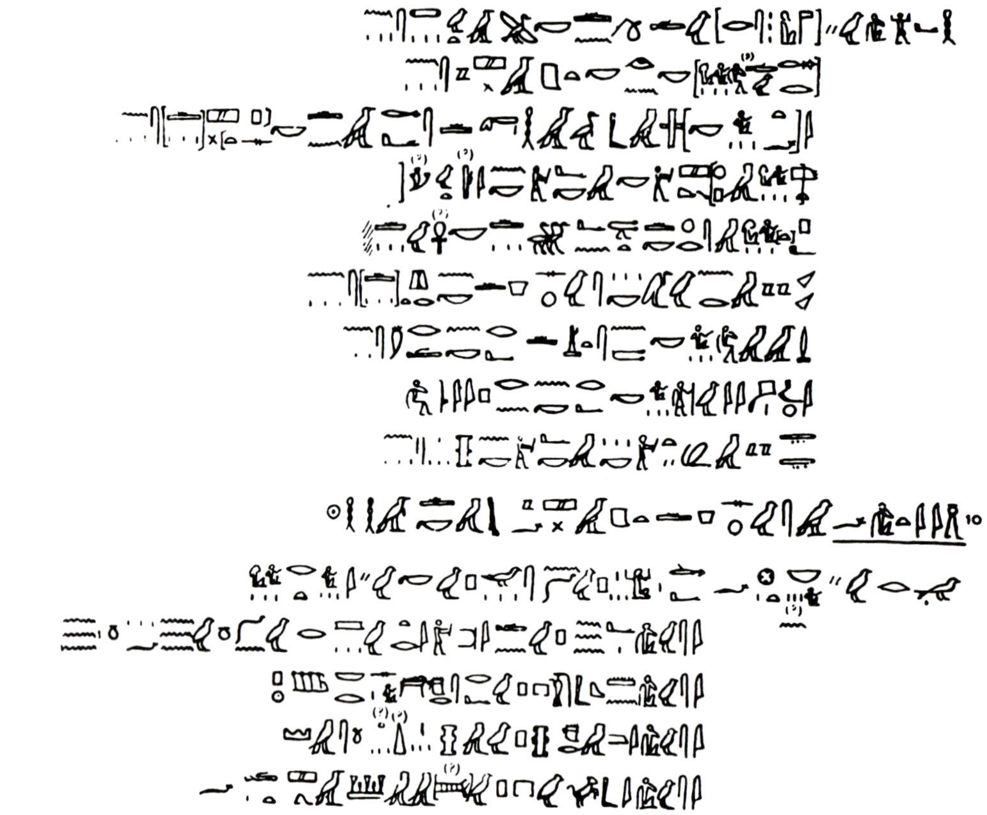

512 ICONOGRAPHIA GYNIATRICA

Fig. 19-1. A page from the Kahoun Papyrus. It was discovered during excavations near Faiyum, Upper Egypt in the late nineteenth century by Sir Flinders Petrie. Its date is variously estimated at 2200 to 1950 BC. This papyrus, consisting of only three pages, contained 34 instructions, all dealing with diseases of women including urinary disorders during pregnancy, varicose veins, genital cancer, sterility, contraception, pregnancy diagnosis, and determination of fetal sex. Subsequent Egyptian manuscripts, known as the Edwin Smith Papyrus, the Carlsburg Papyrus, the Ebers Papyrus, and the Berlin Papyrus, likewise contained a series of obstetric and gynecologic prescriptions, so strikingly similar as to strongly suggest a common source. The uterus was pictured as a free organ in the abdomen. To treat it required attracting it to its proper place by fumigations of turpentine and dried excreta placed under the standing woman. See also Fig. 16-67.

the "Rosengarten," Rösslin's work was translated into English, French, Spanish, Italian, Dutch, Polish, Czech, and Latin, enjoying the popularity of about 100 editions and remaining a bestseller for 200 years. Thus the obstetric teaching of Soranus was perpetuated for 1500 years.

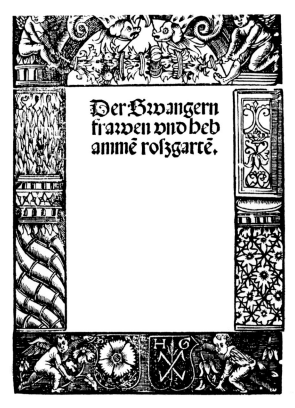

Fig. 19-2. Title page of one of the three first editions (1513) of Rösslin's "Rosengarten." A woodcut border of Renaissance style frames the three lines of the title. In the upper cross-piece appear two angels holding garlands above which are two dolphins. In the lower cross-piece one angel holds a sprig of flowers, and another holds a coat-of-arms bearing the letters H and G, the initials of the publisher Henricus Gran.

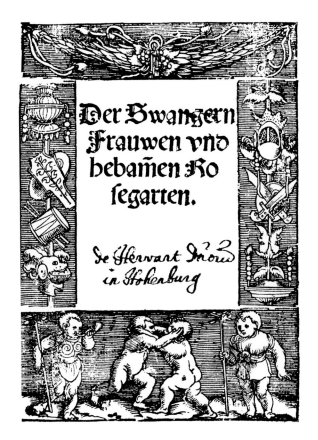

Fig. 19-3. Title page of one of the three first editions (1513) of Rösslin's "Rosengarten." The side borders enclosing the four lines of the title contain figures of some of the accouterments of war: a shield, drum, swords, and helmets. The scuffling nude boys at the bottom are flanked by two other boys, each bearing a pinwheel, one also blowing a horn.

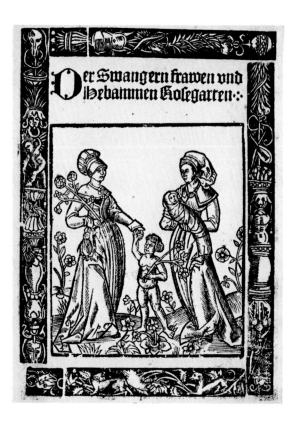

Fig. 19-4. Title page of one of the three first editions (1513) of Rösslin's "Rosengarten." An ornamental woodcut border encloses the title and a figure of two women in a rose garden, one carrying a swaddled infant, the other holding a nude boy by the hand.

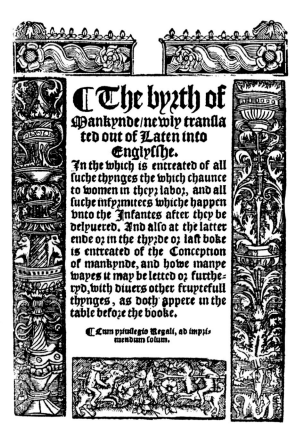

Fig. 19-5. Title page of *The Byrth of Mankynde*, 1540 English translation of Rösslin's "Rosengarten." Published by Thomas Raynalde, the translation was made by Richard Jonas from the Latin version *De partu hominis*.

DE CONCEPTV
ET GENERATIONE
HOMINIS: DE MATRICE ET EIVS
PARTIBVS, NEC NON DE CONDITIONE IN-
FANTIS IN VTERO, ET GRAVIDARVM CVRA ET OFFICIO:
De partu & parturientium infantiumq; cura omnifaria: De differentijs non naturalis partus & earundem curis: De Mola alijsq; falsis vteri tumoribus, simulque de abortibus & monstris diuersis, nec non de conceptus signis varijs: De sterilitatis causis diuersis, & de præcipuis Matricis ægritudinibus, omniumque horum curis varijs, libri sex, opera clarissimi viri IACOBI RVEFFI, Chirurgi Tigurini, quondam congesti.

Nunc denuò recogniti & in plerisq; locis castigati, picturis insuper conuenientissimis fœtus primùm in vtero siti, deinde in partu, mox etiam matricis & instrumentorum ad partum promouendum, & extrahendum pertinentium, illustrati, ornati, & in vsum eorum qui parturientibus, & obstetricibus consulere debent, typis euulgati.

Francoforti ad Mœnum. Anno M. D. LXXX.

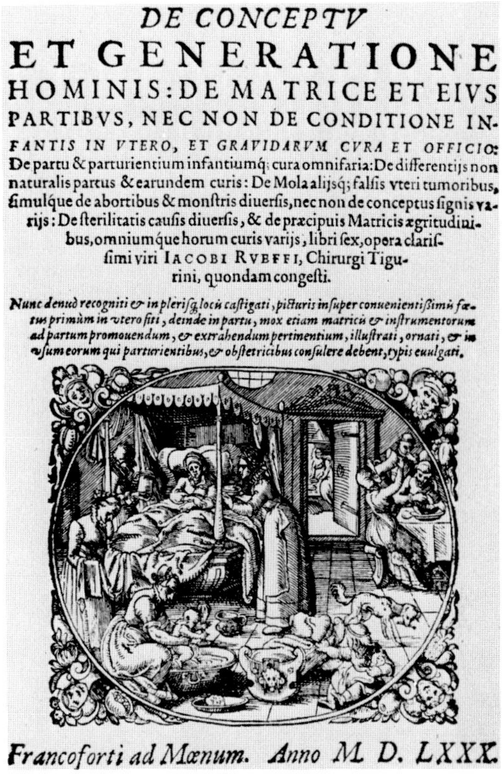

Fig. 19-6. Title page of *De conceptu et generatione hominis,* 1580 edition, by Jacob Rueff (1500–1558), Zürich surgeon and obstetrician. An improved version of Rösslin's "Rosengarten," Rueff's guide for midwives was published originally in 1554 in the German vernacular *(Ein schön lustig Trostbüchle),* but the 1580 edition was the first to contain the woodcuts of Jobst Amman, a principal feature of the work. Pictured in it are the smooth and toothed duck-bill forceps for extracting the dead fetus, used long before by the early Arabians.

LA COMARE,
ORICOGLITRICE
DI SCIPIONE MERCVRI
CITTADINO ROMANO,
Medico della Magnifica Communità di Lendenara,
DIVISA IN TRE LIBRI.
Nel primo si tratta del parto naturale dell'huomo, e dell'officio della Comare, che in esso è necessario.
Nel secondo del parto preternaturale, illegitimo, e vitioso, e di quei modi, con i quali può la Comare aiutare così le madri, come le creature.
Nel terzo delle principali infirmitadi, che accadono & alle Impagliolate, & a i fanciulli, e de i rimedij loro.
Al molto Ill. & Eccell. Sig. Bartolomeo Malmignati Dottore dell'vna, e l'altra legge, e mio Signore.
CON PRIVILEGIO.
IN VENETIA,
Appresso Gio. Battista Cioti. M D XCVI.

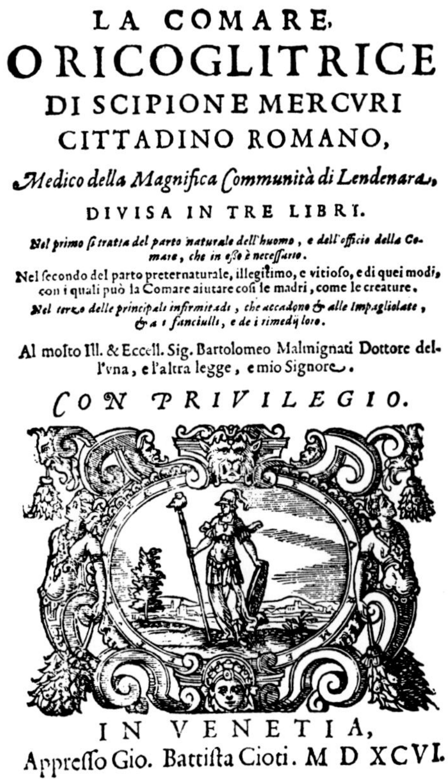

Fig. 19-7. Title page of *La Comare* by Scipione Mercurio (1540–1615), Venice, 1596. Its title later spelled *La Commare,* this first Italian text for midwives was divided into three parts or *books,* the first dealing with natural labor, the second with malpresentations, and the third with diseases of the parturient and newborn. Pelvic contraction was mentioned for the first time as an indication for cesarean section on the living woman. The operation was described and illustrated in each of the 20 editions, in Chapter 29 of Book II. The second and third parts of the first edition are dated 1595, but the volume was not published until the following year. Only four known copies remain.

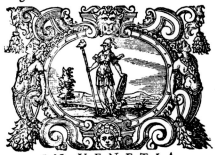

Fig. 19-8. Title page of the 1655 edition of *Armamentarium chirurgicum* by Johann Schultes, called Scultetus (1596–1645) (first edition, Ulm, 1653). Published posthumously by his nephew Scultetus the Younger, this work, translated from the Latin into French, German, and English, catalogued all the known surgical operations and instruments of the time, described the multiple-tailed binder named for the author, pictured bivalve and trivalve vaginal speculums, and gave directions and original illustrations for a number of gynecologic therapeutic procedures.

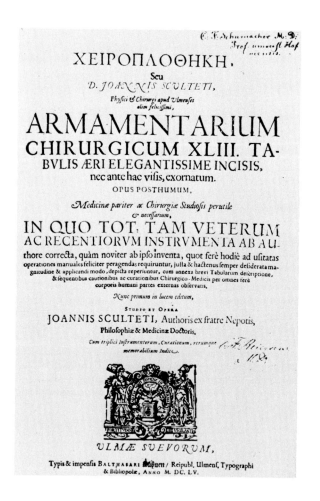

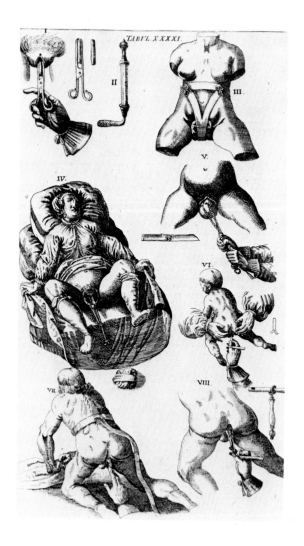

Fig. 19-9. Page of illustrations from Scultetus' *Armamentarium chirurgicum* (Table 41.) (I) Shortening the clitoris. (II) Uterine syringe. (III) Truss for vaginal medication. (IV) Use of the vaginal speculum. (V) Dead child being extracted with crooks, when it "cannot be driven forth with horsestones... or by drinking the milk of another woman."

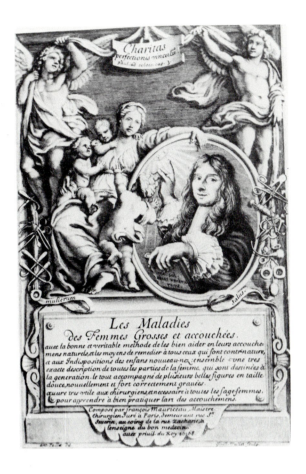

Fig. 19-10. Frontispiece from *Les maladies des femmes grosses*, 1668, by François Mauriceau (1637–1709). He was a barber-surgeon of Saint-Côme and became the most accomplished accoucheur of his day in France and the dominant figure in obstetrics of the seventeenth century. This text which went into many editions and was translated into English, German, Dutch, Italian, Latin, and Flemish helped establish obstetrics as a specialty. The third edition, published in 1681, contains a description of the technique for breech delivery and extraction of the aftercoming head, subsequently known as the *Mauriceau maneuver*.

The major obstetric texts of the next century included the "Novum lumen" of Hendrik van Deventer (1651–1724) (*Operationes chirurgicae novum lumen exhibentes obstetricantibus*, 1701) which pointed out the unyielding nature of woman's bony pelvis during labor; *A Treatise on the Theory and Practice of Midwifery* (1752–1764) of William Smellie (1697–1763) edited if not actually written by his friend Tobias Smollett, the well-known poet and author, a work distinguished by its accurate and clear description of the mechanism of labor; and *An Introduction to the Practice of Midwifery* (1795) of Thomas Denman (1733–1815) the third edition of which H. R. Spencer called

"the most splendid work on midwifery in the English language, whether regarded from the point of view of the format, paper, printing and illustrations of the work; the learning and knowledge it exhibits; or the ordered, lucid, and judicial manner in which that knowledge is presented."

Also gracing the medical literature of the eighteenth century was the general surgical text *Chirurgie* of Lorenz Heister (1683–1758), one of the foremost surgeons of his time. This systematic surgical treatise encompassed gynecology which had not yet grown to an independent specialty. First published in German in 1718, Heister's work appeared in numerous later editions as well as translations into Latin, English, Spanish, French, Italian, and Dutch. Two of its copper plate engravings (Figs. 19-11 and 19-12) are of special obstetric and gynecologic interest.

518 ICONOGRAPHIA GYNIATRICA

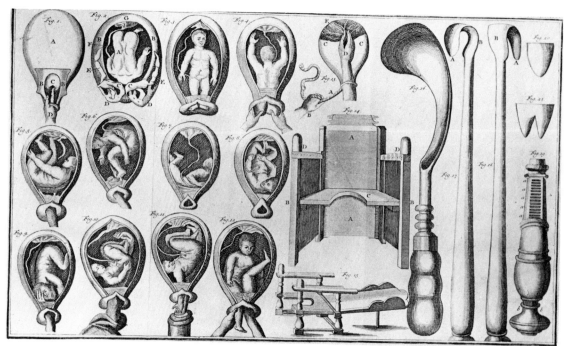

Fig. 19-11. Plate of obstetric illustrations from the early eighteenth century *Chirurgie* of Lorenz Heister. It contains the first illustration of digital examination of the cervix (Fig. 1) and shows fetal positions in utero, breech extraction, version, manual removal of the placenta, birth chairs, and the obstetric forceps and hooks.

Fig. 19-12. Plate of gynecologic illustrations from Heister's *Chirurgie*. These show avulsion of a growth from the uterine fundus, prolapse of the uterus, a douche bag, removal of a vaginal tumor, a variety of pessaries, a vaginal speculum, and a device for blowing tobacco smoke into the rectum.

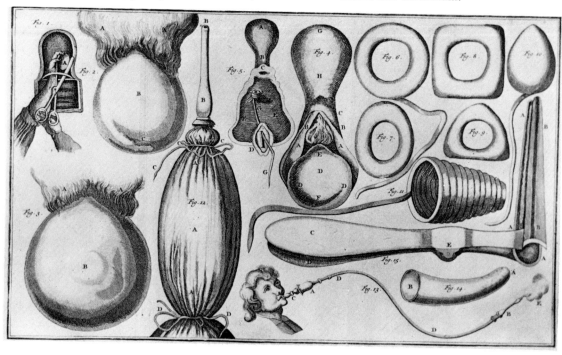

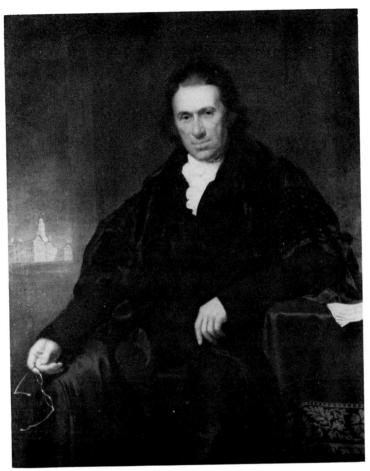

Fig. 19-13. Samuel Bard (1742–1821). He was founder of King's College Medical School and of the New York Hospital, President of the College of Physicians and Surgeons, 1813–1821, author of A *Compendium of the Theory and Practice of Midwifery,* 1807, the first textbook of obstetrics by an American physician.

Medical textbooks in America consisted mainly of European imports in the form of *American editions* or translations from France, Germany, and England until the late nineteenth century. The first textbook of obstetrics by an American author appeared in 1807, *A Compendium on the Theory and Practice of Midwifery* by Samuel Bard (1742-1821). In it Bard wrote, "There is greater safety in this branch of medicine from modest unassuming ignorance, than from a meddling presumption which frequently accompanies a little learning." Five editions were published, the last in 1819.

Popular in the United States during the mid nineteenth century were textbooks of obstetrics and gynecology by William P. Dewees, Professor of Midwifery in the University of Pennsylvania, and Charles D. Meigs, Professor of Midwifery and the Diseases of Women and Children in Jefferson Medical College. From Lea and Carey, his publishers, Dewees received $21,000 in royalties over a period of 14 years, a large sum for that era. Surpassing all previous efforts by American obstetric authors was the work of Dewees' successor at the University of Pennsylvania, Hugh Lenox Hodge (1796–1873) whose *Principles and*

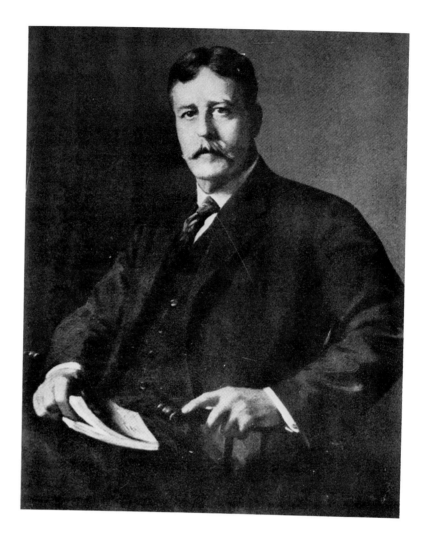

Fig. 19-14. John Whitridge Williams (1886–1931). Williams was Professor of Obstetrics in Johns Hopkins University and author of America's most popular obstetric text, first published in 1903. Painting by Thomas Cromwell Corner (1865–1938).

Practice of Obstetrics, dictated from memory because of the author's blindness and published in 1864, became one of the classics of American obstetrics. John Whitridge Williams referred to it as late as 1903 as "a model of scrupulous observation...the most original work that had appeared in America and, with few modifications, still retaining its value." In it Hodge clearly described the pelvic types, directed attention to the inadequacy of external pelvimetry, urged more frequent resort to the forceps in cases of dystocia, and introduced a placental forceps for the completion of abortion. Gynecologic counterpart of Hodge's obstetric text was *The Principles and Practice of Gynaecology* (1879) of Thomas Addis Emmet (1829–1919), surgeon to New York's Woman's Hospital, characterized by

Howard A. Kelly as "the first thoroughly scientific, comprehensive work on this subject in English."

In none of the obstetric treatises of the mid nineteenth century was a word to be found on the subject of antepartum care. Medical consultation was sought by women before the onset of labor only for such obvious complications as bleeding or convulsions.

A new standard of excellence for obstetric scholarship was established by *Williams Obstetrics,* first published in 1903 by John Whitridge Williams (1866–1931), Professor of Obstetrics in Johns Hopkins University, in an attempt "to set forth ... the scientific basis for and the practical application of the obstetrical art." Subsequently updated by Henricus J. Stander, then by Nicholson J. Eastman, *Williams Obstetrics* is now in its fourteenth edition (1971) under the editorship of Doctors Louis M. Hellman and Jack A. Pritchard. Presenting the science as well as the art of obstetrics with full consideration of its theoretical as well as its practical aspects and emphasizing its potentialities for fruitful research, Williams' first edition contained more than 1,100 references to the original literature, in contrast to the virtual absence of such citations from predecessor works.

In 1913 *Williams Obstetrics* was joined by *The Principles and Practice of Obstetrics* of Joseph B. DeLee (1869–1942), Professor of Obstetrics in Northwestern University, a meticulously prepared volume profusely illustrated with 906 figures. Under the later editorship of J. P. Greenhill, DeLee's book has undergone repeated metamorphosis and in 1965 went into its thirteenth edition.

In addition to the obstetric and gynecologic tomes for professional readers—medical students, physicians, nurses, and midwives—volumes have been published for the laity in every generation since at least as early as 1495. Many of these treatises of the eighteenth and nineteenth centuries, although written ostensibly to instruct women in matters of so-called feminine hygiene, the symptoms and treatment of disease, and the care of the newborn, served actually as not so subtle advertising for their authors or for the promotion of their patent medicines, inventions, and secret remedies.

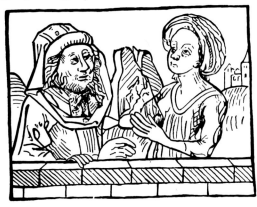

Fig. 19-15. Title page of a German guidebook for expectant mothers. This book was published in Ulm about 1495 by a Dr. Ortolf, a Bavarian physician.

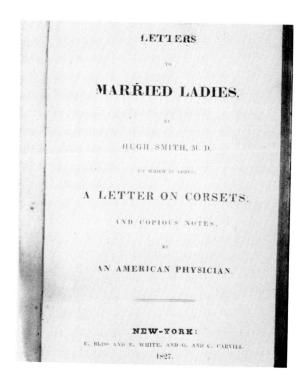

Fig. 19-16. Title page of an American edition, 1827, of the long popular *Letters to Married Ladies* by Hugh Smith, a London physician. In this small volume first published in 1767 under the title *Letters to Married Women,* a plea was made for maternal breast feeding; birthmarks, miscarriage, and old age were also discussed.

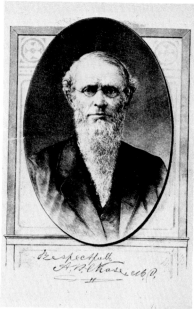
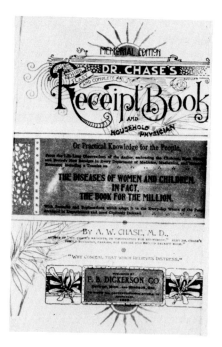

Fig. 19-17. Frontispiece and title page of *Dr. Chase's Receipt Book,* 1893, including "a treatise on the diseases of women and children." Medical manuals for the layman were popular during the second half of the nineteenth century, the heyday of American medical diploma mills and an era of depressed medical ethical standards.

The level of obstetric literature for nonmedical readers was elevated in the twentieth century by several authoritative handbooks. Outstanding among them was Nicholson J. Eastman's *Expectant Motherhood,* first published in 1940. During the next three decades nearly three million copies were produced in five editions, the last under the co-authorship of Dr. Keith P. Russell.

PICTORIAL CREDITS AND SOURCES

Aartsbisschoppelijk Museum, Utrecht (*2-27*); *Actas Cibas* (*11-16B* from La operación cesarea, 1952); *Acta Hist. Sci. Natur. Med.* (*4-15, 11-5* from V. Møller-Christensen, Middelalderens Laegekunst I Danmark, 1944); *Aesculape* (*4-73, 15-22, 15-28* from vol. 19, 1929; *8-71* from P. Huard and O. Zansetsou, L'Obstétrique Japonaise à la période préméija, 1962); Alinari, Florence (*1-61, 2-19, 4-36–4-39, 4-44, 4-86, 6-3, 8-5, 12-15, 14-2, 14-7, 14-8, 14-16, 14-17, 16-13, 16-22, 17-2*); American Heritage Publishing Co., New York (*13-20* from M. B. Davidson, ed., *The Horizon Book of Lost Worlds*, 1962); *Am. J. Med. Sci.* (*17-29* from J. M. Sims, A new uterine elevator, 1858; *17-53* from J. M. Sims, On the treatment of vesico-vaginal fistula, 1852); *Am. J. Obstet.* (*9-15* from J. W. McLane, The Sloane Maternity Hospital, 1891; *17-60* from I. S. Stone, The pedicle in hysterectomy, 1891); *Ann. Gynec.* (*8-82* from A. Couvelaire, Traitment chirurgical des hémorrhagies utero-placentaires, 1911; *9-29* from Champetier de Ribes, De l'accouchement provoqué, 1888); *Ann. NY. Acad. Sci.* (*8-4* from A. Plaut, Historical and cultural aspects of the uterus, 1959); *Ann. Ostet. Ginec.* (*11-1, 11-22, 11-32, 15-42* from P. Gall, L'iconografia del taglio cesareo, 1936); *L'Anthropologie* (*1-58* from H. Meige, L'infantilisme, le féminisme, et les hermaphrodites antiques, 1895); Appleton-Century-Crofts, New York (*1-36, 1-38* from H. A. Kelly, *Gynecology*, 1928; *8-90* from N.J. Eastman, *Williams Obstetrics*, 1956; *17-25, 17-27, 17-57, 17-58* from A. J. C. Skene, *Treatise on the Diseases of Women*, 1889); *Arch. Geschichte Med.* (*17-1* from K. Sudhoff, Mutterrohr und Verwandtes im medizinischen Instrumentarium der Antike, 1926); *Arch. Gynaek.* (*1-29* from A. Mackenrodt, Ueber die Ursachen der normalen und pathologischen Lagen des Uterus, 1895; *8-57* from G. Leopold and Spörlin, Die Leitung und regelmässigen Geburten nur durch äussere Untersuchung, 1894; *12-5* from C. S. Credé, U e b e r Erwärmungsgeräthe für frühgeborene und schwächliche kleine Kinder, 1884; *17-56* from G. Leopold, Die operative Behandlung der Uterusmyome, 1890); *Archiv. Gynaek.* (*5-44* from P. Zweifel, Ueber Extrauteringravidität und retrouterine Hämatome, 1891); *Arch. Klin. Chir.* (*17-72* from W. Meyer, Ueber die Nachbehandlung des hohen Steinschnittes sowie über Verwendbarkeit desselben zur Operation von Blasenscheidenfisteln, 1884); *Arch. Prov. Chir.* (*17-39* from H. Dayot, Enorme Kyste de l'ovaire chez une jeune fille de 17 ans, ablation, guérison, 1893); Archives Photographiques, Paris (*1-60, 9-54, 16-28, 18-1*); Artia Publishers, Prague (*16-29* from J. Poulik, *Kunst der Vorzeit*, 1956); Aukland Institute and Museum (*6-7*); J.B. Baillière et Fils, Paris (*14-4, 14-10, 14-14, 14-15, 14-23, 15-40, 15-54* from I. Geoffroy Saint-Hilaire, *Histoire générale et particulière des anomalies de l' organisation chez l' homme et les animaux*, 1857; *17-5* from J. H. Guilbert, *Considérations pratiques sur les certaines affections de l' utérus*, 1826; *17-14* from F. W. de Scanzoni, *Traité pratique des maladies de organes sexuels de la femme*, 1858); Bale & Danielsson, London (*16-76, 16-77* from M.C. Stopes, *Contraception: Its Theory, History and Practice*, 1923); Johann Ambrosius Barth Verlagsbuchhandlung, Leipzig (*1-2, 4-40, 5-2, 5-4, 5-31, 5-34* from K. Sudhoff, *Ein Beitrag zur Geschichte der Anatomie im Mittelalter speziell der anatomischen Graphik nach Handschriften des 9. bis 15. Jahrhunderts. Studien zur Geschichte der Medizin*, 1908; *19-15* from K. Sudhoff, *Deutsche Medizinische Inkunabeln*, 1908); Bechet & Labé, Paris (*8-80, 9-49* from J. P. Maygrier, *Nouvelles démonstrations d'accouchements*, 1840); Berger-Levrault, Paris (*18-4, 18-6* from M. Fosseyeaux, *L'Hôtel Dieu de Paris au XVIIe et au XVIIIe siècle*, 1912); J. F. Bergmann, Munich (*5-5, 6-38, 8-16, 8-18, 8-58, 9-2, 9-16* from P. Diepgen, *Die Frauenheilkunde der alten Welt*, in W. Stoeckel, *Handbuch der Gynäkologie*, 1937); J. F. Bergmann, Wiesbaden (*15-33* from F. Schatz, *Die Griechischen Götter und die Menschlichen Missgeburten*, 1901); Biblioteca Ambrosiana, Milan (*1-14* courtesy of *Ciba Symposia*, formerly published by Ciba Pharmaceutical Co.); Biblioteca Medicea-Laurenziana, Florence (*13-23*); Bibliothèque de l'Academie Royale de Médicine de Belgique, Brussels (*15-4*); Bibliothèque de l'Arsenal, Paris (*11-11, 15-18, 15-62*); Bibliothèque Municipale, Amiens, France (*2-25*); Bibliothèque Nationale, Paris (*1-43*,

2-31, 4-8, 4-14, 4-72, 4-82, 4-84, 4-85, 4-101, 4-96, 11-10, 11-12, 11-13, 12-21, 13-35, 13-41, 14-13, 15-16, 15-24, 18-3); Black, Edinburgh (*8-61, 8-62* from J. M. Duncan, *Contributions to the Mechanism of Natural and Morbid Parturition,* 1875); Blakiston, Philadelphia (*11-25, 11-28, 11-30, 17-4, 17-34, 17-41, 17-42, 17-66, 17-69* from J. V. Ricci, *The Development of Gynaecological Surgery and Instruments,* 1949); *12-4* from A. M. Fullerton, *A Handbook of Obstetrical Nursing for Nurses, Students and Mothers,* 1893); The Boston Globe (*3-11*); The British Museum, London (*11-6, 12-17, 13-7, 16-35, 16-73*); The Brooklyn Museum, Brooklyn (*12-12, 16-26, 16-27, 16-47–16-49, 16-57*); *Bull. Gen. Thérap.* (*17-22* from L. Lefort, Nouveau procédé pour la guérison du prolapsus utérin, 1877); *Bull. Hist. Med.* (*17-75* from J. Friedenwald and S. Morrison, The history of the enema, 1940; *17-80* from T. G. H. Drake, Antique pewter of medical interest, 1955, courtesy of Mrs. Nina Drake); *Bull. Med. Library Assn.* (*4-29* from G. E. Mestler, A galaxy of old Japanese medical books, 1954); *Bull. N. Y. Acad. Med.* (*18-15* from A. Vogl, Six hundred years of medicine in Vienna, 1967); J. E. Bulloz, Paris (*6-1*); Dr. Stanley M. Bysshe (*9-48*); Cambridge University Press, Cambridge (*2-16, 6-12, 6-14, 6-16, 6-17, 6-22, 6-23, 6-39* from J. Needham, *A History of Embryology,* 1959; *9-1, 14-12, 15-35* from A. B. Cook, *Zeus: A Study in Ancient Religion,* 1925); Campo Santo, Pisa (*15-15*); Carnegie Institution of Washington, Baltimore (*6-35, 6-36*); Carré et Naud, Paris (*9-46* from P. Bar, *Le Professeur S. Tarnier, 1828-1897*); Casanatense Library, Rome (*17-70*); Chambers, St. Louis (*8-44–8-46, 8-51–8-53, 8-55* from G. J. Engelmann, *Labor Among Primitive Peoples,* 1883); *La Chronique Médicale* (*12-14* from H. Villard, La circoncision dans l'art, 1909; *12-16* from Origines de l'imprimerie en France, 1907; *12-19* from 1905 edition); John Churchill, London (*9-40* from J. H. Aveling, *The Chamberlens and the Midwifery Forceps,* 1882; *17-24* from G. J. Crosse, *An Essay, Literary and Practical, on Inversio Uteri,* 1847; *17-54* from H. Savage, *The Surgery, Surgical Pathology and Surgical Anatomy of the Female Pelvic Organs,* 1870); Ciba Symposia (*4-23, 8-42, 16-25, 16-53, 16-54* from R. F. Spencer, Primitive obstetrics, 1949-1950; *6-11* from M. F. A. Montagu, Early history of embryology, 1949; *8-17* from E. G. Wakefield and S. C. Dellinger, Diseases of prehistoric Americans of South Central United States, 1940; *16-52* from I. Stevenson, Twins, 1941; *18-16* from A. Castiglioni, The medical school of Vienna, 1947); *Ciba Symposium* (*5-32, 6-8, 8-59, 15-17* from L. C. MacKinney, Childbirth in the Middle Ages, 1960); *Ciba Z.* (*4-32, 16-33* from H. Buess, Die Anfänge der Geburtshilfe, 1950; *13-43* from H. Buess and G. Mamlock, Die Milch in der Therapie der neueren Zeit, 1948); Cleveland Health Museum (*6-10, 15-9*); *Clin. Ostetr.* (*4-94* from P. Gall, Il parto di Alcmena, 1936); *Clin. Pediat.* (*4-17* from T. E. Cone, Jr., Emerging awareness of the artist in the proportions of the human infant, 1962); Colchester and Essex Museum, The Castle, Colchester, England (*16-20*); Compagnie des Libraires, Paris (*6-41* from F. Mauriceau, *Traité des maladies des femmes grosses*); Czermak, Vienna (*8-78* from L. Bandl, *Über Ruptur der Gebärmutter und ihre Mechanik,* 1875); Roger Dacosta, Paris (*1-5, 1-7, 1-12, 1-28, 1-40, 1-63, 1-71, 1-72, 6-9, 17-79* from A. Pecker, *Hygiène et maladies de la femme au cours des siècles,* 1961; *2-23, 4-7, 4-53, 11-8, 11-12, 15-13* from A. Pecker and H. Rouland, *L'accouchement au cours des siècles,* 1958; *17-15* from P. Huard and M.D. Grmek, *Le premier manuscrit chirurgical Turc,* 1960); F. A. Davis Co., Philadelphia (*7-21, 9-47* from J. C. Ullery and M. A. Castallo, *Obstetric Mechanisms and Their Management,* 1957; *12-7, 18-25* from H. Speert, *The Sloane Hospital Chronicle,* 1963; *17-40* from D. T. Gilliam, *A Text-book of Practical Gynecology,* 1907; *18-19, 18-20* from C. E. Heaton, *The New York Obstetrical Society,* 1963, collection of Dr. Claude Heaton); F. B. Dickerson Co., Detroit (*19-17* from A. W. Wood, *Dr. Chase's Receipt Book and Household Physician,* 1893); Dornan, Philadelphia (*17-51* from American Gynecological Society, *Album of the Fellows,* F. E. Keene, ed., 1930); O. Doin, Paris (*1-35, 12-6* from P. C. Budin and E. Crouzat, *La pratique des accouchements à l'usage des sage-femmes,* 1898); Mrs. Nina Drake (*13-59*); Dresden Gemäldegalerie (*13-56* courtesy of Deutsche Fotothek Dresden); Dumbarton Oaks, Washington, D. C. (*8-15* from Robert Woods Bliss Collection); *Edinburgh Med. J.* (*8-21, 8-26–8-37, 11-20* from R. W. Felkin, Notes on labour in Central Africa, 1884; *9-11* from A. R. Simpson, On a delivery-pan in use at the present time in Spain, 1895); Egyptian Museum, Cairo (*4-33, 4-35, 16-24*); Elsevier Publishing Company, Amsterdam (*15-26, 15-27* from J. Smalbraak, *Trophoblastic Growths,* 1957); Ferdinand Enke Verlag, Stuttgart (*1-74, 6-13* from E. Holländer, *Wunder Wundergeburt und Wundergestalt,* 1921; *2-6, 2-7, 4-95, 15-23* from E. Holländer, *Die Karikatur und Satire im der Medizin,* 1905; *2-13, 2-14, 4-9, 11-2, 16-8, 16-40* from E. Hollander, *Plastik und Medizin,* 1912; *2-36, 4-16, 4-113, 4-51, 4-70, 8-85, 11-15, 12-20, 15-14, 15-19, 18-2* from E. Holländer, *Die Medizin in der klassischen Malerei,* 1913; *4-25–4-27, 4-45–4-50, 4-54–4-58, 4-66, 8-6, 9-53, 12-9, 12-10, 15-15, 15-21* from R. Müllerheim, *Die Wochenstube in der Kunst,* 1904; *13-42, 13-44, 13-48, 13-49, 13-65* from H. Brüning, *Geschichte der Methodik der Künstlichen Säuglingsernährung,* 1908; *17-12* from A. Hegar and R. Kaltenbach, *Die Operative Gynäkologie,* 1881); Andreas Feininger (*16-44*); Benno Filser Verlag, Augsburg (*16-41* from R. Kriss, *Das Gebärmuttervotiv,* 1929); *Fisiol. e Med.* (*9-39* from S. Baglioni, Conoscevano gli antichi l'uso del forcipe ostetrico? 1937); Galleria Borghese, Rome (*4-88, 4-89* Photo Anderson); Galleria Pitti (*1-47*); Gallerie dell' Academia, Venice (*4-102* Photo Osvaldo Böhm); Gamut

Press, New York (*16-70, 16-72, 16-73* from N. E. Himes, *Medical History of Contraception,* 1963); Gemäldegalerie Alte Meister, Dresden (*4-115*); Germanisches Nationalmuseum, Nürnberg (*4-110, 4-114* formerly, *9-8, 12-23–12-25, 16-82*); Giraudon, Paris (*1-1, 1-42, 4-31, 4-64, 10-8, 11-9, 13-2* permission ADAGP 1968 by French Reproduction Rights, Inc., *15-18*); Glasgow University Library, Glasgow, Scotland (*4-99*); Glyptothek, Munich (*16-61*); Grant Sanger, M.D. (*16-75*); William Green, Edinburgh (*14-32, 15-48* from J. W. Ballantyne, *Manual of Antenatal Pathology and Hygiene*); T. Grieben, Leipzig (*8-8, 8-9* from E. Bischoff, *Die Kabbalah,* 1917); Groeninge Museum, Bruges (*4-52*); Grunow, Leipzig (*8-60* from F. Ahlfeld, *Lehrbuch der Geburtshilfe,* 1894); Guido Calza (*4-10*); Gurney & Jackson, London (*8-67, 8-68* from G. Barger, *Ergot and Ergotism,* 1931); Harcourt, Brace & World, New York (*4-3, 4-4* from J. Thorwald, *Science and Secrets of Early Medicine,* 1962); George G. Harrap & Co., London (*1-55* from E. Grillot de Givry, *Witchcraft, Magic, and Alchemy,* 1963); Harvard College Library, Theater Collection, Cambridge, Mass. (*1-75*);Hawthorn Books, New York (*9-21* from J. Starobinski, *A History of Medicine,* 1964); Karl Hechter-Schulz (*16-58, 16-59*); Wm. Heinemann, London (*2-37, 4-6, 4-20, 4-78* (codex Borbonicus), *4-103, 4-108, 4-111, 4-112, 5-38, 5-39, 8-10–8-14, 8-19, 8-25, 8-47, 8-50, 8-63, 8-64, 9-3, 9-9, 9-31, 11-14, 13-8, 13-10, 13-30–13-33, 13-39, 15-2, 15-3, 15-12, 15-25, 16-9, 16-55, 16-61, 16-80, 16-81, 16-83* from H. Ploss, M. Bartels, and P. Bartels, *Woman,* 1927); The Hermitage, Leningrad (*13-15*); Hestia Verlag, Bayreuth (*18-11–18-13* from G. Jaeckel, *Die Charité. Die Geschichte des Berühmtesten Deutschen Krankenhauses,* 1965); Stephen Higgons Collection, Paris (*4-90*); Hirmer Fotoarchiv München (*14-1*); Hirschwald, Berlin (*2-28, 7-17, 12-27* from G. E. Curàtulo, *Die Kunst der Juno Lucina in Rom,* 1902); *Hist. Med.* (*17-76* from M. Rousseau, *Les bains de vapeur,* 1965); Holbein-Verlag, Basel (*2-10* from H. B. Bandi and J. Maringer, *Kunst der Eiszeit,* 1952); Iraq Museum, Baghdad (*16-6*); *Isis* (*6-29* from G. Sarton, The discovery of the mammalian egg); Istanbul Archaeological Museum (*1-56*); *J.A.M.A.* (*14-11* courtesy of Dr. Joseph L. Roberge; *16-65* from I. C. Rubin, The nonoperative determination of patency of fallopian tubes by means of intra-uterine inflation with oxygen and the production of artificial pneumoperitoneum, 1920); *J. Chir. Augen.* (*17-68* from von Alten, Der im chirurgische-augenärztliche Clinico zu Berlin eingeführte Operationstisch, 1820); *J. Hist. Med.* (*8-2* from L. H. Wells, Iconographic origins of some early anatomical diagrams: A further suggestion, 1962); *J. Warburg and Courtauld Inst.* (*16-37, 16-38* from A. A. Barb, Diva Matrix, 1953); Jansson-Waesberg, Amsterdam (*9-42* from L. Heister, *Institutiones Chirurgicae,* 1747); *Jenaer Med. Hist. Beitr.* (*16-34* from T. Mayer-Steineg, Darstellungen normaler und Krankheit veränderter Körperteile, 1912); Johns Hopkins Press, Baltimore (*17-74* from A. W. Davis, *Dr. Kelly of Hopkins,* 1959; *19-14* from J. M. Slemons, *John Whitridge Williams,* 1935); Marshall Jones, Boston (*4-87, 14-6, 14-19* from W.S. Fox, *Greek and Roman,* in L. H. Gray, *The Mythology of All Races,* 1916); Jordon, Chicago (*4-75* from M. Avi-Yonah and A. Malamut, *Views of the Biblical World,* 1959); S. Karger, Berlin (*11-31*); Prof. Robert J. Kellar (*9-38*); *Kinderaerztl.Prax.*(*4-2* from A. Peiper, Die ältesten Bilder von Mutter und Kind, 1963); Königliche öffentliche Bibliothek, Dresden (*15-5*); Koninklijk Museum voor Schone Kunsten, Antwerp (*13-25*); Carl Kuhn, Munich (*4-18, 5-37, 15-49, 19-2–19-5* from G. Klein, *Eucharius Rösslin's "Rosengarten,"* 1910); Kunsthistorisches Museum, Vienna (*14-21*); *Lancet* (*8-81* from J. B. Hicks, On a new method of version in abnormal labour, 1860); H. Lauwereyns, Paris (*17-67* from A. W. L. Leblond, *Traité élémentaire de chirurgie gynécologique,* 1878); Lea & Febiger, Philadelphia (*5-45* from J. B. Sutton, *Surgical Diseases of the Ovaries and Fallopian Tubes Including Tubal Pregnancy,* 1891; *8-84* from W. P. Dewees, *A Compendious System of Midwifery,* 1830; *9-24* from F. Churchill, *On the Theory and Practice of Midwifery,* 1846; *9-25* from C. D. Meigs, *Obstetrics: The Science and the Art,* 1849; *12-2, 12-3* from E. B. Cragin, *Obstetrics,* 1916; *13-34, 14-22, 14-26* from B. C. Hirst and G. A. Piersol, *Human Monstrosities,* 1891; *15-58* from E. P. Davis, *A Treatise on Obstetrics,* 1896; *17-9, 17-46* from T. A. Emmet, *The Principles and Practice of Gynaecology,* 1879; *17-13, 17-32, 17-65, 17-73* from F. H. Davenport, *Diseases of Women,* 1898; *17-28, 17-38* from R. Barnes, *A Clinical History of the Medical and Surgical Diseases of Women,* 1874; *17-31* from H. L. Hodge *On Diseases Peculiar to Women, Including Displacements of the Uterus,* 1860; *17-50* from F. Churchill, *Diseases of Females,* 1844); The Lehman Collection, New York (*2-21*); Library of the College of Physicians of Philadelphia (*15-20*); R. Lier & Co., Florence (*1-17, 1-18, 1-21, 1-23, 5-7* from C. Singer, *The Fasciculo di Medicina, Venice, 1493,* 1925); Lindsey & Blakiston, Philadelphia (*2-40* from A. Meadows, *A Manual of Midwifery,* 1871; *17-20* from C. Clay, *The Complete Handbook of Obstetric Surgery,* 1874); J. B. Lippincott Co., Philadelphia (*17-7* from J. Y. Simpson, *Obstetric Memoirs and Contributions,* 1855); *17-43* from A. Schachner, *Ephraim McDowell,* 1921; *17-49* from J. M. Keating and H. C. Coe, *Clinical Gynecology, Medical and Surgical,* 1895); Little, Brown & Company, Boston (*14-20* from E. Hamilton, *Mythology*); London, (*5-24* from T. J. Pettigrew, *Medical Portrait Gallery,* 1838-1840); Longmans, Green & Co., London (*17-37, 17-81* from Obstetrical Society of London, *Catalogue and Report of Obstetrical and Other Instruments,* 1867); Toni Lynn Maternities (*2-42*); *Lyon Medical* (*4-60* from Les sages-femmes de la nativité et leurs figurations à Lyon, 1936); Macmillan Company, New York (*5-20, 5-30* from H. Speert, *Obstetric and Gynecologic*

Milestones; 8-74 from W. E. Fothergill, *Manual of Midwifery,* 1896; *17-55, 18-21–18-23* from S. Harris, *Woman's Surgeon,* 1950); Macmillan & Co., Ltd., London (*10-7* from R. J. Godlee, *Lord Lister,* 1917); W. Malende, Leipzig (*1-62, 1-67* from M. Hirschfeld, *Geschlechtsübergänge, Misschungen männlicher und weiblicher Geschlechtscharaktere,* 1905); Librairie Maloine, Paris (*1-50, 2-41* from G. J. Witkowski, *Anecdotes historiques et religieuses sur les seins et l'allaitement*); Dr. James P. Marr (*17-52*); Maternity Center Association, New York (*8-1* from R. L. Dickinson and A. Belskie, *Birth Atlas,* 1962; *15-8*); Pierre Matisse Gallery, New York (*4-5*); The Mauritshuis, the Hague (*2-4* given on loan to Gemeentemuseum, Arnhem); *M. D. Newsmagazine* (*4-71,* 1963); Mead Johnson Laboratories, Elkhart, Ind. (*13-27, 13-53–13-55, 13-57, 13-58, 13-60–13-64*); *Med. Hist.* (*8-66* from F. Guerra, Aztec medicine, 1966); *Med. Mschr.* (*4-92, 15-34, 15-41* from H. K. Hofmeier, Widernaturliche und zweite Geburten in der altgriechischen Mythologie, 1964); *Med. Times Gazette* (*17-47* from J. Clay, Adhesion clamp: A new instrument for aiding the removal of ovarian tumours, etc., 1862); James Mellaart (*4-32, 16-2, 16-3, 16-30, 16-31*); *Memoires de l'académie imperiale de médecine* (*17-48* from E. Koeberle, De l'ovariotomié, 1863); Metropolitan Museum of Art, New York (*2-18, 2-20, 4-91, 12-1, 14-18, 16-12, 16-32, 16-39, 16-45, 16-46*); Méquignon, Paris (*9-36* from J. L. Baudelocque, *L'art des accouchemens,* 1807); Éditions Albin Michel, Paris (*1-69, 1-70, 2-2, 2-11, 3-13, 4-10, 4-13, 4-21, 5-33, 5-35, 12-13, 16-14, 17-45, 17-77, 18-3* from M. Laignel-Lavastine, *Histoire générale de la médecine, de la pharmacie, de l' art dentaire et de l'art vétérinaire,* 1938); Miller Library of the History of Medicine, Richmond Academy of Medicine, Richmond, Va. (*11-18*); *Modern Medicine* (*15-32* Lawrence Katzman); *Mschr. Geburt. Frauen.* (*17-36* from G. Simon, Operationen an den weiblichen Geschlechtstheilen, 1859); *München. Med. Wschr.* (*6-32* from R. Kohnz, Mikroskopie im Mittelalter); Musée des Beaux-Arts, Beaune, France (*12-8*); Musée de Dejon, France (*1-13*); Musée de l'Homme, Paris (*8-72*); Musée Guimet, Versailles, France (*4-67, 4-68*); Musée de l' Assistance Publique, Paris (*13-37*); Musée Carnavalet, Paris (*18-5*); Musée de Chatillon-sur-Seine, France (*16-14*); Musée de Cluny, France (*16-80*); Musée du Louvre, Paris (*1-59, 2-26, 4-80, 4-81, 8-3, 8-7, 9-52, 9-54, 13-5, 13-20, 13-21, 13-24, 13-36, 16-5, 16-7–16-11, 16-21*); Musée d'Unterlinden, Colmar, France (*4-62, 4-65, 12-22, 13-17*); Musée Royaux des Beaux-Arts de Belgique, Brussels (*4-42*); Musei Capitolini, Rome (*13-46, 16-22*); Museo Archeologico, Florence (*13-8, 16-13, 16-36*); Museo Nazionale, Florence (*4-107* Photo Bertoni); Museo Nazionale, Naples (*17-2*); Museo Nazionale di Villa Giulia, Rome (*16-42*); Museo Poldi-Pezzoli, Milan (*13-16*); Museum der Bildenden Künste, Leipzig (*17-78* formerly); **Museum für Indische Kunst,** West Berlin (*11-4*); Museum für Völkerkunde, West Berlin (*13-22, 13-28, 13-39* formerly, destroyed in W. W. II, *16-56*); Museum of the History of Science, University of Ghent, Belgium (*15-38*); Museum of Medical Art, Hospital of Santo Spirito, Sassia, Rome (*15-7, 15-39*); The Museum of Modern Art, New York (*14-3*); Museum of Primitive Art, New York (*16-50*); Museum of San Marco, Italy (*15-37*); Museum of Science and Industry, Chicago (*5-13*); Museum of the Tavera Hospital, Toledo, Spain (*1-73* from Dr. John B. Sears); Museum voor de Geschiedenis van de Wetenschappen, Rijksuniversiteit Gent (*9-43*); National Archaeological Museum, Athens (*1-57, 2-15, 2-38, 2-33, 4-104–4-106, 6-4, 16-15*); Nationalbibliothek, Vienna (*8-65, 15-17*); Reproduced by courtesy of the trustees, the National Gallery, London (*2-35, 4-61, 13-3, 13=12, 13-14*); National Library of Medicine, Bethesda, Maryland (*3-12*); *Natural History* (*6-5* from H. Arbman, Bronze age seen in granite, courtesy of Lee Boltin; *13-47* from Per-Olle Stackman); Naturhistorisches Museum, Vienna (*16-1*); Neufeld & Henius Verlag, Berlin (*2-32* from H. Ploss, M. Bartels, and P. Bartels, *Das Weib in der Natur und Völkerkunde,* 1927; New Haven (*9-4* from *A Collection of Early Obstetrical Books,* 1952); The New York Academy of Medicine (*7-11, 7-14, 10-5, 17-3, 18-17*); The Society of the New York Hospital (*19-13*); © 1963 by The New York Times Company. Reprinted by permission (*6-2*); Open Court Publishing Co., Chicago (*16-16, 16-17* from E. A. W. Budge, *The Gods of the Egyptians,* 1904); Oriental Institute, University of Chicago (*16-4*); Peter Owen, London (*16-69, 16-71* from B. E. Finch and H. Green, *Contraception Through the Ages,* 1963); Oxford University Press, New York (*4-11* from H. E. Sigerist, *A History of Medicine,* vol. 2, 1961); Robert Percival (*9-41*); Jean Perrot, Centre de recherches préhistoriques français de Jérusalem (*16-43*); Phaidon Press, London (*13-15* from L. Goldscheider, *Leonardo da Vinci,* 1943); The Philadelphia Museum of Art (*4-109* courtesy of Smith, Kline, and French Laboratories); Pierpont Morgan Library, (*2-5*); The Population Council, New York (*16-78*); Prestel Verlag, Frankfort (*1-64* from *Collection of Greek Drawings,* 1929); *Proc. Brit. Acad.* (*16-2, 16-3, 16-30, 16-31* from J. Mellaart, Çatal Hüyük, a neolithic city in Anatolia, 1965); G. P. Putnam's Sons, New York (*6-6* from H. R. Hays, *In the Beginnings, Early Man and His Gods*); B. Quaritch, London (*16-67* from F. L. Griffith, *The Petrie Papyri,* 1898); Rascher **Verlag,** Zürich (*2-24* from C. G. Jung, *Psychologie und Alchemie,* 1944); *Rev. Gynéc.* (*2-12, 5-41* from F. R e g n a u l t, **La gynécologie dans l' iconographie** antique); *Rev. Méd. Franç. Etrang.* (*17-35* from Colombat, 1828); *Rev. Medicosoc. Enfance* (*13-26* from M. L. Cahen-Hayem, La maternité dans l' art, 1934); Rijksmuseum, Amsterdam (*2-3, 2-29, 6-18, 13-40* on loan to Rubenshuis, Antwerp); Roche Laboratories (*16-1*); Royal Collection, Windsor Castle; copyright reserved (*5-18, 5-19*); The Royal College of Medicine, London (*4-97*); The Royal College of

PICTORIAL CREDITS AND SOURCES 527

Physicians of Ireland (*10-4, 18-7–18-10*); Reproduced by permission of the Treasurer of the Royal College of Physicians of London (*6-15*); The Royal College of Surgeons of Edinburgh (*3-15*); The Royal College of Surgeons of England (*15-57*); Copyright, The Royal Society, London (*6-19, 6-21*); Library, The Royal Society of Medicine, London (*4-98*); I. C. Rubin, M. D. (*16-66*); S. S. Oceanic, Home Lines, Riviera Deck (*13-9*); Sansoni, Florence (*4-1* from P. Graziosi, *L' arte dell' antica età della Pietra*, 1956); W. B. Saunders Co., Philadelphia (*5-46, 11-19, 13-29, 15-46, 15-55, 15-56* from G. W. Gould and W. L. Pyle, *Anomalies and Curiosities of Medicine*, 1897; *7-18, 8-23, 8-48, 8-77, 8-83, 8-87, 9-27, 9-50* from J. B. De Lee, *The Principles and Practice of Obstetrics*, 1913; *10-3* from I. S. Cutter, *Obstetrics and Gynecology*, A. H. Curtis, ed., 1933; *17-21* from C. B. Penrose, *A Text-book of Diseases of Women*, 1908; *17-33* from J. C. Webster, *A Textbook of Diseases of Women*, 1907; Dr. David C. Schechter (*1-49*); Schindler, Cairo (*11-7, 19-1* from D. C. Joannides, *Esquisse de la gynécologie et de l' obstétrique chex les Egyptiens et les Grecs*, 1934); *Science* (*6-20* from P. E. Klopsteg, The indispensable tools of science, 132:1913-1922, 1960, Copyright 1960 by the American Association for the Advancement of Science); G. D. Searle & Co. (*16-68*); Dr. Landrum B. Shettles (*6-30, 6-31, 6-34*); Shoe String Press, Hamden, Conn. (*9-6* from H. Thoms, *Our Obstetric Heritage*, 1960); Alexander R. Simpson (*9-9*); **Somerset County Museum, Taunton, England** (*15-51*); Copyright SPADEM, Paris, 1964 by French Reproduction Rights, Inc. (*frontispiece*; 1968, *6-33*); Springer Verlag, Berlin (*17-62* from W. A. Freund, *Leben und Arbeit*, 1913); St. Luke's Hospital, New York (*18-24*); Staatliches Museum für Völkerkunde, Munich (*13-38*); Staatliche Museen, East Berlin (*1-41, 8-20, 13-19*); Staatliche Museen, West Berlin (*9-51, 13-4, 13-6*); Staatliche Museen Gemäldegalerie, Berlin-Dahlem (*4-22*); Städelsches Kunstinstitut, Frankfurt a. M. (*13-13*); Städtisches Reiss-Museum, Mannheim, permanent loan from Staatliche Kunsthalle, Karlsruhe (*6-24*); Stanford University Press, Stanford, Calif. (*6-28* from A. W. Meyer, *Human Generation*); Elwin Staude, Osterwieck am Harz (*9-55, 9-56, 12-11, 12-26* from E. Schlieben, *Mutterschaft und Gesellschaft*, 1927); G. Steinheil, Paris (*3-5, 4-100, 10-1, 15-29, 15-30, 16-63* from G. J. Witkowski, *Les accouchements dans les beaux-arts, dans la littérature et au théatre*, 1894; *3-10, 9-5, 9-12, 9-22, 9-26, 9-28, 9-32, 9-33, 9-35, 9-37, 11-17, 16-64* from G. J. Witkowski, *Les accoucheurs et sages-femmes célèbres*, 1891; *4-12, 4-43, 4-76, 4-77, 4-93, 8-38–8-40, 8-49, 8-54, 8-86* from G. J. Witkowski, *Histoire des accouchements chez tous les peuples*, 1887; *4-79, 4-83, 13-45* from G. J. Witkowski, *Les accouchements à la cour*, 1890; *10-2* from H. Carrier, *Origines de la maternité de Paris*, 1888); Steuben Glass, New York (*13-1*); Stuart & Watkins, London (*1-53, 1-54* from T. Burckhardt, *Alchemy*); Suermondt-Museum, Aachen, Germany (*2-34*); *Surg. Gynec. Obstet.* (*8-79* from A. B. Spalding, A pathognomonic sign of intra-uterine death, 1922; *17-23* from T. J. Watkins, Treatment of cases of extensive cystocele and uterine prolapse, 1906); Duke of Sutherland Collection, on loan to the National Gallery of Scotland (*2-30*); Thieme, Leipzig (*8-88* from A. D. Döderlein and B. Krönig, *Operative Gynäkologie*, 1912); Charles C Thomas, Springfield (*8-56* from O. Bettmann, *A Pictorial History of Medicine*, 1956 ; *15-7, 15-36, 15-37, 15-39* from L. Gedda, *Twins in History and Science*, 1961); Professor Dyre Trolle, Copenhagen (*11-3*); Tropenmuseum, Amsterdam (*16-51*); Charles Tuttle Publisher, Rutland, Vt. (*8-41, 8-43, 9-10, 9-19, 9-30, 13-50* from M. W. Standlee, *The Great Pulse*, 1959); Uffizi Gallery, Florence (*1-48, 2-22, 4-59*); University of California Press, Berkley (*12-18, 17-70* from L. MacKinney, *Medical Illustrations in Medieval Manuscripts*, 1965); University of California, Medical Center, San Francisco (*4-24*); University College, Department of Egyptology, London (*16-19*); Urban & Schwarzenberg, Berlin (*8-75* from W. Leipmann, *Der Geburtshilfliche Phantomkurs*, 1922; *8-89* from H. Naujoks, *Winter-Naujoks Lehrbuch der operativen Geburtshilfe*, 1951; *17-64* from E. Wertheim, *Die Erweiterte Abdominale Operation bie Carcinoma Colli Uteri*, 1911); U.S.S.R. Ministry of Health (*6-27*); Vail, New York (*17-8, 17-10, 17-11, 17-26, 17-30, 17-61* from D. B. Hart and A. H. F. Barbour, *Manual of Gynecology*, 1883); The Vatican (*16-60*); Vatican Library, Urbino (*2-17*); Vatican Museum (*15-43*); Victoria and Albert Museum, London (*13-11, 13-18*); F. C. W. Vogel, Leipzig (*17-63* from K. Schroeder, *Handbuch der Krankheiten der Weiblichen Geschlechtsorgane*, 1893); Von Z a h n & Jaensch, Dresden (*1-3, 1-4, 1-6, 1-8, 1-9, 1-11, 1-15, 1-16, 1-22, 1-24, 1-25, 1-27, 1-31, 1-34, 5-1, 5-3, 5-6, 5-8, 5-11, 5-12, 5-14, 5-15, 5-17, 5-36, 15-5, 15-6* from F. Weindler, *Geschichte der Gynäkologisch-Anatomischen Abbildung*, 1908); *The Wall Street Journal* (*15-31*, Bob Weber); The Wellcome Historical Medical Museum, London (*15-52, 16-23*); White, New York (*16-74* from *National Cyclopaedia of American Biography*, 1916); The Williams & Wilkins Co., Baltimore (*1-68* from H. H. Young, *Genital Abnormalities, Hermaphroditism, and Related Adrenal Diseases*, 1937; *10-4, 18-7–18-10* from O. T. D. Browne, *The Rotunda Hospital*, 1947; *16-79* from R. L. Dickinson and L. S. Bryant, *Control of Conception*, 1931); Wm. Wood & Co., New York (*7-16, 15-11* from Carlton Oldfield, *Herman's Difficult Labor*, 1920; *9-34* from W. H. Byford, *A Treatise on the Theory and Practice of Obstetrics*, 1873); *Z. Anat. Entwicklungsgesch.* (*6-40* from R. Herrlinger, *Die frühesten embryologischen Abbildungen in der Geschichte der Medizin*); *Z. Ethnol.* (*15-53* from H. Bab, *Geschlechtsleben, Geburt und Missgeburt in der asiatischen Mythologie*, 1906); *Z. Geburtsh. Gynaek.* (*6-25* from G. L. Moench, *Studien zur Fertilität*); *Zbl. Gynaek.* (*10-6* from 53:1751, 1929)

INDEX

Note: Where figure and legend appear on facing pages, figure page is given.

A-Z test, 44, 48
Abandonment of infants, 332
Abdominal binder, 60-61
Abdominal pregnancy, 186
Abimelech, 437
Abondio, Antonio, 341
Aborigines, Australian, 187
Abortion, 460
Abraham, 324
Abulcasis, 182, 234, 248, 270, 383, 387, 458
Accouchement, 81
Achilles, 287
Acormia, 369-372
Acrisius, King, 369
Adam, 98, 99, 228
   creation of, 98
   Eve and, 188, 189
Adnexa, 13, 19
Adolphe, Jean-Baptiste, 289
Adonis, 298
   birth of, 134-135, 151, 298
Adonis, Pierre, 312
Aedesius, 227
Aeneid, 297
Aftercoming head, delivery of, 77
Agatha, Saint, martyrdom of, 26, 27
d'Agnola, Andrea, 105, 496
d'Agrate, Ferrari, 17
Agrippini, 1
Ahmes, Queen, 97
Ahrimen, 378
Aigremont, Duchess of, 387
Aitken, John, 285
Akerly, S., 253
Akhnaton, 187

Albert, W., 219
Albertus Magnus, 44
Albinus, Bernhard Siegfried, 18
d'Albret, Henri, 124
d'Albret, Jeanne, 124
Alchemy, 31-32
Alcmaeon, 189
Alcmene, 136, 336
Aldobrandin, 67, 191, 348
Aldrovandi, U., 194
Alexander, William, 470
Alexander operation, 471
Alexis, Guillaume, 90
Al-Hariri, Abu Mohammed al-Kissim, 86
Allen, Joseph, 291
Allgemeines Krankenhaus, Vienna, 289, 294, 295, 504
Almänna Barnbördhuset, 289
Altdorfer, Albrecht, 105
von Alten, Herman, 488
Al-Wasiti, 86
Amalthea, 353
Amand, Pierre, 278
Amazon, 28
Amenerdais, temple of, 418
Amenophis IV, 187
American College of Nurse-Midwifery, 74
Amhotep IV, 97
Amine, 118
Amman, Jobst, 158, 515
Amphytryon, 136
Amulets
   birth, 228-230
   fertility, 421-435
   twin, 378, 379, 433

Analgesia in labor, 237
Anarcha, 456
Anatomy, dark ages of, 3
Androgyne, 31
Andromeda, 371
Angé, Marie, 37
Angelica, Fra, 52
Animalculists, 189
Anna. See Anne.
Anne, 102, 104, 106, 349. *See also* Mary, birth of.
   Queen, 271
   of Austria, 125
Anne-Marie-Victoire of Bavaria, confinement of, 126
Annunciation, 51-55, 287
   with Donors and St. Joseph, 51
Antepartum care, 521
Anthemoëssa, 365
Anti-cesarean society, 306
Anti-christ, birth of, 305
Aortic compressors, 263
Aphrodite, 130, 410
Apollo, 297-298, 336, 378
   hymn to, 231
Apulejus, 252
Aquila-Priscilla, 405, 406
Arantius, 211
Arcas, 59
Archbishop of Canterbury, 271
Arcturus, 59
Aretaeus the Cappadocian, 8, 463
Ariosto, Lodovico, 378
Aristotle, 1, 3, 16, 190, 193, 195
Armamentarium chirurgicum, 516
Arnolfini, Giovanni, 62
Arnott, Neill, 280

d'Arras, Jean, 338
Art, department of, as applied to medicine, 19
Artemis, 298, 418
Artificial feeding, 348-349, 357-360
Artificial insemination, 439
Arunta, 187
Aschheim, Selmar, 44, 502
Aschheim-Zondek test, 44, 48
Asclepius. See Asklepios.
Asdrubali, F., thimble of, 220
Asklepios, 190, 297-298
Ass as wet nurse, 356
Association for the Promotion and Standardization of Midwifery, 73
Astarte, 347, 410, 414
Astruc, Jean, 71
Athene, 130, 336, 369, 371, 397
  birth of, 395-396
Átman, 187
Aton, 187
Augustus, Caesar, 362
Aura seminalis, 189
Aurignacian period, 1, 48, 409, 422
Australian aborigines, 187
Autopsy, 1, 3, 182, 289, 294
Auvard, Pierre V. A., 321
Avicenna, 43, 51, 234
Axis of parturition, 217-218
Ayur-Vedas, 187, 289

Baartman, 24
Bacchanal, 338
Bacin, 268
Badianus codex, 253
von Baer, Karl Ernst, 194-197, 203
Bags. See Instruments.
Ballantyne, J. W., 404
Balloons. See Instruments.
Balsamodendron myrrha, 134, 298
Bandl, Ludwig, 171, 259
Baptism, 331, 332
Baquoy, Jean Charles, 142
Barbada, La, 41
Barber-surgeons, 68-70, 497
Bard, John, 185
Bard, Samuel, 48, 72, 249, 519
  portrait of, 519
Barnum, P. T., 42, 408
  Bailey and, Circus, 406
Barry, Martin, 197
Bartholin, Thomas, 367, 403
Bartisch, Georg, 13, 160

Basiotribe. See Instruments.
Baubo, 417
Baudelocque, Jean-Louis, 212-217, 219
  diameter of, 212-217, 219
Bauhin, Caspar, 37
Beach, W., 95
Bear, lesser, 59
Bear mother, 355
Bearded women, 35, 40-42
Beham, Barthel, 262
Bell, The, 378
Bell, Charles, 21
Bellevue Hospital, 506
Belskie, Abram, 192, 223, 224, 382, 383
Belt, chastity, 452-454
Benedetti, Alessandro, 297
Benedict III, Pope, 119
Benjamin, 142
Bennett, Jesse, 307
Ben-oni, 142
Benton, Francies, 38
Berger, George, 254
Berlin Papyrus, 43, 512
Berrettino, Petro, 158
Bes, 225
Betsy, 456
Biddenden Maids, 404
Bidet, 494
Bidloo, Govert, 14
Binder, abdominal, 60-61
Birch, Sampson, 372
Bird-boy, 374, 375
Birnberg, Charles H., 450
Birth
  amulets of, 228
  first, 102
  grief at, 141-148
  of Venus, 130-132
  postures during, 231-234
  practices in, 235-247
Birth control clinics, 448
Birthstools, 231-232, 265-268
Bisj-pole, 432
Blastocyst, 206
Blood-stone, 263
Blundell, James, 291, 451
Blunt, John, 68, 71
Boaistuau, P., 375
Boccaccio, Giovanni, 1, 119
Boehmer, P. A., 184
Boilly, Leopold, 494
Boisdechene, Josephine, 42
Boleyn, Anne, 347

Boltraffio, Antonio, 340
Book of Hours, 101, 112
Bosse, Abraham, 93, 151, 323, 493
Bossi, Luigi Maria, 276
Boston Hospital for Women, 507
Boston Lying-in Hospital, 505, 507
Botticelli, Sandro, 131
Boulanger, Jean, 401
de Bourbon-Montpensier, Marie, 72
Bourdichon, Jehan, 40
Bourgeois, Loyse, 73, 74, 126
Bourgogne, Duke of, birth of, 126
Boursier, Loyse Bourgeois, 72. See also Bourgeois, Loyse.
Boys from Syracuse, 378
Bradlee, Mrs. Timothy, 383
Brahma, 297
Braidwood, Robert J., 411
Brassieres, 60, 64
Braun, Carl, 466
Breast, 22-30, 335. See also Lactation.
  amputation of, 29-30
  as fertility symbol, 422, 423, 430
  binder for, 64
  connection to uterus of, 192
  feeding of adults by, 350-352
  mutilation of, 26-29
  pumps for, 357
Breech presentation, 181, 255-256
  delivery with, 77, 80
von Brekelenkam, Quiringh Gerritsz, 152
Brentel, Frédéric, 341
Brian, Thomas, 43
British Lying-in Hospital, London, 500
Brödel, Max, 19, 20, 490
Brownlow Street Hospital, London, 500
Brueghel, Pieter, 92
Brugsch papyrus, 43, 512
Brunet-Debaines, Alfred-Louis, 499
Brunswick and Lüneberg, Duchess of, 511
Bryant, L. S., 451
Buddha, birth of, 116-117, 297, 299
Budin, Pierre-Constant, 219
Bull, accouchement by, 308
Bumm, Ernst, 502
Bunker brothers, 397, 408
Bureau des nourrices, 350
Burnham, Walter, 482

Byrne's repositor, 468
Byrth of Mankynde, 514

Cadaver, 1-3, 182
Cadogan, William, 323
Caesar, birth of, 302-303
Cain, birth of, 102
Calderón de la Barca, Pedro, 378
Caldwell, William E., 219
Caldwell-Moloy pelvic classification, 222
California Indian birth scene, 91
Calipers, obstetric, 217
Callisto, 59, 60
Callixtus, Nicephorous, 109
Campin, Robert, 51, 339
Cancer of cervix, 473, 484
Canova, Antonio, 370
Cantelupe, Eugene B., 287
Cap, cervical, 449
Capote anglaise, 449
Caritas, 344
Carnot, Sadi, 296
da Carpi, Giacomo Berengario, 3, 6, 10, 11
Carus, Carl Gustav, 218
de las Casas, Bartolomé, 352
Casserius, Julius, 6
Castor, 125, 129
Castro, Roderigo a, 67
Catherine of Cleves, 101
Cavallini, Joseph, 455
Cavallini, Julia, 316
Cave drawings, 1
Cazotte, Marc, 373
Cellini, Benvenuto, 369
Centaur, 361
Centeotl, 231
Cephalotribe. See Instruments.
Cervix, 171
    amputation of, 455, 474
    cancer of, 473, 484
    digital examination of, 518
    prolapse of, 474
Cesarean section, 297-316
    classical, 314-316
    dressings for, 313-314
    first monograph on, 310
    first in United States, 307
    incision for, 306, 310-313
    instruments for, 312-313
    position during, 310-312
    postmortem, 298-306
Cesarean-hysterectomy, 316
C'est un Fils, Monsieur!, 142

Chagall, Marc, 334
Chair
    birth, 231-232, 265-269
    gynecologic examining, 487-488. See also Table, gynecologic examining.
Chaldeans, 361, 373, 409
Cham, 394
Chamberlen, Peter, 281
Chamberlen family, 270-273
    forceps of, 270-273, 281
Chang, 397, 408
Chapman, Edmund, 272
Charité Hospital, 502-503
Charity, Roman, 351
Charles I, King, 3, 271
Charr, William, 42
Chase, Dr., Receipt Book of, 522
Chastity girdle, 452-454
de Chauliac, Guy, 9, 458
Chevalier, Étienne, 115
Chiara, Domenico, 257
Chicago Hospital for Women and Children, 507
Childbirth, god of, 411
Childebert I, King, 495
Chinese birth scene, 89
Christ. See Jesus; Nativity.
Christine and Millie, 407
Chulkhurst twins, 404
Cicero, 361
Cignaroli, Bettino, 142
Cihuapatli, 253
Childbirth, death in, 142, 148
Cimon, Pero and, 352
Cinyras, 134
di Cione, Andrea, 103
Circumcision, 114, 324-330
Clamp
    for vesicovaginal fistula, 480
    hysterectomy, 485
    ovariotomy, 478-479
Clark, John G., 486, 490
Clay, Charles, 466
Clay, John, 479
Clément, Jules, 126
Cleopatra, 209
    accouchement of, 122
Clofullia, Madame Fortune, 42
Clothing, maternity, 60-66, 340
Clytemnestra, 129
Cochen, Michael, 31
Codex Badianus, 253
Coiter, Volcher, 209
Coitus, 191, 192

Cole, B., 407
College of Physicians and Surgeons
    in Baltimore, 505
    in New York, 510
Collins, Robert, 292, 500
Collision, twins, 384
Colloredo, Lazarus-Joannes Baptista, 403
Colostrum, 348
Colpeurynter, 466. See also Instruments.
Colpocleisis, 463, 466
Colporrhaphy, 463
Columbat, Marc, 473
Columbia-Presbyterian Medical Center, 510
Columna lactaria, 332
Comadre, 67
Comare, La. See *Commare, La.*
Comedy of Errors, 378
Commare, La, 13, 64, 176, 234, 310, 311, 515
Compaction, twins, 384
Comparaison du Bouton de Rose, 23
Comstock, Anthony, 447
Conceptu, de, 515
Condom, 444-445
Confinement, cunicular, of Mary Toft, 136-140
Congenital malformation, 361-376
Conjugate
    diagonal, 212-217, 219-220
    internal, 212-217, 219-220
Constantius, 68
Consultation Indiscréte, 46
Consultation des Piqûres, 47
de' Conti, Bernardo, 341
Contraception, 441-451
    devices for
        intrauterine, 450
        vaginal, 449
    prescriptions for, 441-442
Contracted pelvis, 214-216, 221, 255
Cooper, Astley Paston, 25-26
Cord, umbilical, prolapse of, 258
Coriander seed, 252
Corinthian vase, 82
Corner, Thomas Cromwell, 520
Coronis, 297-298
Corpus Hermeticum, 31
da Cortona, Pietro Berettini, 349
Cot, obstetric, 269
Council of Ephesus, 102

de la Courvée, J. C., 285
Cousin, Jean, 262
Coutouli, pelvimeter of, 219
Couvelaire, Alexandre, 260
Couvelaire uterus, 260
Cow as wet nurse, 353
Cragin, Edward Bradford, 510
Cranach, Lucas, 344
Cranioclast. See Instruments.
Craniopagus, 397
Craniotomy, 274
Crawford, Jane, 455-456, 477
Creation
    of Adam, 98
    of Eve, 99-101
    of Man, 98-101
    of Man and of the World, 99
Credé, Carl Siegmund, 248, 320, 502
Credulity, superstition, fanaticism and, 138
Cross, devotion to the, 378
Crosse, John Green, 467
Crotchet. See Instruments.
Cruikshank, William Cumberland, 194
Cullen, Thomas S., 490
Cummater, 67
Cunicular confinement of Mary Toft, 136-140
Cuniculari or the Wise Men of Godalming, 137
Cup-and-stem pessary, 469
Cupid, birth of, 133
Curette, 463. See also Instruments.
Curve of Carus, 218
Cuspidate fetus, 366
Cuvier, Georges, 24
Cyclopes, 362
Cyclops, 362-364
Cynocephali, 374
Cypris, 31
Cyst, ovarian, 475-479
Cytherea, 130

Dagmar, Queen, 302
Dalenpatius, 189, 200
Dallin, Cyrus E., 75
Danaë, 369
Dariri, Mustafa b. Yusuf b. Omer Erenzi, 118
D'Arras, Jean, 338
Daumier, Honoré, 48, 141
Davenport, F. H., 487
David, 52

Dayot, H., 475
Death
    in childbirth, 142, 148
    of Rachel, 142-143
Debata idup, 435
Decidua, 184
Delaune, Étienne, 385
DeLee, Joseph B., 234, 521
Delivery table, 266, 269
Delos, 231
Denman, Thomas, 257, 492, 517
Deschi da parto, 90, 286
Deutsch, Niklaus Manuel, 41
van Deventer, Hendrik, 212, 267, 517
Devéria, Eugène François, 124
Devotion to the Cross, 378
Devy, G., 126
Dew, Harvie J., 319
Dewees, William P., 519
Diagonal conjugate, 212-217, 219-220
Diana, 59, 60, 378
    Callisto and, 59, 60
    of Ephesus, 347
Dicephalus dipus, 399
Dickens, Charles, 70
Dickinson, Robert L., 192, 223-224, 382, 383
    sterilization and, 451
Dieties, fertility, 409-420
Dilators, 455, 460-462, 482. See also Instruments.
Dione, 130
Dionis, Pierre, 182, 465, 497
Dionne quintuplets, 383
Dionysus, 297, 397, 400, 401, 402
Dioscuri, 129, 378
Diprosopus, 368
Dishes for parturient, 286-288
Disproportion, feto-pelvic, 218-219, 234, 255. See also Contracted pelvis.
Dissection, 1-3, 208
Dog-boy, 375
Dollinger, Johann, 119
Dolls, fertility, 421, 432, 436
Dominic, Saint, birth of, 116
Donatello, Donato di Betto Bardi, 338
Dorothea, 383
Douche, 443, 491, 494
Douglas, James, 70, 137
Douglas, John C., 257
Dress, maternity, 60-66, 340

Dryander, Johannes, 6, 12, 180
Dryden, John, 75
Dublin Lying-in Hospital, 500, 501
Dubuffet, Jean, 81
Duct, lactiferous, 26
Dürer, Albrecht, 329, 492
Dugong, 367
Duncan, James Matthews, 250
    mechanism of, 250
Dutch cap, 449
Duverney, J. G., 183
Dysmenorrhea, 460
Dystocia, 236, 237, 243-246, 252-264. See also Uterine inertia.

East of Eden, 378
Eastman, Nicholson J., 521, 522
Ebers papyrus, 8, 442, 463, 512
Eckarth, 69
Écraseur, 483, 484
Ectopic pregnancy, 182-186
Ed-Din, Charaf, 464
Eden, east of, 378
Edinburgh Royal Infirmary, 499
Effigies, obstetric, 232
Egg, 16, 189. See also Ovum.
Eichmann, J., 6
Eileithyia, 265, 395
Eleazar, circumcision of, 326
Elisha, 318
Elizabeth, 56, 58, 106, 114. See also Visitation, the; John, birth of.
Emaillattement, 323
Emboîtement, 189-190
Embryotome. See Instruments.
Embryotomy, 275
Emmet, Thomas Addis, 456, 481, 520
    water dilator of, 461
Enema, 491-494
Enfant à la bouillie, 359
Eng, 397, 408
Engelbrechtsen, Cornelius, 61
Engelmann, George J., 231, 247
Entrée dans la Vie, 141
Envie de femme grosse, 48
Epidemics, puerperal fever, 289-296, 497
Epigenesis, 190, 195
Erechtheus, 130
Ergot, 253-254
Erichthonios, birth of, 130
Eros, 34

Erziehung des Jupiter, 353
Esau, 42, 378
Esau and Jacob, birth of, 384-386
Estienne, Charles, 5, 157, 306, 381
État Sauvage, 40
Euryle, 369
Eusebia, 68
Eustachio, Bartolommeo, 1, 18
Evans, John, 279
Eve, 228
    creation of, 99-101
Ewell, Thomas, 72
Examination
    gynecologic, 455
    obstetric, 248, 289-291, 294
Extractors. See Instruments.
Extrauterine pregnancy, 182-186
van Eyck, Huybrecht, 188
van Eyck, Jan, 53, 62, 188, 340

da Fabriano, Gentile, 111
Fabricius, Hieronymus, 1, 6, 16, 17, 161, 458
Fall of the House of Usher, 378
Fallopian tube, 12, 14, 17
Falloppio, Gabrielle, 1, 12, 16, 444
Family planning, 441-451
Fanaticism, credulity, superstition and, 138
Fasbender, H., 78
Fatio, Johann, 456
Fécondateur, 439
Feeding, artificial, 348-349. See also Nursing paraphernalia.
Feeding vessels, 357-360
Felkin, Robert, W., 235-239, 308
Female
    semen of, 189
    testis of, 2, 16, 189, 190, 208
Femme Enceinte et Barbue, 41
Femme à sa Toilette, 494
Ferdinand II, Duke of Alcalá, 41
Fermentation, 296
Fertility goddess, 409, 411, 412, 420. See also Astarte, Artemis, Baubo, Diana, Hathor, Ishtar, Isis, Venus.
Fetishes, fertility, 421-435
Fetus, 207-210
    circulation of, 207
    cuspidate, 366
    positions of, 172-181, 380, 381, 384
Ficquet, Etienne, 76
Ficus religiosa, 116

Fièvre de lait, 289
dei Filipepi, Allesandro di Mariano, 131
Firdausi, 300
Fistula, vesicovaginal, 456, 480-482
Flémalle, Master of, 339
Fluhmann, C. Frederic, 470
Follicle, ovarian, 190-196
Font, baptismal, 332
Forceps, obstetric, 74, 254, 270-273, 281-284
    Chamberlen, 270-273, 281
Fores, S. W., 68
Fothergill, William Edward, 463
Fouguet, J., 115
France, Anatole, 511
della Francesca, Piero, 112, 226
Franceschini, 298
Francis Joseph Charles, Napoleon II, 128
Frank, Peter, 152
Frankenhäuser, Ferdinand, 21
Frappa, José, 350
Freak of nature, 361
Free Hospital for Women, Boston, 507
Freund, Wilhelm Alexander, 485
Fried, Johann Jacob, 496
Friedman test, 46, 48
Friedrich III, 74
Friedrich the Great, 502
Friedrich Wilhelm III, 502
Fünfbilder, 153, 154
Fumigation, 236, 459
    vaginal, 240, 245, 455, 463, 492

Gabriel, 52, 54, 300. See also Annunciation.
Gaddi, Taddeo, 110
Gaea, 130
Galbiati, Gennaro, 285
Galen, 3, 12, 164, 189, 322, 455, 469
Galileo, 199
Gamp, Mrs., 70
Ganglion, uterocervical, 21
Gauss's aortic compressor, 263
Gautier-d'Agoty, Jacques-Fabien, 7
Ge, 130
Gemini, 125
General Lying-in Hospital, London, 500
Generation, Australian aboriginal theory of, 193
Genital malformations, 32

George I, King, 136, 137
Gerard of Cremona, 51, 173
Gibelin, Esprit-Antoine, 87
Gigli, Leonardo, 285
    saw of, 285
Gigon, 417
Gilberta, Fraw, 118
Gilliam, D. Tod, 476
Girdle
    chastity, 452-454
    maternity, 60-61, 66
Glanvil, B., 100
Gnostic gems, 425
Goat as wet nurse, 349, 356
God of childbirth, 411
Goddess
    fertility, 409, 411, 412, 415, 420. See also Artemis, Astarte, Baubo, Diana, Hathor, Ishtar, Isis, Venus.
    motherhood, 412
    pregnant, 410
Gonadotrophic hormone, 44, 379
Goodell, William, 460, 462
Gordon, Alexander, 291
Gorgippus of Thasos, 40
Gorgons, 369-371
Gozzoli, Benozzo, 317, 386
de Graaf, Reinier, 17, 183, 190, 202, 491
Graafian follicle, 14, 190-196. See also Ovarian follicle.
de Gradi, Gian Matteo, 17
Gräfenberg, Ernst, 450
Great Bear, 59
Greenhalgh, Robert, 470
Greenhill, J. P., 521
Grief at birth, 141-148
Grünewald, Mathias, 113
Guelders, Duke of, 101
Guidi, Tommaso, 90, 286
Guillemeau, Jacques, 70, 77, 310
Gusserow, Adolf, 502
Guy's Hospital, 291

Hadrian, 70
Haggadah, 384, 390
Hall, Herbert H., 450
von Haller, Albrecht, 32
Hair, 40-42, 355
Hamilton, Alexander, 185
Hamilton, G., 264
Hamilton, James, 254
Hanging-legs position, 234
Hanks, Tracy, 462

Hannah, 437
Harelip, 373
Hartsoeker, Niklaas, 189, 200
Harvard Medical School, 293
Harvey, William, 164, 189, 190, 195, 196, 197, 224
Harvie, John, 249, 250
Hathor, 426, 427
Hebamme, 67
Heberden, William, 323
Hebosteotomy, 285
Hebotomy, 285
Hebrews, 67
van Heemskerck, Marten, 386
Hegar, Alfred, 460
    dilators of, 462
Heister, Lorenz, 30, 517, 518
Helen, 129
Helen of Rome, 68
Hélène, Judith and, 407
Hélie, L. T., 16
Hellenistic-Roman period, 31
Hellin, Dionys, 379
    law of, 379
Hellman, Louis M., 521
Helmas, King, 338
Helvetius, 30
Hemolytic streptococcus, 296
Hemorrhage, postpartum, 263-264, 268. See also Oxytocics.
Henneberg, Countess of, 392, 393
Henrietta Maria, Queen, 124, 271
Henry IV, King, 124-125
Henry VIII, King, 347
Hephaistos, 130, 395
Hera, 59, 400
    nursing Heracles, 336
Heracles
    birth of, 136
    suckled by Hera, 336
Herbiniaux, George, 280, 473
Hercules. See Heracles.
Hermaphrodite, 31-39, 361, 374
Hermaphroditos, 31, 35, 36
Hermes, 31, 265, 369, 395
    Dionysus and, 400, 401
    women honoring, 438
Hermes Trismegistos, 31
Hermetic Androgyne, 31, 33
Herodotus, 324
Hersent, Louis, 352
Hertwig, Oskar, 197
Hesiod, 370, 395
Heyms, Hermann, 175, 381
Hicks, John Braxton, 260

Hieroglyphs, Egyptian, 80, 245
Hildegard, Saint, visions of, 194
Himes, Norman E., 409, 441
Hippocrates, 9, 28, 40, 43, 70, 189, 208, 224, 289, 455, 460
Hirsutism, 40-42, 355
Hoboken, Nicolaas, 164
Hodge, Hugh Lenox, 469, 519, 520
    pessary of, 471
Hogarth, William, 137, 138
Holbein, Hans, the Younger, 63
Holmes, Oliver Wendell, 293, 295, 357
Homer, 130, 231, 362, 365, 395
Homunculus, 189, 201
van Hoogstraten, Samuel, 43
Hooks. See Instruments.
van Horne, Jan, 17, 190
Hormone, gonadotrophic, 44, 379
Horner, D. A., 259
Horns of uterus, 12
Horus, 335-336, 411, 416
Hosack, David, 254
Hospital
    American, 505-510
    for Poor Lying-in Women, Dublin, 499, 500
    of Santa Maria della Scala, Siena, 495
Hôtel-Dieu, Lyon, 495
Hôtel-Dieu, Paris, 289, 290, 495-499
Hottentot apron, 21
Hottentot Venus, 24
Hours
    book of, 101, 112
    of the Virgin, 46
Houstoun, Robert, 477
Howard, John, 136, 137
Hundt, Magnus, 10
Hunter, John, 184, 439
Hunter, William, 70, 162, 168-170, 181
Hut, parturition, 235, 242
Hutchinson, Anne, 72, 75
Hydatidiform mole, 372, 392-393
Hygeia, 190
Hymn to Apollo, 231
Hyrtl, Joseph, 19
Hysterectomy, 455, 463, 482, 484-486

Ice age, 79
Impressions, maternal, 376
Inanna, 412

Inclined position, 489-490
Incubators, 320-321
India, monstrous races of, 374
Indians, American, 378
Induction of labor, 240, 246
Infants, abandonment of, 332
Infection, puerperal, 289-296, 497, 500
Infertility, 437-440
Infirmary of St. James, Westminster, 496
Innervation of female pelvic organs, 21
Innocent III, Pope, 495
Insemination, artificial, 439
Instruments, 270-285, 457-485
Insufflation, tubal, 440
Interlocking twins, 384
Internal conjugate, 212-217, 219-220
International Confederation of Midwives, 74
Interposition operation, 463, 467
Intersex, 31-39
Intrauterine devices, 450
Inversion of uterus, 261, 467-469. See also Uterus, displacements.
Irvine, 408
Ischiopagi, 398
Ishihama, Atsumi, 450
Ishmael, 324
Ishtar, 410, 413
Isis, 335, 336, 410, 416, 417

Jacob, 67, 106, 143, 378, 437
    Esau and, birth of, 384-386
Jacobi, Ludwig, 439
Janiceps, 368
Jansen, Tryn, 72
Janssen, Zacharias, 199
Janus, 368
Japanese birth scene, 94
Jeremiah, 437
Jesus, 52, 56, 58, 80, 131, 227, 339-341, 411
    baptism of, 331
    birth of, 108-113, 339
    circumcision of, 327, 328
    nursed by Mary, 340-341
Jeu de nature, 361
Jeune femme allaitant son enfant, 344
Joachim, 349
Joan, Pope, parturition of, 118-121

Joanna of Aza, 116
Job, 187
de Jode, Geerhardt, 396
John, Saint, 57, 131
  birth of, 114, 115
John VIII, Pope, 119
Johns Hopkins Hospital, 38, 39
Johnston, George, 295, 500
Jonas, Richard, 514
Jones, Churchill, 480
Joseph, Saint, 54, 55, 108, 110, 341
  See also The Nativity.
Joseph II, Emperor, 504
Jotze dofan, 298
Journals, obstetric-gynecologic, 511
Joy at birth, 141, 142
Judith, Hélene and, 407
Julian the Apostate, 68
Juliet, weaning of, 346
Julius Obsequens, 362
Jumi gokoto, 356
Juno, 84

Kagawa, Genetsu Shigen, 268
Kagawa, Genteki, 277
Kahoun papyrus, 441, 511, 512
Kaisei-jitsu, 273
Kalkar, Jan, 3
Kamm, Johann Peter, 288
Kasim, Abul, 300
Katwame, 433
Katzman, Lawrence, 394
Kelchner, Ernst, 305
Kelly, Howard Atwood, 490, 507 520
Kennedy, Evory, 171, 500
Kensington Hospital, Philadelphia, 507
Kerckring, Theodore, 208
Ketham, 9
King of Rome, birth of, 128
Kiowa Indian birth scene, 91
von Kirchheim, Johannes, 9
Kirke, 365
Kiwai Papuans, 378
Klein, Johann, 294
Knee-chest position, 242, 246, 456, 481
Kobelt, George Ludwig, 18
Kolletschka, Jakob, 294
Kollwitz, Käthe, 148
Kondo, Gaksiu, 256
Koras, George, 344
Ktesias, 374

von Kulmbach, Hans, 105
Kumaz, 452
Kursie el-wilada, 265
Kyesteine pellicle, 44

Labia minora, 21
Labor
  complications of, 252-264. See also Dystocia.
  induction of, 240, 246
  onset of, 224
  scenes, 231-247
Lacombe, Georges, 95
Lactation, 26, 289, 334, 335, 351-356. See also Breast.
Lactiferous duct, 26
Ladies, married, letters to, 522
Lafosse, 289
Laloo, 403
Laminaria, 460, 482
Lancelot, 287
Lanfranc of Milan, 29
Lara, birth of seven sons of, 391
Latona, 231, 378
Laughlin, E. O., 495
Lavoisier, Antoine L., 497
Lavrate, 71
League of Awakened Magyars, 452
Leah, 437
Lebas, Jean, 314
Leda and the Swan, 129
Lee, Robert, 21
Leeches, 455, 463
van Leeuwenhoek, Antoni, 189, 198-200
Le Fort, Léon, 466
Lenses, 199
Leo IV, Pope, 119
Leopold, Gerhard, 248
  maneuvers of, 248
Lesser Bear, 59
Letters to Married Ladies, 522
Léveillé, J. B., 482
Lever, 279
Levret, André, 165, 166, 212, 217
  forceps of, 283
Lex caesarea, 299
Lex regia, 299
Liber chronicarum, 374
Liber Scivias, 194
Liceti, Fortunio, 376
Lichas, 297
Lichtenberger, Johannes, 88
Ligament
  broad, 14

Ligament *(Cont.)*
  cardinal, 15, 463
  round, 14, 470
Lilith, 69, 228, 229
Lillie, Frank, 31
Lime, chlorinated, 292, 293, 295
Lippes, Jack, 450
Lippi, Lorenzo, 27
Lister, Joseph, 295-296
Lithopedion, 185, 262
Litta, Conte, 340
Litzmann, Carl Conrad, 215, 217
Lochia, 289
Lombardi, Lorenzo, 116
Lonicer, Adam, 253
Louis XI, King, 497
Louis XII, King, 374
Louis XIII, King, 124
  birth of, 125
Louis XIV, King, 491
  birth of, 125
Louis XVI, King, 492
Lucina, 124
Lucy, 456
Lugalgirra, 378
Lüneberg, Brunswick and, Duchess of, 511
Lusus naturae, 361
Lycaon, 59
Lycosthenes, 375
Lyedet, Loyset, 303
Lymphatics, female urogenital, 20

McClintock, Alfred H., 270, 500
McDowell, Ephraim, 455-456, 477
McLane, James W., 284, 505, 510
Macbeth, 40
Mackenrodt, Alwin, 15
Madonna Litta, 340
Madonna del Parto, 226, 227
Magdalen, Mary, 61
Magi, 109
Magyars, Awakened, League of, 452
Maia, 370
Maiestas Domini, 287
Mains de fer, 272, 282
Maisonneuve, Jacques-Gilles-Thomas, 476
Maitani, Lorenzo, 99, 100
Majolica plates, 233, 286, 298
Majzlin, Gregory, 450
Maladies des femmes grosses, 517
Malformations
  congenital, 361-376
  fantastic, 374-376

Malformations (Cont.)
  genital, 31-32
Malthus, Thomas Robert, 441-443
Mamma, ectopic, 347
Man, birth of, 194
Manas, 187
Manatee, 367
Manchester operation, 463
Mandeville, Sir John, travels of, 374
Manfredini, Gaetano, 381
Man-midwives, 68-70, 74, 79, 497
Manningham, Richard, 137, 496
Margaret, Saint, 62, 227
Margulies, Lazar C., 450
Marie Thèrèse, 127
Marion Street Maternity, 505, 507
de Marne, Jean Louis, 394
Married ladies, letters to, 522
Marstrand, Wilhelm Nicolai, 150
Martin, Eduard, 502
Marvels of the East, 374
Mary, 52, 55, 56, 58, 102, 108-109, 115, 131, 149, 226, 227, 339-341, 411. *See also* Annunciation; Visitation.
  birth of, 102, 103-107, 349
  nursing Jesus, 340-341
Masaccio, 90, 286
Mascherini, Marcello, 337
Masculinization, 40
Master of Flémalle, 51
Mater Matuta, 415
Maternal impressions, 376
Maternité, 1914, 334
Maternité Hospital, 72, 291
Maternity
  garb of, 60-66, 340
  girdle of, 60, 66
Maternity Center Association, 73
Mating, 192
Matrisalus cap, 449
de Mattos, Dona Rachel Teicheira, 142
Mauriceau, François, 7, 70, 77, 210, 265, 266, 271, 274, 497, 517
  maneuver of, 77, 517
Maya, 299
de'Medici, Catherine, 270
de'Medici, Marie, 72
  birth of, 124
Medici family, 109
Medicine, department of art as applied to, 19
Medusa, 369, 371

Meigs, Charles D., 275, 519
Mellaart, James, 96, 377, 410, 422, 423
Melli, Sebastiano, 234
Melusine, 338
Memling, Hans, 54
Mercurialis, Hieronymus, 289
Mercurio, Scipione, 13, 64, 176, 234, 272, 310, 311, 515
Mermaids, 365-367
Meslamtaea, 378
Mesnard, Jacques, 269, 313, 357
Mesonephros, 18
Metis, 395
Metreurynter, 482
Metrotome, 475
Meunier, M., 368
Meyer, Robert, 502
Meyer, Willy, 490
Michael, 300
Michaelis, Gustav Adolf, 217, 221
Michal, 437
Michelangelo, 3, 98, 99
Michell, W., 254
Microscope, 198, 199
Midwives
  Colonial, 72
  early, 67-72
  New York, 73
  puerperal fever and, 291-294
  regulation of, 71-72
  training of, 68-72, 497
  United States, 72-74
da Milano, Giovanni, 103
Milk fever, 289. *See also* Puerperal fever.
Milky Way, origin of, 334
Mill, John Stuart, 443
Millie, Christine and, 407
Minerva, 395
Mirandula, Franciscus Picus, 383
Mishnah, 298
Mizpah cap, 449
Mizuhara, Yoshihiro, 94
Moé, Amédéé C. H., 394
Moench, G. L., 202
Moeurs conjugales, 48
Mohammed, birth of, 118
Mohel, 325, 330
Mole, hydatidiform, 372, 392, 393
Molière, Jean-Baptiste P., 491
Moloy, Howard C., 219
Momburg's tourniquet, 263
Le Monde Renversé, 41

de Mondeville, Henri, 2, 9
Mondino, Carlo, 381
Mondino dei Luzzi, 10, 11, 12
Monocoli, 374
Monopodia, 366
Monsters, 361-376
  double, 395-408
Monstrous races of India, 374
Montagu, Ashley, 40
di Montalbano, Rinaldo, 387
de Montauban, Renaud, 387
Moore, John George, Jr., 510
Moreau, J. L., 14, 21
Moreau, Jean Michel, the younger, 142
Moschion, 172, 174-179, 265, 380, 511
Mosse, Bartholomew, 499-500
Mother, Child and, 333
Motherhood, goddess of, 412, 415
Mound Builders, 232
Muelder, D., 364
Multiple pregnancy, 372, 377-408
Mundinus, 10, 11, 12
Murdoch, Iris, 378
Muses, 326
Myoma, uterine, 483, 484
Myomectomy, 483-484
Myometrium, 16
Myrrha, 134, 298

Naegele, Franz Carl, 215, 231
Naegele pelvis, 215
Naissance de l'Homme, 95
Nanno, 40
Napoleon I, 128
Napoleon II, birth of, 128
Nativity, 108-113, 339
Naturspiel, 361
Navel. *See* Umbilicus.
Needham, Joseph, 207, 208
de Negker, Jobst, 156
Nero, Emperor, 1
Nerves, female pelvic organs, 21
Nestorian Christians, 102
Netsuke, 350
New York Academy of Medicine, 72-73
New York Almshouse, 505, 506
New York Asylum for Lying-in Women, 505, 507
New York Hospital, 455
New York Lying-in Hospital, 505
Newborn
  baptism of, 331-332

Newborn *(Cont.)*
   circumcision of, 114, 324-330
   resuscitation of, 317-321
   swaddling of, 322-323
Niddah, 298
Nihell, Elizabeth, 74
Nile, Father, 437
Nipple
   human, 25
   inverted, 357
   nursing, 358
Northeastern Hospital for Women and Children, Boston, 507
Novarini, Antonius, 6
Novum lumen, 212, 517
Nuck, Anton, 20
Nürnberg Krankenhaus, 496
Numa Pompilius, 298-299
Nunc Dimittis, 327
Nuremberg Chronicle, 374
Nurse-midwifery, 73-74
Nursing paraphernalia, 357-360
Nut, 410
Nyssa uniflora, 460

Obnayim, 265
Oceanus, 337
Obsequens, Julius, 362
Obstetric instruments, 270-285
Obstetric stool, 231-232
Odysseus, 362, 365, 366
Oeuf de Paques, 394
Olhaf, Joachim, 372
von Olshausen, Robert, 502
Omphalopagus twins, 405, 407, 408
Omphalos of Delphi, 190
Onna-ishi, 434
Oophorectomy, 455-456
Opodymus, 368
Oppenheimer, W., 450
Orcagna, Andrea, 103
Organ of Rosenmüller, 18
Origin of the Milky Way, 334
Orlando Furioso, 378
Ormazd, 378
Ortolf, Dr., 521
Osiander, Friedrich Benjamin, 21, 269
Osiris, 411
Osler, William, 3
Ospedale di Santo Spirito, Rome, 495
Osteomalacia, 211, 215
Ota, Tenrei Takeo, 450
Ould, Fielding, 500

Ovarian cyst, 455-456, 475-479
Ovarian follicle, 14, 16, 17, 190-196, 202, 208
Ovariotomy, 455-456, 477-479
   clamp for, 478-479
Ovary, 16-19
   blood supply to, 19
   fetal, 18
Ovid, 35, 59, 136
Oviduct, 12, 14, 17
Ovists, 189
Ovulists, 189
Ovum
   human, 204-206
   quest for, 190-197
Oxytocics, 253-254

Pacher, Michael, 328
Pajot, Charles, 439
Paleolithic era, 49
Palfyn, Jean, 272, 282
Palissy, Bernard, 343
Pallas, 395. See also Athene.
Pan, parturition, 268
Pantzer, M. E. C., 248
Pap boats. See Nursing paraphernalia.
Papyrus
   Brugsch (Berlin), 43, 512
   Carlsburg, 512
   Ebers, 8, 442, 463, 512
   Edwin Smith, 512
   Kahoun, 441, 511, 512
   Petrie, 441, 511, 512
Paracelsus, 201
Parasitic fetus, 372
Paré, Ambroise, 61, 70, 72, 76, 265, 310, 362, 374
Paris, 287
Parovarium, 18
Partera, 244
Parthenos, Maiden, 395
De partu hominis, 514
Parturient
   dishes for, 286-288
   protectors of, 224-227
   visit to, 152
Parturition
   axis of, 217-218
   house for, Japanese, 241
   hut for, 235, 242
   pan for, 268
Partus caesareus, 299
Pasteur, Louis, 296
Paulus, Julius, 332
Peaslee, E. R., 456

Pech-Merle, caves of, 48
Peillon, Gabriel, 192
Pelvic band of Dr. Protheroe Smith, 65
Pelvimeters, 219, 221
Pelvimetry, 212-217, 219
Pelvis
   contracted, 214-216, 221, 255
   obstetric, 211-222
   rhachitic, 166
   types of, 222
Penis, amputation of, 39
Pennsylvania Hospital, 505
Pépin, 373
Perce-crâne. See Instruments.
Persephone, 134
Perseus, 369-371
Perugino, Pietro, 326
Pessaries, 455, 463, 466, 469, 470, 471, 518. See also Instruments.
Peter, Saint, 26
Petrie papyrus, 441, 511, 512
Phaetusa, 40
Pharaohs, 67, 324
Pharez and Zarah, birth of, 386
Phenol spray, 296
Philadelphia Almshouse, 505
Phocomelia, 373
Pica, 48
Picasso, Pablo, 205
Pierre, Adam, 352
Pineau, S., 207, 285
del Piombo, Sebastiano, 26
Pippi, Giulio, 57
Pisano, Giovanni, 99, 110
Pisano, Nicola, 109
Piss-prophet, 44
Place, Francis, 443, 446
Placenta, 63, 207, 336.
   abruption of, 260-261
   basket for, 251
   delivery of, 248-249. *See also* Schultze mechanism; Duncan mechanism.
   in multiple pregnancy, 166
   relations in twin pregnancy, 382
   retained, 238-240
   separation of, 250
Placenta previa, 170, 259-260
Planned Parenthood-World Population, 447
de Plantades, François, 189
Plato, 31
Plazzoni, Francesco, 21

Plexus, uterocervical, 21
Plicae palmitae, 14
Pliny, 361, 374
Podalic version, 76
Poe, Edgar Allen, 378
Polin, Frank E., 314
Pollux, 129
Polydectes, King, 369, 371
Polyphemus, 362-364
Polyp, uterine, 473
Pomeroy, M. P., 246
de Pompadour, Madame, 491
Pompilius, Numa, 298-299
Population control, 437-451
Porro, Edoardo, 316
 operation of, 316
Portal, Paul, 497
Porter, Katherine Anne, 378
Poseidon, 59
Position
 fetal, 172-181
  knee-chest, 242, 246, 456, 481
  Trendelenburg, 489-490
Postpartum hemorrhage, 268
Posture, birth, 231-234
Poullet, Jules, 278
Pousser des cris de Mélusine, 338
de Predis, Ambrogio, 340
Preformation, 203, 189-190
Pregnancy
 abdominal, 186
 diagnosis, 43-48
 extrauterine, 182-186
 garb, 60-66, 340
 multiple, 372, 377-408
 pride of, 49
 scenes of, 48-60
 tests for, 43-48
Presbyterian Hospital, New York, 455, 510
Prescott, Oliver, 254
Pritchard, Jack A., 521
Pro Race cervical cap, 449
Prolapse, uterine, 455, 463, 464-466, 518
Protectors of the parturient, 224-227
Pseudo-Apuleius, 343
Ptolemy, 28
Puah, 68
Puerperal feast, 152
Puerperal fever, 289-296, 497, 500
Puerperium, 149
Pugh, Benjamin, 283
Pulvis parturiens, 253

Pygopagus twins, 407
Pytheus of Abdera, 40

Qěb, 410
Quadruplet pregnancy. *See* Multiple pregnancy.
Queen Charlotte's Lying-in Hospital, London, 500
Quintianus, 26
Quintuplets, 383. *See also* Multiple pregnancy.

Rabbits delivered by Mary Toft, 136-140
Rachel, 67, 142-143, 437
Radical hysterectomy, 486
Raguenot, Jean-Baptiste, 498
Raguenot, Nicolas, 498
Ramazzini, Bernardino, 266
Rashi, 452
Raskolniki, 29
Raymond of Poitiers, 338
Raynalde, Thomas, 514
Re, birth of, 97, 122
Rebekah, 384
Récamier, Joseph C. A., 463
Redon, Odilon, 132, 363
Reichstadt, Duke of, 128
Reis, Emil, 486
Remmelin, Johann, 4
Remus, 354, 378
Renaissance, 3, 109, 131, 189, 339
Renoir, Pierre Auguste, 344
Repositors. *See also* Instruments.
 umbilical cord, 258
 uterine, 468-470
Resuscitation, 317-321
Retraction ring, 171, 259
Retroversion of uterus, 469-470
de Ribera, José, 41
de Ribes, Champetier, 277
Richelieu, 125
Rickets, 166, 211, 214, 215
Riemenschneider, Tilman, 341
Riolan, Jean, 182
Rise, Anna, 389
Rita-Christina, 399
Rite de passage, 325
Ritho, 97
Riverius, Stephanus, 157
Rixens, André, 296
della Robbia, Andrea, 322
Robert, Heinrich Ludwig, 216
Robert pelvis, 216
Robinson, Ralph, 450

Robusti, Jacopo, 106, 334
Roe, H. V., 448
Roemer septuplets, 392
Roentgen pelvimetry, 219
Rösslin, Eucharius, 71, 88, 136, 176-179, 511-515
Roger of Salerno, 489
Roland of Parma, 489
Roman charity, 351
Romano, Giulio, 57
Romulus and Remus, 354, 378
Ronsee, Boudewijn, 306
van Roonhuyze, Hendrik, 313, 456
van Roonhuyze, Rogier, 272, 279
 forceps of, 282
Roosendaal, Kniertje, 390
Rosengarten, 71, 88, 136, 176-179, 511
 title pages of, 513-514
Rosenmüller, Johann, 18
 organ of, 18
Ross, Russell R., 268
Rotunda Hospital, 292, 295, 499-501
Rousseau, Jean Jacques, 348-349
Rousset, François, 310
Rowlandson, Thomas, 70
Rubens, Peter Paul, 124, 125, 352, 354, 371
Rubin, I. C., 440
Rudabe, Queen, 301
Rueff, Jacob, 6, 44, 68, 89, 158, 161, 193, 271, 515
Russell, Keith P., 522
Rustan, birth of, 300-301
Ryckaert, David, 201
Ryff, Walther Hermann, 156, 160
van Rymsdyck, Jan, 168

Sacombe, Jean, 306, 307
Saemann, Johann Christian, 280
Sänger, Max, 314-316
Saenredam, Jan Pietersz, 60
Saf-T-Coil, 450
Sage-femme, 67
Sage-femme de Campagne, 71
Sage-femmes en culottes, 70
Sagittarius, 124
St. André, Nathaniel, 137
Saint-Aubin, Gabriel Jacques, 23
St. Bartholomew's Hospital, London, 495
Saint-Esprit, 495
Saint-Hilaire, Geoffroy, 372
St. Landry, Bishop of Paris, 495
St. Léger, Bishop, 439

St. Luke's Hospital, New York, 509
Salmacis, 35
Salome, 108
Sammangelof, 228
Samson, 287
San-Senori, 228
da San Severino, Giacomo Salimbeni, 114
da San Severino, Lorenzo, 114
San twins, 406
Sanger, Margaret Higgins, 447
Sansovino, Jacopo, 227
Sarah, 437
del Sarto, Andrea, 105, 496
Sauromatae, 28
Sauvage, Nicolas, 398
Savage, Steele, 371
Savonarola, Giovanni Michele, 43, 265, 266
Scanzoni, Friedrich Wilhelm, 295
Schalcken, Godfried, 46
Schedel, Hartmann, 374
Schön, Erhard, 36, 511
Schröder, Carl, 502
Schultes, Johann. See Scultetus.
Schultze, Bernhard Sigmund, 250, 318
  mechanism, 250
Sciapodae, 374
Scissors. See Instruments.
Scultetus, 29, 273, 311, 357, 373, 516
Sekiyen, Toriyama, 148
Sella perforata, 265
Selz, Peter, 81
Semele, 297, 400
Semen, 12, 187-189, 193, 197
  female, 189
Semmelweis, Ignaz Philipp, 294-295, 504
Semites, 324, 410
Seneca, 189
Senoi, 228
Sériceps, 278
Servetus, Michael, 32
Sex determination, 189
Shadow-feet, 374
Shakespeare, William, 346, 378
Sheila-na-gig, 417
Ship of Fools, 378
Shiphrah, 68
Shippen, William, Jr., 72, 505-506
Siamese twins, 397, 404-408
Sick Lady, 45
Siddhartha, 116

Siebold, Adam Elias, 502
Siegemundin, Justine Dittrichin, 74, 257, 267
Sigurlykkja, 229
Silver sutures, 456
Silvester, Henry R., 320
Simeon, 327
Simon, Gustav, 474
Simpson, Alexander R., 268, 283
Simpson, James Young, 280, 482
  metrotome of, 475
  uterine sound of, 459
Sims, James Marion, 456, 480-482, 484, 507
  repositor of, 470
  uterine guillotine of, 474
Simurgh, 301
Sirenia, 367
Sirenomelia, 366
Sirens, 365-367
Skutsch, F., 221
Slaves, 208, 456
Sloane, Emily Thorn Vanderbilt, 510
Sloane, William Douglas, 510
Sloane Hospital for Women, 293, 496, 505. See also Sloane Maternity Hospital.
Sloane Maternity Hospital, 269, 321, 510. See also Sloane Hospital for Women.
Smellie, William, 70, 74, 78, 167, 255, 256, 257, 258, 274, 517
  forceps of, 282
Smith, Hugh, 522
Smith, Kathleen and Lexie, 397
Smith, Protheroe, 65
Smollett, Tobias, 517
Smyly, William, 500
Solomons, Bethel, 500
Song of Mary, 56
Soranus of Ephesus, 61, 70, 172, 265, 322, 348, 511
Sound, uterine, 459, 469. See also Instruments.
Spacher, Stephan Michael, 4
Spalding, Alfred B., 259
  sign of, 259
Spallanzani, Lazaro, 439
Spanheim, F., 121
Spanish windlass, 261
Speculum, vaginal, 455, 456-459, 518. See also Instruments.
Spencer, H. R., 517

Spermatozoa, 11, 189, 197, 198, 200, 202, 204
Spermists, 189
Spes Nostra, 58
Spiegel, Adrian, 158
Spielart, 361
Splitting of the cell, 205
Sponges, 460
Spontaneous evolution, 257
Sport, 361
Squaw-belt, 246
Stander, Henricus J., 521
Stearns, John, 253-254
Steen, Jan, 359, 493
Stein, Georg Wilhelm, 269
Steinbeck, John, 351, 378
Steinfurth, Hermann, 353
Steller's sea cow, 367
Stenson, Niels, 17, 190
Stephanus, Carolus, 5
Sterilization, tubal, 451
Steven of Bourbon, 119
Stheno, 369
Stoeckel, Walter, 502
Stone, Martin L., 450
Stone figures, 1
Stool, obstetric, 231-232, 265-266
Stopes, Marie Carmichael, 448
Streptococcus, 296
Studdiford, William Emery, 510
Striae gravidarum, 182
Stromayr, Caspar, 464-465, 489
Suction-tractor, 280
Suddhodano, Prince, 116
Suetonius Tranquillus, 309
Sumerians, 409
Sun god Aton, 187
Supernumerary mammae, 347
Superstition, credulity, fanaticism and, 138
Surrey Wonder, 139
Susruta Samhita, 211
Süss, Hans, 105
Sutures
  for cesarean section, 314-316
  silver, 456
Swaddling, 322-323
Swammerdam, Jan, 16, 17, 190, 439
Sylvius, 1
Symelia, 366
Symphysiotomy, 285
Sympodia, 365-367
Syringes, 491, 494. See also Instruments.

Tables
　delivery, 266, 269
　examining, 487. *See also* Chair, gynecologic examining.
　operating, 488, 490
Tait, Lawson, 461
Talmud, 187, 298, 452, 456
Tamar, 67, **386**
Tanganki, 277
Tarnier, Étienne Stéphane, 275, 276, 321
　forceps of, 283
Tarnowska, Valeria, 370
Tarnowska Perseus, 370
Taurt, 225
Tavernier, Melchior, 323
Taylor, Howard C., Jr., 510
Telephus, 354
Tenadora, 244
Tennyson, Alfred, 361
Tent, tupelo, 460, 482
Teratology, 361-376
Tertullian, 276
Testes, female, 2, 16, 189, 190, 208
Tests, pregnancy, 43-48
Tethys, 337
Textbooks, American, 519-521
Thalidomide, 373
Theophrastus, 31
Thomas, T. Gaillard, 456
　hysterectomy clamp of, 485
Thompson, George, 333
Thoracopagus twins, 405, 406, 408
Thoth, 31
Tibaldi, Pellegrino, 363
Time the Best Doctor, 47
Il Tintoretto, 106, 334
Tire-tête, 272. *See also* Instruments.
Titus, Emperor, birth of, 123
Tlacolteotl, 123
Tlacuatzin, 253
Tlazoltéotl, 231
Tocci brothers, 407
Toft, Mary, cunicular confinement of, 136-140
Tornabuoni, Giovanni Francesco, 146-147
Toueris, 419
Tourniquet, Momburg's, 263
Trajan, Emperor, 70, 332
Transverse lie, 256
Trautmann, Jeremias, 307
Trendelenburg, Friedrich, 490
　position of, 489-490
Triplet pregnancy, 377-408

Tristan, 287
Triumph of Venus, 287
Trocars, 476
Troglodytes, 374
Troilus, 287
Tubal insufflation, 440
Tubal pregnancy, 182-185
Tube, uterine, 12, 14, 17
Tuberculosis, 211
Tubules of Kobelt, 18
Tupelo tent, 460, 482
Tweedy, Ernest Hastings, 500
Twelfth Night, 378
Twin goddess, 377, 378
Twinning, incomplete, 368, 395-408
Twins, 67, 298, 377-408. *See also* Multiple pregnancy.
　conjoined, 37, 397-408
　of Melusine, 338
Tyndareus, King, 129
Tyndaridae, 129

Ubame, 148
Umbilical vessels, 164
Umbilicus, 190
　of Adam and Eve, 102, 189
Urethra, 12, 13
Urhsheihsze Heaou, 351
Uroscopy, 43-46
Ursa major, 59
Urslerin, Barbara, 42
Usher, house of, fall of, 378
Uteroplacental apoplexy, 260
Uterus, 9
　bimanual compression of, 264
　blood supply to, 13, 18, 19, 169
　connection to breasts of, 192
　displacements of, 455, 463-472, 518
　double, 14
　early views of, 8-13
　ex-voto, 424, 427, 428
　as fertility symbol, 426
　horns of, 12
　inertia of, 252
　innervation of, 21
　musculature of, 16
　myomas of, 482-484
　pregnant, 160-171
　relation to breasts of, 335
　repositors for, 463-469
　retraction ring for, 259
　seven cells doctrine of, 8-12
　suspension operations for, 463-469, 471, 472

Uterus *(Cont.)*
　sympathies of, 469

Vacuum extractor, 280
Vallée, Antoine, 77
Vande Wiele, Raymond L., 510
Vanderbilt Clinic, 510
Vagina, 12-14, 19
Varnier, Henri-Victor, 219
Vauchelet, Theophile Auguste, 102
Vecellio, Tiziano, 59
Vectis. *See* Instruments.
Velpeau, A. L. M., 331, 456
Venter equinus, 201
Ventura, Magdalena, 41
Venus, 35, 133, 287, 410, 421
　birth of, 130-132
　of Willendorf, 409
Verkolje, Johannes, 198
del Verrocchio, Andrea, 146-147
Version, 256, 260
　extraction and, 257-258
　podalic, 76
Vertue brothers, 139
Vesalius, Andreas, 1, 3, 4, 5, 11, 12, 16, 158, 211
Vesicovaginal fistula, 456, 480-482
Vespasianus, Flavius Sabinus, birth of, 123
Vestal virgins, 378
de la Vigne, André, 391
Vincent, Tom, 333
da Vinci, Leonardo, 3, 55, 129, 162-163, 192, 207, 340
Virchow, Rudolph, 295
Virgil, 297
Virgin, the. *See* Mary.
Virgin and Child Before a Fire Screen, 339
Virgin of Lucca, 340
Visitation, 56-57
Völter, C., 94, 312
Vogtherr, Heinrich, 157, 454
van der Vondel, Joost, 134
Votives, fertility, 421, 424-436
Vulva, ex-voto, 428

Walcher, Gustav Adolf, 234
　position of, 234
Ward, W., 291
Watkins, Thomas James, 467
Watson, Benjamin P., 293, 510
Watson, Thomas, 292
Weber, Bob, 394
Webster, John Clarence, 472, 484

Wells, Thomas Spencer, 455
Wertheim, Ernst, 486
Westminster Lying-in Hospital, London, 500
Wet nurse, 338, 348-351, 356
White, Charles, 291
  repositor of, 468
William Rufus, King, 404
Williams, John Whitridge, 173, 521
  portrait, 520
Williams Obstetrics, 521
Wise Men of Godalming, Cuniculari or, 137
Wolf, Joannes, 120
Wolf as wet nurse, 354
Wolff, Caspar Friedrich, 190, 203
Wolffhart, Conrad, 375
Wolffian body, 18
Woman and Death, 148
Woman's Hospital of the State of New York, 456, 496, 507-509
Women's Hospital of the State of Illinois, 507
Woods, John, 376
Woyerkowski, Roch, 478

Xochiquetzal, 378

Yonge, James, 280
Young, Hugh H., 38
Yuncan birth scene, 82

Zachariah, 56, 114. *See also* John, birth of.
Zacharias. *See* Zachariah.
Zakheim, Bernard Borouch, 91
Zarah and Pharez, birth of, 386
Zeitblom, Bartholomäus, 104
Zelemi, 108
Zenobius, Saint, 317
Zephyrina, Princess, 127
Zerbi, Gabriele, 351
Zervan, 378
Zeus, 59, 129, 130, 136, 196, 265, 297, 336, 353, 362, 365, 369, 370, 371, 378
  birth of Athene and, 395-396
  Dionysus and, 400, 401
Zipper, Jaime, 450
Zipporah, 326
Zondek, Bernhard, 44, 502
Zoomyle, 372
Zweifel, Paul, 184
Zwierlin, Conrad Anton, 349